Cardiology
1983

Cardiology: 1983

Printed in the United States of America

First Edition

International Standard Book Number: 0-914316-36-2

International Standard Serial Number: 0275-0066

Cardiology
1983

WILLIAM C. ROBERTS, MD, Editor
Chief, Pathology Branch
National Heart, Lung, and Blood Institute
National Institutes of Health, Bethesda, Maryland, and
Clinical Professor of Pathology and Medicine (Cardiology)
Georgetown University, Washington, D.C.
Editor-in-Chief, The American Journal of Cardiology

CHARLES E. RACKLEY, MD
Professor and Chairman
Department of Medicine
Georgetown University Medical Center
Washington, D.C

DEAN T. MASON, MD
Director, Cardiac Center
Cedars Medical Center
Miami, Florida
Editor-in-Chief, American Heart Journal

JAMES T. WILLERSON, MD
Professor of Medicine
Chief, Division of Cardiology
Department of Medicine
University of Texas Health Science Center
Dallas, Texas

ROBERT B. KARP, MD
Professor of Surgery
Department of Surgery
University of Alabama Medical Center
Birmingham, Alabama

ALBERT D. PACIFICO, MD
Professor of Surgery
Department of Surgery
University of Alabama Medical Center
Birmingham, Alabama

THOMAS P. GRAHAM, JR, MD
Professor of Pediatrics
Chief, Division of Pediatric Cardiology
Department of Pediatrics
Vanderbilt University
Nashville, Tennessee

 YORKE MEDICAL BOOKS

Contents

5. Valvular Heart Disease   287

6. Myocardial Heart Disease   337

9. Miscellaneous Topics 423

Preface

The number of contributors to this year's edition has been increased, and the number of articles summarized by each contributor is listed below. Rackley's submissions were from *Circulation*; Willerson's, from *The American Journal of Cardiology*, and Mason's, from *The American Heart Journal*. The other contributors summarized articles from more than one journal. The summaries from each contributor were then submitted to me, at which time they were edited and organized into the various chapters.

CARDIOLOGY 1983

AUTHOR	CHAPTER NUMBER									TOTALS	
	1	2	3	4	5	6	7	8	9		
WCR	55	38	40	40	27	29	10	11	33	283	(39.2%)
CER	38	23	20	8	9	6	2	6	17	129	(17.9%)
JTW	39	19	26	1	13	3	2	10	9	122	(16.9%)
DTM	14	13	21	5	10	3	4	11	7	88	(12.2%)
RBK	9	2	5	0	8	0	0	0	10	34	(4.7%)
ADP	0	0	0	0	5	0	28	0	0	33	(4.6%)
TPG Jr	2	0	4	0	1	1	24	0	0	32	(4.5%)
TOTALS	157	95	116	54	73	42	70	38	76	721	(100.0%)

Special thanks go to Ann K. Bradley, Vivian Young, Margaret M. M. Moore, Barbara Winterrowd, Tamsin Wolff, Leslie Silvernail and Mary McMahon for their superb efforts in behalf of this task. Gay C. Morgulas, Director of Yorke Medical Books, again coordinated publication of this book with her usual finesse and expertise.

WILLIAM C. ROBERTS, MD
EDITOR

Coronary Heart Disease

Prevalence and magnitude of ST-segment and T-wave abnormalities in normal men during continuous ambulatory electrocardiography

Armstrong and associates[1] from Indianapolis, Indiana, studied 50 asymptomatic normal male volunteers to determine the prevalence and magnitude of ST-segment and T-wave changes during continuous ambulatory ECG monitoring. Transient ST-segment depression ≥1.0 mm was recorded in 15 (30%) of individuals studied and labile T-wave inversion ≤3 mm in an additional 18 (36%). ST changes during monitoring did not correlate with daily activity status, heart rate, or age. There was no correlation with ST-segment response or work performance during treadmill exercise testing. ST-segment depression and T-wave inversion are commonly observed during ambulatory ECG monitoring in normal men. Therefore similar changes observed in patients with CAD should be interpreted with caution.

Implications of an early positive treadmill exercise test

Schneider and associates[2] from Durham, North Carolina, studied 80 men (group A) with CAD who underwent coronary arteriography irrespective of symptoms and previous therapy because they had a positive treadmill exercise test at a low work load (stage I or II by a Bruce protocol) and 34 men (group B) who also had an early positive treadmill test because they had disabling angina pectoris despite medical therapy. Left main CAD ≥50% was found in 28% of patients in group A and 35% of those in group B (NS). Only 10% of other patients undergoing cardiac catheterization with treadmill tests that were not positive at a low work load had LM CAD (p < 0.001). Fifty-four patients in group A without LM CAD ≥50% were treated medically; 85% of these patients had 2 or 3 major coronary arteries ≥75% stenosis. These patients had a 36-month survival rate of 89%. These data suggest that a treadmill test positive at a low work load identifies patients with an increased likelihood of having LM CAD ≥50%, even if they have few symptoms. The data also indicate that in those patients without LM CAD most can be treated medically with a relatively low mortality during a subsequent 3-year interval.

Effect of medical or surgical treatment on exercise-induced hemodynamic and ECG abnormalities

In a retrospective study, Sarma and Sanmarco[3] from Downey, California, assessed the long-term effects of medical management or CABG on serial exercise testing in patients with exertional hypotension. Forty patients (35 men, 5 women) who experienced hypotension during maximal symptom-limited exercise tests were retested after a 12-month interval. The mean age of the patients was 53 years and all had multiple vessel CAD; 17 had CABG because of disabling angina and 23 patients without disabling angina had medical management only. At entry, there were no significant differences in age, LV function, or exercise performance between the medical and surgical groups. At follow-up, the surgical group had an average increase in exercise duration of 2.2 min, maximal heart rate of 17 beats/min, maximal systolic BP 26 mmHg, and maximal rate-pressure product of 60. These measurements did not change significantly in the medically treated group. Thus, exercise-induced hypotension is apparently caused by ischemic LV dysfunction, since in most patients it is reversible after successful CABG. This observation is supported by the lack of improvement in a comparable group of patients managed medically with CABG.

Systolic blood pressure during exercise testing

Weiner and associates[4] from Boston, Massachusetts, studied 47 patients to determine the reproducibility and prognostic significance of an exercise-induced decrease in systolic BP. These 47 patients manifested a reduction in systolic BP below the preexercise standing level and were selected from a consecutive series of 436 patients undergoing treadmill exercise testing and cardiac catheterization during a 3-year period. The prevalence of this abnormal finding was 11% in the total group, but 21% in the 124 patients with 3-vessel or LM CAD. Patients with an exercise-induced reduction in systolic BP were more likely to be men, have typical angina pectoris with class III or IV functional limitation, and to have had a prior AMI (p < 0.05). Most of these 47 patients had severe ischemic responses, and 14 (30%) showed complex repetitive ventricular arrhythmias. Of the 47 patients, 24 received medical treatment and 23 underwent CABG. With repeat exercise testing in 42 patients, a decrease in systolic BP during exercise was consistently present in the group receiving medical therapy (17 of 20), but entirely absent (0 of 22) in a group that had undergone CABG. The mean treadmill time, peak heart rate, and systolic BP were not significantly different in the initial and repeat exercise tests in patients subsequently treated medically; however, in patients undergoing CABG all of the variables were significantly higher in the repeat test (p < 0.001). After a mean follow-up time of 37 months, the total cardiac mortality rate was 8% in the group treated medically and 4% in the group that had had CABG. These data suggest that a decrease in systolic BP during exercise testing is reproducible and may be reversed by CABG.

Exercise treadmill test performance in severe left main coronary narrowing

The exercise treadmill test performance of 60 patients with angiographically documented LM CAD was analyzed by Stone and colleagues[5] from San Francisco, California, to determine the spectrum of exercise treadmill test response in this subset of CAD patients. Location and extent of CAD also was determined to assess its effect on exercise response in patients having LM CAD. The ST-segment response indicated ischemia in 46 patients (77%), and only 1 patient (2%) achieved a maximum predicted heart rate with a negative ST-segment response. During exercise treadmill test, exertional hypotension developed in 6 patients (10%), frequent VPC in 19 patients (32%), and ST-segment elevation occurred in 5 patients (8%). A markedly positive exercise treadmill test response, defined as either ≥2.0 mm ischemic ST-segment depression, a positive ST-segment response in stage I of the Bruce protocol, termination of the exercise test in stage I or II, or the development of exertional hypotension, was observed in 53 patients (88%). A benign treadmill test response, defined as either a negative test at the maximum predicted heart rate or the ability to exercise at least to stage IV, was observed in only 4 patients (7%). Patterns of coronary anatomy were divided into group I (9 patients) in which only portions of the myocardium were in jeopardy of ischemia (patients with an obstruction in the LM but with a normal dominant right coronary artery), and group II (51 patients) in which the entire myocardium was in jeopardy (patients with LM CAD and either a dominant left coronary artery or a dominant right coronary artery that was obstructed). There was a significantly higher prevalence in group II -vs- group I of exercise-induced frequent VPC (19 patients -vs- 0 patients), termination of the treadmill test in stage I (28 patients -vs- 0 patients), and marked ischemic ST-segment depression ≥2.0 mm (30 patients -vs- 2 patients). Thus, patients with LM CAD have a very high prevalence of a markedly positive ischemic exercise treadmill test response and only rarely exhibit a benign response. The degree of LV jeopardy exerts a major adverse effect on treadmill test performance in patients with LM CAD.

Effect of propranolol on left ventricular performance

The effect of oral propranolol on LV performance during early upright exercise was evaluated by ear densitography in patients with arteriographic CAD by Sugiura and associates[6] from Worcester, Massachusetts. Measurments of systolic time intervals differentiated 10 unmedicated patients with CAD (group 1) and 15 patients with CAD taking propranolol (group 3). The patients in group 3 had less shortening of preejection period (PEP) at 1 minute and 4 minutes of exercise than group 1 patients ($p < 0.0001$ and $p < 0.005$, respectively), with propranolol appearing to prevent the abnormal shortening of PEP observed in the unmedicated group. Group 3 patients, in contrast to group 1 patients, had reduced heart rate and heart rate-BP product both at rest and during exercise. Furthermore, PEP/LV ejection time (ET) and percentage change in PEP/LV ET from control responses were similar to those of subjects free of CAD (group 2). These results indicate that propranolol effects a favorable change in LV performance by postponing early exhaustion of cardiac reserve, despite significant CAD. There was relatively large overlap in percent change in PEP/LV ET from control between group 2 and group 3 in contrast to the clear separation among unmedicated patients. Thus, the excellent diagnostic accuracy of systolic time intervals recorded during exercise is greatly reduced by beta adrenoceptor blockade.

Relation of P-S₄ interval to left ventricular end-diastolic pressure

Previous reports suggested that the interval between P-wave onset and the fourth heart sound (P-S_4 interval) reflects changes in LV myocardial stiffness. Schapira and associates[7] from Stanford, California, made simultaneous measurements of the P-S_4 or atrial electrogram to S_4 (A-S_4) interval and LV pressure in 19 patients with CAD who were studied before and after atrial pacing. Thirteen patients developed angina accompanied by significant rises in their end-diastolic pressure and a consistent decrease in P-S_4 or A-S_4 interval; whereas the 6 patients who had atrial pacing without the development of angina had no changes in end-diastolic pressure, P-S_4, or A-S_4 interval. The resting data showed an inverse correlation between LV end-diastolic pressure and the P-S_4 interval. In addition, the P-S_4 interval allowed discrimination between patients with normal and abnormal (>15 mmHg) end-diastolic pressures.

Echo detection of left main coronary obstruction

Since CABG improves life expectancy in patients with LM coronary obstruction, a practical noninvasive procedure is needed for detecting or excluding lesions in the LM coronary artery. Rink and associates[8] from

Indianapolis, Indiana, reported on advances in 2-D echo which have improved the prospects for using this technique to detect LM obstruction. Using an echo that had digital gray scale, a 3 MHz transducer and strobe-freeze frame capability and reviewing recordings on an off-line videotape-videodisc analyzer, these investigators retrospectively examined the LM in 72 patients who underwent coronary cineangiography. Angiography showed ≥50% stenosis of the LM in 7 patients. All 7 had high intensity echo in the walls of the LM. The high intensity echo was irregularly located in the artery and partially occluded the vessel. LM could frequently be recorded proximal and distal to the obstruction. The blind observer reviewed 28 randomly selected patients from this group and correctly identified the 4 patients with LM obstruction. There was 1 true and 2 questionably false positive diagnoses. In a prospective study of 31 patients, 2 independent observers correctly identified the 3 patients with LM coronary obstruction. There were no false negatives and 1 observer had 1 false positive. All of the false positives were in patients with proximal LAD coronary artery lesions. Thus, echo may be a practical means of identifying patients with LM coronary obstruction.

Angiographic and histologic morphology of localized coronary stenoses

Levin and Fallon[9] from Boston, Massachusetts, correlated postmortem coronary angiographic morphology with histologic sections of 73 localized subtotal coronary artery stenoses to determine whether complicated or uncomplicated atherosclerotic lesions could be detected angiographically. Lesions were divided into 2 types according to angiographic morphology. Type 1 stenoses had smooth borders and hourglass configuration and no intraluminal lucencies. Type 2 stenoses had irregular borders or intraluminal lucencies. Histologic sections also were divided into 2 types: "uncomplicated" stenoses and fatty or fibrous plaques with intact intimal surfaces and no superimposed thrombus; "complicated" stenoses manifested plaque rupture, plaque hemorrhage, superimposed partially occluding thrombus, or recanalized thrombus. Among the 35 lesions with type 1 angiographic morphology, 4 were complicated lesions histologically. Among the 38 stenoses demonstrating type 2 angiographic morphology, 30 were complicated lesions. Postmortem angiography demonstrated a sensitivity of 88% and a specificity of 79% for detecting complicated stenoses on the basis of irregular borders or intraluminal lucencies. Thus, the complicated lesions represent a greater risk for AMI or sudden death than do uncomplicated lesions. These observations suggest that coronary stenoses characterized angiographically by irregular borders or intraluminal lucencies are probably the clinically more dangerous complicated type.

Significant narrowing isolated to the left anterior descending coronary artery

Brooks and associates[10] from London, England, summarized angiographic and clinical findings in 218 patients with significant narrowing confined to

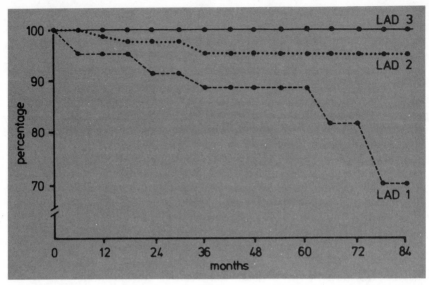

Fig. 1-1. Survival curves of patients classified according to site of most proximal anterior descending artery obstruction. Reproduced with permission from Brooks et al.[10]

the LAD coronary artery. The LAD was divided into 3 segments: from its origin to the origin of the first septal branch (LAD1), from the first septal to the first diagnonal branch (LAD2), and the remaining distal LAD (LAD3) (Fig. 1-1). Cardiogenic shock occurred only in patients with LAD1 narrowings, but apart from this the clinical presentation bore no consistent relation to the site of narrowing in the LAD. Patients with proximal LAD narrowings were more likely to have a "positive" exercise test, had more severely impaired LV function, and had a worse prognosis than those with more distal narrowings. Nonvisualization of collateral arteries in patients with LAD narrowing was associated with extensive AMI, and patients who presented with AMI had more severely impaired LV function than those who presented with angina pectoris and subsequently had AMI. LV function was poor at the time of angiography in 11 of 12 of those who subsequently died.

Effect of cough on coronary perfusion pressure

Coughing is frequently employed as a means of interrupting bradycardia or arterial hypotension after selective coronary angiogram. To evaluate the effect of coughing after coronary angiography on the perfusion gradient and the clearing of contrast medium from the coronary circulation, Little and associates[11] from Birmingham, Alabama, studied the effect of a single forceful cough on the coronary perfusion pressure (CPP), calculated as diastolic aortic minus RA pressure. During coughing before angiograms in 12 normotensive subjects, RA pressure increased more than aortic pressure increased, causing the CPP to decrease by 17 mmHg. Immediately after the cough, aortic pressure was less than before and CPP was decreased by 9 mmHg. Increased central venous pressure in coughing was not transmitted beyond the thoracic and abdominal exits. The effects of coughing in 23 patients after coronary angiogram when aortic pressures were as low as 28 mmHg were similar to those in normotensive subjects. The CPP decreased by 21 mmHg during coughing and was decreased by 7 mmHg after coughing. To examine the cause of these effects further, 200 forceful coughs in 9 normal subjects were studied with simultaneous transesophageal M-mode echo and Doppler brachial artery pulse velocity recordings. Coughing during diastole did not open the aortic valve but produced a peak of diastolic brachial arterial flow velocity. Flow velocity in the beat after coughing was less than control. Thus, these investigators concluded that in normal subjects, coughing displaces aortic volume peripherally without producing cardiac output in diastole and prevents venous outflow causing the CPP to be decreased during and after the cough. Cough produces similar decreases in CPP in patients with moderate hypertension after coronary angiogram. Thus, if coughing helps to clear the coronary arteries of contrast medium in such patients, the maneuver does not achieve this by increasing the CPP.

Myocardial metabolic alterations after contrast angiography

Wisneski and associates[12] from San Francisco, California, evaluated whether contrast media used during angiography produces transient alterations in cardiovascular physiology. Sixteen patients with symptoms of CAD undergoing left ventriculography and coronary arteriography were studied. Coronary sinus and arterial blood samples were obtained for free fatty acids, glucose, and lactate before and after performing left ventriculography with Renografin-76. Coronary blood flow was determined by the thermodilution technique. Five minutes after ventriculography, the arterial level of free fatty acids had decreased by $18 \pm 5\%$ (mean $\pm$ SD) from baseline values, $p < 0.001$. Associated with this decrease in arterial free fatty acids was an increase in the myocardial uptake of the substrate. Five minutes after left ventriculography, the free fatty acid uptake had increased $48 \pm 33\%$ compared with the baseline value, $p < 0.001$. After injection of contrast medium, there were no significant changes in the arterial levels of glucose or lactate. However, significant decreases in myocardial uptake of lactate and glucose could be demonstrated at 5 minutes. These changes in arterial free fatty acids and in myocardial uptake of various substrates persisted for at least 20 minutes after ventriculography. Thus, these data demonstrate that contrast medium significantly alters myocardial metabolism and that these alterations persist longer than hemodynamic changes induced by contrast angiography.

"Missing" coronary artery or congenital coronary anomalies detected angiographically

Donaldson and Raphael[13] from London, England, studied 8,235 patients without associated congenital heart disease by coronary angiography and found that 75 (0.9%) had at least 1 coronary artery arising from an abnormal location (Table 1-1). Symptoms attributable to the aberrant artery were present in 19 of the 75 patients. Failure to recognize the coronary anomalies

TABLE 1-1. *Angiographic findings. Reproduced with permission from Donaldson et al.*[13]

VARIANTS OF CORONARY ANATOMY	# PATIENTS
Missing left anterior descending (LAD)	
Separate origin LAD and LCx in left sinus of Valsalva	8
Origin LAD from right sinus of Valsalva or from RCA	4
LAD from PA	2
Missing left circumflex artery (LC)	
Separate origin LAD and LCx in left sinus of Valsalva	8
Origin LCx from right sinus of Valsalva or RCA	26
Missing right coronary artery (RCA)	
RCA and LCA from left sinus of Valsalva (2)	
RCA from LCA (1)	7
Extreme left dominance (4)	
Separate origin RCA and long conus artery	12
Missing left coronary artery (LCA)	
LCA from right sinus of Valsalva	2
LCA from RCA	1
LCA from PA	13

prolonged angiographic procedures and led to repeated cardiac catheterizations in 28 (37%) of the the 75 patients.

Angiographic prevalence of myocardial bridging

Although frequently noted in necropsy, the prevalence of angiographically demonstrable myocardial bridging was determined by a retrospective review of 465 consecutive coronary angiograms by Irvin[14] from Charleston, South Carolina. Bridging was present in 35 arteriograms (7.5%) and involved exclusively in the LAD coronary artery. The prevalence of bridging of the LAD was 10% in the arteriograms in which the LAD artery was adequately visualized. Only 8 of the 35 cases with myocardial bridging had been noted in the initial catheterization reports, a prevalence of 2%, which is similar to that previously reported. The higher frequency of bridging reported here is believed to reflect its increased recognition.

Exercise thallium-201 myocardial scintigraphy in women and correlation with coronary angiography

Friedman and associates[15] from Philadelphia, Pennsylvania, studied 60 women suspected of having CAD with thallium-201 and exercise and coronary arteriography. Thirty-two patients had no significant CAD; 28 patients had severe CAD defined as ≥70% diameter narrowing of 1 vessel (14 patients) or multiple vessels (14 patients). The exercise ECG was abnormal in 17 patients (9 with and 8 without CAD), negative in 16 patients (3 with and 13 without CAD), and equivocal in 27 patients (16 with and 11 without

CAD). The exercise thallium-201 scintigram showed exercise-induced defects (reversible ischemia) in 21 patients with CAD, a fixed defect in 1 patient with 1-vessel disease and no previous AMI, but was normal in the remaining 6 patients with 1-vessel disease. The exercise thallium-201 scintigrams in patients with no CAD were normal in 28, showed an exercise-induced defect in 1, and a fixed defect in the remaining 3 patients. The fixed defects involved the anterolateral segment in the anterior projection and were considered to be due to attenuation of activity by overlying breasts. The sensitivity of the exercise ECG was 32% and the specificity 41%, whereas, the sensitivity of exercise thallium-201 scintigraphy was 75% and specificity 97% if exercise-induced defects were considered abnormal and 79 and 88%, respectively, if all fixed defects were considered abnormal. The data suggest that exercise thallium scintigraphy is useful in women suspected of having CAD; attenuation of activity by the breast may affect the specificity but not sensitivity.

Influence of location of left anterior descending coronary aertery stenosis on left ventricular function during exercise

The presence and magnitude of exercise-induced LV dysfunction in an individual patient with CAD might result from a number of factors: age, sex, history of prior AMI, level of exercise stress achieved, level of exercise conditioning, magnitude of intravascular blood volume, extent of collateral supply, and magnitude and location of coronary stenoses. Leong and Jones[16] from Durham, North Carolina, evaluated the hypothesis that a stenosis located proximally caused a greater amount of exercise-induced LV dysfunction than a stenosis of similar magnitude located more distally. Twenty-six patients with isolated LAD coronary artery lesions documented by angiography were studied by RNA at rest and during exercise on a bicycle ergometer. Thirteen patients demonstrated a proximal lesion of the LAD averaging 91% of the luminal diameter (designated group 1), and 13 patients had a distal lesion averaging 88% of the lumen (designated group 2). The EF in group 1 decreased from 63–55%. LV end-diastolic volume (EDV) increased from 130 to 174 ml and LV end-systolic volume (ESV) increased from 49–80 ml during exercise. In group 2 the EF and the ESV showed no significant change during exercise and in the same group, the EDV increased from 117–140 ml with exercise. Although the 2 groups reveal no significant hemodynamic difference during the rest studies, group 1 revealed a significantly lower EF and higher EDV and ESV during exercise. Thus, these observations confirm that a stenotic lesion located at a more proximal level of the coronary arterial system reduces blood flow in the larger area of myocardium, resulting in a more pronounced ischemic response to exercise than a similar lesion located more distally.

Assessment of jeopardized myocardium with 1-vessel disease

The size of the perfusion defect of the LV myocardium was assessed from a quantitative analysis of exercise thallium-201 images by Iskandrian and colleagues[17] from Philadelphia, Pennsylvania. Quantitative analysis was determined by measuring the area and the perimetry of the perfusion defect and expressing this as a percentage of the total LV perimeter in 3 projections. Fifty patients with 1-vessel disease of >50% diameter narrowing were studied. The planimetric and perimetric methods correlated well. In 11 patients with <70% narrowing, only 1 patient had an abnormal exercise thallium-201 image. In the remaining 39 patients with ≥70% narrowing, 35 had an abnormal exercise image. Defects were larger in patients with LAD CAD (33 ± 10%) than in patients with LC CAD (19 ± 14%) or right CAD (17 ± 11%). There was significant variation in the sizes of the defects in the 3 projections in patients with LC and right CAD but not in patients with LAD CAD. Patients with LAD CAD with collaterals had smaller defects than their counterparts without collateral. The investigators concluded that in patients with 1-vessel disease, the quantitative size of the perfusion defect during exercise is highly variable. Patients with LAD CAD have larger defects than patients with LC or right CAD. The significantly lower quantitative thallium-201 scores in patients with LAD CAD and collaterals suggests that collaterals have a protective role during exercise in these patients.

Right ventricular thallium-201 rest imaging following dipyridamole-induced coronary vasodilation and relation to right coronary anatomy

The relation of coronary anatomy to RV appearance on serial thallium-201 myocardial imaging following dipyridamole-induced coronary vasodilation was examined by Brown and colleagues[18] from Boston, Massachusetts, in 71 consecutive patients undergoing coronary angiography for the evaluation of chest pain. Transient defects of the right ventricle were found in 18 patients. All had significant stenosis of the proximal right coronary artery. Nonvisualization of RV activity occurred in 13 patients; 6 had proximal right narrowing (compared with transient defects). Normal RV appearance was seen in 40 patients, of whom only 6 (15%) had proximal right coronary narrowing (compared with transient defects). The RV appearance was not affected by significant LAD or LC narrowing, or by the LV thallium-201 uptake. Thus, with serial (initial and delayed) thallium imaging following dipyridamole: 1) a transient RV defect appears to indicate significant proximal right coronary narrowing; 2) normal RV appearance suggests the absence of proximal right coronary disease; and 3) nonvisualization of the right ventricle appears to be nondiagnostic of right coronary narrowing.

Myocardial blood flow in multivessel coronary disease

Chen and associates[19] from New York City investigated the relation between resting LV myocardial blood flow (MBF) and hemodynamic determinants of myocardial oxygen consumption (MVO$_2$) in 15 patients with multivessel CAD and in 10 patients with normal coronary arteriograms. Mean LV MBF per unit mass of tissue was measured with a multicrystal scintillation camera from the regional clearance rates of xenon-133 injected into the LM coronary artery. Peak LV wall stress, mean velocity of circumferential fiber shortening (Vcf), rate of ejection during the first third of systole, LV EF, and the ratio of peak LV systolic pressure to LV end-systolic volume were measured by contrast left ventriculography. Mean LV MBF per unit mass was significantly reduced in patients with multivessel CAD. However, none of the patients with CAD experienced chest pain or had ECG evidence of myocardial ischemia during the resting measurements. Ejection phase indexes were lower in the patients with CAD. LV wall thickness and LV mass index were significantly increased in patients with CAD, accounting for the reduction in peak LV wall stress observed in these patients. Multiple regression analysis indicated that indexes of 3 of the major determinants of MVO_2 explained 65% of the variation in MBF in patients with CAD. These determinants were peak LV stress, mean Vcf, and heart rate. After adjustment for these 3 indexes, the average LV MBF rates were not significantly different in the 2 groups. In both groups, resting MBF/beat correlated most highly with LV wall stress. Thus, the reduction in LV MBF per unit mass observed in patients with multivessel CAD at rest is related to lower levels of hemodynamic variables that determine MVO_2. This clinical study confirms in patients with CAD that peak LV wall stress is the most important hemodynamic variable determining the level of resting MBF.

Thallium-201 myocardial imaging after dipyridamole infusion and utility in detecting coronary stenoses and relation to regional wall motion

After a 4 minute intravenous dipyridamole infusion, Leppo and colleagues[20] from Boston, Massachusetts, obtained serial thallium scan in 60 patients undergoing cardiac catheterization: 40 patients had >50% stenosis CAD, 20 had normal coronary arteries or insignificant lesions. Damages were graded qualitatively for thallium activity by 3 observers. The sensitivity and specificity of the thallium study were not affected by the extent of CAD, the presence of Q waves, or propranolol therapy. Of 37 patients, 27 who had initial defects had complete thallium redistribution of 1 or more defects. Patient by patient analysis using a regression model of all patients showed that the fate of a segmental thallium defect predicted abnormal wall motion by angiography better than ECG Q waves. The presence of propranolol therapy or collaterals did not significantly affect the thallium redistribution result. These investigators conclude that qualitative interpretation by multiple observers of thallium images after dipyridamole infusion is a highly sensitive and specific test for CAD. After dipyridamole infusion, as with exercise stress, the extent of thallium redistribution is related to the degree of myocardial wall motion abnormality.

Ejection fraction response to exercise with chest pain from coronary narrowing but normal resting ventricular function

Gibbons and associates[21] from Durham, North Carolina, examined the EF response to upright exercise using first-pass RNA in 281 patients with chest pain, significant CAD, and normal ventricular function. A wide range of resting function for heart rate and EF and exercise function measured as heart rate, EF, and peak work load was recorded. The EF response to exercise varied widely, ranging from a decrease of 36% to an increase of 26%. Twenty-eight clinical catheterizations and RNA variables were examined to determine the relation of the EF response to exercise. Considered individually, the variables showing the strongest relation were resting pulse rate, positive exercise ECG changes, and adequate exercise. Multivariable analysis identified resting pulse pressure, adequate exercise, resting EF, the change in end-diastolic volume index with exercise, positive exercise ECG changes, and, to a lesser degree, the number of diseased vessels as variables that were significant independent predictors of the EF response to exercise. These observations indicate that the EF response to exercise is complex, influenced by many pathophysiologic variables in the presence of CAD, and several of these variables are not related to the extent of anatomic CAD.

Radionuclide angiography for diagnosis of CAD

Austin and associates[22] from Durham, North Carolina, prospectively evaluated the accuracy of rest and exercise radionuclide ventriculography (RVG) in detecting CAD in 221 consecutive patients who also had undergone cardiac catheterization. Multivariate analysis of patients with angiographically normal coronary arteries provided a formula from which to predict normal exercise LV EF response in a given patient. The presence of CAD was indicated by 1 or more of the following abnormalities in the RVG measurements: 1) rest LV EF <0.50; 2) exercise LV EF at least 0.06 less than the predicted value; 3) exercise increase in LV end-systolic volume >20 ml, and 4) exercise-induced LV wall motion abnormality. The absence of significant CAD was indicated by the absence of all 4 abnormalities. Applying these criteria to the 221 consecutive patients analyzed indicated that the sensitivity of the RVG was 0.87 and the specificity 0.54. These data suggest that RVG is of value in screening patients for consideration for cardiac surgery. No patient with significant LM coronary narrowing and only 4 of 65 with 3-vessel CAD were misdiagnosed. However, the relatively poor specificity of the test limits its overall usefulness in the evaluation of large numbers in patients with cardiovascular disease.

Right ventricular thallium-201 imaging after exercise and its relation to narrowing of the right coronary artery

Brown and associates[23] from Boston, Massachusetts, evaluated the usefulness of the appearance of the right ventricle on serial thallium-201 myocardial imaging in predicting coronary arterial abnormalities accurately in 88 consecutive patients undergoing exercise thallium-201 scintigraphy for the evaluation of chest pain. Transient defects in the right ventricle were found in 8 patients and all had high grade (>90% diameter reduction) stenosis of the proximal right coronary artery. Nonvisualization of the right ventricle occurred in 10 patients; 9 of them had significant (≥50% stenosis) narrowing of the proximal right coronary artery and 7 had high grade stenoses. The right ventricle appeared normal in 70 patients: 29 (41%) of them had significant proximal right CAD. The appearance of the right ventricle was not affected by the presence or absence of narrowing in the LAD or LC artery or by the appearance of the left ventricle. Thus, these data suggest that with serial RV thallium-201 myocardial imaging after exercise: 1) transient defects in the right ventricle suggest the presence of high grade proximal right coronary artery stenosis, 2) nonvisualization of RV activity also predicts significant proximal right coronary disease, and 3) the right ventricle frequently appears normal despite proximal right CAD; therefore this finding does not exclude significant right CAD.

Relation of phase image to patterns of contraction and conduction

One of the interesting digital computer manipulations of blood pool scintigraphy is the color coded EF image with a phase contraction display. Botvinick and colleages[24] from San Francisco, California, determined the relation of phase changes and abnormalities of ventricular contraction and conduction by performing phase image analysis of blood pool scintigrams in 29 patients. Eleven patients had no evidence of blood pool contraction or ECG conduction abnormalities, 4 had contraction abnormalities, 7 had abnormal conduction, 7 had abnormalities of both variables. The phase delay generally related to the degree of contraction abnormality. The mean phase delay in hypokinetic segments differed from that of normokinetic segments in the same patient. The phase delay of akinetic and dyskinetic segments differed from that in normokinetic segments and the phase delay in dyskinetic segments differed from that in the akinetic segments. However, there was a significant overlap in the phase delay in normal and hypokinetic segments. The investigators also observed in patients with conduction abnormalities that the minimal associated regional phase delay presented a phase dispersion and a pattern of contraction consistent with a pattern of conduction and different from normal. Thus, a single study performed both at rest and with stress demonstrated the effect of heart rate on phase assessment and confirmed the independent effects of contraction and conduction on phase delay. The acquisition and analytic methods should add significantly to the resolution of the phase method.

Coronary collateral vessels

Fifty-six patients undergoing CABG had transmural myocardial tissue samples obtained from myocardium perfused from the LAD coronary artery during open heart surgery. Schwarz and associates[25] from Heidelberg, West Germany, determined whether coronary collateral vessels protected LV myocardium. Microscopic morphometry was performed using myocardial tissue samples from 56 surgically treated patients with CAD. Stenosis of the

LAD coronary artery was determined from preoperative angiography. Patients in group A comprised those with <75% area reduction of the LAD coronary artery, whereas those in group B had >95% area reduction without collateral supply as determined by arteriography. In contrast, patients in group C had >95% reduction in the area of the LAD coronary artery with collateral supply. Myocardial fibrosis averaged 17% in patients in group A, 68% in patients in group B, and 29% in patients in group C (p < 0.001 as compared with group B). Thus, these data suggest that collateral coronary vessels to regions supplied by severe coronary stenosis do protect the myocardium.

Kolibash and associates[26] from Columbus, Ohio, studied the physiologic significance of coronary collateral vessels in 91 patients with stable CAD. Four physiologic variables were assessed in the distribution areas of 101 totally occluded coronary arteries associated with angiographically defined collateral vessels. These variables included myocardial perfusion at rest and during stress, LV wall motion, and the presence or absence of healed myocardial infarction. One hundred and one collateralized areas of myocardium were classified into 2 major groups on the basis of normal (43 areas) or abnormal (58 areas) myocardial perfusion at rest. Among the 43 areas with normal perfusion at rest, 3 or more variables were normal in 37 instances (86%) and all variables were normal in 17. In the 58 areas with abnormal perfusion at rest, 3 or more variables were abnormal in 47 (81%), and all 4 variables were abnormal in 32. Although the results were generally concordant when all variables were assessed as a group, significant discrepancies existed if each variable were compared individually with rest perfusion. In the 43 areas with normal resting perfusion, 14 (33%) had stress defects, 15 (35%) had wall motion abnormalities, and 5 (12%) showed ECG evidence of myocardial infarction. In 58 areas with abnormal resting perfusion, 5 (9%) had normal stress perfusion, 16 (18%) had normal wall motion, and 22 (38%) lacked ECG evidence of infarction. Thus, the presence or absence of significant CAD distal to the origin of a collateral vessel, the extent of CAD in all coronary vessels, and the angiographic appearance of collateral vessels were not helpful in defining the physiologic significance of a collateral vessel.

These data indicate that the functional significance of collateral vessels varies considerably. In many patients collateral vessels are effective in maintaining myocardial perfusion and LV function and preventing infarction. However, in others collateralization may be of no significance.

Regional myocardial perfusion was measured by Horwitz and colleagues[27] from San Antonio, Texas, in 12 normal subjects and in 34 patients with CAD at rest and during infusion of isoproterenol. Increments in regional flow normalized for change in heart rate times systolic product were 91 ± 28% in normal subjects, 71 ± 44% in normal regions in diseased hearts, 58 ± 33% in regions supplied by 50%–70% stenosed arteries, 35 ± 32% in regions supplied by arteries stenosed by more than 70%, and 16 ± 27% in regions supplied by collateral vessels only. In 3 of 14 regions perfused entirely via collateral pathways, regional perfusion decreased with isoproterenol. Therefore the extent to which coronary flow reserve estimated with isoproterenol was compromised varied directly with the severity of anatomic coronary artery lesions, and, in some regions entirely perfused by collateral vessels, an increase in heart rate times systolic pressure product was accompanied by a decrease in perfusion below resting levels. Thus, collateral vessels effectively maintain flow rates at normal levels at rest, but tend to be inefficient at delivering blood when myocardial oxygen demand is increased.

Transcardiac 1-norepinephrine response during cold pressor test

Mueller and colleagues[28] from St. Louis, Missouri, determined whether an increase in cardiac sympathetic activity can enhance coronary vasomotor tone and lower the VF threshold in 40 patients with normal coronary arteries and in 23 patients with significant CAD before and during cold pressor tests. Baseline hemodynamic data did not differ in the 2 patient groups except for LV end-diastolic pressures. LV end-diastolic pressure was 10 ± 3.7 (mean $\pm$ SD) and 15 ± 4.5 mmHg in patients with normal and abnormal coronary arteries. Baseline 1-norepinephrine contents averaged 295 ± 152 in those with normal coronary arteries and 250 ± 134 pg/ml in patients with CAD in arterial blood and 273 ± 152 and 250 ± 115 pg/ml, respectively, in the coronary sinus. Hemodynamic responses during cold pressor stimulus were similar in both groups. Cold pressor-induced increases in arterial and coronary sinus 1-norepinephrine contents were balanced in patients with normal coronary arteries, averaging 19 ± 30 and $17 \pm 37\%$, respectively. In patients with CAD, however, a $26 \pm 58\%$ increase in arterial 1-norepinephrine content was associated with a $58 \pm 62\%$ increase in coronary sinus 1-norepinephrine content ($p < 0.02$), suggesting myocardial 1-norepinephrine net release. These data suggest that transcardiac 1-norepinephrine responsiveness during cold pressor is enhanced in patients with significant CAD.

PROGNOSIS

Survival of medically treated patients in the Coronary Artery Surgery Study (CASS)

Mock and colleagues[29] from several USA cities evaluated the impact on survival of the anatomic extent of obstructive CAD and 2 measures of LV performance. The study is based on 20,088 patients without previous CABG enrolled in the Registry of the National Heart, Lung, and Blood Institute CASS from 1975–1979. The cumulative 4-year survival of medically managed patients was analyzed to determine the survival of specific subsets of patients with obstructive CAD. The vital status of 99.8% of the patients was known. The 4-year survival of medically treated patients with no significant obstructive disease was 97% in contrast to 92%, 84%, and 68% in patients with 1-,

2-, and 3-vessel disease, respectively. The presence of LM coronary disease decreased survival significantly. The 4-year survival decreased from 70%–60% in patients with 3-vessel disease when significant obstruction of the LM coronary artery was also present. Furthermore, patients with significant CAD who had an EF of 50%–100%, 35%–49%, and 0%–34% had a 4-year survival of 92%, 83%, and 58%, respectively. Segmental wall motion of the left ventricle was assessed in 5 selected segments and graded on the basis of 1–6, 1 being normal and increasing to 6 if an aneurysm was present. In a patient with normal LV contraction in all 5 segments of the ventriculogram, the LV score is 5. Patients with an LV score of 5–11, 12–16, and 17–30 had 4-year survivals of 90%, 71%, and 53%, respectively. Patients with good LV function (a score of 5–11) had a 4-year survival of 94%, 91%, and 79% for 1-, 2-, and 3-vessel disease, respectively. Patients with poor LV function (score of 17–30) had a 4-year rate of 67%, 61%, and 42% in 1-, 2-, and 3-vessel disease, respectively. Thus, this very large, carefully collected study reports that LV function is a more important predictor of survival than the number of diseased vessels.

Asymptomatic or mildly symptomatic coronary patients

Kent and associates[30] from Bethesda, Maryland, evaluated 147 asymptomatic or mildly symptomatic patients with CAD who did not have LM coronary occlusion and who did have an LV EF >20%. These patients were followed for 6–67 months (average, 25). Of the 147 patients, 28% had significant 1-vessel disease, 31% had 2-vessel disease, and 41% had significant 3-vessel CAD. An LV EF ≥55% was present in 69% of the patients. There were 8 deaths during the follow-up period. The annual mortality rate was 3% for the entire group, including 1.5% for patients with 1- and 2-vessel CAD and 6% for those with 3-vessel CAD. Exercise testing helped to classify the patients with 3-vessel disease further. Specifically, 25% of the patients with 3-vessel stenoses had poor exercise capacity on exercise testing. Forty percent of these patients either died (20%) or had progressive symptoms requiring operation (20%); the annual mortality rate in these patients was 9%. In those patients with good exercise capacity, only 22% either died (7%) or had progressive symptoms (15%); the annual mortality rate was 4% in this group. These data suggest that prognosis is good in patients with mild or no symptoms who have 1- or 2-vessel CAD. Patients with 3-vessel CAD with good exercise capacity documented by objective testing have an annual mortality rate of 4%. Patients with 3-vessel disease and poor exercise capacity have a poor prognosis with continued medical therapy.

Survival after a strongly positive exercise test

Patients who develop ST decrease of 2 mm or more during a GETT are generally presumed to have a poor prognosis. Dagenais and colleagues[31] from Quebec, Canada, assessed the prognosis of patients with a strongly positive exercise ECG. The 5-year cumulative survival rate was computed for

220 medically treated patients. Of these, 107 had coronary arteriograms, which comprised group A, and 113 did not have arteriography, group B. All patients demonstrated horizontal or down sloping ST decrease >2 mm during a multistage Bruce protocol GETT. In group A, the overall 5-year survival was 74%. Survival decreased with decrease in duration of exercise. All patients who achieved stage IV (≥541 s) survived, whereas the survival rate was 86% when the patients terminated their exercise during stage III (361–540 s), 73% survival when dropping during stage II (181–360 s), and only 52% survived when exercise was stopped during state I (<180 s). Mortality was associated with more severe CAD, and sudden death was the main cause of death. Patients in group B had a longer mean exercise duration than those in group A and as expected a higher survival of 91%, which also varied according to the exercise duration. Thus, among patients with a strongly positive exercise ECG, the duration of exercise identifies subsets that have different survival rates.

PROGRESSION OF CORONARY NARROWING BY ANGIOGRAPHY

To determine the effect of progression of CAD on LV function, Buda and associates[32] from Toronto, Canada, studied 47 patients who had 2 cardiac catheterizations 3–92 months (mean, 25) apart without intervening surgery. Of them, 35 had CAD and 12 had normal or near normal coronary arteries by angiography. Progression of CAD was seen more often in patients with initial CAD than in those without (66% -vs- 25%, p <0.02). The LV EF decreased in patients with CAD progression (0.63 ± 0.03–0.51 ± 0.04, p <0.01), but was unchanged in patients without progression (0.58 ± 0.04–0.50 ± 0.03, p = NS). Interval AMI was the major cause of deteriorating LV function. The rate or degree of CAD progression did not predictably change global LV function, and progression in individual arteries did not predictably alter regional LV function. The presence or development of collateral vessels did not significantly alter LV performance.

EFFECT OF PHYSICAL TRAINING

Ehsani and associates[33] from St. Louis, Missouri, evaluated the influence of prolonged exercise training in 8 men with CAD, mean age 52 ± 3 years, using echo. Training consisted of endurance exercise 3 times a week at 50%–60% of the maximal measured oxygen uptake for 3 months followed by exercise 4–5 days/week at 70%–80% of maximal oxygen uptake for 9 months. Maximal oxygen uptake capacity increased by 42% with exercise training, p < 0.001. Heart rate at rest and submaximal heart rate and systolic BP at a given work rate were significantly lower after training. Systolic BP at the time of maximal exercise increased after training. LV end-diastolic diameter was increased after 12 months of training from 47 ± 1 to 51 ± 1 mm, p < 0.01. LV fractional shortening and mean velocity of circumferential shortening decreased progressively in response to graded isometric exercise before training but not after training. At comparable levels of BP during static exercise, mean velocity of circumferential shortening was significantly higher after training. No improvement in echocardiographically determined or exercise variables was observed over a 12-month period in 5 patients who did not exercise. Thus, these data suggest that prolonged and vigorous exercise training in selected patients with CAD can result in beneficial cardiac adaptations.

Conn and associates[34] from Durham, North Carolina, performed treadmill exercise tests before and after physical conditioning in 10 patients with a prior AMI and a LV EF at rest of <27% as determined by radionuclide ventriculography. All patients participated in the supervised exercise program with a follow-up from 4–37 months (mean, 13). Although 2 patients died during the study period, there was no exercise-related morbidity or mortality. Baseline exercise capacity showed marked variability, ranging from 4.5–9.4 (mean, 7.0 ± 1.9) METS, and improved to 5.5–14 (mean, 8.5 ± 2.9) METS after conditioning (p = 0.05). The oxygen pulse (maximal oxygen uptake/maximal heart rate) before and after conditioning was used to assess a training effect and increased significantly from 12.8 ± 2.0 to 15.7 ± 3.2 ml/beat (p < 0.01). These data are consistent with the notion that selected patients with severely impaired LV function can participate safely in conditioning programs and achieve some cardiovascular training.

LIPIDS

Prevalence of CAD and serum lipids in subjects aged 45–64 years (Speedwell study)

Bainton and associates[35] from Bristol and London, England, performed a longitudinal study to examine the incidence of CAD and its associations with serum lipoproteins and their subfractions. Cross-sectional data were available on 283 men and on 68 women aged 45–64 years. These numbers represented 85% of the available population randomly selected from lists of 16 general practitioners. Reproducibility of the measurements of total serum cholesterol, triglyceride, and LDL cholesterol was acceptable. The reproducibility of some of the other serum lipid fractions, for example HDL cholesterol, was less good, in part because of the small range of the values found for these components. Univariate associations of physical and behavioral characteristics and serum lipoproteins of men and women, with and without CAD, disclosed small and statistically nonsignificant differences except for levels of BP. In particular, there was no significant difference in mean levels of serum HDL cholesterol between men with CAD (0.91 mmol/liter) and men without it (0.94 mmol/liter).

Serum lipoproteins and susceptibility of men of Indian descent to CAD in Trinidad

Population migration from the Indian subcontinent to other parts of the world dates from 1834, when over 3 years about 7,000 men and women sailed from Calcutta to settle in Mauritius. Emigration to the West Indies commenced soon afterward, with many thousands of Indians arriving, mainly in Trinidad and Guyana, between 1844 and 1917. Whether they settled in Africa, Europe, the Americas, or other parts of Asia, the rate of CAD is much higher in Indian people than in their compatriots of other ethnic descent. This susceptibility has been thought to be due possibly to a high prevalence of diabetes mellitus or to high serum cholesterol concentrations. Miller and associates[36] from Trinidad and London, England, compared the prevalence of CAD and fasting serum lipoprotein concentrations in ethnic groups in Port of Spain, Trinidad. In a total community survey of 1,416 men aged 35–69 years, angina pectoris, a history of possible AMI, and major Q waves on the ECG were significantly more common in men of Indian descent than in other ethnic groups (relative risk about 3/1). Indians had significantly lower HDL cholesterol concentrations and significantly higher LDL cholesterol concentrations than other groups. After allowance for age and ethnic group, men with major Q waves or a history of possible AMI had a significantly greater ratio of LDL/HDL cholesterol than men without either. Comparison of surveys in the Caribbean suggests that in this region CAD is prevalent only in communities in which a sizeable proportion of men have an LDL/HDL cholesterol ratio >6 and an LDL concentration >5 mmol/liter.

Total serum cholesterol level and risk of death from cancer in men aged 40–69 years

The association between circulating total serum cholesterol level and 10-year cancer mortality was investigated in 61,567 men aged 40–69 years from 11 population studies in 8 countries.[37] Those dying of cancer within 1 year of cholesterol determination had mean cholesterol levels 24–35 mg/dl lower on the average than the rest of the men. For years 2–5 and 6–10, the inverse association diminished markedly, with differences in mean cholesterol levels of only 4–5 mg/dl and 2 mg/dl, respectively. Lung cancer mortality was inversely associated with cholesterol level only in the first year, and no significant association was seen with colonic cancer. These findings are consistent with the hypothesis that lower cholesterol levels in cancer decedents are due to the effect of undetected disease on cholesterol level.

In an accompanying editorial, Levy[38] made several points in considering the relation between lower levels of serum cholesterol and noncardiovascular mortality: 1) a number of population-based studies worldwide have shown a high cholesterol level and higher consumptions of saturated fat with increased noncardiovascular mortality, particularly cancer mortality. 2) The population-based studies that have described the low cholesterol and noncardiovascular disease relation have dealt with free living subjects followed prospectively without drug or diet intervention to lower cholesterol levels. No study has linked diet change with cancer. 3) Five studies have suggested a link between cancer and lowered levels of cholesterol. The combined results of the studies are consistent with the hypothesis that the cholesterol-lowering diets do not influence cancer risk. 4) When one compares the cholesterol and cardiovascular disease to the cholesterol and cancer association using the criteria for assessing etiologic significance of epidemiologic association, the differences are striking. The strength, graded nature, temporal sequence, coherence, independence, and predictive capacity of the cholesterol and cardiovascular disease relation are all present and far more striking. The article by the International Collaborative Group, however, throws new doubt on the etiologic significance of the cancer and cholesterol relation. With cholesterol and cardiovascular mortality, the evidence of a temporal sequence is strong. With cholesterol and cancer, suggestive evidence is available that the cancer precedes the association.

What, then, do we now do with the cardiovascular disease and high cholesterol association and the suggested association between colonic cancer and low cholesterol levels? Clearly, we need to continue to review population-based data to try to understand better the low cholesterol and noncardiovascular association, tenuous as it may be. We should also be mindful of the 1981 panel's overall assessment of the public health implications of the data they reviewed. "It was the unanimous opinion of the panelists that the data did not preclude, countermand or contradict the current public health message which recommends that those with elevated cholesterol levels seek to lower them through diets lower in saturated fat and cholesterol."

The observations made by the International Collaborative Group do not totally explain why the cholesterol and cancer relation, inconsistent as it has been, was observed in subjects with cholesterol levels only <190 mg/dl and only in men. In this group, it is possible that the lower cholesterol may be a biologic "marker," possibly genetic in origin. As additional data are collected in this area of considerable complexity, it is important to review continually and update the scientific evidence and to be wary of dramatic headlines and sporadic reports. At present, the facts on hand support the position of such organizations as the American Heart Association and the National Heart, Lung, and Blood Institute that the reduction of cholesterol and saturated fats in the American diet represents a prudent step in our attempt to reduce the incidence of CAD in the USA.

Search for an optimal serum cholesterol

Kannel and Gordon[39] from Boston, Massachusetts, and Washington, DC, wrote a piece defending the proposition (I think—WCR) that there is a gradient for CAD risk with increasing serum cholesterol levels. From their Framingham data both 10-year and 20-year incidences of de novo CAD for Framingham men aged <50 at the beginning of follow-up did increase, as did the level of serum cholesterol. The measure of serum cholesterol used was the average of determinations at examinations 2 and 3, done 2 years apart. In these data there was a distinct gradient of risk, the gradient being sharper at lower levels of serum cholesterol than at higher levels. Even when the effect of age, systolic BP, and cigarette smoking was taken into consideration, a distinct gradient of risk still remained with the serum cholesterol level. The univariate logistic regression coefficients for the 20-year incidence of AMI, angina pectoris as the first manifestation of CAD, and sudden CAD death without previous clinical evidence of AMI shows the association of serum cholesterol level with sudden CAD death to be stronger, as evidenced by the larger coefficient than that with other manifestations of CAD, but in general the association of serum cholesterol level with all manifestations of CAD was similar.

Kannel and Gordon made 3 interesting statements: 1) "Serum cholesterol is not a strong risk factor for CAD, in the sense that BP is a strong risk factor for stroke or cigarette smoking is a risk factor for lung cancer. There is . . . no such truly powerful CAD risk factor." Hence, Kannel and Gordon would anticipate that random variation would take its toll of regularity. I would disagree with this statement. It has to do with what level one considers the total serum cholesterol abnormal. If one picks 150 mg/dl, it is extremely rare to see fatal or nonfatal coronary events at levels below that number. 2) "CAD is a multifactorial disease. Thus, the relation of serum cholesterol to CAD will be modified by the distribution of other associated risk factors in a population; and this may differ from one population to another." I would also disagree with this statement. Systemic hypertension is rampant in Africa but CAD is virtually nonexistent in the black population. Cigarette smoking is extremely common in many countries where CAD is virtually nonexistent. If the total serum cholesterol, however, is >150 mg/dl, systemic hypertension, cigarette smoking, and the other so-called risk factors become extremely important, but only when the total cholesterol level is >150. 3) "Coronary atherosclerosis probably reflects the person's lifetime history." I do not know what this statement means. 4) "Serum cholesterol is not a pure CAD risk factor. Its effect will depend on its lipoprotein concentration." The last point, of course, has to do with the HDL component of the total cholesterol. The higher the HDL, the less the likelihood that CAD will be present, and the higher the LDL cholesterol the greater the likelihood that CAD will be present. Their final statement concerns their regret that there does not seem to be a gradient of CAD risk at low levels of serum cholesterol.

Relation of serum total cholesterol and triglyceride levels to amount and extent of coronary narrowing in CAD

Cabin and Roberts[40] from Bethesda, Maryland, determined the amount of cross-sectional area (XSA) narrowing by atherosclerotic plaques histological-ly in each 5 mm segment of the entire lengths of the right, LM, LAD, and LC coronary arteries in 40 patients with fatal CAD and known fasting serum total cholesterol and triglyceride levels. The patients were divided into 4 groups based upon the serum total cholesterol and triglyceride levels: group

I, total cholesterol of ≤250 mg/dl, triglyceride of ≤170 mg/dl; group II, total cholesterol of ≤250, triglyceride of >170; group III, total cholesterol of >250, triglyceride of ≤170; group IV, total cholesterol of >250, triglyceride of >170. The number of 5 mm segments of coronary artery narrowed severely (76–100% in XSA) by atherosclerotic plaques in each group was as follows: 172 (34%) of 505 5 mm segments from group I; 242 (69%) of 353 segments from group II; 120 (41%) of 295 from group III, and 425 (48%) of 884 segments from group IV. The mean percent of 5 mm segments narrowed severely was significantly greater in group II than in group I (p < 0.005) or group III (p < 0.01). Additionally, the mean number of 4 coronary arteries per subject severely narrowed and the number of subjects with severe narrowing of the LM coronary artery were significantly greater in groups II and III than in group I. The mean percent of 5 mm segments narrowed severely correlated significantly with the serum triglyceride level (p < 0.03). Although it correlated with the number of severely narrowed coronary arteries per subject, the serum total cholesterol level did not correlate with the percent of 5 mm segments of coronary artery with severe narrowing.

Value of measuring high density lipoproteins in assessing risk of cardiovascular disease

A depressed level of plasma HDL has been shown to be an independent risk factor in CAD and low levels of HDL also have been found in patients with peripheral vascular and cerebrovascular disease. Certain experimental findings have demonstrated that HDL has a cholesterol-mobilizing effect and may inhibit the development of atherosclerotic arterial disease. Most previous studies have been based on measurement of the blood concentration of HDL, but recent studies have suggested that a more critical measure is the percent of HDL to total lipoprotein or the percent of HDL cholesterol to total cholesterol. Several different lipoprotein assays have been used. First, most epidemiologic studies have measured HDL cholesterol by measuring cholesterol in the supernatant after precipitating the other lipoproteins with heparin and manganese chloride. This method has the advantage of simplicity, but it loses accuracy in the presence of hypertriglyceridemia and is subject to technical error if the proper conditions of precipitation are not rigorously maintained. Second, lipoproteins can be measured by electrophoresis, using a lipid or enzymatic stain, followed by densitometric scanning. These methods require special equipment but provide a convenient, quantitative profile of cholesterol and other lipids in the major lipoproteins. Third, lipoprotein cholesterol can be measured after separating the lipoproteins by ultracentrifugation. This remains the reference method for HDL-cholesterol, but is too impractical for routine clinical use.

Lipinska and Gurewich[41] from Boston, Massachusetts, evaluated HDL measurement as a clinical discriminator for cardiovascular disease in individual subjects. Three laboratory methods were compared, 2 electrophoretic and 1 heparin-manganese precipitation, and the HDL results were expressed both as a percent and as an absolute concentration. In phase 1 of the study, the optimal method and the best cutoff point were identified. In phase 2, these were applied to a larger population who were assigned, on the basis of clinical criteria, to a CAD and to a control group. The overall probability of correct classification of an individual by the HDL result was calculated. When HDL was expressed as a percent and determined by gel electrophoresis, 83% of control subjects and 83% of patients with CAD were classified correctly using the optimal cutoff point of 23.5%.

Treatment of ambulatory type-1 diabetics with the subcutaneous insulin pump and its effect on HDL cholesterol

Patients with type I diabetes mellitus (DM) have accelerated atherosclerosis. To control glucose levels better and possibly slow down the rate of atherosclerosis, Falko and associates[42] from Columbus, Ohio, treated 12 ambulatory patients (mean age, 29 years) with type 1 DM by a continuous subcutaneous open loop insulin pump. Hemoglobin A, mean blood glucose, total cholesterol, total triglycerides, LDL cholesterol (LDL-C), HDL cholesterol (HDL-C), and the total cholesterol/HDL-C ratio were assessed monthly before and after glucoregulation from 5–14 months (mean, 9). Mean HDL-C level ratios increased significantly (52 ± 4–60 ± 5 mg/dl); mean total cholesterol/HDL-C levels decreased significantly (4.46 ± 0.43–3.89 ± 0.39). Mean values for triglycerides, total cholesterol, and LDL-C, all initially normal, did not change. Both mean hemoglobin A_1 levels and glucose levels fell from 11.2% ± 0.5%–9.8% ± 0.5% and 177 ± 15–128 ± 12 mg/dl, respectively. Insulin requirements decreased from 0.80 ± 0.08–0.61 ± 0.05 units/kg/24 hours. These results may favorably alter the prediction for development of accelerated atherosclerosis in type 1 diabetics.

High density lipoprotein cholesterol in marathon runners

Dressendorfer and associates[43] from Davis, California, Honolulu, Hawaii, San Francisco, California, and Royal Oak, Michigan, measured plasma HDL cholesterol and lipid levels in 12 male marathon runners (mean age, 40 years) who ran an average of 28 km/day for 10 days, rested 70 hours, then ran for 8 more days, covering a total distance for both running periods of 500 km. Blood samples were obtained on 8 mornings. After 1 week of running, HDL cholesterol levels increased 18% and triglyceride levels decreased 22%. However, the 3-day rest period reversed these changes. As running resumed, HDL cholesterol levels again increased and triglyceride levels decreased. There were no significant changes in total cholesterol, body weight, or skinfold thickness, despite an average caloric intake of 4,800 kcal/day. Heavy beer drinking had no discernible effect on HDL cholesterol levels, but may have caused mild hepatic injury, as suggested by significantly increased serum alanine transferase and γ-glutamyl transferase values. This study demonstrates that HDL cholesterol levels increase with higher running mileage and decrease within days of stopping exercise when caloric and alcohol intake remain elevated.

High density lipoprotein cholesterol levels in Japan

Ueshima and associates[44] from Osaka, Akita, and Ibaraki, Japan, measured HDL cholesterol levels of 6 Japanese population groups with different lifestyles (1,804 men and 1,561 women). They found the HDL cholesterol levels of the Japanese men aged 40–69 years to be approximately 55 mg/dl, or about 10 mg/dl higher than those of American men of similar age.

Frequency of apolipoprotein E-ND phenotype and hyperapobetalipoproteinemia in normolipidemic subjects with xanthelasma of the eyelids

Apolipoprotein E isomorphs in VLDL and apolipoprotein B of LDL were measured in the plasma of normolipidemic patients with xanthelasma of the eyelids and in appropriate control subjects by Douste-Blazy and associates[45] from Montreal, Canada. All patients tested in the experimental group had an apolipoprotein E11/E111 ratio typical of the heterozygous state for familial dysbetalipoproteinemia or both. Some patients had concomitant atherosclerosis. This is the first report of an increased frequency of the apolipoprotein E-ND phenotype in nomolipidemic xanthelasma. This condition should not be dismissed as benign; tissue lipid deposition in the absence of hyperlipidemia might be related to the presence of lipoproteins of abnormal composition with an enhanced atherogenic potential.

Familial deficiency of apolipoproteins A-I and C-III and precocious coronary artery disease

The inverse relation between CAD and the concentration of HDL cholesterol in blood suggests that this lipoprotein is an important factor in the pathogenesis of atherosclerosis. Low levels of HDL cholesterol have been associated with an increased frequency of CAD, even at an HDL level <50% of "normal." Yet in Tangier disease, an inherited disorder of cholesterol metabolism in which HDL cholesterol is about 8% of "normal," the frequency of symptomatic atherosclerosis is not increased. Norum and associates[46] from Toronto, Canada, studied 2 sisters aged 29 and 31 years who had skin and tendon xanthomas, corneal clouding, and severe coronary atherosclerosis. Histologic examination disclosed collections of lipid-laden histiocytes in the skin. The patients' plasma cholesterol concentrations were 177 and 135 mg/dl (4.58 and 3.49 mmol/liter). Levels of HDL cholesterol were 4 and 7 mg/dl (0.1 and 0.2 mmol/liter). Only traces of apolipoprotein A-I were detected in whole plasma. The plasma density fraction from 1.06–1.21 g/ml contained no HDL on high pressure liquid chromatography, no apolipoprotein A-I on sodium dodecyl sulfate electrophoresis, and only traces of apolipopotein A-I on radioimmunoassay. Apolipoprotein C-III also was not detectable. The activity of lecithin cholesterol acyltransferase was 40% of normal. The half-life of infused normal HDL was 3 days (normal, 5.8 days). The parents and children of these 2 patients had low levels of HDL cholesterol and apolipoprotein A-I. Thus, these cases support the hypothesis that low concentrations of HDL promote atherosclerosis.

Myelomatosis with type III hyperlipoproteinemia

Pronounced hyperlipidemia is an infrequent but well-documented finding in myelomatosis. Hyperlipidemia also is an occasional finding in other disorders associated with hypergammaglobulinemia. The metabolic bases of immunoglobulin-induced hyperlipidemias are of considerable interest. Autoimmune mechanisms, including inhibition of the lipoprotein lipase system and antibodies to lipoprotein, have been considered. Since receptor-mediated catabolism of lipoproteins depends on the recognition of their apolipoproteins, impairment of lipoprotein interconversion and degradation due to blocking of recognition sites by immunoglobulins could be responsible. Cortese and associates[47] from Marburg, Federal Republic of Germany, and Harrow, England, investigated the metabolism of IDL (1.006–1.019 g/ml) and LDL (1.019–1.063 g/ml) in 2 men with type III hyperlipoproteinemia associated with myelomatosis. In vivo kinetic studies using radiolabeled autologous lipoproteins demonstrated a greatly reduced fractional catabolic rate of IDL, relative to control values (patients -vs- normal, 0.006 and 0.025/h -vs- 0.20 ± 0.08/h [mean ± SEM]) and a greatly prolonged IDL to LDL conversion time (45 and 17 h -vs- 5.4 ± 1.6 h). In studies in vitro, LDL from both patients failed to bind to the LDL receptor of normal blood lymphocytes, whereas LDL from subjects with familial type III bound normally to the receptor. In 1 patient, immunoglobulin was associated with IDL and LDL. Thus, hyperlipoproteinemia reflected an impaired metabolism of IDL, probably secondary to the binding of immunoglobulin to the lipoproteins. A similar impairment of receptor-mediated LDL catabolism did not elevate the plasma LDL concentration because of the low IDL to LDL conversion rate.

Lipoprotein remnant formation in chronic renal failure

It is generally accepted that patients undergoing long-term dialysis for chronic renal failure are at increased risk for CAD. One postulated risk factor is hyperlipidemia, which occurs commonly, although the moderate degree of hypertriglyceridemia, the most usual abnormality, would only marginally increase the risk in an otherwise healthy population. It is possible, however, that the specific type of lipoprotein particle that characterizes this disorder is potentially highly atherogenic. Since it is likely that certain remnants derived from the catabolism of triglyceride-rich lipoproteins, such as the remnants that accumulate in type 3 hyperlipoproteinemia (HLP), do lead to atherosclerosis, Nestel and associates[48] from Melbourne, Australia, analyzed the lipoproteins of 11 patients receiving maintenance dialysis and looked for evidence of apoproteins that might indicate accumulated remnant particles. The authors found several abnormalities in lipoproteins and lipids: enrichment of IDL and LDL with triglyceride; the presence of apoprotein B48 (a "marker" for intestinal lipoproteins) in VLDL; an increased concentration of aproprotein AIV (a protein related to chylomicron transport); the presence of AIV in VLDL, IDL, and LDL; and the presence in LDL of apoproteins C and E (proteins not normally found in LDL). These findings strongly suggest accumulation of remnants of triglyceride-rich lipoproteins in patients with chronic renal failure who are undergoing peritoneal dialysis or hemodialysis, and they may explain in part the increased incidence of CAD deaths among these patients.

Effect of exercise on plasma lipoproteins (The National Exercise and Heart Disease Project)

As part of the National Exercise and Heart Disease Project, 223 men, aged 30–64 years, all of whom had had an AMI 2–36 months (mean, 14) before entry, were randomly assigned to moderate exercise or control groups and reported by LaRosa and associates[49] from Washington, DC. Levels of total plasma cholesterol, HDL and LDL cholesterol, and triglycerides were measured. At baseline, alcohol intake, weight, and skinfold thickness but not treadmill work capacity correlated with triglyceride or HDL cholesterol levels (Table 1–2). After 1 year, no clinically important change in lipid levels was observed in either group. Using multiple regression analysis of the combined groups, changes in several independent variables, including work capacity change, were not predictive of changes in lipid levels. Thus, changes in levels of fitness and/or regular exercise did not substantially influence HDL cholesterol or other lipid levels.

Plasma lipid and lipoprotein levels after exercise

Since high levels of LDL cholesterol are related to increased risks of CAD and high levels of HDL cholesterol may protect against CAD, Brownell and associates[50] from Philadelphia, Pennsylvania, and Baltimore, Maryland, measured levels of HDL cholesterol and other lipids and lipoprotein in 24 men and 37 women before and after a 10-week exercise program. The program involved 3 sessions of aerobic exercise each week with 15–20 minutes of activity at 70% maximal heart rate. Men and women demonstrated significantly different lipid patterns in response to exercise despite equivalent increases in maximal oxygen uptake. Men displayed 5% increase in HDL cholesterol, a 6% decrease in LDL cholesterol, and a 12% increase in HDL/LDL ratio. In contrast, women had a 1% decrease in HDL cholesterol, a 4% decrease in LDL cholesterol, and no significant change in the HDL/LDL ratio. A number of exercise sessions correlated positively with HDL/LDL changes in men and correlated negatively with HDL/LDL changes in women. Thus, these findings suggest that moderate exercise may have different effects on men and women.

TABLE 1-2. *Baseline and 1-year means of various lipid measurements.* * *Reproduced with permission from LaRosa et al.*[49]

GROUP	SUBJECTS	MEAN (± SEM) AT BASELINE	P	MEAN (± SEM) AT 1 YEAR	ADJUSTED MEAN (± SEM)† AT 1 YEAR	P
Cholesterol, mg/dL						
Exercise	110	222.5 (3.3)	—	226.8 (3.4)	226.1 (2.3)	—
Control	113	220.2 (3.3)	0.62	230.7 (3.1)	231.3 (2.2)	.10
LDL,‡ mg/dL						
Exercise	108	150.1 (3.1)	—	154.1 (2.2)	153.1 (2.2)	—
Control	113	145.5 (3.1)	0.28	156.2 (2.1)	156.2 (2.2)	.32
HDL,‡ mg/dL						
Exercise	110	43.9 (1.0)	—	45.2 (1.2)	45.3 (0.9)	—
Control	113	44.4 (1.0)	0.79	44.8 (1.2)	44.7 (0.9)	.61
Triglyceride, mg/dL						
Exercise	110	143.4 (5.8)	—	138.4 (7.0)	138.9 (5.5)	—
Control	113	145.5 (7.1)	0.82	155.8 (7.6)	155.3 (5.4)	.04

* Levels for each group at baseline and at 1 year are presented. No significant differences are apparent at baseline. At 1 year, however, triglyceride levels are significantly lower in the exercise group.
† Adjusted for baseline differences in age at entry, time from qualifying myocardial infarction to randomization, baseline lipid value, weight, and work capacity.
‡ LDL indicates low-density lipoprotein; HDL, high-density lipoprotein.

Effect of diet on serum lipoproteins in a population with a high risk of CAD

The population of North Karelia, a county in Finland, has a high rate of CAD. It also has a high prevalence of hypercholesterolemia, but whether the latter reflects a diet rich in animal fat or is a result of genetic factors is unclear. Ehnholm and associates[51] from Helsinki, Finland, studied the effect on serum lipoproteins of a low fat diet with a high ratio of polyunsaturated to saturated fatty acids in 54 middle-aged volunteers in North Karelia. Total serum cholesterol decreased, from 263 ± 8 mg/dl (mean, ± SE) to 201 ± 5 mg/dl in men (p < 0.0001) and from 239 ± 8–188 ± 8 mg/dl in women (p < 0.0001), along with LDL cholesterol and apoprotein B (Table 1–3). High density lipoprotein cholesterol decreased from 54 ± 2–44 ± 2 mg/dl in men (p < 0.0001) and from 56 ± 3–47 ± 2 mg/dl in women (p < 0.0001). A small but significant reduction occurred in serum apoprotein A-I, whereas apoprotein A-II increased slightly. The individual changes in LDL cholesterol correlated with those in HDL cholesterol. The changes in serum lipids and apoproteins were reversed when the participants returned to their original diets. These results suggest that the hypercholesterolemia characteristic of this population is due at least in part to dietary factors.

Treatment of homozygous familiar hypercholesterolemia in childhood by a high glucose diet

Homozygous familiar hypercholesterolemia (HFH) is refractory to standard dietary or drug therapy. Recent studies, however, suggest that a high carbohydrate/low fat diet may reduce circulating cholesterol levels in normal or hyperlipidemic subjects. Accordingly, Stacpoole and associates[52] from Nashville, Tennessee, treated a 9-year-old boy with HFH with a liquid formula diet containing 82%–90% of total calories as glucose. The diet was given as a constant nasogastric infusion or as intermittent daytime drinks followed by a nighttime infusion. Plasma total and LDL cholesterol fell from basal levels of 719 and 676 to 456 and 434 mg/dl, respectively, after 1 week of therapy. After approximately 14 weeks of treatment, plasma total and LDL cholesterol levels were 311 and 277 mg/dl, each representing approximately a 58% decrease from basal levels. The fall in circulating cholesterol levels was accompanied by a regression of xanthomatous skin lesions, a rise in plasma insulin levels, and no change in plasma glucose or glucagon concentrations. No adverse effects of therapy occurred. Thus, high carbohydrate diets may be a safe and effective adjunct in the treatment of HFH.

Protection of myocardium by coronary collaterals after total occlusion of major company arteries in familial hypercholesterolemia

Kuo and colleagues[53] from Piscataway, New Jersey, evaluated 11 in a group of 21 asymptomatic patients with heterozygous familial hypercholes-

TABLE 1–3. *Total serum cholesterol, triglycerides, and HDL cholesterol concentrations at ends of study periods.* *Reproduced with permission from Ehnholm et al.*[51]

	BASE-LINE PERIOD	INTERVENTION PERIOD	SWITCH-BACK PERIOD
		mg/dl	
Men (n = 30)			
Total cholesterol	263 ± 8†	201 ± 5	259 ± 7†
LDL cholesterol	185 ± 8†	137 ± 5	183 ± 7†
HDL cholesterol	54 ± 2†	44 ± 2	55 ± 2†
Triglycerides	124 ± 18	96 ± 9	99 ± 11
Women (n = 24)			
Total cholesterol	239 ± 8†	188 ± 8	231 ± 10†
LDL cholesterol	164 ± 7†	125 ± 7	156 ± 9†
HDL cholesterol	56 ± 3†	47 ± 2	60 ± 2†
Triglycerides	91 ± 12	76 ± 6	76 ± 7

* Data are presented as means ± S.E.M. To convert values for cholesterol and triglycerides to millimoles per liter, multiply by 0.02586 and 0.01129, respectively. † Significantly different from value for intervention period (P < 0.0001 by paired comparison test).

terolemia and progressive CAD to assess the role of compensatory mechanisms, especially coronary collaterals, in providing adequate blood supply to the myocardium, following complete occlusion of ≥1 major coronary arteries. Diet colestipol, nicotinic acid treatment decreased the plasma total cholesterol and LDL cholesterol (mg/dl, mean ± SEM) from 443 ± 26 and 363 ± 24, respectively, to 231 ± 12 and 185 ± 14, respectively, for 6–9 years. The initially stenotic lesions of these 11 patients slowly progressed to complete occlusion, while the patients remained free of myocardial ischemia or infarction and exhibited no abnormality on 24-hour ambulatory ECG monitoring, exercise stress, and thallium-201 stress tests. Thus, coronary occlusion can be retarded in patients with familial hypercholesterolemia by strenuous hypocholesterolemic therapy to allow the development of compensatory mechanisms, including coronary collaterals. Apparently, the angiographically visible collaterals combined with subendocardial anastomosis can give adequate myocardial blood supply to such patients with familiar hypercholesterolemia following occlusion ≥1 major coronary artery.

Efficacy of colestipol -vs- clofibrate in type IIa hyperlipoproteinemia

Vecchio and associates[54] from Kalamazoo, Michigan, sumarized findings in a multiclinic study comparing colestipol hydrochloride, clofibrate, and placebo in 245 patients with type IIa hyperlipoproteinemia (HLP). Eighty-five subjects took colestipol hydrocholride in progressive doses of 15, 20, and

30 g/day; 87 took 2.0 g/day of clofibrate; and 73 took placebo over the 6 months of study. Colestipol lowered total cholesterol level 21% in comparison with clofibrate (14%) (statistically significant at months 3, 5, and 6), and lowered LDL cholesterol level 29% in comparison with clofibrate (15%) (significant at months 2, 4, and 6, all times measured). High-density lipoprotein cholesterol level remained unchanged in all groups. Clofibrate lowered total triglyceride levels 23%, compared with an increase of 13% in the colestipol group and 11% in the placebo group (significant at all time intervals). Colestipol was more effective than clofibrate in lowering the cholesterol fractions associated with increased cardiovascular risk.

Serum estrogen level

Klaiber and associates[55] from Shrewsbury and Worcester, Massachusetts, assessed the serum estradiol and serum estrone levels in 29 men with AMI, in 17 men with unstable angina pectoris, in 14 men in whom AMI was ruled out, in 12 men without apparent CAD but hospitalized in an intensive care unit, and in 28 men who were not hospitalized and who acted as controls. (The 12 men who were hospitalized but who did not have CAD were included to control for physical and emotional stress of a severe medical illness.) Ages ranged from 21–56 years. Age, height, and weight did not differ significantly among groups. Blood samples were obtained in the patient groups on each of the first 3 days of hospitalization. The serum estrone level was significantly elevated in all 4 patient groups when compared with that in the control group. Estrone level did not differentiate patients with and without CAD. Serum estradiol levels were significantly elevated in the groups with AMI, unstable angina, and in the group in whom AMI was ruled out. However, estradiol levels were not significantly elevated in the group in the intensive care unit without CAD when compared with the level in the normal control group. Serum estradiol levels, then, were elevated in men with confirmed or suspected CAD, but were not elevated in men without CAD even under the stressful conditions found in an intensive care unit. Serum estradiol levels were significantly and positively correlated (p < 0.03) with serum total creatinine phosphokinase levels in the patients with AMI. The 5 patients with AMI who died within 10 days of admission had markedly elevated serum estradiol levels. The potential significance of these serum estradiol elevations is discussed in terms of estradiol's ability to enhance adrenergic neural activity and the resultant increase in myocardial oxygen demand.

Recent studies have reported higher plasma estradiol levels in male survivors of AMI. This finding has raised the possibility that hyperestrogenemia may constitute a separate coronary risk factor. In 443 men, aged 30–60 years, Lindholm and associates[56] from Copenhagen, Denmark, assessed the relation between plasma levels of estradiol, testosterone, and testosterone-binding globulin and coronary risk factors: fasting plasma concentrations of triglyceride, total cholesterol, and HDL cholesterol, BP, cigarette smoking, and leisure time physical activity patterns. Plasma estradiol concentrations correlated significantly with body weight. After adjustment for this association, the authors found that the mean plasma estradiol concentration still was significantly higher in smokers than in nonsmokers. No other correlation could be established between plasma hormone levels and coronary risk factors. The relative hyperestrogenemia reported in men with previous AMI may be due to an effect of smoking, but may also reflect the relation between body weight and plasma estradiol levels.

OTHER RISK FACTORS

Familial aggregation of CAD and its relation to known genetic risk factors

Ten Kate and associates[57] from Seattle, Washington, studied 145 white male survivors of AMI, 145 age-matched white male blood donors, and the first-degree relatives of both groups to determine whether the familial aggregation of CAD is explained by familial clustering of coronary risk factors. Risk factors, including serum cholesterol, triglyceride, and fasting blood glucose levels, BP, and cigarette smoking were determined in patients and control subjects. Relatives were interviewed and if the person had died, a copy of the death certificate was obtained. Risk factors, with the exception of high BP, were significantly more frequent in patients than in control subjects. In first-degree relatives of survivors of AMI 16% had had an AMI compared with 9% of relatives of control subjects. The frequency of CAD among the first-degree relatives of patients and control patients was 21% and 15%, respectively. Statistical analyses that eliminated the role of the various known genetic risk factors by data stratification according to confounding risk variables and subsequent calculation of a pooled relative risk estimate indicated an approximately 2-fold relative risk for AMI among families of survivors of AMI. Risk factors did not predict familial occurrence. These data suggest that familial aggregation of CAD is not entirely explained by the familial clustering of currently known risk factors.

Significance of family history and cigarette smoking as risk factors for CAD in adults ≤50 years

Chesebro and associates[58] from Rochester, Minnesota, reviewed 435 consecutive white patients aged ≤50 years who had coronary arteriography from July 1975–June 1977 at the Mayo Clinic because of typical or atypical chest pains. The patients were divided into 2 groups: 335 patients with CAD (median and mean ages 46 and 45 years, respectively, 88% men) who had at least 1 coronary artery narrowed >50% in diameter (138, or 41%, had previous AMI) and 100 patients (median and mean ages 44 and 43 years, respectively, 58% men) who had angiographically normal coronary arteries,

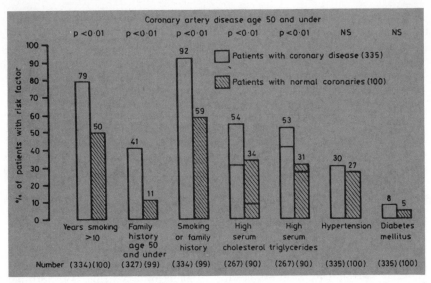

Fig. 1-2. Univariate analysis of risk factors in young patients with CAD and those with normal coronary arteries. Serum cholesterol and serum triglycerides were taken at ≥80th centile for age and sex (top of bar) and 95th centile (solid line in bar). Not shown is current smoking status for CAD (26%) and normal coronary (22%) patients. Each risk factor except diabetes, hypertension, and current smoking status was significantly (p < 0.01) more frequent in patients with CAD than in those without. Number of patients in each risk factor subgroup is shown below each bar. Patients in whom a risk factor was unknown were excluded from analysis: smoking 1, family history 8, cholesterol and triglycerides 68 (CAD), and 10 (normal). Reproduced with permission from Chesebro et al.[58]

no previous AMI by history or ECG criteria, and no clinical evidence of peripheral arteriosclerosis obliterans as judged by normal arterial pulses and absence of claudication and bruits. Patients with coronary narrowings <50% in diameter and associated valvular, congenital, or cardiomyopathic heart diseases were excluded. The number of "packet-years" (number of packs, of 20 cigarettes, per day times number of years smoked) of smoking was determined from the patient and the number of first-degree relatives who had family histories of CAD (AMI, sudden death, angina pectoris, or coronary narrowing documented by coronary angiography), aged ≤50 years were determined (Fig. 1–2). In addition, the number of patients with hypercholesterolemia and hypertriglyceridemia (defined as ≥95th or 80th percentile for age and sex) were determined (Fig. 1–2). In addition, the frequency of systemic hypertension (BP 160/95 mmHg) was made before arteriography. The presence of diabetes mellitus was defined as 2 fasting plasma glucose values ≥120 mg/dl or insulin dependence. By univariate analysis, each risk factor except systemic hypertension and diabetes mellitus was significantly more frequent in patients with CAD than in those without. By multivariate analysis of all risk factors in patients with and without CAD, the patient with CAD could best be identified by the strong family history, cigarette smoking history, and age- and sex-corrected serum cholesterol. The percentage of patients with CAD when the 3 risk factors were present was 95%; 2 factors, 88%; 1 factor, 67%; and none of the 3 factors, 25%; strong family history alone, 90%; cigarette smoking alone, 66%; and serum cholesterol >80th percentile alone, 52%.

Hemostatic factors associated with CAD in men aged 45–64 years (Speedwell study)

Baker and associates[59] from Cardiff, Bristol, and Portsmouth, UK, measured various hemostatic factors that might contribute both to thrombogenesis and atherogenesis in the same population of patients used by Bainton and associates,[35] namely, 283 men and 68 women, aged 45–64 years. Fibrinogen and plasma viscosity were positively associated with the prevalence of CAD. Antithrombin III was negatively associated with the prevalence of CAD. These associations were statistically significant (p < 0.001). The negative association of "clottable" fibrinogen and the positive association of plasma viscosity with the prevalence of CAD were confirmed and both were statistically significant (p < 0.05). Apart from age, the independent association of the other variables with CAD did not achieve statistical significance. Fibrinogen measured nephelometrically and by a clotting method had positive and statistically significant associations with serum total cholesterol, but no associations with serum total triglycerides, cigarette smoking, or alcohol consumption. "Clottable" fibrinogen had an inverse and statistically insignificant association with serum HDL cholesterol. The observed associations support the concept of the involvement of some hemostatic factors in the etiology of CAD.

Benefits and risks of running

To estimate better the rates of certain benefits and risks of recreational running, Koplan and associates[60] from Atlanta, Georgia, sent questionnaires to 1,250 randomly selected male and 1,250 female registrants for a 10 km road race. The response rate was 55% for men and 58% for women. Telephone interviews of a randomly selected group of nonrespondents indicated that the only significant differences between respondents and nonrespondents were that 1) respondents were older than nonrespondents, 2) more male nonrespondents had stopped running during the year after the race, and 3) more male nonrespondents had been hit by thrown objects. One year after the race, 89% of male and 79% of female respondents were still running regularly. Eighty-one percent of men and 75% of women who smoked when they began running had stopped smoking after beginning recreational running. Giving up smoking was significantly more common for current runners than for "retired" runners. Weight loss was commonly associated with running and was greater in those persons who were overweight when they began running. More than a third of respondents had a musculoskeletal injury attributed to running in the year after the race and about one-seventh of all respondents sought medical consultation for their injury. The risk of injury increased with increasing weekly mileage. This study used epidemiologic methods to quantify some of the benefits and risks of running. This study is important because of the strong association of running with weight reduction and smoking cessation, both of which, of course, are desirable lifestyle changes. Weight loss was greater among those who began running to lose weight.

CAD in blacks

Examination of CAD in blacks by Gillum[61] from Minneapolis, Minnesota, showed that CAD is the leading cause of death among black Americans (57,999 deaths in 1977) despite the widely held belief that CAD is uncommon in blacks. CAD death rates were lower in black men than in white men in the USA in the 1940s, but rose rapidly until they exceeded those of white by 1968. Since 1968, CAD death rates in blacks have fallen (by approximately 30%) to levels similar to whites, but still higher than 1940 rates. Black women have higher CAD mortality than white women. The few population studies of AMI in the 1970s suggest similar or lower age-specific incidence in black than white men but higher case fatality and more out of hospital deaths. Trends in death certification practice and access to medical care may be of particular importance in these differences between blacks and whites.

Fire fighting and CAD

Some reported studies suggest that fire fighters are at a higher risk of developing CAD than are men in the general population. Dibbs and associates[62] from Boston, Massachusetts, followed 1,646 men for 10 years to determine the incidence of CAD. Subjects were participants of the Normative Aging Study, a longitudinal study of aging. Comparison of fire fighters (n, 171) and nonfire fighters (n, 1,475) revealed no significant difference in the incident rates of CAD. Comparison of the groups regarding baseline risk factors also demonstrated no significant differences.

Dietary fiber and 10-year mortality from CAD, cancer, and all causes (Zutphen study)

A prospective study among 337 middle-aged men in London, England, found that a high intake of dietary fiber from cereals was associated with a low risk of CAD. An inverse relation between dietary fiber intake and cancer, especially colonic cancer, also has been suggested. Case control studies of this relation, however, have had inconsistent results. Kromhout and associates[63] from Leiden, The Netherlands, collected usual food intake information in 1960 on 871 middle-aged men in the town of Zutphen, The Netherlands, in a survey of risk indicators, including diet, for CAD. The food intake information was collected for 6–12 months before the interview by cross-check dietary history method. During 10 years of follow-up, 107 men died from all

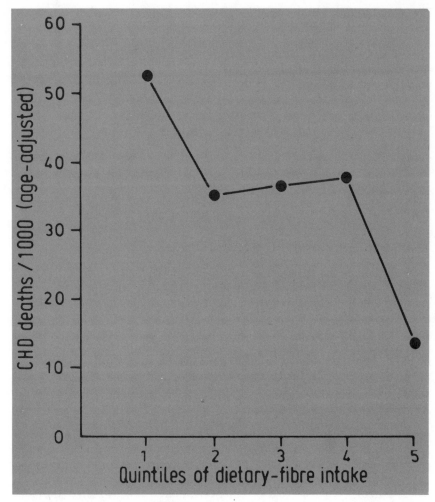

Fig. 1-3. Relation between quintiles of dietary fiber intake at baseline and 10-year CAD death rates. Reproduced with permission from Kromhout et al.[63]

causes, 37 from CAD, and 44 from cancer. Mortality from CAD was about 4 times higher for men in the lowest quintile of dietary fiber intake than for those in the highest quintile, but this inverse relation disappeared after multivariate analysis (Fig. 1–3). Rates of death from cancer and from all causes were about 3 times higher for men in the lowest quintile of dietary fiber intake than for those in the highest quintile, and these relations persisted after multivariate analysis. Thus, a diet containing at least 37 g/day dietary fiber may be protective against certain chronic disease in the Western world, including CAD.

Cardiovascular death and serum selenium

Salonen and associates[64] from Kuopio and Helsinki, Finland, investigated the association between serum selenium and risk of death from acute CAD, as well as risk of fatal and nonfatal AMI in case control pairs from a population of 11,000 persons examined in 1972 from 2 counties in eastern Finland, an area with an exceptionally high mortality from cardiovascular diseases. The patients were aged 35–59 years and had died of CAD or other cardiovascular disease or had a fatal AMI during a 7-year follow-up. Controls were matched for sex, age, daily tobacco consumption, serum cholesterol, diastolic BP, and history of angina pectoris. The mean serum selenium concentration for all cases was 52 μg/liter and for all controls, 55 μg/liter (p < 0.01). Serum selenium 45 μg/liter was associated with an adjusted relative risk of CAD death of 2.9, a relative risk of cardiovascular disease death of 2.2, and a relative risk of fatal and nonfatal AMI of 2.1.

Multiple Risk Factor Intervention Trial

The Multiple Risk Factor Intervention Trial (MRFIT) was a randomized primary prevention trial to test the effect of a multifactor intervention program on mortality from CAD in 12,866 high risk men aged 35–57 years.[65] Men were randomly assigned either to a special intervention (SI) program consisting of stepped care treatment for hypertension, counseling for cigarette smoking, and dietary advice for lowering blood cholesterol levels, or to their usual sources of health care in the community (UC). Over an average follow-up period of 7 years, risk factor levels declined in both groups, but to a greater degree for the SI men (Fig. 1–4). Mortality from CAD was 17.9 deaths per 1,000 in the SI group and 19.3/1,000 in the UC group, a statistically nonsignificant difference of 7.1% (90% confidence interval, −15–25%). Total mortality rates were 41.2/1,000 (SI) and 40.4/1,000 (UC). Three possible explanations for these findings are considered: 1) the overall intervention program, under these circumstances, does not affect CAD mortality; 2) the intervention used does affect CAD mortality, but the benefit was not observed in this trial of 7 years' average duration, with lower than expected mortality and with considerable risk factor change in the UC group; and 3) measures to reduce cigarette smoking and to lower blood cholesterol levels may have reduced CAD mortality within subgroups of the SI cohort, with a possibly unfavorable response to antihypertensive drug therapy in certain but not all hypertensive subjects. This last possibility was considered most likely, needs further investigation, and lends support to some preventive measures while requiring reassessment of others.

This large and complex trial was operationally successful. The recruitment phase was completed in a 28-month period and exceeded the design goal in numbers recruited. Randomization proceeded without incident, the 2 randomized groups being well balanced on numerous relevant characteristics. The completeness of follow-up exceeded expectations, with 91% of those alive returning for the sixth annual visit. For mortality end points, require-

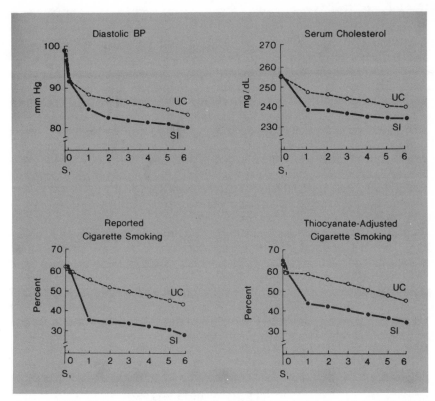

Fig. 1-4. Mean risk factor levels by year of follow-up for Multiple Risk Factor Intervention Trial Research Group participants. SI indicates special intervention; UC, usual care; S_1, first screening visit. Reproduced with permission from the Multiple Risk Factor Intervention Trial Research Group.[65]

ments of thorough documentation of all deaths and "blinded" classification of causes of death were met.

Intervention accomplishments in the SI group, which have been reported in detail, were substantial: smoking cessation was much more successful than had been expected, the BP reduction in the SI group exceeded the desired drop in diastolic BP, and the effect on cholesterol lowering was considerable, but less than had been sought. A notable achievement of the intervention program was a continued decline in mean risk factor levels after the substantial drop in the first year.

Risk factor changes also were observed in the UC group, although to a lesser degree. Whereas it had been projected on the basis of the best information available 10 years ago that this group would exhibit over 6 years no important changes in BP and serum cholesterol levels, and only minimal change in smoking habits, the actual findings were very different. Sizable reductions occurred in the levels of all 3 risk factors for UC men. Thus, over 6 years, reported cigarette smoking declined from 59%–46%, the diastolic BP from a baseline value of 91–84 mmHg, and plasma cholesterol levels from 241–233 mg/dl. Also, 47% of the UC men were receiving antihypertensive medication at the end of the sixth year compared with 19% at baseline.

In conclusion, the MRFIT showed that it is possible to apply an intensive long-term intervention program against 3 coronary risk factors with considerable success in terms of risk factor changes. The overall results do not show a beneficial effect on CAD or total mortality from this multifactor intervention. These results are accompanied by an apparent heterogeneity of effects among sizable subgroups, but there must be caution in reaching conclusions from such subgroup data. It may be relevant that multifactor intervention received a less than optimal test owing, in part, to unexpected declines in risk factor levels and, in part, to lower than expected mortality in the UC group. In regard to the former, the UC men thus constituted to a considerable extent a "treated" group.

The SI-UC comparisons indicate that among men with normal baseline ECGs, the MRFIT intervention program may have a favorable effect on CAD mortality. The data also suggest that men with hypertension, primarily those with resting ECG abnormalities, had no favorable, and possibly an unfavorable, response to intervention. More study is required to clarify this issue and its possible relation to antihypertensive treatment. Findings also include the within-group observation that men who stopped cigarette smoking had lower CAD and total mortality than those who continued to smoke.

PLATELETS and CAD

Platelet function during exercise in normal and CAD patients

Platelet function parameters as influenced by exercise stress were evaluated by Mehta and Mehta[66] from Gainesville, Florida, in 22 patients with CAD and in 13 normal subjects. Upon exercise stress, 14 CAD patients had positive tests and 8, negative tests. Platelet counts during exercise increased similarly in normal and CAD patients. Platelet aggregation response to adenosine diphosphate was unaffected by exercise both in normal subjects and CAD patients. Platelets from 7 of the 14 CAD patients with positive stress tests and increased sensitivity to endoperoxide analog (U-46619) defined as <200 ng/ml U-46619 required for 50% platelet aggregation. Resting plasma β-thromboglobulin (BTG) levels, an index of in vivo platelet activation, were significantly higher in CAD patients compared with normal subjects (74 and 41 ng/ml, respectively). During exercise plasma BTG levels increased in normal subjects to 60 ng/ml. In contrast, BTG levels increased to 102 ng/ml in CAD patients. These increases were transient and BTG declined to preexercise values soon after exercise. Of 12 CAD patients with positive exercise stress tests, 11 had increases in plasma BTG levels, whereas only 3 of the 8

CAD patients with negative stress tests had any increase. These observations of increased platelet activation in certain CAD patients during exercise appear to be related to exercise-induced myocardial ischemia.

Platelet release and thromboxane synthesis in CAD

DeBoer and colleagues[67] from Hamilton, Canada, evaluated the incidence and significance of platelet activation in myocardial ischemia by serial measurments of plasma thromboxane B_2 (TXB_2) and β-thromboglobulin (BTG) in plasma and urine in 98 patients admitted to a coronary care unit with chest pain. All measurements were normal in the 26 patients with nonspecific chest pain. Mean TXB_2 and BTG concentrations, but not urine BTG concentration, were elevated in the 25 patients with AMI and the 47 patients with angina pectoris. The BTG levels remained normal in 61% of the patients with angina or AMI. The TXB_2 levels were significantly higher in patients with recurrent episodes of angina at rest and those without ischemic episodes following admission. There was a weak correlation between TXB_2 and plasma BTG and between plasma and urine BTG. The results indicate that platelets are frequently activated with myocardial ischemia or AMI. However, as these investigators caution, the measurement of BTG and TXB_2 is of limited value in detecting or differentiating myocardial ischemia from AMI and therefore lacks clinical value in the management of patients with CAD.

Effects of propranolol on platelet release and prostaglandin generation in CAD

Suppression of platelet function is currently believed to be a mechanism of propranolol's beneficial action in angina pectoris. To examine the effects of propranolol on platelets, Mehta and Mehta[68] from Gainsville, Florida, measured plasma β-thromboglobulin and plasma thromboxane B_2 (TXB_2) levels by radioimmunoassay as indexes of platelet α-granule and thomboxane A_2 (TXA_2) released, respectively. Platelet TXA_2 generation in vitro in response to arachidonate and thrombin also was quantitated of 29 patients with CAD, 15 not taking propranolol (group A), 14 on propranolol (group B), and of 15 normal subjects. Plasma β-thromboglobulin levels were increased in group A and B patients compared with normal subjects. Plasma TXB_2 were similar in group A and B patients and in normal subjects. Arachidonate-induced platelet TXA_2 generation was significantly higher in group A patients than in normal subjects. In contrast, platelets from group B patients had very low TXA_2 generation compared with platelets from group A patients than in normal subjects. Similar results were obtained using thrombin. These data show that propranolol therapy does not affect platelet-released β-thromboglobulin or TXA_2 at rest, but significantly reduces the capability of platelets to generate TXA_2 in vitro. Thus, these investigators concluded that reduction in platelet TXA_2 generation may be an important mechanism of the action of propranolol in patients with CAD.

ANGINA PECTORIS

Diurnal variation in exercise responses

Joy and associates[69] from Surrey, UK, investigated 30 men with stable angina pectoris. They were divided into 3 groups: 1 of 9 patients on no treatment who underwent symptom-limited exercise ECG at 8:00 am, 12:00 noon, and 4:00 pm on the same day. Their heart rates and ST-segment displacements at 4:00 pm were significantly greater than at 8:00 am. The same phenomenon was seen in the second group of 9 patients who were receiving propranolol 40 mg 4 times a day. The third group of 12 patients on no treatment had a similar effect for ST-segment displacement but not for heart rate when tested at 8:00 am and 4:00 pm on separate days 2–3 weeks apart. Nine normal control subjects showed no diurnal variation in heart rate and their heart rate responses at 4:00 pm were reduced by propranolol. Thus, these observations show a circadian variation in the ST-segment response to exercise in patients with angina and a possible training effect on heart rate with multiple exercise testing on the same day. This is associated with a reduction in vagal parasympathetic tone to the heart and should be taken into account in the assessment of patients with angina and in particular when comparing responses to treatment.

Continuous ECG monitoring in unstable angina

In patients with unstable angina pectoris, transient ST-segment alterations occurring with or without chest pain serve as reliable evidence of periodic episodes of myocardial ischemia. ST-segment alterations occurring on 12-lead ECG during chest pain help to identify those with poor long-term prognosis, and the magnitude of such ST alterations by 12-lead ECG is related to the extent of underlying CAD. Johnson and associates[70] from Dallas, Texas, assessed the value of 2-channel Holter monitoring during the initial hours of hospitalization in patients with unstable angina pectoris to identify those with severe CAD, variant angina, and/or poor prognosis over the next 3 months. The 116 unstable angina patients had Holter monitoring for an average of 27 (range, 12–50) hours after hospitalization. Of these, 24 evolved AMI during monitoring and 92 did not. Transient ST-segment alterations occurred in 21 of the 92. Of these 4 had variant angina, were treated with calcium antagonists, and did well. Each of the remaining 17 had severe CAD (LM or 3-vessel; n, 12) and/or poor prognosis over the 3 months after discharge as manifested by death (n, 1), AMI (n, 3), and/or severe angina (n, 3). In contrast, 71 patients did not demonstrate transient ST-segment alterations: none had variant angina, 9 had LM or 3-vessel CAD, and 50 were alive and well 3 months after discharge. Ventricular tachycardia was demonstrated by Holter monitor in 5 of the 92 patients: 4 had 3-vessel CAD and the other had severe persistent angina. Thus, in patients hospitalized with unstable angina, transient ST-segment alterations and/or VT on Holter monitor are specific predictors of high risk subgroup unstable angina patients with LM or 3-vessel CAD, variant angina, and/or impaired 3-month prognosis.

Detection by a new exercise test

Elamin and associates[71] from Leeds, England, tested the ability of a new exercise test to detect accurately the presence and severity of CAD in 206 patients with angina pectoris, including patients on beta blockers or with concomitant cardiac lesions. From recordings of 13 ECG leads during exercise, the maximal rate of progression of ST-segment depression relative to increases in heart rate (maximal ST/HR slope) was obtained and used as an index of myocardial ischemia. The maximal ST/HR slope and results of coronary arteriography were independently obtained and the 2 sets of data compared. The ranges of the maximal ST/HR slopes in the 38 patients with no significant CAD, 49 with 1-vessel, 75 with 2-vessel, and 44 patients with 3-vessel CAD were different from each other and there was no overlap in the data between adjacent groups; there were no false positive, false negative, or indeterminate results. Thus, the maximal ST/HR slope can be used reliably to predict the presence or absence and severity of CAD in individual patients presenting with anginal pain in a hospital.

Influence of R-wave analysis upon diagnostic accuracy of exercise testing in women

Exercise ECG in women with chest pain is associated with a high frequency of false positive ST-segment depression. Recently, it was observed that changes in R-wave amplitude during exercise also can be used diagnostically to improve the value of stress testing in women. Ilsley and associates[72] from London, England, reviewed the results of 12-lead treadmill exercise tests and coronary angiography in 62 women (mean age, 51 years) presenting with "angina" without previous AMI. These results were compared with exercise results in 14 healthy asymptomatic volunteers (mean age, 26 years). In addition to conventional ST analysis, R-wave amplitude changes during exercise, measured in leads II, III, aVF, and V4–6, were examined. Although the sensitivity and specificity of ST and R-wave changes were similar at about 67%, their combined interpretation was helpful. If both ST and R-wave criteria were negative, the predictive accuracy for normal coronary angiography was 94% (17 of 18). Alternatively, in tests showing both ST depression and an abnormal R-wave response, coronary angiography was always abnormal (13 of 13). None of the normal volunteers developed ST-segment depression and 93% (13 of 14) had a normal R-wave response. If both were positive, however, coronary angiography was always abnormal (13 of 13). Although stress test interpretation in women is difficult, R-wave analysis is a useful adjunct to ST change and can improve the predictive accuracy of the test in a significant number of patients.

Vasospastic ischemic mechanism of asymptomatic transient ST-T changes during continuous ECG monitoring in unstable angina

Asymptomatic episodes of ST-segment and/or T-wave changes are often reported during Holter monitoring in patients with angina pectoris. The interpretation of such changes is debated relative to silent myocardial ischemia. Biagini and associates[73] from Pisa, Italy, studied 11 patients admitted to the coronary care unit because of frequent episodes of unstable angina and who had undergone repeated periods of Holter monitoring with asymptomatic episodes of ST-segment and/or T-wave changes associated with less frequent typical anginal attacks. In 89 days of Holter monitoring, the patients had 520 episodes of transient ECG changes, including 180 of ST elevation, 73 of ST depression, and 267 of T-wave alterations. Only 12% of episodes were symptomatic. Coronary injection during asymptomatic ST-T changes was performed in 8 patients; in 6 spontaneous coronary spasm was observed. In 7 patients, ergonovine administration induced anginal pain, ST-T changes, and coronary spasm. In all patients, the anginal attacks completely disappeared with medical treatment, and the asymptomatic episodes were abolished in 6 and reduced in 4. These findings support the hypothesis that in certain selected unstable anginal patients, transient asymptomatic ECG changes are caused by acute myocardial ischemia.

Collateral circulation in unstable angina

Of 218 consecutive patients with unstable angina (defined as ischemic cardiac pain at rest associated with transient ECG changes) studied by Plotnick and associates[74] from Baltimore, Maryland, 106 (49%) had collaterals by coronary angiography. The presence of collaterals correlated with the extent and severity of the CAD but not with age, sex, or risk factors. Among patients with comparable severity of narrowings, the presence of collaterals did not appear to protect against abnormal wall motion or abnormal Q waves on ECG. In patients with 1-vessel CAD, collaterals also did not appear to protect against transient ST-segment elevation during ischemia.

Spontaneous angina in the coronary care unit

Madias[75] from Boston, Massachusetts, studied serial ECGs of 16 patients with repetitive attacks of spontaneous angina in the coronary care unit. Transient repolarization ECG changes occurring during unprovoked angina included ST-segment elevation and depression, alterations of T-wave amplitude and polarity, and pseudonormalization of previously inverted T waves. QRS complexes, altered transiently during chest pain, included augmentation or reduction of amplitude of R and S waves, widening of QRS complexes, and a merging of R waves with the elevated ST segments. Occasionally, the ECG during attacks of angina did not change. Between attacks of spontaneous angina, the ECG either returned to baseline or had minor ST-segment shifts, and/or T-wave alterations. Such changes became either persistent or were replaced in the late course of hospitalization by ECG alterations diagnostic of AMI. Twelve of the 16 patients had an AMI. Four died within 1 month of admission. During follow-up of the 12 surviving patients, amelioration of T-wave changes occurred in patients who remained asymptomatic, but new ischemic alterations were seen in patients who had recurrent angina or were readmitted to the hospital for evaluation.

Segmental wall motion abnormalities in unstable angina by 2-D echo

To determine the value of real-time 2-D echo in unstable angina, regional wall motion on serial short-axis 2-D echo recordings was analyzed by Nixon and associates[76] from Dallas, Texas. The summed segment scores of abnormal motion were compared and classified according to each patient's clinical status 12 weeks after hospital discharge. Nineteen men who fulfilled criteria for unstable angina and responded to medical therapy underwent 2-D echo study within 48 hours of admission and discharge. Of 11 patients with abnormal 2-D echo scores on admission, 5 had reduced scores and 6 had similar or increased scores at discharge. Six of 8 patients who had scores of 0 on admission had scores of 0 at discharge. At follow-up, 11 patients had minimal or no angina pectoris (group 1) and 8 patients had worsening angina or recurrent unstable angina (group 2). At discharge, 2-D echo studies showed that all group 1 patients had reduced or 0 scores, whereas group 2 patients retained or increased their abnormal scores. This study shows that in patients with unstable angina both transient and persistent abnormalities can be identified by 2-D echo. Abnormal segmental wall motion was transient or absent in patients with a good outcome and worsened or remained abnormal in patients with a poor outcome.

Treatment with isosorbide dinitrate

Thadani and associates[77] from Kingston, Canada, evaluated the effects of different doses of oral isosorbide dinitrate administered acutely and 4 times daily during sustained therapy in 12 patients with angina pectoris. Thirty, 60, and 120 mg isosorbide dinitrate resulted in an average plasma concentration that was higher during sustained than during acute therapy. Systolic BP was greater during acute than during sustained therapy ($p < 0.001$) and the reduction in systolic BP was dose related, persisting for 8 hours during acute therapy but was not dose related and demonstrable for only 4 hours after sustained therapy. Exercise duration to the onset of angina and to the development of moderate angina increased significantly after each dose of isosorbide dinitrate for 8 hours during acute therapy, but for only 2 hours during sustained therapy. Acute therapy with a single dose of 15–30 mg isosorbide dinitrate produced similar improvement in exercise tolerance as did a dose of 60 or 120 mg. During sustained therapy (15 mg 4 times/day), exercise tolerance increased to the same magnitude as with doses of 30, 60, or 120 mg 4 times daily. In most patients, near maximal improvement in exercise tolerance occurred after a dose of 15 or 30 mg 4 times daily. These data suggest that partial tolerance to the antianginal and circulatory effects of isosorbide dinitrate develop during sustained therapy with this agent.

Treatment with beta blockers

Experimental studies suggest that propanolol favorably alters myocardial blood flow (MBF) to ischemic areas and improves performance of ischemic regions. These favorable changes with propanolol have been attributed to alteration of myocardial oxygen requirements, since propanolol was observed to have no effect on MBF when administered in a dose that did not alter hemodynamics. Rainwater and associates[78] from Denver, Colorado, studied the effects of propanolol on LV EF and MBF during exercise in men with CAD. In 30 men with arteriographically demonstrated CAD and exercise limited by angina, 15 without prior AMI and 15 with AMI, the LV EF was measured with a scintillation probe and MBF distribution was determined with thallium-201 imaging. Exercise was performed as control and after 1 week of treatment with propanolol, 40 mg 4 times daily orally. Propanolol improved the exercise LV EF in men without AMI from 0.37–0.45 and in patients with previous AMI from 0.30–0.36. Propanolol also increased MBF during exercise in men without AMI, but no changes were demonstrated after propanolol in men with previous AMI. Changes in exercise LV EF and MBF appeared related, since MBF improved with 17 men with propanolol treatment and LV EF was increased in 15 of these. Propanolol was associated with a worsening of MBF in 5 men and all had no change in exercise LV EF. The beneficial effect of propanolol on EF during exercise was more apparent in men without prior AMI, and these individuals had a normal EF in rest. In the patients with prior AMI and depressed EF only 7 of 15 had improvement in EF during exercise. The results suggest that propanolol can favorably alter MBF and LV EF in men with CAD, particularly in those without prior AMI.

Propranolol remains an effective antianginal agent and the daily dosage is usually administered in 4 divided portions. In a double-blind crossover study in 20 patients with stable angina pectoris, the effects of long-acting propranolol 160 mg administered once daily for 4 weeks were compared with those of standard propranolol 40 mg give 4 times daily for 4 weeks by Parker and associates[79] from Ontario, Canada. The patients had no adverse effects when they were switched between treatment schedules. The average number of episodes of angina during the 4 weeks on long-acting propranolol was 7.3 and on standard propranolol, 6.3. The average nitroglycerin ingestion was 5.8 and 4.9 tablets during therapy with these 2 programs. Resting values for heart rate (HR), systolic BP (SBP), and rate-pressure product (RPP) remained similar when determined 25 hours after a dose of long-acting propranolol and 10 hours after standard propranolol. When the patients were exercised, individuals on long-acting propranolol and standard propranolol had similar walking times to the onset of angina and to the development of moderate angina. Again, values for HR, SBP, and RPP remained similar at rest and during exercise during the 2 treatment programs. Thus, long-acting propranolol administered in a dose of 160 mg daily is as effective as 40 mg of standard propranolol given 4 times/day.

Taylor and associates[80] from Leeds, England, compared the effects of 4 intravenous beta adrenoreceptor antagonists with different ancillary properties on LV function in 24 patients with CAD without CHF but presumably with angina pectoris. All 4 depressed the relation between LV filling pressure and cardiac output at rest and during exercise. Practolol and oxprenolol, which have intrinsic sympathomimetic activity, induced significantly less depression of LV function than either propranolol or metoprolol, which do not have this activity. Cardioselectivity, a property of both practolol and metoprolol, had no discernible hemodynamic advantage. Thus, beta blocking drugs that have intrinsic sympathomimetic activity appear to be more effective in maintaining cardiac function than drugs without this property, when given intravenously to patients with CAD.

Gagnon and associates[81] from Montreal, Canada, evaluated the influence of labetalol, an alpha and beta receptor blocking agent, in 11 patients with stable angina pectoris from CAD. The mean dose of labetalol was 1.5 mg/kg (range, 1–2 mg/kg). Cardiovascular effects began within 1 minute after injection and were maximal within 10 minutes. Specifically, mean arterial pressure decreased from 105 ± 13–81 ± 10 mmHg, heart rate from 70 ± 10–66 ± 7 beats/minute, and the rate-pressure product from $10,322 \pm 2,344$–$7,717 \pm 1,650$. Cardiac output and pulmonary wedge pressure did not change significantly. Mean PA pressure decreased from 20 ± 3–16 ± 2 mmHg after labetalol. Coronary sinus flow increased from 107 ± 26–118 ± 25 ml/minute and coronary vascular resistance decreased from 1.0 ± 0.2–0.77 ± 0.1 mmHg/ml/minute. These data suggest that labetalol may be a useful addition to the pharmacologic agents available to treat angina pectoris because it diminishes myocardial oxygen requirements and improves coronary blood flow.

Acebutolol, a relatively cardioselective beta adrenergic blocking drug, was administered to 20 men with CAD and angina pectoris by Steele and Gold[82] from Denver, Colorado. A 3-month double-blind crossover (placebo and acebutolol) design was used following a 12-week placebo phase and a 6-week dose titration phase. During the crossover phase, acebutolol (400 mg in 19 men and 300 mg in 1, orally 3 times/day) increased the duration of treadmill exercise (placebo, 6.8 ± 0.5 min average $\pm$ SEM; acebutolol, 8.1 ± 0.6 min; $p < 0.05$) and decreased the frequency of ST-segment depression during exercise (placebo, 20 of 20 men; acebutolol, 6 of 20 men). The heart rate times systolic BP product ($\times 10^{-2}$) was decreased both at rest (placebo, 105 ± 4; acebutolol, 84 ± 3; $p < 0.01$) and during exercise (placebo, 199 ± 10; acebutolol, 144 ± 8; $p < 0.05$). Acebutolol treatment decreased the frequency of angina (placebo, 9.0 ± 2.4 episodes per week; acebutolol, 6.4 ± 2.2 episodes per week; $p < 0.05$) and decreased the consumption of nitroglycerin (placebo, 9 ± 4 tablets per week; acebutolol, 7 ± 4 tablets per week; $p < 0.05$). Thus, acebutolol increases exercise performance and decreases the occurrence of angina in men with CAD.

The therapeutic efficacy of propranolol has been demonstrated for many years in the treatment of CAD but some of the adverse effects on bronchial and smooth muscle as well as glucose metabolism have stimulated interest in identifying other more cardioselective beta blocking agents. Thus, Di-Bianco and colleagues[83] from Washington, DC, Los Angeles, California, and Houston, Texas, compared the effects of oral acebutolol, a cardioselective beta adrenergic blocking agent with partial agonist activity, to those of oral propranolol, a noncardioselective agent devoid of partial agonist activity, on the exercise tolerance and anginal pattern in 46 men with chronic stable angina pectoris. A 28-week, multicenter, placebo controlled, randomized double-blind, crossover study design was employed. Each double-blind treatment phase was followed by a 2-week gradual drug withdrawal phase and a placebo control drug-free week. Angina frequency, nitroglycerin (TNG) consumption, and symptom-limited exercise tests were assessed throughout the study. Acebutolol and propranolol produced comparable levels of beta blocade at 1,650 and 219 mg/day, respectively, as confirmed by a significant reduction in resting and peak exercise heart rates and rate-pressure products. Compared with placebo, acebutolol produced a greater reduction in systolic, mean, and diastolic BP and a similar reduction in resting heart rate than propranolol, presumably reflecting its partial agonist and cardioselective properties during similar dose titration phases. Exercise duration and exercise work improved similarly with each agent. Acebutolol and propranolol significantly and comparably reduced angina frequency 56% and 54%, respectively, and weekly TNG consumption 57% and 47%, respectively, compared with the placebo. No clinical or laboratory side effects of acebutolol or propranolol necessitated drug withdrawal. Thus, acebutolol is a well-tolerated and safe beta adrenergic blocking agent that possesses cardioselective and mild sympathomimetic activities and compares favorably with propranolol in antianginal efficacy in patients with chronic stable angina.

Silke and associates[84] from Leeds, England, compared the immediate hemodynamic dose response effects of beta blockade (propranolol, 2–16 mg) with those of combined alpha beta blockade (labetalol, 10–80 mg) in a randomized study of 20 patients with stable angina pectoris. After control measurements, the circulatory changes induced by 4 logarithmically cumulative intravenous boluses of each drug in equivalent beta blocking doses were evaluated at rest, after which comparison of the effects of the maximum cumulative dose of each was undertaken during a 4-minute period of supine bicycle exercise. Propranolol, at rest, induced significant dose-related reductions in heart rate and cardiac output, with reciprocal increases in the systemic vascular resistance and PA pressure; systemic arterial pressure was unchanged. Labetalol was followed by significant dose-related increases in systemic BP and vascular resistance associated with a significant increase in cardiac output; heart rate and PA pressure were unchanged. The slope of the LV pumping function curve relating output to filling pressure from rest to exercise was significantly depressed by propranolol but unchanged after labetalol. The less deleterious effects on LV hemodynamic performance after alpha beta blockade in contrast to beta blockade alone in CAD may be attributable to the concomitant reduction in LV afterload associated with the alpha blocking activity of labetalol.

Treatment with calcium channel blockers

Pine and colleagues[85] from Long Beach, California, compared verapamil and a placebo in patients with stable effort induced angina. The investigators followed a double-blind crossover protocol with dosages of verapamil of 240, 360, and 480 mg every day in 18 patients. In the patients receiving verapamil, exercise duration increased from 348 ± 127 seconds to 494 ± 182 seconds, but did not change with the placebo. In comparison to placebo, verapamil reduced the weekly number of anginal episodes from 4.5 to 2.4 and similarly reduced nitroglycerin consumption from 3.46 to 1.55 tablets per week. In 26 patients who completed the single-blind dose titration, 16 were improved at a dosage of 240 or 360 mg daily. No patient improved on 480 mg daily who had not already improved on a lower dose. Side effects occurred in 7 patients receiving 480 mg of verapamil daily. Side effects consisted of new rhythm disturbances, CHF, and noncardiac complications of constipation, nausea, vomiting, and headaches with paresthesias. Thus, verapamil is an effective antianginal agent that appears most efficacious at a dose of 360 mg every day. Side effects are common at daily doses of 400 mg.

Tan and associates[86] from Sydney, Australia, evaluated the effect of oral verapamil (320 mg/day) on LV function in 12 patients with stable angina pectoris. Ventricular function was evaluated at rest and during exercise with gated equilibrium radionuclide ventriculography. During verapamil therapy, patients had a lower heart rate-BP product at each work load than with placebo. Anginal threshold increased by 28 ± 19 watts ($p < 0.005$), and maximal exercise capacity increased by 20 ± 14 watts ($p < 0.001$) with verapamil, but the rate-BP product at the onset of angina and at maximal exercise was unchanged. The LV EF at rest during verapamil was the same as with placebo. During exercise, the EF decreased from 40 ± 9–35 ± 11 with placebo, whereas during verapamil the LV EF did not decrease during exercise. These data suggest that oral verapamil is effective treatment for effort angina and may prevent the decrease in LV EF due to exercise-induced ischemia.

Weiner and Klein[87] from Boston, Massachusetts, evaluated clinical and exercise response to therapy with verapamil in 26 patients with stable exertional angina using a double-blind, placebo-controlled randomized crossover study design. Verapamil, 480 mg daily, reduced the frequency of angina (5.6 ± 7.3–2.2 ± 3.0 attacks per week, $p < 0.001$) and number of nitroglycerin tablets consumed (3.4 ± 4.9–1.2 ± 2.5 tablets per week, $p < 0.05$), and increased exercise duration (6.4 ± 2.1–7.5 ± 1.8 min, $p < 0.001$) (mean $\pm$ SD), compared with placebo. These beneficial effects of verapamil were related to significant reduction in heart rate-systolic BP product during submaximal exercise. The primary side effect resulting from verapamil therapy was constipation. These data suggest that verapamil is a highly effective and safe drug for the treatment of stable, effort-related angina pectoris.

Scheidt and associates[88] from New York City evaluated clinical responses to 12-months treatment with verapamil in 63 patients with stable and unstable angina pectoris in whom the effectiveness of verapamil had been established in short-term, double-blind placebo-controlled randomized studies. In 41 patients with effort-related angina, long-term responses were sustained for periods >1 year. Twenty patients were evaluated by clinical history and showed a sustained reduction in frequency of anginal attacks and consumption of nitroglycerin with verapamil compared with initial placebo-controlled periods. The magnitude of benefit was similar to that observed during double-blind treatment with the drug. Twenty-one patients were evaluated by serial treadmill exercise testing and showed sustained improvement in exercise duration after 4, 8, 16, 24, and 52 weeks of verapamil. Withdrawal of the drug resulted in a deterioration of exercise performance to levels similar to those before initiation of therapy. Twenty-two patients with unstable angina at rest received verapamil and had an amelioration of angina that was sustained in most patients for >1 year. However, these patients continued to have a high frequency of death and AMI similar to that previously reported in large clincal studies using either combination of verapamil and nitrates, nifedipine and propranolol, or propranolol and nitrates. Thus, calcium antagonists may decrease the number of patients requiring CABG for relief of refractory angina, but they do not appear to alter the natural history of CAD.

The acute effects of nifedipine on LV systolic and diastolic function were studied in 32 patients by Ludbrook and associates[89] from St. Louis, Missouri. The observations were stratified with respect to baseline LV function before and 30 minutes after nifedipine (20 mg sublingually) with a randomized single-blind protocol. Nifedipine was administered to 19 patients and 13 received a placebo. No change occurred in any variable after placebo. Nifedipine lowered LV after load, reflected by significant decreases in systolic mean and diastolic arterial BP of 13%, 10%, and 17%, respectively. LV systolic pressure fell by 13%; EF, mean normalized systolic ejection rate, and the end-systolic pressure volume (ESPV) ratio increased by 14%, 25%, and 19%, respectively. Cardiac index rose by 16%. Overal diastolic LV function did not change. Diastolic pressures, early diastolic relaxation, diastolic exponential pressure volume and elasticity relation, and end-diastolic stiffness remain constant. Among patients stratified according to baseline LV function (group I end-diastolic volume [EDV] < 90 ml/m^2, end-diastolic pressure [EDP] < 20 mmHg; group II EDV > 90 ml/m^2, EDP > 20 mmHg) striking differences were evident. Group II patients after nifedipine showed decreased LV systolic and EDP while EDP and ESV and systemic and pulmonary vascular resistances all declined significantly. The EF was enhanced greater in group II patients than in patients with normal baseline LV function. Relaxation and diastolic stiffness properties were insignificantly changed in both groups. These results show that nifedipine has significant clinically favorable effects due predominantly to reduction of LV afterload in patients with impaired baseline LV function. Nifedipine reduced myocardial oxygen requirements, enhanced diastolic performance, and improved systemic and pulmonary hemodynamics, LV EF, and cardiac output.

Gerstenblith and associates[90] from Baltimore, Maryland, assessed the efficacy of adding nifedipine to the conventional treatment of unstable angina pectoris in 138 patients in a prospective, double-blind, randomized, placebo-controlled trial. There was no difference between the 2 groups in the dose of conventional antianginal medication or in age prior to AMI, EF, or other risk factors. Failure of medical treatment (defined as sudden death, AMI, or CABG within 4 months) occurred in 43 of 70 patients given placebo and in 30 of 68 given nifedipine. Kaplan-Meier survival-curve analysis of the number and time dependence of treatment failures demonstrated a benefit of nifedipine over placebo (p = 0.03) (Fig. 1-5). The benefit was particularly marked in patients with ST-segment evaluation during angina (p = 0.02). Side effects (transient hypotension or diarrhea) required withdrawal of the drug in 4 patients given nifedipine and in 1 given placebo. Thus, the addition of nifedipine to conventional therapy is safe and effective in patients with unstable angina.

Fig. 1-5. Effect of nifedipine on cumulative probability of no failure of medical therapy in patients with ST-segment elevation during angina. Reproduced with permission from Gerstenblith et al.[90]

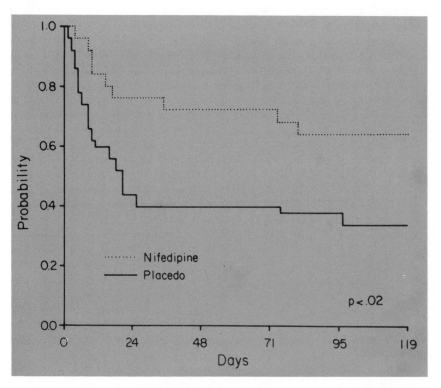

Majid and DeJong[91] from Amsterdam, The Netherlands, studied the acute hemodynamic effects of nifedipine in 20 patients with angiographically proved CAD. Eight patients were examined during exercise-induced pain. There was an expected abnormal increase in pulmonary wedge pressure accompanying the chest pain and ST decrease on the ECG. Pacing stress was utilized in 6 patients and increased LV end-diastolic pressure from 16–26 mmHg, end-diastolic volume from 63–81 ml/m^2, end-systolic volume from 26–47 ml/m^2, and depressed EF from 0.60–0.44 compared with control values. In both groups, nifedipine, 20 mg sublingually, significantly shortened the duration of pain, reduced ST decrease on the ECG, and reversed all hemodynamic abnormalities. In another group of 6 patients with recent AMI and moderately severe LV dysfunction at rest, nifedipine reduced LV end-diastolic pressure from 21–12 mmHg, end-diastolic volume from 109–95 ml/m^2, end-systolic volume from 41–31 ml/m^2, while the EF improved from 0.43–0.58. Thus, this investigation has demonstrated that the antianginal effect of nifedipine is associated with improved systolic emptying and reduced diastolic filling of the heart. Nifedipine appeared to have no measurable adverse effects in patients with depressed LV function.

The efficacy of nifedipine in patients with angina refractory to maximum tolerated conventional therapy has not been extensively studied. Therefore Stone and colleagues[92] from Boston, Massachusetts, reported their experience using nifedipine in the treatment of 3 subsets of patients with refractory angina pectoris. One hundred twenty-seven patients with Prinzmetal's variant angina and documented coronary vasospasm were treated with nifedipine after experiencing an inadequate response to conventional therapy. Nifedipine, 40–160 mg daily, reduced the mean weekly rate of angina attacks from 16 to 2. In 63% of patients, complete control of angina attacks was achieved, and in 87% the frequency of angina was reduced by at least 50%. Nifedipine therapy was well tolerated, and the beneficial response persisted for the 9 months of follow-up. Nifedipine therapy was added to a second group of 11 consecutive patients with refractory episodes of recurrent rest ischemia following AMI. Before AMI all the patients had a history of exertional angina only; yet following AMI, episodes of recurrent ischemia occurred at rest in spite of maximal medical management with beta blockers and/or nitrate preparations. With maximum tolerated conventional therapy, the heart rate was lowered to a mean of 65 beats/minute and the BP to a mean of 109/70 mmHg. The episodes of rest ischemia were prevented in all but 1 patient by the addition of nifedipine (mean daily dose, 60 mg; range, 40 to 120 mg) without causing a change in heart rate or BP. Two patients continued to have myocardial ischemia with minimal exertion, although resting pains were abolished, and they underwent CABG for relief of exertional pain. Only 1 patient continued to have episodes of ischemia at rest, and CABG was necessary for pain relief. The other 8 patients were managed medically for a mean of 5.4 months and remained pain-free on combined regimens of nifedipine, beta blockers, and/or nitate preparations. The third group of patients treated with nifedipine was composed of 239 patients with severe classic exertional angina pectoris without a suspicion of superimposed coronary vasospasm. The anginal episodes in these patients were refractory to maximum tolerated conventonal therapy; however, the addition of nifedipine (mean daily dose, 60 mg; range, 40 to 120 mg) reduced the mean weekly anginal attack rate from 21–6. Although only 11% of patients had complete prevention of angina during nifedipine therapy, 70% experienced a reduction in angina frequency ≥50%. Thus, the addition of nifedipine may provide further benefit for patients with angina pectoris refractory to maximum tolerated conventional therapy.

Zacca and associates[93] from Houston, Texas, studied the effects of nifedipine on LV function and regional myocardial perfusion using exercise radionuclide ventriculography and thallium-201 scintigraphy before and 90 minutes after the oral administration of 20 mg of nifedipine The patients studied had stable angina and angiographically proved CAD without evidence of coronary spasm. Exercise tolerance increased after the administration of nifedipine from 343 ± 42 seconds to 471 ± 50 seconds (p < 0.01), although the peak exercise double product remained essentially unchanged. The LV EF improved significantly at rest (49 ± 4–52 ± 3%, p < 0.05) and at peak exercise (42 ± 3–47 ± 4%, p < 0.05). Administration of nifedipine also resulted in improved segmental wall motion. Thallium-201 perfusion studies suggested that an improved exercise perfusion occurred in 5 of 11 patients and in 7 of 28 segments with reversible hypoperfusion. These data suggest that nifedipine administration is associated with improved global and regional LV function in patients with CAD and stable angina pectoris.

Subramanian and associates[94] from Harrow, England, evaluated 32 patients with chronic stable angina in a randomized, double-blind crossover trial to compare the antianginal actions of verapamil (120 mg 3 times daily) and nifedipine (20 mg 3 times daily). These investigators determined the efficacy of each intervention using exercise testing and 24-hour ambulatory monitoring for ST-segment shifts. Twenty-eight patients completed the trial. Both nifedipine and verapamil increased mean exercise time to angina from 5.7 ± 0.3 minutes (mean ± SEM) to 7.9 ± 0.5 minutes for nifedipine and 10.0 ± 0.7 minutes for verapamil. Similar improvement was found in other objective variables. Verapamil produced a mild bradycardia and nifedipine a mild tachycardia. Four patients noticed palpitations and angina after nifedipine and were shown by ambulatory ECG monitoring to have tachycardia and persistent ST depression. These data suggest that both calcium antagonists are effective in the treatment of chronic stable angina pectoris, but that each has certain side effects and should be selected for appropriate patients with care.

Diltiazem (DL) is a slow-channel blocking drug effective in treatment of chronic stable angina pectoris. Wagniart and associates[95] from Quebec, Canada, evaluated the therapeutic efficacy 3 hours after a single dose of 120 mg of DL. Twelve men with chronic stable angina pectoris performed a maximal exercise test on a bicycle ergometer after ingesting either placebo or DL administered in a double-blind fashion. During submaximal exercise, at a fixed work load, DL decreased the average heart rate response from 119–107 beats/minute, systolic BP from 182–175 mmHg, and the rate-pressure product from 22–19 × 10^{-3} units. The average submaximal work load at which significant ST decrease first appeared was increased from 355 to 525 seconds after DL. At peak exercise, after DL, the average depth of ST decrease in any one lead and the extent of myocardial ischemia observed in all 12 ECG leads were decreased even though the average work load was increased by 29%. Peak heart rate, systolic BP, and rate-pressure product were similar with placebo and DL. The plasma DL concentration was 139 ng/ml 3 hours after ingestion and was significantly related to the increased time to the onset of important ST decrease and to the decrease in the extent of myocardial ischemia observed in all ECG leads compared with placebo. Thus, DL is effective in treating chronic stable angina pectoris. The drug decreases myocardial oxygen requirements during upright exercise and appears to increase myocardial oxygen delivery.

Comparison of calcium channel to beta blockers or new treatment with one while already receiving the other

Using multigated equilibrium cardiac blood pool imaging and single-blind placebo crossover protocol, the effects of oral verapamil (480 mg/day) were compared by Josephson and colleagues[96] from Los Angeles, California, with those of oral propranolol (320 mg/day) on the LV EF and regional wall motion abnormalities at rest and during supine bicycle exercise in 15 CAD patients. During exercise on placebo before verapamil, the mean LV EF fell from the resting value of 0.54–0.47; on verapamil the corresponding values were 0.54 and 0.53. On placebo before propranolol, exercise reduced LV EF from 0.54–0.48; on propranolol, the resting LV EF was 0.54 and exercise LV EF 0.52. Both drugs reduced the exercise-induced regional wall motion abnormality and ST-segment depression, but the changes were only significant with verapamil. Propranolol attenuated the exercise-induced increase in heart rate by 25%, in systolic BP by 13%, in diastolic pressure by 9%, and in heart rate times BP product by 35%. Verapamil reduced exercise heart rate response by 10%, systolic pressure by 5%, diastolic pressure by 8%, and the heart rate times BP product by 15%. These data indicate that verapamil and propranolol exhibit comparable potency in reducing the ischemic consequences of exercise stress in CAD patients. With propranolol, the beneficial effect was accountable in terms of reduction in oxygen demand; with verapamil, additional mechanisms, such as those involving myocardial metabolism or primary changes in perfusion, may be involved.

Subramanian and associates[97] in Harrow, England, evaluated the comparative efficacy of verapamil (360 mg/daily) and propranolol (240 mg daily) in the control of chronic stable angina pectoris in 22 patients. This evaluation was a placebo-controlled, double-blind, crossover study with 4 weeks on each active phase. Fourteen patients still had angina despite active drug therapy, and they were evaluated further with a combination of verapamil and propranolol for 4 weeks. Both propranolol and verapamil increased mean exercise time and the combination of the 2 further increased mean exercise time from 4.8 ± 0.22 minutes with placebo and 10.1 ± 0.88 with combination therapy. Electrocardiographic ambulatory monitoring showed no evidence of conduction defects and mean hourly heart rates were similar with combined therapy to those found with propranolol alone. The LV function indexes were not significantly different from those obtained with propranolol alone. Thus, combination therapy with verapamil and propranolol is efficacious in the treatment of selected patients with severe chronic stable angina pectoris, but these patients need to be monitored carefully for adverse effects.

Although drugs that block slow-channel activity in cardiac and vascular smooth muscle are being used with increasing frequency in cardiac disease, there has been reluctance to combine therapy with calcium antagonists and beta blocking agents because of concern over additive detrimental cardiac responses. Packer and associates[98] from New York City administered 40, 80, 120 mg doses of verapamil orally to 15 patients with angina pectoris who were receiving high doses of propranolol or metroprolol. Verapamil produced dose-dependent decreases in cardiac performance: with 120 mg dose of verapamil, cardiac index decreased by 0.38 liter/minute/m^2, stroke index decreased by 2.8 ml/beat/m^2, and heart rate decreased by 6 beats/minute associated with increases in pulmonary capillary pressure and RA pressure. Two patients had marked but asymptomatic hypotensive reactions. In contrast, repeat administration of 120 mg doses of verapamil 24–30 hours after withdrawal of beta blockade produced no significant cardiodepressant effects despite significantly higher plasma levels of verapamil than during propranolol therapy. Thus, verapamil does produce significant negative inotropic and chronotropic effects in patients treated with beta adrenergic antagonists, and combination therapy should be used with caution in patients with angina pectoris.

To evaluate the effects of verapamil on LV systolic function and diastolic filling in patients with CAD, Bonow and associates[99] from Bethesda, Maryland, performed gated RNA at rest and during exercise in 16 symptomatic patients before and during oral verapamil therapy (480 mg/day). Twelve patients also were studied during oral propranolol therapy (160–320 mg/day). LV EF at rest was normal in 13 patients but abnormal diastolic filling at rest, defined as peak filling rate (PFR) <2.5 end-diastolic volume (EDV) per second or time to PFR >180 msec, was present in 15 patients. During verapamil, resting EF decreased but resting diastolic filling improved: PFR increased and time to PFR decreased. Exercise EF did not change during verapamil but exercise PFR increased and exercise time to PFR decreased. In contrast, propranolol did not alter EF, PFR, or time to PFR at rest or during exercise. Thus, LV EF is decreased by verapamil at rest but is unchanged during exercise. Although LV systolic function is not improved by verapamil, LV diastolic filling is enhanced by verapamil, both at rest and during exercise.

Frishman and colleagues[100] from New York City evaluated 20 patients with stable angina pectoris to determine the effects of withdrawal of long-term treatment with propranolol and verapamil. Patients received placebo for 2 weeks, then increasing doses of propranolol (60–320 mg/day) or verapamil (240–480 mg/day) for 3 weeks. Patients were then abruptly withdrawn from drug to placebo for 1 week, followed by crossover to the other drug regimen and the second withdrawal period. All 20 patients were withdrawn from verapamil without evidence of a rebound increase in frequency of angina, BP, heart rate, the rate-pressure product, and without a rebound deterioration in exercise tolerance. In contrast, with propranolol withdrawal, 2 patients (both with the highest baseline angina attack rate) had a severe exacerbation of their angina and could not undergo formal exercise testing. The remaining 18 patients were withdrawn without incident. Therefore it appears that rebound phenomenon from either propranolol or verapamil withdrawal are uncommon, but may be slightly more common with propranolol than with verapamil.

Subramanian and colleagues[101] from Harrow, England, evaluated the effectiveness and safety of verapamil, nifedipine, and placebo in patients with chronic stable angina pectoris in 2 double-blind randomized crossover trials. Nifedipine (10 mg 3 times/day) was compared with placebo in 24 patients with chronic effort-related angina pectoris, and in a second study verapamil (120 mg 3 times daily), nifedipine (20 mg 3 times daily), and placebo were compared in 32 patients with chronic stable angina using a double-blind crossover study design. Nifedipine (10 mg 3 times daily) was not found to be superior to placebo in altering exercise performance. Nifedipine in increased dosage (20 mg 3 times/day) and verapamil prolonged exercise duration (5.7 ± 0.3 min with placebo, 7.9 ± 0.5 min with nifedipine [$p < 0.001$], and 10.0 ± 0.7 min with verapamil [$p < 0.001$]), but the improvement with verapamil was greater than that found with nifedipine ($p < 0.01$). Seven patients had increasing angina with nifedipine, but none did with verapamil. The exacerbation of angina in some patients with nifedipine appeared related to an increase in heart rate while on nifedipine. These data indicate that in the doses used, verapamil was more effective and better tolerated than nifedipine in patients with chronic stable angina pectoris.

Parodi and associates[102] from Pisa, Italy, compared the efficacy of verapamil and propranolol in the treatment of unstable angina pectoris in 17 patients enrolled in a randomized, triple crossover study. Both verapamil and propranolol reduced the number of episodes of angina at rest (from 3.0–1.7/day with propranolol, $p < 0.05$, and to 0.2/day with verapamil, $p < 0.001$) (Fig. 1-6). The degree of improvement with verapamil was superior to that found with propranolol ($p < 0.005$). In 10 patients with rest angina evaluated in a single-blind multiple crossover trial, the number of ischemic events was reduced significantly only by verapamil (5 ± 1 episode/48 hours) but not by placebo or propranolol (25 ± 3 and 23 ± 3 episodes/48 hours, respectively) (Fig. 1-7). These data confirm the effectiveness of verapamil in the management of patients with angina at rest. They also suggest that propranolol may be of some use in patients with this syndrome, but that it is inferior to verapamil in this clinical setting.

Winniford and associates[103] from Dallas, Texas, evaluated the combined use of a beta adrenergic blocking agent and a calcium antagonist in 26

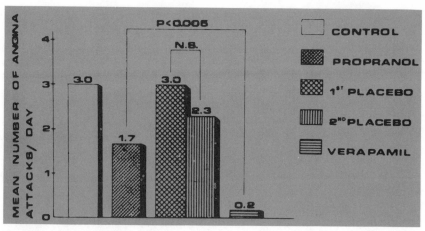

Fig. 1-6. Overall results of double-blind single crossover study of propranolol -vs- verapamil in 18 patients with unstable angina.

patients with severe angina by studying the hemodynamic and electrophysio-logic effects of verapamil or nifedipine in patients receiving oral propranolol. The patients with stable angina were receiving oral propranolol 234 ± 230 mg/day, mean ± SD) at time of cardiac catheterization. Cardiac output, mean arterial pressure, LV dP/dt, coronary sinus blood flow, and the A-H interval were measured at baseline and 5 to 10 minutes after 1) intravenous saline, 2) intravenous verapamil, 0.15 mg/kg body weight to a maximal dose of 10 mg, and 3) sublingual nitroglycerin, 10 mg. Cardiac output was unchanged after saline solution and verapamil, but increased with nifedipine (4.3 ± 1.1–5.0 ± 1.4 liters/min, $p < 0.05$). Mean arterial pressure did not change with saline solution or nifedipine, but decreased with verapamil. Peak positive LV dP/dt was reduced only by verapamil (from 1,086 ± 175–926 ± 167 mmHg/s, $p < 0.05$). Coronary sinus blood flow determined by thermodilution was not altered by saline solution, nifedipine, or verapamil. Verapamil reduced the heart rate from 63 ± 8–60 ± 9 beats/minute, $p < 0.05$, and increased the A-H interval from 108 ± 14–129 ± 23 ms, $p < 0.05$. Nifedipine increased the heart rate 65 ± 8–71 ± 8 beats/minute, $p < 0.05$, but did not change the A-H interval. LV EF determined by radionuclide ventriculography was not changed by saline or verapamil but increased with nifedipine from 0.52 ± 0.13–0.57 ± 0.13, $p < 0.05$. These data suggest that nifedipine improves cardiac output and LV EF without altering filling pressures or AV conduction when administered to patients receiving oral propranolol with normal or only mildly depressed LV function. In contrast, verapamil diminishes LV contractility and slows AV conduction when administered to similar patients. Thus, the combination of verapamil and propranolol should be used with caution in patients with underlying LV dysfunction or conduction system disease.

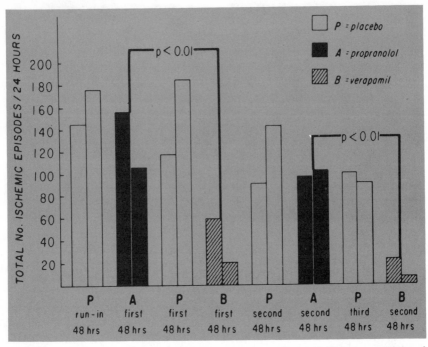

Fig. 1-7. Overall results of single-blind double crossover study in which propranolol (A) and verapamil (B) were compared in 10 patients with frequent ischemic attacks at rest. Every 48 h period of treatment with each active drug is matched and compared with 48 h placebo period (P).

Operative treatment

Hultgren and associates[104] from Palo Alto, California, performed a prospective, nonrandomized data bank study of the effect of medical -vs- surgical management of patients with unstable angina seen at 1 hospital during an 8-year period. The patients were entered into the study after an initial 5-day period of medical management, and entry characteristics were similar in 104 surgically and 124 medically treated patients. The mean follow-up was 52 months. Operative mortality rate was 2% (2 of 104) and the incidence of perioperative AMI was 13% (13 of 104). Twenty-seven medically treated patients had late surgery for progressive angina without an operative death. The 7-year survival was 65% for the medical group and 85% for the surgical group as analyzed by initial treatment (p = 0.01) (Fig. 1-8). When crossover medical patients were followed up to the date of surgery, similar results in survival were found (p = 0.008) (Fig. 1-9). Compared with survivors, nonsurvivors had an age >60 years, borderline systemic arterial hypertension, ST-T changes on resting ECG, 3-vessel disease, an elevated LV end-diastolic pressure at rest, and an elevated LV end-diastolic pressure at

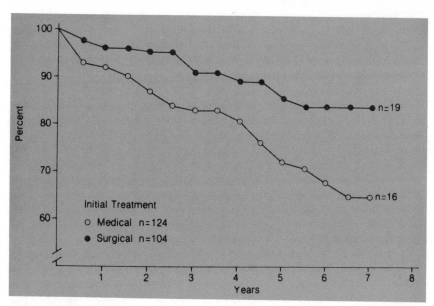

Fig. 1-8. Survival curves for patients according to initial treatment. Mantel-Haenszel test at 7 years, p = 0.012.

exercise. The incidence of delayed AMI during the first 5-year follow-up was 17% in the medical and 22% in the surgical group; however, 13% of AMIs occurring in the surgically treated patients occurred in proximity to the operation. In the operated patients, 62% had no angina and only 8% had severe angina compared with 37% and 24%, respectively, in the medically treated group. The data obtained suggest that surgical intervention in selected patients with unstable angina reduces mortality and morbidity compared with results obtained in medically treated patients.

Previous reports of the European Coronary Surgery Study Group, a prospective randomized study, reveal a gradually increasing difference in survival between the medically and surgically treated groups. The projected minimum follow-up time of 5 years for all patients is now completed. The present report[105] compares final results of survival and symptomatic changes in the 2 treatment groups. In addition, prognostic factors other than treatment were examined with respect to survival. The study included 768 men aged <65 years with mild to moderate angina pectoris, ≥50% stenosis in at least 2 major epicardial coronary arteries, and good LV function. Of the 768 men, 395 were randomized to CABG and 373 to no treatment. One patient in the surgery group was lost to follow-up. These original groups were compared, whatever subsequently happened to the patients. Survival was improved significantly by CABG in the total population, in patients with 3-vessel disease, and in patients with stenosis in the proximal third of the LAD coronary artery constituting a component of either 2- or 3-vessel disease,

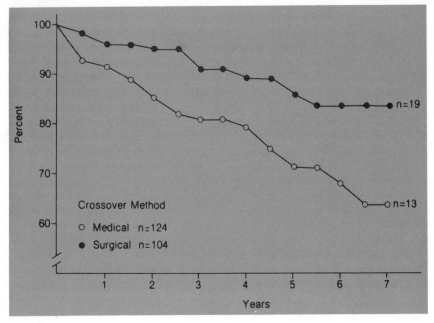

Fig. 1-9.   Survival curves for patients analyzed by crossover method (medical patients included only to date of surgery). Total deaths. Mantel-Haenszel test at 7 years, p = 0.008.

and nonsignificantly in patients with LM coronary narrowing (Figs. 1-10–1-14). An abnormal ECG at rest, ST-segment depression ≥1.5 mm during exercise, peripheral arterial disease, and increasing age independently pointed to a better chance of survival with surgery. In the absence of these prognostic variables in patients with either 2- or 3-vessel disease, the outlook was so good that early surgery was unlikely to increase the prospect of survival. In terms of anginal attacks, use of beta adrenergic blockers and nitrates, and exercise performance, the surgical group did significantly better than the medical group throughout the 5 years of follow-up, but the difference between the 2 treatments tended to decrease.

Rodgers and Wysham[106] from Portland, Oregon, followed for 6.5–10.3 years 100 consecutive patients who had CABG (1.8 graph per person) for angina pectoris at rest. At operation, their ages ranged from 42–78 years (mean, 61) and 75 were men. Preoperatively, an average of 2.1 major coronary arteries were significantly narrowed per patient. Eight years postoperatively, 89 of the 100 patients were alive. The mortality rates were 1.4%/postoperative year, or 2.2 times that of normal subjects of the same age. Angina was usually satisfactorily relieved, but a second CABG was performed in 20 patients. Of the 99 patients who survived the first CABG, 91 resumed work, and 52, at an average age of 61 years, were working 8 years later.

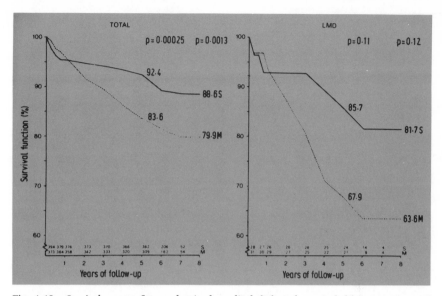

Fig. 1-10. Survival curves for randomized medical (M) and surgical (S) groups in total population, and in subset of patients with left main disease (LMD). Reproduced with permission from the European Coronary Surgery Study Group.[105]

Fig. 1-11. Survival curves for subsets of patients with 3-vessel disease (3VD) and 2-vessel disease (2VD). Reproduced with permission from the European Coronary Surgery Study Group.[105]

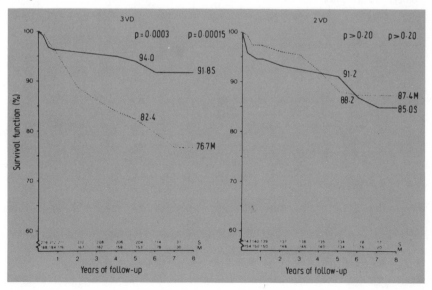

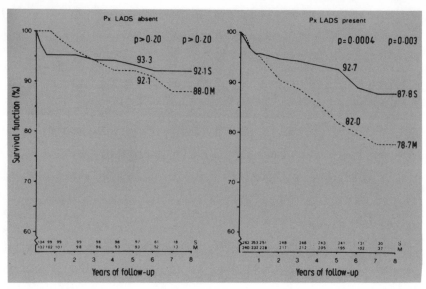

Fig. 1-12. Survival curves for 2 subsets of patients defined by absence or presence of stenosis in proximal segment of left anterior descending artery (Px LADS) as component of 2- or 3-vessel disease. Reproduced with permission from the European Coronary Surgery Study Group.[105]

Fig. 1-13. Survival curves for subset of patients with exertional ST-segment depression by 0–1 mm and subset with ≥1.5 mm ST depression. Reproduced with permission from the European Coronary Surgery Study Group.[105]

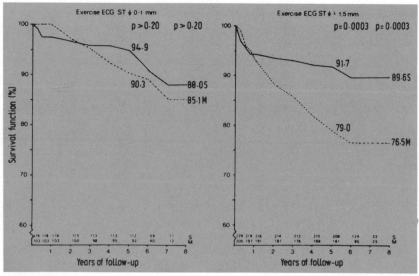

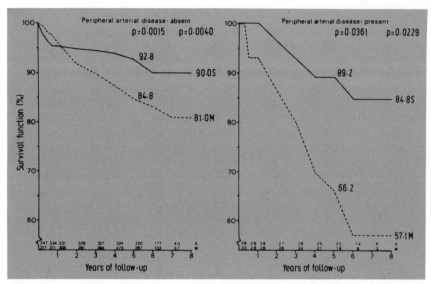

Fig. 1-14. Survival curves for subsets of patients with and without peripheral arterial disease. Reproduced with permission from the European Coronary Surgery Study Group.[105]

Other treatment

Mohr and associates[107] from Tel Aviv, Israel, studied the effect of 10° reverse Trendelenburg tilt of the bed in 10 patients with refractory nocturnal angina pectoris on 2 consecutive nights before CABG. For the control night, the bed was placed in the semiorthopneic position and for the test night it was put in the reverse Trendelenburg position. The latter position significantly reduced the central venous pressure, diastolic PA pressure, the number of isosorbide dinitrate tablets taken sublingually, and the number of angina episodes per night. Reverse Trendelenburg tilt of the bed therefore seems effective for relief of nocturnal anginal pain in some patients.

VARIANT ANGINA and/or CORONARY SPASM

Frequency of provoked spasm in patients undergoing coronary angiography

Coronary artery spasm plays a major role in the mechanism of variant angina and possibly may contribute to chest pain in patients with fixed atherosclerotic lesions. Bertrand and associates[108] from Lille, France, established the incidence of coronary artery spasm provoked by 0.4 mg of methylergonovine in 1,089 consecutive patients undergoing coronary arteriography. The test was performed after routine coronary arteriography. Subjects included individuals with angina, both typical and atypical, and those with recent AMI and either valvular disease or dilated cardiomyopathy. Patients with spontaneous spasm, LM narrowing, or severe 3-vessel CAD were excluded. One hundred and thirty-four patients had focal spasm. Focal spasm was uncommon in patients with atypical precordial pain (1%), angina of effort (4%), valvular disease (2%), or cardiomyopathy (0%). Coronary artery spasm occurred most often in patients with angina at rest, less frequently in patients with angina both at rest and induced by exercise. Spasm was provoked in 20% of patients with recent transmural infarction, but in only 6% in patients studied later after infarction. Spasm was superimposed on fixed atherosclerotic lesions in 60% of the patients. No serious complications were encountered in the present study. Although the patients who underwent provocation tests were not representative of all patients with CAD, spasm occurred in 20% of patients who had experienced a coronary event and 15% of patients who complained of chest pain.

Exercise testing

In the original description of variant angina, Prinzmetal did not describe exercise-induced ST-segment changes. Although exercise-induced ST segment increase has been reported in patients with typical variant angina, the significance of these ECG changes has remained unclear. Waters and colleagues[109] from Montreal, Canada, reported on exercise treadmill testing (GETT) in 82 patients with variant angina and 67 also underwent exercise thallium-201 scans. The GETT produced ST increases in 25 patients (30%), ST decreases in 21 (26%), and no ST segment abnormality in 36 (44%). The ST segment increase during exercise occurred in the same ECG leads as during spontaneous attacks at rest and was always associated with a large perfusion defect on the exercise thallium-201 scan. In contrast, exercise-induced ST decrease often did not occur in leads that exhibited ST increase during episodes at rest. The exercise-induced ST segment changes did not accurately predict coronary anatomy. Coronary stenoses >70% were observed in 14 of 25 patients with ST increase, in 13 of 21 with ST decrease, and in 14 with no ST abnormality. The extent of disease activity did correlate with the results of the exercise test: ST increase occurred during exercise in 11 of 14 patients who experienced an average of ≥2 spontaneous attacks per day, in 12 of 24 who had between 2 attacks per day and 2 per week, and in only 2 who had <2 attacks per week. Exercise-induced ST increase was reexamined in 12 patients during treatment with calcium antagonist drugs and in 10 of the 12 ST increase did not occur with the second test. Over an average follow-up period of 20 months, death or AMI occurred in 3 of the 25 patients with ST increase, in none of 21 with ST decrease, and in only 2 of 36 with no ST abnormality. Thus, in variant angina patients, the results of an exercise test correlated well with the degree of disease activity but not with coronary anatomy and thus did not define a high risk subgroup.

Complicated by myocardial infarction or sudden death

Waters and associates[110] from Montreal, Canada, evaluated 132 consecutive patients hospitalized in a 5-year period because of active variant angina. Eighteen patients died or had an AMI within 1 month. In 4 patients an episode of pain and S-T elevation unrelieved by calcium antagonist drugs and intravenous nitroglycerin persisted for >1 hour, including cardiogenic shock and death before the appearance of Q waves and elevated serum enzyme levels. In the remaining 14 patients, AMI developed in the ECG leads in which ST-segment elevation had occurred during attacks of variant angina. In the 18 patients with complications, clinical features were not helpful in distinguishing them from the other 114 individuals. Angina at rest had been present for <1 month in 7 of the 18 with AMI compared with 31 of 114 in the other group. Before AMI, the artery presumed to be perfusing the involved myocardium at risk had a fixed stenosis of ≥70% of luminal diameter in 8 of 14 patients with complications who had coronary arteriograms compared with 50 of 112 in the other patients. In 13 of the 18 patients, complications occurred despite large doses of calcium antagonists. In 11 of these 13 patients, attacks of variant angina were monitored for 3–17 days before and during treatment; all 11 had fewer attacks with treatment and 5 had no attacks. Daily attacks of variant angina decreased from 4.6 ± 4.3–0.5 ± 0.7 (mean ± S.D.) with therapy. These data suggest that in patients with variant angina of recent onset AMI occurs frequently and unpredictably. AMI may occur in the absence of fixed coronary lesions and in spite of apparent clinical improvement following the administration of calcium antagonists.

After hospital discharge, 114 patients with variant angina were followed by Miller and colleagues[111] from Montreal, Canada, for a mean period of 26 months. Six died suddenly, and 13 others were resuscitated from cardiac arrest. The extent of CAD and the prevalence of LV dysfunction in these 19 sudden death patients were similar to those in the patients who did not have sudden death. During spontaneous episodes of ST increase recorded in the hospital, 56 of the 114 patients had serious arrhythmias, VF in 2, VT in 28, ventricular couplets or bigeminy in 17, 2 or 3° AV block in 6, and asystole in 3. Patients with and without these arrhythmias during attacks were similar with respect to extent of coronary disease, LV function, and most other clinical variables. The maximal ST increase was higher in the arrhythmia group. Serious arrhythmias were detected in 16 of the 19 sudden death patients compared with 36 of the 86 survivors. Sudden death occurred during follow-up in 15 of the 36 patients with VF, VT, high degree AV block, or asystole during attacks compared with only 4 of 69 patients without these arrhythmias. Thus, variant angina patients with serious arrhythmias during spontaneous attacks differ from other variant angina patients only in the degree of ischemia during attacks as reflected by maximal ST increase but are at a much higher risk for sudden death.

Roberts and associates[112] from Bethesda, Maryland, Gainesville, Florida, and Washington, DC, described clinical and necropsy findings in 3 patients who had angina pectoris at rest, S-T segment elevation on ECG during chest pain, coronary arterial spasm on angiography, and sudden death. Although significant "fixed" coronary narrowing (i.e., narrowing due to atherosclerotic plaques) was appreciated by angiography in 1 of 3 patients, necropsy disclosed in all 3 patients severe fixed coronary narrowings involving particularly the artery in which spasm had been demonstrated during life. Additionally, examination of each 5 mm segment of the coronary artery that had been spastic during life (2 patients) disclosed several focally spastic segments at necropsy, indicating that spasm persisted after death. Although most previously described patients with Prinzmetal's angina had some fixed coronary narrowing, underlying fixed narrowing may be difficult to identify angiographically, as demonstrated by the 3 patients in this study.

Treatment with calcium channel blockers and/or comparison with nitrates

To assess the efficacy of the new calcium channel blocker, diltiazem, for prophylaxis of Prinzmetal's angina, Schroeder and associates[113] from Stanford, California studied 48 patients in a randomized, multiple crossover multiclinic study (2 weeks single blind, 8 weeks double blind). Diltiazem dosage in 1 crossover phase was 120 mg/day, and in the other, 240 mg/day. Therapeutic response was measured by patients' diary records of angina frequency and nitroglycerin tablet consumption. Treatment with 120 mg/day diltiazem reduced angina by 41% from the entry placebo period and 20% from the paired placebo period (p < 0.005). Treatment with 240 mg/day diltiazem reduced angina frequency by 68% from the entry placebo period and 43% from the paired placebo period (p < 0.01). There were similar reductions in nitroglycerin consumption. Adverse experiences that may have been related to the medication were noted in only 5% of the patients. There were no alterations in BP or heart rate. The PR interval increased 3% at the 240 mg dosage level. Thus, diltiazem is an effective and safe agent for control of symptoms of Prinzmetal's angina.

Winniford and associates[114] from Dallas, Texas, studied 27 patients to compare the effectiveness of placebo, verapamil, and nifedipine. Comparisons between placebo and verapamil were part of a long-term, randomized, and double-blind study of 9 months' duration. At the end of this study, 23 patients were treated with nifedipine in a nonblind fashion for 2 months. Verapamil reduced the frequency of angina, nitroglycerin usage, transient episodes of ECG S-T segment deviation as assessed by 2-channel Holter monitoring, and hospitalization for clinical instability. In the 23 patients treated with nifedipine for 2 months, this agent exerted a similar beneficial effect (Fig. 1–15). Thus, these data demonstrate that long-term verapamil and nifedipine are superior to placebo and are of similar efficacy in treating patients with variant angina.

Freedman and associates[115] from Sydney, Australia, evaluated 37 patients with coronary artery spasm and minor coronary atherosclerosis or normal

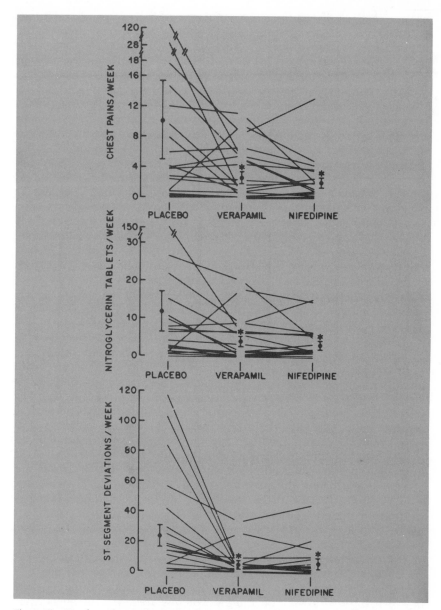

Fig. 1-15. Number of anginal episodes per week (top panel), nitroglycerin tablets consumed per week (middle panel), and transient S-T segment deviations by 2-channel ambulatory ECG monitoring (lower panel) during placebo (left), verapamil (middle), and nifedipine (right) in 23 patients with variant angina pectoris. Each line represents data from 1 patient, and the means ± SEM are shown for each treatment period. In comparison with placebo, both verapamil and nifedipine reduced frequency of all 3 variables, and there was no difference between the 2 drugs. Asterisks indicate p < 0.05 in comparison with placebo.

coronary arteries to determine the long-term effects of verapamil and nitrate treatment for coronary artery spasm. All patients had angina at rest, 32 had nocturnal angina, and 13 had a positive exercise test with ST elevation. Three had a previous subendocardial AMI; 10 had serious arrhythmias causing syncope in 7. After a mean of 21 months of therapy (range, 1–61 months), 27 patients continued on verapamil, 314 (120–600) mg/day; 4 who did not respond to verapamil were taking nifedipine, 58 (30–80) mg/day; and 16 were also taking isosorbide dinitrate, 41 (20–80) mg/day. In 31 patients on therapy, 21 were asymptomatic, 9 were improved (1–4 attacks/month), and 1 had an average of 8 anginal attacks per month. The remaining 6 had stopped therapy and 5 were asymptomatic at a mean of 10 (3–18) months after discontinuing the medication. Exercise tests became negative in all 12 patients tested on therapy, although 3 required nitrates in addition to verapamil or nifedipine. Withdrawal of the calcium antagonists was performed under supervision in 26 patients in the hospital at a mean of 15 (1–55) months on therapy. Ten developed angina in <48 hours. Angina recurred in all 6 unsupervised, patient-initiated withdrawals. Failure to stop smoking was positively associated with recurrence of angina on treatment withdrawal. These data suggest that long-term treatment of coronary arterial spasm with verapamil or nifedipine together with isosorbide dinitrate is well tolerated and effectively relieves angina. No serious arrhythmias, syncopal episodes, AMI, or death occurred in these patients during follow-up.

Ginsburg and associates[116] from Stanford, California, evaluated 12 patients who were entered prospectively into a randomized double-blind study comparing the efficacy of nifedipine and isosorbide dinitrate in the treatment of variant angina pectoris due to coronary artery spasm. Using the diary technique, both anginal episodes and nitroglycerin tablets consumed were recorded during the pretrial no drug period and during both active drug phases. During the baseline pretrial period, an average of 1.1 anginal episodes a day occurred with reduction to 0.28/day during nifedipine treatment and 0.39/day during isosorbide treatment. Headache was the major side effect during isosorbide treatment, occurring in 9 of 11 patients, and nonheart failure-related pedal edema during nifedipine treatment, occurring in 4 of 12 patients. Intolerable side effects necessitating cessation of treatment occurred in 2 patients during nifedipine treatment and in 3 patients during isosorbide treatment. Patients preferred nifedipine over isosorbide because of increased efficacy and fewer uncomfortable side effects. Thus, both nifedipine and isosorbide are effective for coronary spasm, but nifedipine is more effective, and more preferred, in most patients.

Hill and associates[117] from Gainesville, Florida, compared the influence of nifedipine and isosorbide dinitrate on the frequency of angina and consumption of nitroglycerin in 19 patients with coronary arterial spasm. Studies were performed in a double-blind manner with optimal titration of a dose for each patient. One patient was unable to tolerate isosorbide dinitrate and 1 patient dropped out of the study prematurely. In the remaining 16 patients, the mean frequency of angina was less during therapy with both nifedipine (0.69 episodes/day, p < 0.05) and isosorbide dinitrate (0.77 episodes/day, p < 0.05) than during the control period (1.71 episodes/day). The mean frequency of angina was similar in the nifedipine and isosorbide dinitrate treatment periods. A ≥50% decrease in frequency of angina compared with that occurring during the control period occurred in 13 of 18 patients during treatment with nifedipine and in 10 of 16 during isosorbide dinitrate. In the 15 patients who completed treatment with both agents, 7 showed greater improvement with nifedipine than with isosorbide dinitrate, whereas 6 other patients showed greater improvement with isosorbide dinitrate. Three patients had a <50% difference in frequency of angina with the 2 drugs. Thus, both nifedipine and isosorbide dinitrate are effective in some patients with coronary arterial spasm, but neither drug is clearly superior.

Treatment with nitroglycerin

Hill and colleagues[118] from Gainesville, Florida, examined segmental left coronary artery responses to nitroglycerin in 17 variant angina patients and in 34 nonvariant angina patients using a quantitative angiography technique. In those patients with LAD vasospasm, there was a marked exaggeration in the degree of dilation to nitroglycerin in those segments that at other times were involved with spasm. This observation was consistent when these segments were compared to 1) other left coronary segments in the same patient, 2) the same left coronary segments in nonvariant angina patients, and 3) the same left coronary segments in patients with right coronary spasm. These data suggest that a localized disorder in coronary vasomotion is present in patients with coronary spasm that is not limited to construction but also involves increased dilation in response to nitroglycerin.

Treatment with propranolol

Using a double-blind protocol, Robertson and associates[119] from Nashville, Tennessee, investigated the use of propranolol in patients with coronary artery spasm assessed by subjective and objective variables at low dosages (40 mg every 6 hours) and high dosages (160 mg every 6 hours). Propranolol significantly prolonged the duration of angina attacks but did not increase the frequency. These investigators concluded that propranolol in dosages up to 160 mg every 6 hours as single therapy is frequently detrimental in angina pectoris due to coronary artery spasm and should not be used as a sole treatment of this disorder.

Treatment with prostacyclin

Prostacyclin (PGI$_2$), an arachidonic acid metabolite produced by the vascular endothelial cells and by the lungs, exerts powerful vasodilating and antiplatelet effects in vitro and in vivo. A lack of PGI$_2$ production due to atherosclerosis may play a role in the pathophysiology of some clinical manifestations of CAD and, in particular, coronary vasospasm. Chierchia and associates[120] from London, England, evaluated the effects of intravenous PGI$_2$ in 9 patients with variant angina and 6 normal volunteers. In the normal subjects, PGI$_2$ (infused at 2.5, 5, 10, and 20 ng/kg/min) had significant antiplatelet effects, caused a dose-dependent decrease in both systolic and diastolic arterial pressure, and a decrease in pulmonary vascular resistance. Heart rate increased in a dose-dependent manner but no consistent effects in myocardial contractility by echo determination were observed. Although producing obvious antiplatelet and vasodilatory effects, PGI$_2$ did not affect the number, severity, and duration of spontaneous ischemic episodes due to coronary vasospasm in 5 patients and ergonovine-induced coronary spasm in 3 individuals. However, the number of ischemic episodes was consistently reduced in 1 patient during 4 consecutive periods of PGI$_2$ infusion, alternated with placebo. In this patient, a severe prolonged ischemic episode with ST increase on ECG and chest pain was consistently observed every time PGI$_2$ was discontinued. Side effects were negligible and readily reversible. These consisted of skin flushing, especially marked on the face and the palms, accompanied by a sensation of warmth in the same areas. Two subjects complained of headaches, 3 of restlessness, 3 experienced nausea, and 1 vomited. Thus, in the appropriate environment, PGI$_2$ can be administered safely to patients with CAD. Occasionally, PGI$_2$ may result in a complete disappearance of ischemic episodes due to coronary spasm. These conflicting results could be related to different causes of coronary spasm and chest pain.

Treatment by percutaneous transluminal coronary angioplasty

Among the first 83 patients treated with PTCA by David and colleagues[121] from Montreal, Canada, typical variant angina was recognized beforehand in 5 cases and discovered within 4 months of PTCA in 6 others. All patients had a significant proximal LAD coronary stenosis and only 1 had coronary narrowing >50% in other coronary arteries. Before PTCA, all patients were premedicated with calcium antagonist drugs. Of the 15 angioplasties, 13, including 3 or 4 repeat procedures, were technically successful. However, variant angina recurred after successful PTCA in 3 of the 5 patients in whom it was documented beforehand and in an additional 2 of 2 patients with variant angina before a successful repeat PTCA. Overall, among the 9 patients with variant angina after successful PTCA, 5 had restenosis at the site of PTCA and 2 others developed severe lesions adjacent to the site of the PTCA within 4 months of the procedure. Three patients without restenosis had been treated with calcium antagonist drugs and remained angina free. Thus, the observations suggest that PTCA is technically feasible in patients with variant angina who have organic stenotic lesions, but symptoms due to coronary spasm usually persist or recur, often with restenosis of the vessel.

PERCUTANEOUS TRANSLUMINAL CORONARY ANGIOPLASTY

Report of registry of the National Heart, Lung, and Blood Institute

Kent and associates[122] from The Registry of the NHLBI for studying PTCA collected data from 34 centers in the USA and Europe where such technical procedures are performed. This procedure was carried out in 631 patients, with an average age of 51 years in whom 80% had 1-vessel CAD, 17% had 2- or 3-vessel CAD, and 3% had stenosis of the LM coronary artery. Coronary angioplasty was successful in 59% of the stenosed coronary arteries with a resulting >20% decrease in the severity of coronary stenosis. The mean degree of stenosis was reduced from 83%–31%. Emergency coronary artery surgery was required in 6% of the patients (40 patients). AMI occurred in 29 patients (4%); in-hospital death occurred in 6 patients (1%). Follow-up has been possible for at least 1 year in 91 patients after PTCA. In these patients, 83% appeared improved clinically. These data suggest that initial satisfactory results may be obtained in many different centers by PTCA in selected patients with CAD.

Left ventricular function after successful PTCA

Percutaneous transluminal coronary angioplasty clearly improves the angiographic appearance of coronary artery stenoses and generally leads to improvements in symptoms of myocardial ischemia. Kent and associates[123] from Bethesda, Maryland, evaluated 59 consecutive patients with CAD undergoing PTCA by RNA at rest and during exercise before angioplasty and afterward if the procedure was successful. Of the 59 patients, 38 (64%) had an angiographically successful procedure (Figs. 1-16 and 1-17). Three (5%) had coronary occlusion as a complication. Arterial stenosis was reduced from $74 \pm 2\%$–$31 \pm 3\%$ (mean, $\pm$ SEM). The mean EF was $55 \pm 2\%$ at rest and $51 \pm 3\%$ during exercise before the procedure. After successful angioplasty, the EF was unchanged at rest but increased to $62 \pm 2\%$ ($p < 0.001$) during exercise (Fig. 1-18). Regional dysfunction was present during exercise in 94% of the patients before the procedure and in only 8% after successful angioplasty. Of the 38 patients in whom the procedure was successful, 19 had sustained improvement for >6 months, and 8 for 3–6 months (Fig. 1-17). Eleven patients had recurrence of symptoms; the second angioplasty was initially successful in 9. In 24 patients remaining asymptomatic for 6 months (19 after the first procedure and 5 after the second), the LV EF during exercise remained stable or improved.

Sigwart and colleagues[124] from Lausanne, Switzerland, evaluated ventricular function in 7 consecutive patients 1 day before and 6 months after PTCA

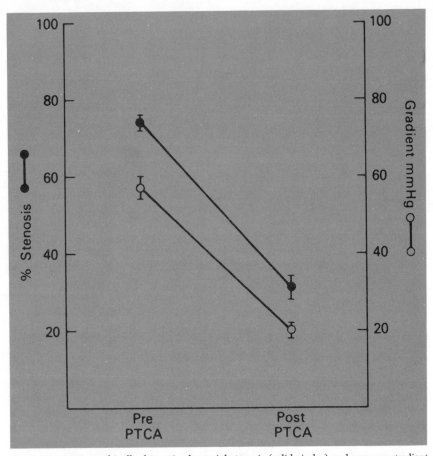

Fig. 1-16. Angiographically determined arterial stenosis (solid circles) and pressure gradient across the stenosis (open circles) before successful percutaneous transluminal coronary angioplasty (PTCA) and immediately afterward in 38 patients. Bars denote SEM. Reproduced with permission from Kent et al.[123]

for subtotal proximal stenosis of the LAD coronary artery. Before angioplasty, all patients had obvious LV dysfunction during exercise, and after PTCA, their clinical condition was improved significantly. Following PTCA, LV end-diastolic pressure was normal at rest and decreased from a mean ($\pm$SE) 34 $\pm$ 2–19 $\pm$ 0.05 mmHg on exercise. The LV EF (measured by gated radionuclide ventriculography) improved with exercise from 46 $\pm$ 5%–69 $\pm$ 1%. Cardiac output and stroke volume index improved significantly with exercise after angioplasty. Thus, these data suggest that improvement in LV function may occur after PTCA in patients with proximal LAD coronary artery stenosis.

Left ventricular diastolic filling is abnormal at rest in many patients with

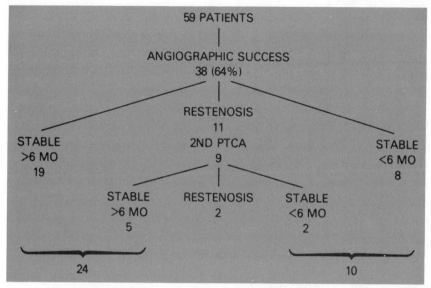

Fig. 1-17. Clinical results in patients undergoing initial and subsequent angioplasty (PTCA) procedures. Figures denote numbers of patients. Reproduced with permission from Kent et al.[123]

CAD even when other parameters of LV systolic function may be normal. To assess the effects and improved myocardial perfusion on impaired LV diastolic filling, Bonow and colleagues[125] from Bethesda, Maryland, studied 25 patients with 1-vessel CAD by high resolution RNA before and after PTCA. No patient had ECG evidence of a previous AMI. Despite normal regional and global LV systolic function in all patients, LV diastolic filling was abnormal in 17 of 25 patients. Twenty-three patients had abnormal LV systolic function during exercise. After successful PTCA, LV EF and heart rate at rest were unchanged but LV EF during exercise increased from 52%–63%; LV diastolic filling at rest improved also. Peak filling rate increased from 2.3–2.8 end-diastolic volume/second and time to peak filling rate decreased from 181 to 160 ms. Thus, a reduction in exercise-induced LV systolic dysfunction after PTCA, reflecting a reduction in reversible ischemia, was associated with improved LV diastolic filling at rest. The data from this investigation suggest that in many patients with CAD, without previous AMI and normal resting LV systolic function, abnormalities of resting LV diastolic filling are not fixed but appear to be reversible manifestations of impaired coronary blood flow.

Scholl and associates[126] from Montreal, Canada, evaluated the diagnostic value of exercise ECG and thallium scintigraphy in 54 of 70 patients who underwent PTCA both in the initial assessment and serial follow-up. Of the 45 patients who had successful PTCA, 36 had complete noninvasive studies performed before and 1 month after the procedure. Of these 36, 33 were asymptomatic 1 month after PTCA; the number of patients with an

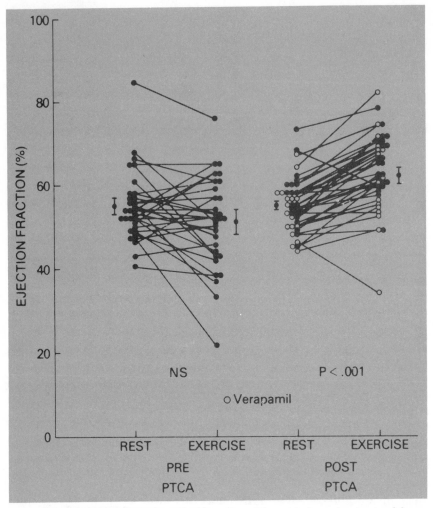

Fig. 1-18. Ejection fractions as determined by radionuclide ventriculography at rest and during exercise before angioplasty (PTCA) and afterward. Open circles denote patients receiving verapamil (120 mg every 8 hours) after angioplasty. Solid circles and vertical bars denote mean ejection fraction of group at rest and during exercise before and after angioplasty ($\pm$S.E.M.). Before angioplasty, data were obtained from patients who subsequently had successful procedures and could exercise without medication. After angioplasty, all patients who had successful procedures exercised for 1–14 days after the procedure (average, 2 days). NS denotes not significant. Reproduced with permission from Kent et al.[123]

abnormal exercise ECG decreased from 20 to 7 and with an abnormal thallium scintigram from 21 to 6. The number of patients who had at least 1 of the 2 tests positive decreased from 26 to 10. The average treadmill time increased from 448–618 second and the average rate-pressure product increased from 20 to 31 units. Of the 10 patients with a positive test, 2 had a partial restenosis >50% but <70% on the 6-month control angiogram. Six months after PTCA, a control angiogram was performed in 20 asymptomatic patients; 18 had an excellent result and 2 had a partial restenosis >50% but <70%. Stress test results were normal in patients with a successful 6-month PTCA and abnormal in the 2 patients with a partial restenosis. Ten patients developed angina within 3 months of PTCA, 9 developed a restenosis and 1 had a 90% circumflex stenosis that could not be dilated or grafted. Six of the 10 patients had a normal exercise ECG and scintigram at 1 month that became abnormal when symptoms reappeared. Thus, these clinical symptoms in conjunction with the exercise ECG and myocardial scintigram provide important short-term data on the angiographic evolution of PTCA results. The noninvasive tests may be useful in determining guidelines for repeat coronary angiography in patients who have undergone PTCA.

Operative transluminal angioplasty

Mills and Doyle[127] from New Orleans, Louisiana, reported their experience using operative transluminal angioplasty (OTA) as an adjunct to CABG. Twenty-four patients underwent OTA. Twenty-nine lesions were dilated: 17 distal lesions in a primary coronary artery limiting runoff, 6 tandem lesions that would otherwise not warrant separate grafts, and 6 lesions in coronary branches not large enough to accept a bypass graft. After coronary arteriotomy the angioplasties were performed using a 20 mm long 2 mm diameter balloon. Dilation was performed with saline inflated balloons using a 2.5 ml syringe and held for 10 seconds. The end point was successful passage of a 1.5–2 mm probe across the lesion that before dilation had not accepted a 1 mm probe. Of 29 lesions in the 24 patients, 25 were successfully dilated. The 4 failures were in long lesions (20–40 mm) that could not be crossed with a dilating catheter. Calcific deposits in the lesions did not determine the success of dilation. The patients were followed 1–12 months and none died. No perioperative AMI resulted, although 1 patient sustained a perioperative AMI in an area far from a distal LAD lesion dilated at operation. Repeat cardiac catheterization was performed on 8 patients 10 days to 4 months postoperatively. Seven patients improved, 1 did not, and there were no closures, extravasations, or aneurysms. The authors recommend OTA for lesions in tandem in an artery to be grafted or for lesions downstream to improve runoff in a saphenous vein or internal mammary graft.

CORONARY ARTERIAL BYPASS GRAFTING

Carotid bruit and the risk of stroke in elective surgery

The finding of a carotid artery bruit before elective surgery leads to a variety of actions among different physicians. Some recommend angiography or noninvasive carotid artery studies followed by endarterectomy if appropriate; others recommend study only in candidates for CABG or operations anticipated to involve large blood losses, and many consider the bruit to be an unimportant risk factor for perioperative or intraoperative stroke. Ropper and associates[128] from Boston, Massachusetts, studied prospectively 735 unselected patients undergoing elective surgery to determine the frequency of carotid bruit and postoperative stroke. Of the 104 patients (14%) who were found to have bruit, only 1 had a stroke within 3 days postoperatively. Of the 631 patients without a bruit, 4 had a stroke within 3 days after operation. Thus, the overall incidence of stroke was 0.7% and was not different in patients with and without bruits. All the strokes occurred in patients undergoing CABG and were thought to be embolic in nature.

For severe left main stenosis with total right occlusion

Rittenhouse and associates[129] from Seattle, Washington, studied 69 patients with severe ($\geq$70%) diameter narrowing of the LM coronary artery and occlusion of the right coronary artery who underwent CABG from December 1970 through December 1978. Preoperatively, 41% of patients were functional class III and 55%, class IV; 96% had a positive ECG test. Coronary bypass-grafting was accomplished in all patients. An average of 2.7 grafts/patient were placed. The hospital mortality rate was 4% and an additional 4% of patients died before the end of the first year. CHF was a significant predictor of postoperative mortality ($p > 0.05$). An intraaortic balloon was not inserted in 64 patients. Postoperative treadmill test was negative in 92% of patients studied. In patients surviving 1 year postoperatively, 89% were in functional class I and 8%, in class II. These data suggest that these patients may be operated on with a surgical mortality rate comparable to that of patients with LM coronary stenosis alone and a significantly better survival rate than that occurring in similar patients treated medically as reported in other studies.

Combined with endarterectomy

Halim and associates[130] in Harefield, England, evaluated 400 patients between October 1969 and December 1979 who had diffuse CAD and were treated with combined endarterectomy and CABG. This represented 42% of all patients operated on at the same institution during this time period. In these patients, 608 endarterectomies were performed; 329 of these were on the right coronary artery, 227 on the LAD, and 42 on the LC coronary artery. The early mortality rate was 4.3% and late mortality was 9% during a mean follow-up period of 47 months. The perioperative AMI rate was 15%. Of the survivors, 95% were asymptomatic or in improved condition. Only 11 patients were lost to follow-up. Three hundred fourteen patients (71%) were reevaluated with coronary and graft arteriography 1 month to 8 years postoperatively. The early patency rate of grafts to the endarterectomized vessels was 85%, the late patency rate was 77% at ≥1 year. The authors concluded that endarterectomy is a valuable additional procedure in the management of patients with diffuse CAD.

In diabetes mellitus

Diabetes mellitus (DM) is a well-established risk factor for CAD, but its effects on the conduct and results of CABG have not been well documented. Accordingly, Johnson and colleagues[131] from Milwaukee, Wisconsin, identified 261 (12%) diabetics among 2,192 patients operated upon from August 1972 through December 1977. All patients were surveyed, in identical manner, during January 1981. There were 51 (20%) dead, 7 (3%) lost to follow-up, and 7 (3%) residing in foreign countries in whom follow-up was not attempted. The 261 patients were divided into 3 groups by severity of DM: drug therapy 106 (41%), diet therapy 60 (23%), and borderline 95 (36%). Severity of DM had no effect on any of the factors investigated. Compared with nondiabetics, those with DM had the same average age, a higher proportion of women, the same number of grafts per patient, slightly worse ventricular function, and a higher surgical and late mortality. Frequency of preoperative angina was slightly higher in DM patients. Relief of angina was essentially the same in both groups. There were 54 serious complications that occurred in 45 (17%) patients; of these 20 (8%) died in the hospital. The only factors reaching statistical significance were the proportion of women and the surgical mortality with good ventricular function. Thus, the presence of DM does increase the morbidity and mortality associated with CABG, but only to a relatively small degree, and controlled DM is not sufficient reason to avoid CABG.

Sex, physical size, and operative mortality after CABG

The Collaborative Study in Coronary Artery Surgery (CASS) is a large multi-institutional study of the results of medical and surgical treatment of CAD. From August 1975–May 1980, 6,258 men and 1,153 women underwent isolated CABG. The operative mortality in men was 1.9% and in women, 4.5% (p < 0.0001). These results were reported by Fisher and colleagues[132] from several USA cities. Size of the patient, including coronary artery diameter, helped to predict operative mortality (Fig. 1-19). Furthermore, the smaller patient, male or female, had an increased risk in surgical mortality after allowing for differences in other risk factors (Fig. 1-20). Angina was more severe and more likely to be unstable in women. Symptoms of CHF were more frequent and more severe in women. The use of diuretics and digitalis also was more frequent in women. There were more women with 1-vessel disease and more men with 3-vessel disease. When adjustment was made for differences in both basic variables (such as angina, use of digitalis) and size variables, the gender variable contributed no predictive information. The patient's sex was not relevant to the risk of surgical death given the

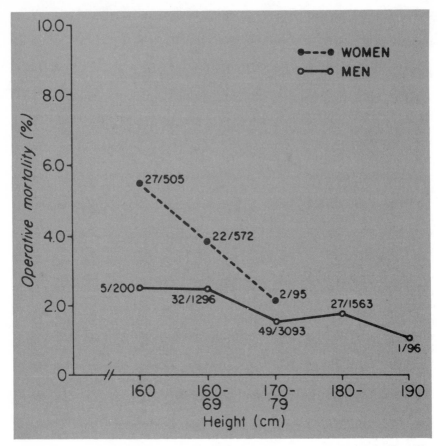

Fig. 1-19. In-hospital operative mortality in the Coronary Artery Surgery Study (CASS) by patient's height and sex. Reproduced with permission from Fisher et al.[132]

information available from clinical and angiograpic risk factors and from knowledge of certain aspects of patient's size. Thus, having done a univariate stepwise regression process, the authors found that height ($p < 0.001$) and average vessel diameter ($p < 0.001$) were predictive for operative mortality. They concluded that 1 possible explanation for the increased risk of coronary operation in women is the smaller stature and smaller diameter of the coronary arteries.

Detection of myocardial injury after CABG using a hypothermic cardioplegic technique

A sensitive and reliable indicator of myocardial necrosis is the release of creatine kinase CK-MB isoenzyme. McDaniel and colleagues[133] from Birmingham, Alabama, studied 50 consecutive patients undergoing isolated CABG.

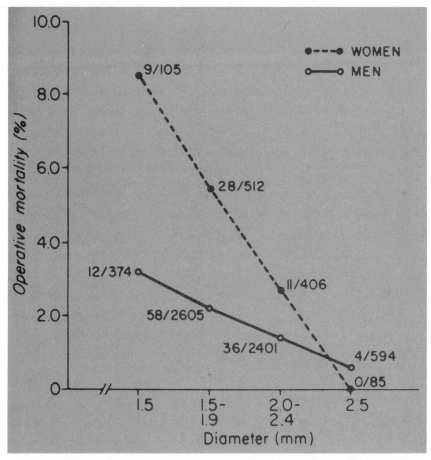

Fig. 1-20. In-hospital operative mortality in the Coronary Artery Surgery Study (CASS) by average diameter (mm) of measured values of distal right, middle and distal LAD, and first obtuse marginal vessel segments shown separately by patient's sex. Reproduced with permission from Fisher et al.[132]

Myocardial protection was induced by a cold cardioplegic solution containing 30 mEq/liter of potassium, 110 mEq/liter of sodium, glucose, calcium, and mannitol to obtain an osmolarity of 320–327 mOsm/liter and a pH of 7.85–7.90 (37°C). This is introduced in clear crystaloid solution at 4°C to obtain electromechanical quiescence and a myocardial septal temperature ≤18°C. The mean duration of aortic clamping was 37 ± 2 minutes, and the average number of arteries grafted was 3.5. Enzymatic and ECG evidence of AMI occurred in 1 patient. Nonspecific ECG changes occurred in 16 patients (32%) and the ECG was unchanged in the remaining 33 patients (66%). In the 49 patients without ECG evidence of AMI, the mean peak plasma CK-MB value that occurred 6 hours after onset of cardiopulmonary bypass was 8 ±

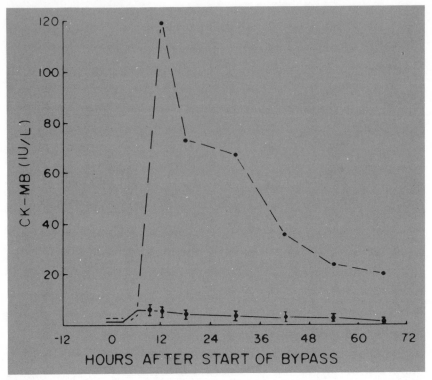

Fig. 1-21.   The CK-MB curve in 49 patients with minimal S-T segment changes or no changes on ECG (solid line) is contrasted with curve from patient with perioperative infarction and new Q waves on ECG (broken line). The bars are 1 standard deviation. Reproduced with permission from McDaniel et al.[133]

0.8 IU/liter and the mean integrated area was 158 ± 20 IU/liter × hours (Fig. 1-21). There was no correlation between CK-MB values and the extent of CAD, number of arteries grafted, or the duration of myocardial ischemia. No patient died. The data demonstrate a low incidence of perioperative myocardial injury with high potassium clear cardioplegic technique. With the exception of the 1 patient in whom ECG evidence of AMI occurred, the CK-MB values in the perioperative period were low. Thus, as judged by the elaboration of plasma CK-MB values after operation, cold clear cardioplegia provides adequate myocardial protection.

Continuous monitoring of left ventricular performance with the computerized nuclear probe during laryngoscopy and intubation before CABG

Giles and associates[134] from New Haven, Connecticut, monitored LV function serially in 25 patients during laryngoscopy and intubation in the anesthetic induction period before elective CABG, using radionuclide labeling of the cardiac blood pool and a computerized probe ("nuclear stethoscope"). Left ventricular ejection fraction was obtained preoperatively, after induction of anesthesia, but before endotracheal intubation, immediately after intubation, and at 1 minute intervals thereafter for 10 minutes. In all patients there was an immediate decrease (mean, 16%) in LV EF accompanying the reflex hypertension and tachycardia occurring during laryngoscopy and endotracheal intubation, and LV EF was significantly depressed for 3 minutes with concomitant hemodynamic changes. In 7 patients, recovery of LV EF did not occur in the time period of monitoring. In 10 healthy patients without known cardiac disease undergoing orthopedic surgery, an identical anesthetic induction, sequence, and intubation resulted in a similar disease in LV EF, but it returned to normal more rapidly. These data demonstrate that there are profound decreases in LV EF in patients with CAD accompanying the reflex hypertension and tachycardia occurring during endotracheal intubation and that in some patients there is persistent depression of LV function.

Perioperative coronary spasm

Buxton and associates[135] from Philadelphia, Pennsylvania, evaluated 6 patients who survived episodes of coronary arterial spasm occurring immediately after CABG and followed them for 15–30 months after operation. Coronary arterial spasm occurred in an unobstructed dominant right coronary artery in all 6 patients and caused inferior transmural ischemia. Hemodynamic collapse occurred in 5 of the 6 patients as a consequence of the coronary spasm. All these patients were treated with nitroglycerin followed by nifedipine. No patient has had recurrent angina or other evidence of spontaneous coronary spasm since CABG. Cardiac catheterization, including ergonovine maleate stimulation, was repeated 3–12 months after CABG in 5 of the 6 patients; in these 5 patients, the right coronary artery and all bypass grafts were patent, but 4 patients had new inferior wall motion abnormalities. Ergonovine provoked coronary artery spasm in the right coronary artery in 1 patient. These data suggest that coronary arterial spasm occurring immediately after CABG can cause severe hypotension and circulatory collapse. These episodes of perioperative spasm can cause myocardial necrosis. Such patients can be treated effectively with nitrates and calcium antagonists.

Bundle branch block following hypothermic cardioplegia in CABG

Hypothermic cardioplegia is a method commonly used for myocardial preservation at the time of aortic cross-clamping during CABG. O'Connell and colleagues[136] from Maywood, Illinois, assessed the frequency and significance of transient BBB in 50 patients undergoing CABG using hypothermic cardioplegia compared to 61 controls (patients undergoing CABG using core hypothermia and VF). All patients had normal QRS complexes on preoperative ECG. Clinical, hemodynamic and operative data were similar in both groups. Seventeen (34%) of the hypothermic cardioplegia group and 4 (6%) of the controls developed postoperative BBB. These changes were transient in all but 3 patients in the hypothermic cardioplegia group. None of the hypothermic cardioplegia patients with transient BBB had evidence of perioperative AMI. Clinical and operative parameters did not provide prediction of development of transient BBB. This study demonstrates that transient BBB in the immediate post-CABG period occurs commonly with the use of hypothermic cardioplegia and does not indicate AMI.

Effect of myocardial infarction during or immediately after CABG on survival

To study the effects of perioperative AMI on long-term survival and symptomatic status after CABG, Gray and colleagues[137] from Los Angeles, California, studied 225 survivors of 227 isolated CABG operations performed at their institution in a 9-month period (November 1975 to July 1976). Their data differed somewhat from that reported from the Seattle Heart Watch study. Their patients were separated into 3 groups. Group I (111 patients) had no postoperative ECG changes; group II (31 patients) had appearance and persistence of new or enlarged Q waves with localized ST elevation; and group III (83 patients) had less specific ECG changes. The frequency of perioperative AMI was 14% (31 of 227 patients). The groups were comparable with regard to age, prior AMI, number of diseased vessels, LM stenosis,

Fig. 1-22. Long-term survival after perioperative MI comparing likelihood of survival of normal group (group 1, triangles) to perioperative infarction (group 2, circles) and intermediate group (group 3, diamonds). Reproduced with permission from Gray et al.[137]

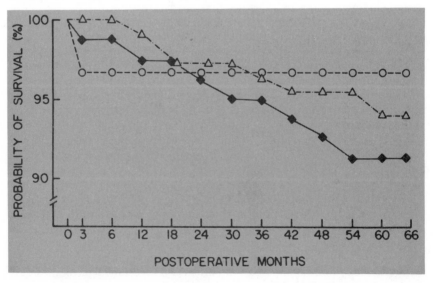

coronary collaterals, LV EF, and number of grafts inserted. However, ischemic time and total pump time were greater in group II than in group I. The 5-year survival rates for group I (94%), group II (97%), and group III (91%) were not significantly different (Fig. 1-22). Late postoperative status regarding relief of angina, dyspnea, level of physical activity, and use of cardiac medications was not different between the groups. Thus, using ECG criteria similar to those used by others, Gray and his colleagues found a 14% incidence of perioperative AMI. In following those patients for a mean of 60 months, the annualized mortality rate for the operative survivors was 1.3%, and there was no difference with regard to survival among the 3 groups of patients.

The effect of perioperative AMI occurring during CABG on hospital mortality, ventricular function, relief of angina, and late survival is controversial. Namay and colleagues[138] from Seattle, Washington, analyzed the effect of AMI (new Q waves) occurring at the time of CABG on late survival. From the Seattle Heart Watch registry, there were 77 patients who sustained AMI compared to 1,790 patients who underwent CABG without perioperative AMI. The actuarial survival probabilities of these 2 groups of surgically treated patients showed significantly poorer survival in patients with perioperative AMI compared with patients without perioperative AMI (Fig. 1–23). The 5-year survival probability was 76% and 90%, respectively (p < 0.001). Operative death rates were not significantly different in the 2 groups, 8 of 77 (10%) in the perioperative AMI group -vs- 89 of 1,790 (5%) in the non-AMI group (p = 0.064). With the exception of the relative paucity of collateral vessels in the patients with perioperative AMI, no baseline or operative

Fig. 1-23. Actuarial survival probabilities of groups of surgically treated patients with and without perioperative infarction. Reproduced with permission from Namay et al.[138]

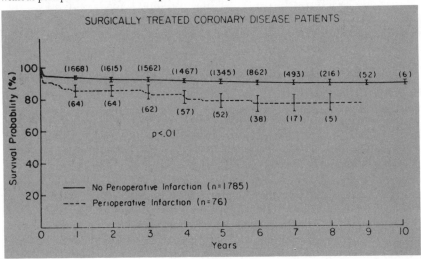

characteristic distinguished between groups. These characteristics included LM stenosis, MR, LV dysfunction, various associated procedures, cardiopulmonary bypass time, aortic cross-clamp time, and number of grafts per patient. Additionally, the authors found that perioperative AMI adversely affected long-term survival, even after adjusting for 7 other variables previously identified as predictive of survival. From this analysis, the risk of death for patients with perioperative AMI is estimated to be 3 times greater than for comparable patients without perioperative AMI.

Comparison of nitroglycerin and sodium nitroprusside for acute hypertension developing after CABG

Systemic hypertension frequently occurs early after CABG and usually requires a vasodilating agent for control. Flaherty and associates[139] from Baltimore, Maryland, tested the hypothesis that intravenous nitroglycerin (TNG) is as effective as sodium nitroprusside (NP) for managing acute hypertension early after CABG. Seventeen patients received both TNG and NP in a randomized crossover study. The infusion rates were increased stepwise to lower mean arterial pressures comparably with each agent. In 14 of 17 patients, similar infusion rates of the 2 vasodilators resulted in equal lowering of both BP and systemic vascular resistance. In the remaining 3 patients, very high infusion rates of TNG were required and achieved only 20%–50% of NPs response in 2 of 3. Hemodynamic responses to the 2 vasodilators were similar except that TNG increased cardiac output more than NP. In contrast, pulmonary gas exchange responses differed in that TNG improved intrapulmonary shunting, whereas NP worsened it. Similarly, TNG resulted in a significantly smaller increase in the alveolar arterial oxygen gradient than did NP. Thus, these results suggest that in most patients, intravenous TNG is as effective as NP in controlling acute hypertension after CABG, and TNG appeared to have a more favorable effect on pulmonary gas exchange. Because TNG has more beneficial effects on intracoronary collateral blood flow in the setting of regional ischemia, this agent may be preferable to NP in patients with CAD.

Factors influencing early patency of coronary artery bypass vein grafts

The expected 5-year patency rate for saphenous vein bypass grafts in CAD is estimated to vary between 60% and 85%. Various factors contribute to loss of vein graft conduit patency, among which are the preparation of the vein during harvesting and storage before grafting. At the present time, the optimal method of saphenous vein preparation is controversial. Catinella and associates[140] from New York City studied 2 methods of saphenous vein preparation. Forty recatheterizations were performed during the postoperative hospital stay (at approximately 10 days) in 2 groups of asymptomatic patients who had undergone isolated CABG. Veins from patients in group I were bathed in autologous, heparinized blood at 20°C and distended to 80 mmHg before grafting. The veins from group II patients were prepared in an identical manner, except that the bathing solution consisted of heparinized electrolyte solution with added papaverine (0.6 mg/ml). Segments of vein from each group were obtained before grafting and preserved in 3% glutaraldehyde for subsequent electron microscopic studies. Comparison of patients in group I and II revealed no significant difference in the number of diseased vessels per patient, the number of grafts per patient, native vessel diameter, or intraoperative graft flows. Early postoperative graft patency in group II patients, however, was 93% -vs- 80% in patients in group I ($p < 0.01$). Electron microscopic analysis revealed severe spasm of venous smooth muscle in the blood-stored veins, causing intraluminal smooth muscle cell cytoplasmic protrusions with resultant endothelial separation and desquamation. These findings were not present in the papaverine solution-treated veins. In view of those ultrastructural findings and the highly significant difference in patency rates, Catinella and associates have abandoned blood storage techniques and now prepare saphenous veins by soaking them in a clear bathing medium with added heparin and papaverine.

The New York group advocated low pressure distention (<100 mmHg) of the vein and use of papaverine. LoGerfo and associates (*Surgery* 90:1015, 1981) have had similar experience using papaverine, a warm crystaloid distention medium, and pressures up to 500 mmHg. They noted no endothelial disruption. However, when cold solutions or blood was used or in the absence of papaverine, high pressure distention resulted in endothelial disruption.

The saphenous vein is but 1 of many factors influencing satisfactory CABG. However, its optimal preparation certainly must lead to better patency and thereby better long-term results after CABG.

Ruptured atheromatous plaque in saphenous vein graft: a mechanism of acute thrombotic graft occlusion

Early occlusion of saphenous vein CABG is usually thrombotic and late occlusion is most often a result of progressive fibromuscular proliferation or atheromatous formation in the implanted veins. Walts and associates[141] from Los Angeles, California, described another mechanism of graft occlusion, namely, atheromatous plaque rupture with superimposed occlusive thrombosis. The authors studied 4 men aged 48–67 who underwent repeat bypass surgery for recurrent angina. Six of 8 vein grafts excised 5–8 years after the original bypass were completely occluded by recent thrombus superimposed on ruptured atheromatous plaques. In a 66 year-old man who died 7 years after CABG, similar findings were present at necropsy in 2 of 3 vein grafts. These lesions were indistinguishable from those that occur in native coronary arteries of patients with AMI.

Effects of sulfinpyrazone, dipyridamole, or aspirin after CABG

Baur and associates[142] from Minneapolis, Minnesota, evaluated the effect of sulfinpyrazone on the incidence of early postoperative closure of saphenous vein bypass grafts compared with placebo in a prospective randomized study of 255 eligible patients. Sulfinpyrazone was given in a dosage of 800 mg/day and started 24 hours after operation in 130 patients; 125 patients received placebo. Graft blood flow was measured at operation in almost all patients. Graft angiography was performed between 7 and 14 days postoperatively. There was no significant difference between the 2 groups in graft blood flow, number and diameter of the grafted arteries, LV filling pressure, or LV EF. In 73 patients, graft angiography could not be performed because of concomitant use of anticoagulant or antiplatelet drugs. The rate of early graft closure in the remaining 182 patients (431 grafts) was 3.8% (8 of 212) in the sulfinpyrazone group and 9.1% (20 of 219) in the placebo group (p < 0.025). The frequency of closure in grafts with a flow of <30 ml/minute did not differ significantly in the sulfinpyrazone and placebo groups. These data suggest that sulfinpyrazone can reduce the frequency of early graft closure in coronary grafts with a flow rate of >30 ml/minute.

Cade and associates[143] from Melbourne, Australia, measured platelet survival and plasma concentrations of beta-thromboglobulin (BTG) and platelet factor 4 (PF4) in 44 patients before and 6 months after CABG. Postoperatively, patients were randomized to receive sulfinpyrazone 800 mg/day or placebo. Preoperatively, platelet survival was significantly shorter than normal and plasma concentrations of both platelet-specific proteins were significantly elevated. Postoperatively, all 3 indexes of platelet function tended to become normal, but these changes were statistically significant only in patients treated with sulfinpyrazone. Postoperative exercise testing correlated significantly with plasma concentrations of BTG and PF4 measured preoperatively and postoperatively. These results are consistent with reports of the effects of sulfinpyrazone on platelet involvement in other conditions and suggest that the drug reduces platelet activation and inhibits actual destruction. The results also demonstrate a relation between abnormalities of platelet function and an index of postoperative myocardial ischemia.

In previous randomized, prospective clinical trials of platelet-inhibiting drugs in patients having CABG, therapy had not been started before the operation and the results have been inconclusive. Chesebro and associates[144] from Rochester, Minnesota, conducted a prospective randomized double-blind trial comparing dipyridamole (instituted 2 days before CABG) plus aspirin (added 7 hours after operation) with placebo in 407 patients. Vein graft angiography was performed in 360 patients (88%) within 6 months of operation (median, 8 days). Within 1 month of operation, 3% of vein graft distal anastomoses (10 of 351) were occluded in the treated patients, and 10% (38 of 362) in the placebo group; the proportion of patients with 1 or more distal anastomoses occluded was 8% (10 of 130) in the treated group and 21% (27 of 130) in the placebo group (Fig. 1-24; Table 1-4). This benefit

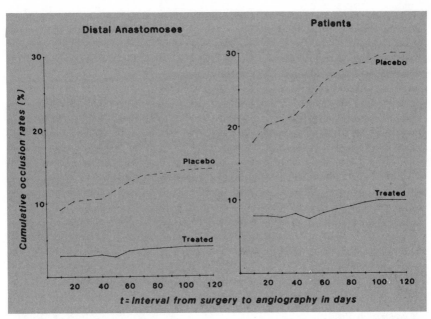

Fig. 1-24. Cumulative rates of occlusion. Left panel shows cumulative percentage of all vein-graft—coronary-artery distal anastomoses occluded in patients who had vein-graft angiography performed by *t* days after operation or sooner. The right panel shows cumulative percentage of all patients who had 1 or more distal anastomoses occluded at vein-graft angiography by *t* days after operation or sooner. Occlusion rates did not change from 120–180 days after operation; only 6 patients underwent angiography during this period. Reproduced with permission from Chesebro et al.[144]

in graft patency persisted in each of more than 50 subgroups. Early postoperative bleeding was similar in the 2 groups. In this trial, dipyridamole and aspirin were effective in preventing graft occlusion early after operation. This study clearly shows that dipyridamole and aspirin are beneficial to patients having CABG. The observation that perioperative antiplatelet therapy can increase CABG patency without increasing bleeding complications has implications for arterial reconstruction in other areas of the body as well, including peripheral vascular disease with or without surgery or transluminal angioplasty. It is hoped, though, that the late follow-up in the Mayo Clinic patients may confirm the favorable therapeutic prospect suggested by these early results.

Left ventricular function after CABG

Whether surgical treatment of symptomatic CAD improves ventricular function has been controversial. Lim and associates[145] from Melbourne, Australia, reported the effect of CABG on LV function assessed by biplane quantitative radionuclide angiography at rest and during sprint maximal

TABLE 1–4. *Frequency of vein graft occlusion in patients having same types of grafts.** *Reproduced with permission from Chesebro et al.*[144]

TYPE OF GRAFT	TREATMENT GROUP		PLACEBO GROUP	
	# with occlusion/total # (percentage occluded)			
Individual grafts only				
Patients with ≥1 occlusion	7/103	(7)	35/101	(35)
Distal anastomoses—grafts with occlusion	7/231	(3)	42/214	(20)
Sequential grafts only				
Patients with occlusion	2/32	(6)	6/38	(16)
Distal anastomoses with occlusion	4/115	(3)	17/143	(12)
Sequential and individual grafts				
Patients with occlusion	7/36	(19)	10/35	(29)
Distal anastomoses with occlusion	7/125	(6)	13/130	(10)
Y grafts and individual or sequential grafts				
Patients with occlusion	1/5	(20)	5/10	(50)
Distal anastomoses with occlusion	1/17	(6)	7/33	(21)
Total # of patients with occlusion	17/176	(10)*	56/184	(30)+
# of distal anastomoses with occlusion	19/488	(4)	79/520	(15)

* Including 1 patient with more than 1 occlusion.
+ Including 17 patients with more than 1 occlusion.

and graded submaximal exercise before and 3 months after CABG. Twenty patients with chronic stable angina were studied. Mean LV EF was unchanged at rest after CABG by both the first-pass ($60 \pm 12\%$ -vs- $60 \pm 12\%$) and equilibrium-gated ($61 \pm 13\%$ -vs- $62 \pm 13\%$) measurements. However, at peak work load (Wmax), mean first-pass LV EF was significantly higher postoperatively than preoperatively ($63 \pm 17\%$ -vs- $53 \pm 17\%$, $p < 0.01$) and a higher Wmax (750 ± 182 -vs- 590 ± 202 kpm/min, $p < 0.001$) and a higher rate-pressure product (302 ± 59 -vs- 222 ± 57 units, $p < 0.001$) was obtained. Similarly, equilibrium-gated LV EF levels during graded exercise was significantly higher postoperatively than preoperatively ($p < 0.001$); at the highest graded work load, they averaged $63 \pm 19\%$ postoperatively and $53 \pm 17\%$ preoperatively. Of the 5 subjects in whom LV EF decreased significantly during exercise postoperatively, all had 1 or more stenosed or occluded grafts. This study documents, by 2 independent radionuclide techniques, an improved LV EF during exercise at an increased maximal work capacity and rate-pressure product 3 months after successful CABG. Preoperatively, however, this group had good LV function.

Various investigators have demonstated improved LV function after CABG. Lindsay and colleagues[146] from Washington, DC, examined the potential of the radionuclide ventriculogram to assess the coronary circulation after CABG. They correlated postoperative coronary arteriography with postoperative multigated nuclear ventriculography. Their study consisted of 3 groups. There were 5 patients in group A in whom all grafts were patent and in whom all native arteries were narrowed <50% and were ungrafted. Group B consisted of 7 patients who had 1 myocardial segment served by a "failed" graft or a native artery narrowed ≥50% in diameter. Group C consisted of 13 patients in whom >1 myocardial segment was served by a "failed" graft or by a native artery narrowed ≥50%. In group A, the resting EF was 0.60 ± 0.03 (Fig. 1-25). Exercise produced an increase in EF in all 5 patients to a mean value of 0.68 ± 0.02 (p < 0.02). In group B, exercise produced a decline in EF in 5 and an increase in 2 patients (Fig. 1-25). As a

Fig. 1-25. Response (R) of LV ejection fraction to exercise (E). All completely revascularized patients (group A) had an increase; 5 of 7 patients with single area of potential ischemia (group B) and 10 of 13 with more than 1 such segment (group C) failed to manifest such an increase. Reproduced with permission from Lindsay et al.[146]

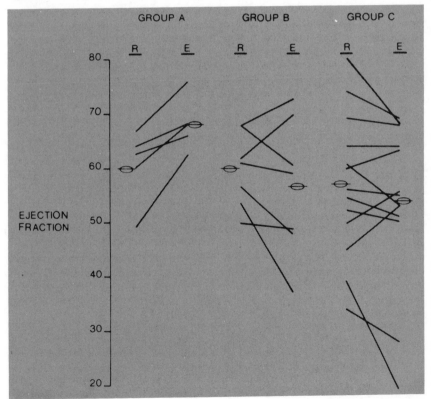

group, the resting EF was 0.60 ± 0.03; during exercise the value was 0.57 ± 0.05. In group C, exercise produced a decline in EF in 9, an increase in 3, and no change in 1 patient (Fig. 1-25). Resting EF of the whole group was 0.57 ± 0.03, and the exercise EF was 0.54 ± 0.03. The authors concluded that the most sensitive single indicator in patients with nonrevascularized myocardial segments was failure of the EF to rise during exercise. No patient who was completely revascularized exhibited a fall in EF with exercise.

Myocardial asynergy is sometimes reversed by CABG, and a noninvasive method of predicting which cases are reversible would be desirable. To assess whether changes in myocardial wall motion observed immediately after exercise can differentiate reversible from nonreversible myocardial asynergy, Rozanski and associates[147] from Los Angeles, California, evaluated 53 patients by RNA before and after exercise and again at rest after CABG. Preoperative improvement in wall motion immediately after exercise was highly predictive of the surgical outcome (average chance-corrected agreement, 91%). At surgery, the asynergic segments that had improved after exercise were free of grossly apparent scarring. The accuracy of these predictions for postoperative improvement was significantly greater (p < 0.01) than that of analysis of Q waves on resting ECG (average chance-corrected agreement, 40%). In contrast, preoperative changes in LV EF after exercise were not predictive of postoperative resting EF. Thus, postexercise RNA can be used to identify reversible resting myocardial asynergy. This test should prove effective in predicting which patients with myocardial asynergy are most likely to benefit from CABG.

Influence of residual narrowing after CABG on the 5-year survival

To determine the independent influence of the extent and sight of residual coronary narrowing on late survival, Lawrie and associates[148] from Houston, Texas, analyzed the fate of 1,448 consecutive patients who had CABG from 1968–1974. Survival was determined at a follow-up of ≥ 5 years. For patients with 2-vessel disease and good ventricular function, survival was similar at 5 years, 89% and 88% for 0 and 1 residual lesion; for those with 2-vessel disease and poor ventricular function; 5-year survival was 84% and 53% for 0 and 1 residual lesion (Fig. 1-26). For those with 3-vessel disease and good ventricular function, survival was 92%, 83%, and 75% for 0, 1, and 2 residual lesions, respectively (Fig. 1-26). With poor ventricular function, the corresponding results were 83%, 72%, and 23%. These rates were all highly significantly different (p < 0.005). Using the Cox multivariate analysis technique, residual disease, age at operation, and LV function were found to be the most important variables affecting survival of patients with 2- and 3-vessel disease. Residual lesions of LAD or LC coronary arteries were the most important predictors of survival; residual lesions of the right coronary artery exerted a lesser influence. Thus, residual narrowing affects survival and contradicts earlier studies suggesting a lack of such influence. Although the authors advocate the concept of complete revascularization, they suggest

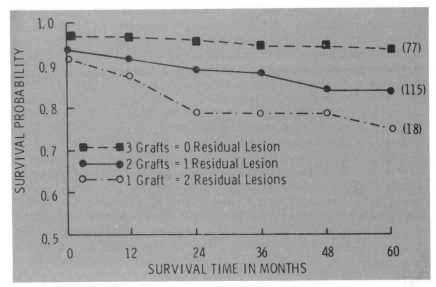

Fig. 1-26. Survival curves for 266 male patients with 3-vessel disease and good ventricular function. Three grafts were placed in 91 patients, 2 grafts in 151 patients and 1 graft was placed in 24 patients. Reproduced with permission from Lawrie et al.[146]

their results indicate that only a maximum of 3 or 4 separate grafts is necessary. Additional benefit from sequential or "snake" techniques will be difficult to demonstrate in patients with good LV function, and they suggest that such techniques may carry unacceptable risks of failure in a 5- to 10-year period after operation.

The authors make a strong case for "complete revascularization." It is controversial as to whether using a maximum of 4 distal anastomoses is equal to or superior to 5, 6, or 7 distal anastomoses.

NONATHEROSCLEROTIC CAD

Coronary aneurysm in Kawasaki disease

Kato and associates[149] from Kurume, Japan, performed aortic or coronary angiography in 290 patients shortly after the acute phase (1–3 months from onset of symptoms) of Kawasaki disease. Coronary aneurysms were found in 43 (15%). Follow-up angiograms 5–18 months after initial study in 42 patients showed: normal arteries in 21 (50%), persistent but small aneurysms in 8 (19%), disappearance or smaller aneurysms with stenosis or complete obstruction in 9 (21%), and regression of aneurysms but fine irregularities of the arterial wall in 4 (10%). Complications included AMI in 6

(14%) with 1 death and 5 complete recoveries, MR in 3 (7%), abnormal LV EF and asynergy in 2 (5%). Echo was used to diagnose correctly aneurysms in 19 of 21 (92%) at initial angiogram and in 8 of 10 (80%) at follow-up angiogram. Thallium studies were normal in 15 of 15 with regression of aneurysms but were also normal in 13 of 19 with abnormal angiograms.

These authors demonstrated the frequency of aneurysms (15%) and the complete regression of aneurysms in 50% of affected patients. Thus, most patients have no significant cardiovascular sequelae, but 1 of 290 (0.3%) died of cardiac problems, 6 of 290 (2%) had AMI, 3 of 290 (1%) developed significant MR, and residual coronary abnormalities were found in 13 of 290 (4%). Aneurysm formation usually can be detected by serial echo beginning on the ninth to the fifteenth day of illness. More data such as these are needed to guide the pediatric cardiologist in managing these patients. All patients with Kawasaki should be placed on aspirin therapy. Echo should be used to detect aneurysms and other cardiovascular abnormalities in the acute stages: 10–14 days from onset of symptoms in the patient without cardiac signs or symptoms (earlier with symptoms). If normal, repeat once in 1–2 months and if normal on second examination, further echo probably is not needed in asymptomatic patients and aspirin treatment can be discontinued 3 months from onset. If echo shows aneurysm, serial echo should be performed, and angiography used to define extent of disease, and aspirin continued indefinitely or until angiograms show complete regression of aneurysms. The few patients with aneurysms undetected by echo do not appear to justify angiography.

Onouchi and associates[150] from Aichi and Kyoto, Japan, performed coronary arteriograms on 30 children aged 4 months to 9 years with Kawasaki disease and coronary aneurysms. The patients were from a group of 86 patients with Kawasaki disease who underwent coronary arteriography; 63 were unselected, consecutive patients and 23 were referred because of severe systemic manifestations or cardiovascular signs and symptoms. The interval between onset of illness and arteriography in the 30 patients with aneurysms was 1 month to 7 years (mean, 1 year). Fifty-three aneurysms were found and number of arteries involved were: 1 in 8, 2 in 11, 3 in 7, and 4 in 4 patients. The left coronary only was involved in 13, left plus right in 13, and right only in 4. Six patients with 9 aneurysms had repeat studies 6 months to 6 years later. Five aneurysms did not change and 4 regressed to smaller size (3 patients) or to a normal appearance (1 patient).

These authors demonstrate excellently the distribution and configuration of coronary aneurysms in Kawasaki disease. The pediatric cardiologist continually is confronted with patients with this disease and the question of whom to study with angiography. Two-D echo is an excellent screening tool and almost certainly indicates coronary aneurysms if present. False negatives, however, are definite possibilities because only the proximal portion of the coronary tree can be visualized. In the series reported, the authors speculated that 9 of the 30 patients had aneurysms that would be difficult to detect by echo. Fortunately, prospective studies of echo -vs- angiographic sensitivity and specificity are underway in Japan. In the meantime, 2-D echo screening probably is satisfactory for most patients. If severe symptoms of the disease are prolonged or other cardiac manifestations detected, angiography may be useful in management.

CAD in systemic lupus erythematosus

Homcy and associates[151] from Boston, Massachusetts, studied 6 patients with systemic lupus erythematosus (SLE) diagnosed at 15–29 years who had ischemic heart disease before age 35. Two patients had coronary arteritis diagnosed at necropsy. In a third patient, alterations in coronary arterial anatomy occurred with angiographic improvement temporally related to the initiation of steroid therapy. The remaining 3 patients had severe diffuse atherosclerotic CAD identified in 2 at necropsy and by clinical course in the third patient who ultimately underwent CABG for relief of angina. These data indicate that both clinically important extramural coronary arteritis and atherosclerosis may occur in young patients with SLE. Coronary artery disease may occur with or without coexisting active extracardiac SLE manifestations.

Origin of the left main from the right coronary artery or from the right aortic sinus with intramyocardial tunneling to the left side of the heart via the ventricular septum: the case against clinical significance of myocardial bridge or coronary tunnel

Several reports in recent years have suggested that tunneling of a major longitudinal coronary arterial trunk into the myocardial wall may cause fatal or nonfatal cardiac dysfunction. Roberts and associates[152] from Bethesda, Maryland, described 2 patients in whom the LM coronary artery arose from the right coronary sinus and tunneled for a distance ≥5 cm within the ventricular septum beneath RV outflow tract to emerge just anterior to the ventricular septum and subsequently divide into the LAD and LC coronary arteries (Fig. 1-27). Neither patient ever had clinical evidence of cardiac dysfunction and death was from noncardiac causes. If an LM coronary artery can be burrowed into ventricular myocardium for a distance ≥5 cm for 34 and 48 years, respectively, in 2 patients, surely burrowing of an LAD coronary artery into LV myocardium for a distance of 2 or 3 cm cannot be implicated as a cause of cardiac dysfunction.

Origin of the right coronary artery from the left sinus of Valsalva and its functional significance

Roberts and associates[153] from Bethesda, Maryland, and Indianapolis, Indiana, described clinical and necropsy findings in 10 patients in whom the

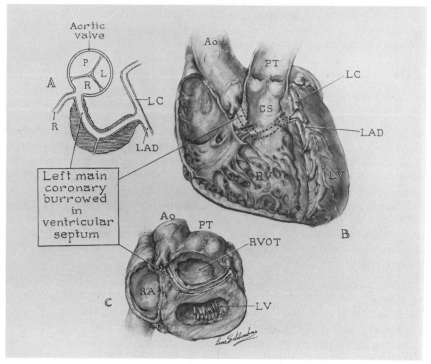

Fig. 1-27. Drawing of heart in 34-year-old man. Left main (LM) coronary artery coursed within ventricular septum beneath RV outflow tract before branching above septum into LAD and LC coronary arteries. Reproduced with permission from Roberts et al.[152]

right coronary artery arose from the left coronary sinus and then passed to the right AV sulcus by coursing between aorta and pulmonary trunk (Fig. 1-28). In 7 of the 10 patients, the coronary anomaly never caused symptoms of cardiac dysfunction. In the other 3, all of whom died suddenly, the coronary anomaly was the only significant abnormality found at necropsy: 1 patient had recurring VT, 1 had typical angina pectoris, and in 1 sudden death was the initial manifestation of cardiac dysfunction. Review of previous angiographic studies during life of 31 patients reported to have origin of the right coronary artery from the left sinus of Valsalva indicated that 9 had symptoms of cardiac dysfunction in the absence of intraluminal coronary narrowing or associated noncoronary cardiac disease. Thus, origin of the right coronary artery from the left sinus may produce cardiac dysfunction that can be fatal.

Isolated dissection of 1 or more coronary arteries associated with eosinophilic cellular inflammation

Robinowitz and associates[154] from Washington, DC, studied at necropsy 8 patients aged 26–47 years who had dissection isolated to ≥ 1 coronary

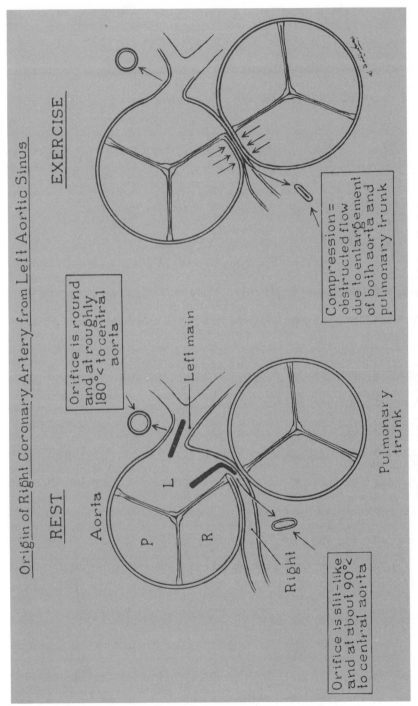

Fig. 1-28. Origin of right coronary artery from left aortic sinus.

arteries. Of the 8 patients, 6 died suddenly and 2 died after the onset of chest pain. All had hearts of normal size and in all the dissections involved the LAD coronary artery. The authors found inflammatory cells in the adventitia of the dissected coronary artery and the cells were predominantly eosinophilic granulocytes. The relation between the eosinophilic inflammatory adventitial infiltrates and the coronary arterial medial dissection is unclear, but the authors speculated that there might be an association.

MISCELLANEOUS TOPICS

Therapeutic and economic value of a normal coronary angiogram

A significant number of patients with severe angina pectoris or intractable atypical chest pain referred for coronary arteriography were found to have normal epicardial coronary arteries. To determine what therapeutic or economic benefit was derived from these studies, Faxon and associates[155] from Boston, Massachusetts, analyzed the data of 72 consecutive patients with normal coronary arteries referred for cardiac catheterization because of severe chest pain. The clinical status and hospitalizations were analyzed for the 2-year period before and the 2-year period after angiography. None died or had AMI. Although 47 were thought to have angina and 25, atypical pain before catheterization, the chest pain was reclassified with only 15 having anginal pain, 40, atypical pain, and 17, no pain. Functional improvement by at least 1 New York Heart Association class occurred in 74% of patients with 36 (50%) having no functional limitation. The use of cardiac medications was also significantly reduced. Despite functional improvement, no change in employment states could be demonstrated. The use of medical facilities was significantly less, the average number of hospital days per patient declining from 17–4 and hospitalization decreasing from 1.5–0.4. The result was a significant decrease in estimated hospital costs. Thus, in patients referred for coronary angiography for severe chest pain, documentation of a normal coronary arteriogram significantly alters the clinical assessment of symptoms, improves functional status, modifies medical therapy, and reduces hospitalization and medical costs. These therapeutic and economic benefits deserve consideration in the evaluation of coronary angiography for its overall effectiveness.

Analysis of coronary responses to various doses of intracoronary nitroglycerin

Feldman and colleagues[156] from Gainesville, Florida, studied the degree of coronary artery dilation resulting from increasing doses of intracoronary nitroglycerin (TNG). Heart rate (HR), aortic pressure, and coronary artery

angiograms were recorded before and after 5, 50, 150, and 250 μg doses of
TNG infused into the LM coronary artery. Coronary artery diameters were
measured by a magnification angiographic technique. After intracoronary
TNG, HR remained unchanged 2 minutes after each dose. Mean aortic
pressure also was unchanged after 5 μg but declined 5 mmHg after 50 μg, 9
mmHg after 150 μg, and 18 mmHg after 250 μg compared with the pressure
before TNG. The maximal increase in diameter occurred after 150 μg and no
additional increase was seen after larger doses. After 5 and 50 μg doses, 67%
and 75% maximal dilation responses, respectively, were observed. Compared
with coronary artery diameter before TNG administration, the 150 μg dose
increased the diameter of the LM coronary artery by 5%, proximal coronary
artery segment by 9%, middle segments by 19%, distal segments by 34%,
collateral-filled coronary arteries by 38%, coronary artery stenoses by 5%,
and small coronary arteries by 54%. Thus, these data indicate that relatively
small doses of intracoronary TNG produce potentially important coronary
artery dilation without important changes in HR and aortic pressure.

Disordered breathing and hypoxia during sleep in CAD

Breathing disorders and hypoxia during sleep were studied by De
Olazabal and associates[157] from Durham, North Carolina, in 17 men with
CAD, demonstrated by angiography, and without symptomatic pulmonary
disease: 13 (76%) had disordered breathing during sleep; 11 had obstructive
apnea, and the other 2 had Cheyne-Stokes breathing. There was an average of
20 episodes of disordered breathing per hour during sleep among the 13
patients, with a mean duration of 24 seconds per episode; significant oxygen
desaturation occurred in 10 of these 13 patients. None had angina pectoris,
AMI, or cardiac arrest. Although cardiac arrhythmias occurred in 12
patients, disordered breathing with hypoxia was not proved to be causative.
Therefore obstructive disordered breathing and nocturnal oxygen desaturation commonly occur during sleep in patients with CAD. Although no
immediate ill effects were noted, the long-term effects are unknown.

Cardiovascular effects of tricyclic antidepressants (imipramine or doxepin) in depressed patients with CAD

Because the tricyclic antidepressants can be cardiotoxic after an overdose,
their use has been considered potentially unsafe in patients with cardiac
disease. The effects, however, of tricyclic antidepressants on ventricular
rhythm and myocardial performance have not been examined in depressed
patients selected for the presence of cardiac disease. Accordingly, Veith and
associates[158] from Seattle, Washington, treated for 4 weeks in a double-blind
trial using imipramine, doxepin, or placebo 24 depressed patients with
cardiac disease (CAD in all, including 8 with CABG and 1 with AVR) to assess
the effects of tricyclic depressants on ventricular function and rhythm. The

tricyclic depressants had no effect on LV EF at rest or during maximal exercise, as measured by RNA obtained before and after treatment; VPC were reduced by imipramine but were not consistently changed by doxepin or placebo. Treatment with imipramine and doxepin, but not placebo, was associated with significant improvement ($p < 0.001$) in standard ratings of depression. These findings underscore the need for a reappraisal of the cardiovascular risks of tricyclic antidepressants and suggest that in the absence of severe impairment of myocardial performance, depressed patients with preexisting heart disease can be effectively treated with these agents without an adverse effect on ventricular rhythm or hemodynamic function.

References

1. ARMSTRONG WF, JORDAN JW, MORRIS SN, McHENRY PK: Prevalence and magnitude of S-T segment and T-wave abnormalities in normal men during continuous ambulatory electrocardiography. Am J Cardiol 50:1638–1642, May 1982.

2. SCHNEIDER RM, SEAWORTH JF, DOHRMANN ML, LESTER RM, PHILLIPS HR, BASHORE TM, BAKER JT: Anatomic and prognostic implications of an early positive treadmill exercise test. Am J Cardiol 50:682–688, Oct 1982.

3. SARMA RJ, SANMARCO ME: Reversal of exercise induced hemodynamic and ECG abnormalities after CABS. Circulation 65:684–689, Apr 1982.

4. WEINER DA, McCABE CH, CUTLER SS, RYAN TJ: Decrease in systolic blood pressure during exercise testing: reproducibility, response to coronary bypass surgery and prognostic significance. Am J Cardiol 49:1627–1631, May 1982.

5. STONE PH, LAFOLLETTE L, COHN K: Patterns of exercise treadmill test performance in patients with left main coronary artery disease: detection dependent on left coronary dominance or coexistent dominant right coronary disease. Am Heart J 104:13–19, July 1982.

6. SUGIURA T, DOI YL, HAFFTY BG, FITZGERALD T, BISHOP RL, SPODICK DH: Effect of oral propranolol on left ventricular performance in patients with ischemic heart disease. Chest 82:576–580, Nov 1982.

7. SCHAPIRA JN, FOWLES RE, BOWDEN RE, ALDERMAN EL, POPP RL: Relation of p-s$_4$ interval to left ventricular end-diastolic pressure. Br Heart J 47:270–276, March 1982.

8. RINK LD, FEIGENBAUM H, GODLEY RW, WEYMAN AE, DILLON JC, PHILLIPS JF, MARSHALL JE: ECG detection of LM coronary artery obstruction. Circulation 65:719–724, Apr 1982.

9. LEVIN DC, FALLON JT: Significance of the angiographic morphology of localized coronary stenosis: histopathologic correlations. Circulation 66:316–320, Aug 1982.

10. BROOKS N, CATTELL M, JENNINGS K, BALCON R, HONEY M, LAYTON C: Isolated disease of left anterior descending coronary artery: angiocardiographic and clinical study of 218 patients. Br Heart J 47:71–77, Jan 1982.

11. LITTLE WC, REEVES RC, COUGHLAN HC, ROGERS EW: Effect of cough on coronary perfusion pressure: does coughing help clear the coronary arteries of angiographic contrast medium? Circulation 65:604–610, March 1982.

12. WISNESKI JA, GERTZ EW, NEESE R, SOO W, BRISTOW JD, ADAMS JR, BEAUDRY JP: Myocardial metabolic alterations after contrast angiography. Am J Cardiol 50:239–245, Aug 1982.

13. DONALDSON RM, RAPHAEL MJ: "Missing" coronary artery: review of technical problems in coronary arteriography resulting from anatomical variants. Br Heart J 47:62–70, Jan 1982.

14. IRVIN RG: The angiographic prevalence of myocardial bridging in man. Chest 81:198–202, Feb 1982.
15. FRIEDMAN TD, GREENE AC, ISKANDRIAN AS, HAKKI AH, KANE SA, SEGAL BL: Exercise thallium-201 myocardial scintigraphy in women: correlation with coronary arteriography. Am J Cardiol 49:1632–1637, May 1982.
16. LEONG K, JONES RH: Influence of the location of left anterior descending coronary artery stenosis on left ventricular function during exercise. Circulation 65:109–114, Jan 1982.
17. ISKANDRIAN AS, LICHTENBERG R, SEGAL BL, MINTZ GS, MUNDTH ED, HAKKI A-H, KIMBIRIS D, BEMIS CE, CROLL MN, KANE SA: Assessment of jeopardized myocardium in patients with one-vessel disease. Circulation 65:242–247, Feb 1982.
18. BROWN KA, BOUCHER CA, OKADA RD, STRAUSS HW, POHOST G: Initial and delayed right ventricular thallium-201 rest-imaging following dipyridamole-induced coronary vasodilation: relationship to right coronary artery pathoanatomy. Am Heart J 103:1019–1024, June 1982.
19. CHEN PH, NICHOLS AB, WEISS MB, SCIACCA RR, WALTER PD, CANNON PJ: LV myocardial blood flow in multivessel coronary artery disease. Circulation 66:537–547, Sept 1982.
20. LEPPO J, BOUCHER CA, OKADA RD, NEWELL JB, STRAUSS HW, POHOST GM: Serial thallium 201 myocardial imaging after dipyridamole infusion: diagnostic utility in detecting coronary stenoses and relationship to regional wall motion. Circulation 66:649–657, Sept 1982.
21. GIBBONS RJ, LEE KL, COBB FR, COLEMAN E, JONES RH: EF response to exercise in patients with chest pain coronary artery disease and normal resting ventricular function. Circulation 66:643–648, Sept 1982.
22. AUSTIN EH, COBB FR, COLEMAN RE, JONES RH: Prospective evaluation of radionuclide angiocardiography for the diagnosis of coronary artery disease. Am J Cardiol 50:1212–1216, Dec 1982.
23. BROWN KA, BOUCHER CA, OKADA ED, STRAUSS HW, McKUSICK KA, POHOST GM: Serial right ventricular thallium-201 imaging after exercise: relation to anatomy of the right coronary artery. Am J Cardiol 50:1217–1222, Dec 1982.
24. BOTVINICK E, DUNN R, FRAIS M, O'CONNELL W, SHOSO D, HERFKENS R, SCHEINMAN M: The Phase Image: its relationship to patterns of contraction and conduction. Circulation 65:551–560, March 1982.
25. SCHWARZ F, SCHAPER J, BECKER V, KÜBLER W, FLAMENG W: Coronary collateral vessels: their significance for left ventricular histologic structure. Am J Cardiol 49:291–295, Feb 1982.
26. KOLIBASH AJ, BUSH CA, WEPSIC RA, SCHROEDER DP, TETALMAN MR, LEWIS RP: Coronary collateral vessels: spectrum of physiologic capabilities with respect to providing rest and stress myocardial perfusion, maintenance of left ventricular function and protection against infarction. Am J Cardiol 50:230–238, Aug 1982.
27. HORWITZ LD, GROVES BM, WALSH RA, SORENSEN SM, LATSON TW: Functional significance of coronary collateral vessels in patients with coronary artery disease. Am Heart J 104:221–225, Aug 1982.
28. MUELLER HS, RAO PS, RAO PB, GORY DJ, MUDD G, AYRES SM: Enhanced transcardiac 1-norepinephrine response during cold pressor test in obstructive coronary artery disease. Am J Cardiol 50:1223–1228, Dec 1982.
29. MOCK MB, RINGQVIST I, FISHER LD, DAVIS KB, CHAITMAN BR, KOUCHOUKOS NT, KAISER GC, ALDERMAN E, RYAN TJ, RUSSELL RO JR, MULLIN S, FRAY D, KILLIP T III: Survival of medically treated patients in the Coronary Artery Surgery Study (CASS) Registry. Circulation 66:562–568, Sept 1982.
30. KENT KM, ROSING DR, EWELS CJ, LIPSON L, BONOW R, EPSTEIN SE: Prognosis of asymptomatic or mildly symptomatic patients with coronary artery disease (CAD). Am J Cardiol 49:1823–1831, June 1983.
31. DAGENAIS GR, ROULEAU JR, CHRISTEN A, RABIA J: Survival of patients with a strongly positive exercise ECG. Circulation 65:452–456, March 1982.

32. BUDA AJ, MACDONALD IL, KWOK KL, ORR SA: Coronary disease progression and its effect on left ventricular function. Chest 82:285–290, Sept 1982.

33. EHSANI AA, MARTIN WH, HEATH GW, COYLE EF: Cardiac effects of prolonged intense exercise training in patients with coronary artery disease. Am J Cardiol 50:246–254, Aug 1982.

34. CONN EH, WILLIAMS RS, WALLACE AG: Exercise responses before and after physical conditioning in patients with severely depressed left ventricular function. Am J Cardiol 49:296–300, Feb 1982.

35. BAINTON D, BURNS-COX CJ, ELWOOD PC, LEWIS B, MILLER NE, MORGAN K, SWEETNAM PM: Prevalence of coronary heart disease and associations with serum lipoproteins in subjects aged 45 to 64 years (the Speedwell study). Br Heart J 47:483–489, May 1982.

36. MILLER GJ, BECKLES GLA, ALEXIS SD, BYAM NTA, PRICE SGL: Serum lipoproteins and susceptibility of men of Indian descent to coronary heart disease. The St. James survey, Trinidad. Lancet 2:200–203, July 24, 1982.

37. INTERNATIONAL COLLABORATIVE GROUP: Circulating cholesterol level and risk of death from cancer in men aged 40 to 69 years: experience of an International Collaborative Group. JAMA 248:2853–2859, Dec 3, 1982.

38. LEVY RI: Cholesterol and disease—what are the facts? JAMA 248:2888–2890, Dec 3, 1982.

39. KANNEL WB, GORDON T: The search for an optimal serum cholesterol. Lancet 2:374–376, Aug 14, 1982.

40. CABIN HC, ROBERTS WC: Relation of serum total cholesterol and triglyceride levels to the amount and extent of coronary arterial narrowing by atherosclerotic plaque in coronary heart disease. Quantitative analysis of 2,035 five-mm segments of 160 major epicardial coronary arteries in 40 necropsy patients. Am J Med 73:227–234, Aug 1982.

41. LIPINSKA I, GUREWICH V: The value of measuring percent high-density lipoprotein in assessing risk of atherosclerotic cardiovascular disease. Arch Intern Med 142:469–472, March 1982.

42. FALKO JM, O'DORISIO TM, CATALAND S: Improvement of high-density lipoprotein-cholesterol levels. Ambulatory type I diabetics treated with the subcutaneous insulin pump. JAMA 247:37–39, Jan 1, 1982.

43. DRESSENDORFER RH, WADE CE, HORNICK C, TIMMIS GC: High-density lipoprotein-cholesterol in marathon runners during a 20-day road race. JAMA 247:1715–1717, March 26, 1982.

44. UESHIMA H, IIDA M, SHIMAMOTO T, KONISHI M, TANIGAKI M, NAKANISHI N, TAKAYAMA Y, OZAWA H, KOJIMI S, KOMACHI Y: High-density lipoprotein-cholesterol levels in Japan. JAMA 247:1985–1987, Apr 9, 1982.

45. DOUSTE-BLAZY P, MARCEL YL, COHEN L, GIROUX J-M, DAVIGNON J: Increased frequency of Apo E-ND phenotype and hyperapobetalipoproteinemia in normolipidemic subjects with xanthelasmas of the eyelids. Ann Intern Med 96:164–169, Feb 1982.

46. NORUM RA, LAKIER JR, GOLDSTEIN S, ANGEL A, GOLDBERG RB, BLOCK WD, NOFFZE DK, DOLPHIN PJ, EDELGLASS J, BOGORAD DD, ALAUPOVIC P: Familial deficiency of apolipoproteins A-I and C-III and precocious coronary-artery disease. N Engl J Med 306:1513–1519, June 24, 1982.

47. CORTESE C, LEWIS B, MILLER NE, PEYMAN MA, RAO SN, SLAVIN B, SULE U, TURNER PR, UTERMANN G, WING AJ, WEIGHT M, WOOTTON R: Myelomatosis with type III hyperlipoproteinemia. Clinical and metabolic studies. N Engl J Med 307:79–83, July 8, 1982.

48. NESTEL PJ, FIDGE NH, TAN MH: Increased lipoprotein-remnant formation in chronic renal failure. N Engl J Med 307:329–333, Aug 5, 1982.

49. LaROSA JC, CLEARY P, MUESING RA, GORMAN P, HELLERSTEIN HK, NAUGHTON J: Effect of long-term moderate physical exercise on plasma lipoproteins. The national exercise and heart disease project. Arch Intern Med 142:2269–2274, Dec 1982.

50. BROWNELL KD, BACHORIK PS, AYERLE RS: Changes in plasma lipid and lipoprotein levels in men and women after a program of moderate exercise. Circulation 65:477–483, March 1982.

51. Ehnholm C, Huttunen JK, Pietinen P, Leino U, Mutanen M, Kostiainen E, Pikkarainen J, Dougherty R, Iacono J, Puska P: Effect of diet on serum lipoproteins in a population with a high risk of coronary heart disease. N Engl J Med 307:850–855, Sept 30, 1982.

52. Stacpoole PW, Swift LL, Greene HL, Slonim AE, Younger RK, Burr IM: Cholesterol reduction by a high-glucose diet in a patient with homozygous familial hypercholesterolemia: a preliminary report. Am J Med 72:889–893, June 1982.

53. Kuo PT, Kostis JB, Moreyra AE: Protection of myocardium by the compensatory mechanism of coronary collaterals after total occlusion of major coronary arteries shown in patients with familial hypercholesterolemia. Am Heart J 104:36–43, July 1982.

54. Vecchio TJ, Linden CV, O'Connell MJ, Heilman J: Comparative efficacy of colestipol and clofibrate in type IIa hyperlipoproteinemia. Arch Intern Med 142:721–723, March 1982.

55. Klaiber EL, Broverman DM, Haffajee CI, Hochman JS, Sacks GM, Dalen JE: Serum estrogen levels in men with acute myocardial infarction. Am J Med 73:872–881, Dec 1982.

56. Lindholm J, Winkel P, Brodthagen U, Gyntelberg F: Coronary risk factors and plasma sex hormones. Am J Med 73:648–651, Nov 1982.

57. ten Kate LP, Boman H, Daiger SP, Motulsky AG: Familial aggregation of coronary heart disease and its relation to known genetic risk factors. Am J Cardiol 50:945–953, Nov 1982.

58. Chesebro JH, Fuster V, Elveback LR, Frye RL: Strong family history and cigarette smoking as risk factors of coronary artery disease in young adults. Br Heart J 47:78–83, Jan 1982.

59. Baker IA, Eastham R, Elwood PC, Etherington M, O'Brien JR, Sweetnam PM: Hemostatic factors associated with ischemic heart disease in men aged 45 to 64 years (the Speedwell study). Br Heart J 47:490–494, May 1982.

60. Koplan JP, Powell KE, Sikes RK, Shirley RW, Campbell CC: An epidemiologic study of the benefits and risks of running. JAMA 248:3118–3121, Dec 17, 1982.

61. Gillum RF: Coronary heart disease in black populations. I. Mortality and morbidity. Am Heart J 104:839–851, Oct 1982.

62. Dibbs E, Thomas HE, Weiss ST, Sparrow D: Fire fighting and CAD. Circulation 65:943–945, May 1982.

63. Kromhout D, Bosschieter EB, De Lezenne Coulander C: Dietary fiber and 10-year mortality from coronary heart disease, cancer, and all causes. The Zutphen study. Lancet 2:518–521, Sept 4, 1982.

64. Salonen JT, Alfthan G, Huttunen JK, Pikkarainen J, Puska P: Association between cardiovascular death and acute myocardial infarction and serum selenium and a matched-pair longitudinal study. Lancet 2:175–179, July 24, 1982.

65. Multiple Risk Factor Intervention Trial Research Group: Multiple risk factor intervention trial. Risk factor changes and mortality results. JAMA 248:1465–1477, Sept 24, 1982.

66. Mehta J, Mehta P: Comparison of platelet function during exercise in normal subjects and coronary artery disease patients: potential role of platelet activation in myocardial ischemia. Am Heart J 103:49–53, Jan 1982.

67. deBoer AD, Turpie AGG, Butt RW, Johnston RV, Genton E: Platelet release and thromboxane synthesis in symptomatic coronary artery disease. Circulation 66:327–333, Aug 1982.

68. Mehta J, Mehta P: Effects of propranolol therapy on platelet release and prostaglandin generation in patients with CAD. Circulation 66:1294–1299, Dec 1982.

69. Joy M, Pollard CM, Nunan TO: Diurnal variation in exercise responses in angina pectoris. Br Heart J 48:156–160, Aug 1982.

70. Johnson SM, Mauritson DR, Winniford MD, Willerson JT, Firth BG, Cary JR, Hillis LD: Continuous electrocardiographic monitoring in patients with unstable angina pectoris: Identification of high-risk subgroup with severe coronary disease, variant angina, and/or impaired early prognosis. Am Heart J 103:4–12, Jan 1982.

71. Elamin MS, Boyle R, Kardash MM, Smith DR, Stoker JB, Whitaker W, Mary Dasg, Linden RJ:

Accurate detection of coronary heart disease by new exercise test. Br Heart J 48:311–320, Oct 1982.

72. ILSLEY C, CANEPA-ANSON R, WESTGATE C, WEBB S, RICKARDS A, POOLE-WILSON P: Influence of R wave analysis upon diagnostic accuracy of exercise testing in women. Br Heart J 48:161–168, Aug 1982.

73. BIAGINI A, MAZZEI MG, CARPEGGIANI C, TESTA R, ANTONELLI R, MICHELASSI C, L'ABBATE A, MASERI A: Vasospastic ischemic mechanism of frequent asymptomatic transient ST-T changes during continuous electrocardiographic monitoring in selected unstable angina patients. Am Heart J 103:13–20, Jan 1982.

74. PLOTNICK GD, FISHER ML, LERNER B, CARLINER NH, PETERS RW, BECKER LC: Collateral circulation in patients with unstable angina. Chest 82:719–725, Dec 1982.

75. MADIAS JE: Spontaneous angina in the coronary care unit: 2. Electrocardiographic changes during and after chest pain. Chest 82:279–284, Sept 1982.

76. NIXON JV, BROWN CN, SMITHERMAN TC: Identification of transient and persistent segmental wall motion abnormalities in patients with unstable angina by 2-D echo. Circulation 65:1497–1503, June 1982.

77. THADANI U, FUNG H, DARKE AC, PARKER JO: Oral isosorbide dinitrate in angina pectoris: comparison of duration of action and dose-response relation during acute and sustained therapy. Am J Cardiol 49:411–419, Feb 1982.

78. RAINWATER J, STEELE P, KIRSCH D, LeFREE M, JENSEN D, VOGEL R: Effect of propranolol on myocardial perfusion images and exercise ejection fraction in men with coronary artery disease. Circulation 65:77–81, Jan 1982.

79. PARKER JO, PORTER A, PARKER JD: Propranolol in angina pectoris. Comparison of long-acting and standard formulation propranolol. Circulation 65:1351–1355, June 1982.

80. TAYLOR SH, SILKE B, LEE PS: Intravenous beta-blockade in coronary heart disease. Is cardioselectivity or intrinsic sympathomimetic activity hemodynamically useful? N Engl J Med 306:631–635, March 18, 1982.

81. GAGNON R, MORISSETTE M, PRESANT S, SALVARD D, LEMIRE J: Hemodynamic and coronary effects of intravenous labetalol in coronary artery disease. Am J Cardiol 49:1266–1269, Apr 1982.

82. STEELE P, GOLD F: Favorable effects of acebutolol on exercise performance and angina in men with coronary artery disease. Chest 82:40–43, July 1982.

83. DiBIANCO R, SINGH SN, SHAH PM, NEWTON GC, MILLER RR, NAHORMEK P, COSTELLO RB, LADDU AR, GOTTDIENER JS, FLETCHER RD: Comparison of the antianginal efficacy of acebutolol and propranolol. A multicenter, randomized, double-blind, placebo-controlled study. Circulation 65:1119–1128, June 1982.

84. SILKE B, NELSON GIC, AHUJA RC, TAYLOR SH: Comparative hemodynamic dose response effects of propranolol and labetalol in coronary heart disease. Br Heart J 48:364–371, Oct. 1982.

85. PINE MB, CITRON D, BAILLY DJ, BUTMAN S, PLASCENCIA GO, LANDA DW, WONG RK: Verapamil versus placebo in relieving stable angina pectoris. Circulation 65:17–22, Jan 1982.

86. TAN ATH, SADICK N, KELLY DT, HARRIS PJ, FREEDMAN SB, BAUTOVICH G: Verapamil in stable effort angina: effects on left ventricular function evaluated with exercise radionuclide ventriculography. Am J Cardiol 49:425–430, Feb 1982.

87. WEINER DA, KLEIN MD: Verapamil therapy for stable exertional angina pectoris. Am J Cardiol 50:1153–1157, Nov 1982.

88. SCHEIDT S, FRISHMAN WH, PACKER M, MEHTA J, PARODI O, SUBRAMANIAN VB: Long-term effectiveness of verapamil in stable and unstable angina pectoris. One-year follow-up of patients treated in placebo controlled double-blind randomized clinical trials. Am J Cardiol 50:1185–1190, Nov 1982.

89. LUDBROOK PA, TIEFENBRUNN AJ, REED FR, SOBEL BE: Acute hemodynamic responses to sublingual nifedipine: dependence on LV function. Circulation 65:489–498, March 1982.

90. GERSTENBLITH G, OUYANG P, ACHUFF SC, BULKLEY BH, BECKER LC, MELLITS ED, BAUGHMAN KL,

Weiss JL, Flaherty JT, Kallman CH, Llewellyn M, Weisfeldt ML: Nifedipine in unstable angina. A double-blind, randomized trial. N Engl J Med 306:886–889, Apr 15, 1982.

91. Majid PA, DeJong J: Acute hemodynamic effects of nifedipine in patients with ischemic heart disease. Circulation 65:1114–1118, June 1982.

92. Stone PH, Turi ZG, Muller JE: Efficacy of nifedipine therapy for refractory angina pectoris. Am Heart J 104:672–681, Sept 1982.

93. Zacca NM, Verani MS, Chahine RA, Miller RR: Effect of nifedipine on exercise-induced left ventricular dysfunction and myocardial hypoperfusion in stable angina. Am J Cardiol 50:689–695, Oct 1982.

94. Subramanian VB, Bowles MJ, Khurmi NS, Davies AB, Raftery EF: Randomized double-blind comparison of verapamil and nifedipine in chronic stable angina. Am J Cardiol 50:696–703, Oct 1982.

95. Wagniart P, Ferguson RJ, Chaitman BR, Achard F, Benacerraf A, Delanguenhagen B, Morin B, Pasternac A, Baurassa MG: Increased exercise tolerance and reduced ECG ischemia with diltiazem in patients with stable angina pectoris. Circulation 66:23–28, July 1982.

96. Josephson MA, Hecht HS, Hopkins J, Guerrero J, Singh BN: Comparative effects of oral verapamil and propranolol on exercise-induced myocardial ischemia and energetics in patients with coronary artery disease: single-blind placebo crossover evaluation using radionuclide ventriculography. Am Heart J 103:978–985, June 1982.

97. Subramanian B, Bowles MJ, Davies AB, Raftery EB: Combined therapy with verapamil and propranolol in chronic stable angina. Am J Cardiol 49:125–132, Jan 1982.

98. Packer M, Meller J, Medina N, Yushak M, Smith H, Holt J, Guererro J, Todd GD: Hemodynamic consequences of combined beta-adrenergic and slow calcium channel blockade in man. Circulation 65:660–668, Apr 1982.

99. Bonow RO, Leon MB, Rosing DR, Kent KM, Lipson LC, Bacharach SL, Green MV, Epstein SE: Effects of verapamil and propranolol on LV systolic function and diastolic filling in patients with coronary artery disease: RNA studies at rest and during exercise. Circulation 65:1337–1350, June 1982.

100. Frishman WH, Klein N, Strom J, Cohen MN, Shamoon H, Willens H, Klein P, Roth S, Iorio L, LeJemtel T, Pollack S, Sonnenblick EH: Comparative effects of abrupt withdrawal of propranolol and verapamil in angina pectoris. Am J Cardiol 50:1191–1195, Nov 1982.

101. Subramanian VB, Bowles MJ, Davies AB, Raftery EB: Calcium channel blockade as primary therapy for stable angina pectoris. A double-blind placebo-controlled comparison of verapamil and propranolol. Am J Cardiol 50:1158–1163, Nov 1982.

102. Parodi O, Simonetti I, L'Abbate A, Maseri A: Verapamil versus propranolol for angina at rest. Am J Cardiol 50:923–928, Oct 1982.

103. Winniford MD, Markham RV, Firth BG, Nicod P, Hillis LD: Hemodynamic and electrophysiologic effects of verapamil and nifedipine in patients on propranolol. Am J Cardiol 50:704–710, Oct 1982.

104. Hultgren HN, Shettigar UR, Miller DC: Medical versus surgical treatment of unstable angina. Am J Cardiol 50:663–670, Oct. 1982.

105. European Coronary Surgery Study Group: Long-term results of prospective randomised study of coronary artery bypass surgery in stable angina pectoris. Lancet 2:1173–1180, Nov 27, 1982.

106. Rogers WR, Wysham DN: Coronary bypass for acute rest angina: 10 year follow-up. Br Heart J 47:365–368, Apr 1982.

107. Mohr R, Smolinsky A, Goor DA: Treatment of nocturnal angina with 10° reverse Trendelenburg bed position. Lancet 1:1325–1327, June 12, 1982.

108. Bertrand ME, LaBlanche JM, Tilmant PY, Thieuleux FA, Delforge MR, Carre AG, Asseman P, Berzin B, Libersa C, Laurent JM: Frquency of provoked coronary arterial spasm in 1089 consecutive patients undergoing coronary arteriography. Circulation 65:1299–1306, June 1982.

109. Waters DD, Szlachcic J, Bourassa MG, Scholl JM, Theroux P: Exercise testing in patients

with variant angina: results, correlation with clinical and angiographic features and prognostic significance. Circulation 65:265–274, Feb 1982.

110. WATERS DD, SZLACHCIC J, MILLER D, THEROUX P: Clinical characteristics of patients with variant angina complicated by myocardial infarction or death within 1 month. Am J Cardiol 49:658–664, March 1982.

111. MILLER DD, WATERS DD, SZLACHCIC J, THEROUX P: Clinical characteristics associated with sudden death in patients with variant angina. Circulation 66:588–592, Sept 1982.

112. ROBERTS WC, CURRY RC JR, ISNER JM, WALLER BF, McMANUS BM, MARIANI-CONSTANTINI R, ROSS AM: Sudden death in Prinzmetal's angina with coronary spasm documented by angiography. Analysis of three necropsy patients. Am J Cardiol 50:203–210, July 1982.

113. SCHROEDER JS, FELDMAN RL, GILES TD, FRIEDMAN MJ, DEMARIA AN, KINNEY EL, MALLON SM, PITT B, MEYER R, BASTA LL, CURRY RC JR, GROVES BM, MACALPIN RN: Multiclinic controlled trial of diltiazem for Prinzmetal's angina. Am J Med 72:227–232, Feb 1982.

114. WINNIFORD MD, JOHNSON SM, MAURITSON DR, RELLAS JS, REDISH GA, WILLERSON JT, HILLIS LD: Verapamil therapy for Prinzmetal's variant angina: comparison with placebo and nifedipine. Am J Cardiol 50:913–918, Oct 1982.

115. FREEDMAN SB, RICHMOND DR, KELLY DT: Long-term follow-up of verapamil and nitrate treatment for coronary artery spasm. Am J Cardiol 50:711–715, Oct 1982.

116. GINSBURG R, LAMB IH, SCHROEDER JS, HU M, HARRISON DC: Randomized double-blind comparison of nifedipine and isosorbide dinitrate therapy in variant angina pectoris due to coronary artery spasm. Am Heart J 103:44–48, Jan 1982.

117. HILL JA, FELDMAN RL, PEPINE CJ, CONTI CR: Randomized double-blind comparison of nifedipine and isosorbide dinitrate in patients with coronary arterial spasm. Am J Cardiol 49:431–438, Feb 1982.

118. HILL JA, FELDMAN RL, PEPINE CJ, CONTI CR: Regional coronary artery dilation response in variant angina. Am Heart J 104:226–233, Aug 1982.

119. ROBERTSON RM, WOOD AJJ, VAUGHN WK, ROBERTSON D: Exacerbation of vasotonic angina pectoris by propanolol: Circulation 65:281–284, Feb 1982.

120. CHIERCHIA S, PATRONO C, CREA F, CIABATTONI G, DE CATERINA R, CINOTTI GA, DISTANTE A, MASERI A: Effects of intravenous prostacyclin in variant angina. Circulation 65:470–476, March 1982.

121. DAVID PR, WATERS DD, SCHOLL JM, CREPEAU J, SZLACHCIC J, LESPERANCE J, HUDON G, BOURASSA MG: Percutaneous transluminal coronary angioplasty in patients with variant angina. Circulation 66:695–701, Oct 1982.

122. KENT KM, BENTIVOGLIO LG, BLOCK PC, COWLEY MJ, DORROS G, GOSSELIN AJ, GRUNTZIG A, MYLER RK, SIMPSON J, STERTZER SH, WILLIAMS DO, FISHER L, GILLESPIE MJ, DETRE K, KELSEY S, MULLIN SM, MOCK MB: Percutaneous transluminal coronary angioplasty: report from the registry of the National Heart, Lung and Blood Institute. Am J Cardiol 49:2011–2020, June 1983.

123. KENT KM, BONOW RO, ROSING DR, EWELS CJ, LIPSON LC, McINTOSH CL, BACHARACH S, GREEN M, EPSTEIN SE: Improved myocardial function during exercise after successful percutaneous transluminal coronary angioplasty. N Engl J Med 306:441–446, Feb 25, 1982.

124. SIGWART U, GRBIC M, ESSINGER A, BISCHOF-DELALOYE A, SADEGHI H, RIVIER J: Improvement of left ventricular function after percutaneous transluminal coronary angioplasty. Am J Cardiol 49:651–657, March 1982.

125. BONOW RO, KENT KM, ROSING DR, LIPSON LC, BACHARACH SL, GREEN MV, EPSTEIN SE: Improved LV diastolic filling in patients with coronary artery disease after percutaneous transluminal coronary angioplasty. Circulation 66:1159–1167, Dec 1982.

126. SCHOLL JM, CHAITMAN BR, DAVID PR, DUPRAS G, BREVERS G, VAL PG, CREPEAU J, LESPERANCE J, BOURASSA MG: Exercise ECG and myocardial scintigraphy in the serial evaluation of the results of percutaneous transluminal coronary angioplasty. Circulation 66:380–390, Aug 1982.

127. MILLS NL, DOYLE DP: Does operative transluminal angioplasty extend the limits of coronary artery bypass surgery? A preliminary report. CV Surgery 1981 (II). Circulation 66:I26–I29, Aug 1982.

128. ROPPER AH, WECHSLER LR, WILSON LS: Carotid bruit and the risk of stroke in elective surgery. N Engl J Med 307:1388–1401, Nov 25, 1982.

129. RITTENHOUSE EA, SAUVAGE LR, MANSFIELD PB, SMITH JC, HALL DG, DAVIS CC, O'BRIEN MA: Severe left main coronary arterial stenosis with right coronary arterial occlusion: results of bypass graft surgery. Am J Cardiol 49:645–650, March 1982.

130. HALIM MA, QURESHI SA, TOWERS MK, YACOUB MH: Early and late results of combined endarterectomy and coronary bypass grafting for diffuse coronary disease. Am J Cardiol 49:1623–1626, May 1982.

131. JOHNSON WD, PEDRAZA PM, KAYSER KL: Coronary artery surgery in diabetics: 261 consecutive patients followed four to seven years. Am Heart J 104:823–827, Oct 1982.

132. FISHER LD, KENNEDY JW, DAVIS KB, MAYNARD C, FRITZ JK, KAISER G, MYERS WO, and the Participating CASS Clinics: Association of sex, physical size, and operative mortality after coronary artery bypass in the Coronary Artery Surgery Study (CASS). J Thorac Cardiovasc Surg 84:334–341, Sept 1982.

133. MCDANIEL H, REVES J, KOUCHOUKOS N, SMITH L, ROGERS W, SAMUELSON P, LELL W: Detection of myocardial injury after coronary artery bypass grafting using a hypothermic, cardioplegic technique. Ann Thorac Surg 33:139–144, Feb 1982.

134. GILES RW, BERGER HJ, BARASH PG, TARABADKAR S, MARX PG, HAMMOND GL, GEHA AS, LAKS H, ZARET BL: Continuous monitoring of left ventricular performance with the computerized nuclear probe during laryngoscopy and intubation before coronary artery bypass surgery. Am J Cardiol 50:735–741, Oct 1982.

135. BUXTON AE, HIRSHFELD JW, UNTEREKER WJ, GOLDBERG S, HARKEN AH, STEPHENSON LW, EDIE RN: Perioperative coronary arterial spasm: long-term follow-up. Am J Cardiol 50:444–451, Sept 1982.

136. O'CONNELL JB, WALLIS D, JOHNSON SA, PIFARRE R, GUNNAR RM: Transient bundle branch block following use of hypothermic cardioplegia in coronary artery bypass surgery: high incidence without perioperative myocardial infarction. Am Heart J 103:85–91, Jan 1982.

137. GRAY RJ, MATLOFF JM, CONKLIN CM, GANZ W, CHARUZI Y, WOLFSTEIN R, SWAN HJC: Perioperative myocardial infarction: late clinical course after coronary artery bypass surgery. Circulation 66:1185–1189, Dec 1982.

138. NAMAY DK, HAMMERMEISTER KE, ZIA MS, DEROUEN TA, DODGE HT, NAMAY K: Effect of perioperative myocardial infarction on late survival in patients undergoing coronary artery bypass surgery. Circulation 65:1066–1071, June 1982.

139. FLAHERTY JT, MAGEE PA, GARDNER TL, POTTER A, MACALLISTER NP: Comparison of i.v. TNG and sodium nitroprusside for treatment of acute hypertension developing after CABG. Circulation 65:1072–1077, June 1982.

140. CATINELLA FP, CUNNINGHAM JN JR, SRUNGARAM RK, BAUMANN EA, NATHAN IM, GLASSMAN EA, KNOPP EA, SPENCER FC: The factors influencing early patency of coronary artery bypass vein grafts. J Thorac Cardiovasc Surg 83:686–700, May 1982.

141. WALTS AE, FISHBEIN MC, SUSTAITA H, MATLOFF JM: Ruptured atheromatous plaque in saphenous vein coronary artery bypass graft: a mechanism of acute thrombolic leg graft occlusion. Circulation 65:197–201, Jan 1982.

142. BAUR HR, VANTASSEL RA, PIERACH CA, GOBEL FL: Effects of sulfinpyrazone on early graft closure after myocardial revascularization. Am J Cardiol 49:420–424, Feb 1982.

143. CADE JF, DOYLE DJ, CHESTERMAN CN, MORGAN FJ, RENNIE GC: Platelet Function in CAD: effects of coronary surgery and sulfinpyrazone. Circulation 66:29–32, July 1982.

144. CHESEBRO JH, CLEMENTS IP, FUSTER V, ELVEBACK LR, SMITH HC, BARDSLEY WT, FRYE RL, HOLMES DR JR, VLIETSTRA RE, PLUTH JR, WALLACE RB, PUGA FJ, ORSZULAK TA, PIEHLER JM, SCHAFF HV,

DANIELSON GK: A platelet-inhibitor-drug trial in coronary-artery bypass operations: benefit of perioperative dipyridamole and aspirin therapy on early postoperative vein-graft patency. N Engl J Med 307:73–78, July 8, 1982.

145. LIM YL, KALFF V, KELLY MJ, MASON PJ, CURRIE PJ, HARPER RW, ANDERSON ST, FEDERMAN J, STIRLING GR, PITT A: Radionuclide angiographic assessment of global and segmental left ventricular function at rest and during exercise after coronary artery bypass graft surgery. Circulation 66:972–979, Nov 1982.

146. LINDSAY J JR, NOLAN NG, KOTLYAROV EV, GOLDSTEIN SA, SCHOOLMEESTER LW, BACOS JM: Radionuclide ventriculography following coronary bypass surgery: correlation with arteriographic findings. Ann Thorac Surg 33:238–243, March 1982.

147. ROZANSKI A, BERMAN D, GRAY R, DIAMOND G, RAYMOND M, PRAUSE J, MADDAHI J, SWAN HJC, MATLOFF J: Preoperative prediction of reversible myocardial asynergy by postexercise radionuclide ventriculography. N Engl J Med 307:212–216, July 22, 1982.

148. LAWRIE GM, MORRIS GC, SILVERS A, WAGNER WF, BARON AE, BELTANGADY SS, GLAESER DH, CHAPMAN DW: The influence of residual disease after coronary bypass on the 5-year survival rate of 1274 men with coronary artery disease. Circulation 66:717–723, Oct 1982.

149. KATO H, ICHINOSE E, YASHIOKA F, TAKECHI T, MATSUNOGA S, SUZUKI K, RIKITAKE N: Fate of coronary aneurysms in Kawasaki disease: serial coronary angiography and long term followup study. Am J Cardiol 49:1758–1766, May 1982.

150. ONOUCHI Z, SHIMAZU S, KIYOSAWA N, TAKAMATSU T, HAMAOKA K: Aneurysms of the coronary arteries in Kawasaki disease: an angiographic study of 30 cases. Circulation 66:6–13, July 1982.

151. HOMCY CJ, LIBERTHSON RR, FALLON JT, GROSS S, MILLER LM: Ischemic heart disease in systemic lupus erythematosus in the young patient: report of six cases. Am J Cardiol 49:478–484, Feb 1982.

152. ROBERTS WC, DICICCO BS, WALLER BF, KISHEL JC, McMANUS BM, DAWSON SL, HUNSAKER JC, LUKE JL: Origin of the left main from the right coronary artery or from the right aortic sinus with intramyocardial tunneling to the left side of the heart via the ventricular septum: the case against clinical significance of myocardial bridge or coronary tunnel. Am Heart J 104:303–305, Aug 1982.

153. ROBERTS WC, SIEGEL RJ, ZIPES DP: Origin of the right coronary artery from the left sinus of Valsalva and its functional consequences: analysis of 10 necropsy patients. Am J Cardiol 49:863–868, March 1982.

154. ROBINOWITZ M, VIRMANI R, McALLISTER HA JR: Spontaneous coronary artery dissection and eosinophilic inflammation: a cause and effect relationship? Am J Med 72:923–928, June 1982.

155. FAXON DP, McCABE CH, KREIGEL DE, RYAN TJ: Therapeutic and economic value of a normal coronary angiogram. Am J Med 73:500–505, Oct 1982.

156. FELDMAN RL, MARX JD, PEPINE CJ, CONTI CR: Analysis of coronary responses to various doses of intracoronary nitroglycerin. Circulation 66:321–326, Aug 1982.

157. DE OLAZABAL JR, MILLER JD, COOK WR, MITHOEFER JC: Disordered breathing and hypoxia during sleep in coronary artery disease. Chest 82:548–552, Nov 1982.

158. VEITH RC, RASKIND MA, CALDWELL JH, BARNES RF, GUMBRECHT G, RITCHIE JL: Cardiovascular effects of tricyclic antidepressants in depressed patients with chronic heart disease. N Engl J Med 306:954–959, April 22, 1982.

Acute Myocardial Infarction and Its Consequences

NECROPSY STUDIES IN HEALED INFARCTION

The percent of LV wall (including ventricular septum) replaced by scar was determined by Cabin and Roberts[1] of Bethesda, Maryland, in 70 necropsy patients with a healed transmural myocardial infarction. The infarct involved 1%–55% (mean, 13) of the LV wall. The ages at death of the patients ranged from 25–82 years (mean, 62) and did not significantly correlate with infarct size ($r = -0.12$). Of the 70 patients, 41 (59%) had unequivocal histories of AMI: the interval from the AMI to death in them ranged from 2–276 months (mean, 50) and correlated negatively with AMI size ($r = 0.32$, $p < 0.05$), and the age at AMI ranged from 26–79 years (mean, 58) and did not correlate with healed infarct size ($r = -0.05$). The 4 major epicardial coronary arteries were examined quantitatively in 56 patients; the number of coronary arteries with severe (>75% in cross-sectional area) narrowing ranged from 1–4 (mean, 2.9) and did not correlate with infarct size ($r = -0.24$). The mean infarct size in the 12 patients with and in the 44 without severe narrowing of the LM coronary artery was

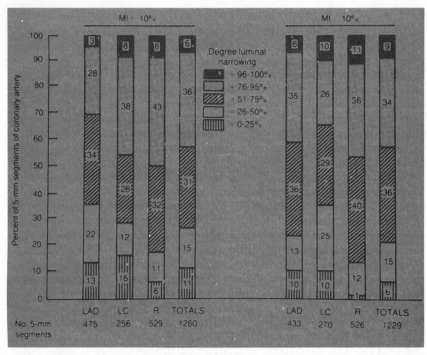

Fig. 2-1. Percent of 5 mm segments of the right (R), LAD, and LC coronary arteries narrowed to various degrees by atherosclerotic plaques in 28 patients with MI involving ≤10% and in 28 with MI involving >10% of the LV wall. Reproduced with permission from Cabin and Roberts.[1]

identical (each 13%). The entire lengths of the right, LAD, and LC coronary arteries in the 56 patients were divided into 5 mm segments and the amounts of cross-sectional area narrowing in each of the resulting 2,489 segments were determined by histologic examination. The percent of 5 mm segments with severe (cross-sectional area narrowing, 76%–100%) narrowing by atherosclerotic plaques in each patient ranged from 3%–93% (mean, 44) and did not correlate with infarct size ($r = -0.20$). When the 28 patients with an infarct involving >10% of the LV wall were compared to those with an infarct involving ≤10%, a similar overall percent of 5 mm segments of coronary artery was severely narrowed (43% -vs- 42%) (Fig. 2-1). In addition, a similar percent of segments was narrowed severely in each of the 3 major epicardial coronary arteries. Thus, in these necropsy patients with healed transmural myocardial infarction, the infarct size correlated with length of survival after the AMI (in patients with definite histories of AMI), but not with age at death or with the amount, location, or extent of coronary arterial narrowing by atherosclerotic plaques.

The amount of cross-sectional area narrowing by atherosclerotic plaque in each 5 mm segment of the entire lengths of the right, LM, LAD, and LC coronary arteries and the size, predominant location, and extent of myocardial scarring were determined by Cabin and Roberts[2] from Bethesda, Maryland, in 59 necropsy patients with healed transmural myocardial infarction. The mean number of the 4 major epicardial coronary arteries narrowed severely (76–100% in cross-sectional area) was 3.0 in the 37 patients with posterior (inferior) infarcts and 2.6 in the 22 patients with anterior infarcts ($p < 0.025$). The mean percent of severely narrowed 5 mm segments from all 4 major coronary arteries was similar in the anterior and posterior infarct groups (38% -vs- 46%) (Fig. 2-2). The patients with anterior infarcts, however, had a higher percent of severely narrowed 5 mm segments of the LAD than of the LC, but not the right coronary artery, 46% -vs- 25% ($p < 0.001$) and 40% (NS). The patients with posterior infarcts had a higher percentage of severely narrowed segments of the right and LC coronary

Fig. 2-2. Percent of 5 mm segments of right (R), LAD, and LC coronary arteries narrowed to various degrees by atherosclerotic plaques in 22 patients with an anterior and 37 with a posterior wall transmural healed MI. Reproduced with permission from Cabin and Roberts.[2]

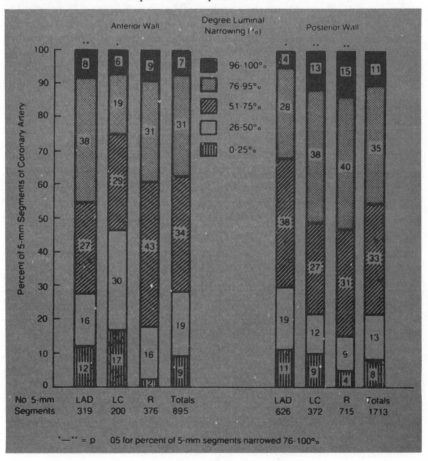

arteries than of the LAD artery, 55% and 51% -vs- 32% (p < 0.05). The anterior infarct group had, on the average, larger LV scars than the posterior infarct group (20% -vs- 9%, p > 0.002) and more frequent scarring of the ventricular septum (16 [73%] -vs- 6 patients [16%], p < 0.001).

Clinical and necropsy observations were described by Cabin and Roberts[3] from Bethesda, Maryland, in 61 patients with a healed transmural myocardial infarction: 33 with and 28 without a clinical history of AMI. There were no significant differences between the 2 groups of patients in mean age, sex, or frequency of angina pectoris, chronic CHF, severe systemic hypertension, sudden coronary death, or fatal AMI. Compared with the patients with clinically recognized AMI, the patients with clinically unrecognized (silent) AMI had a significantly (p < 0.05) higher frequency of diabetes mellitus (43% -vs- 15%), death from noncardiac causes (39% -vs- 9%), posterior (inferior) wall infarcts (82% -vs- 55%), and smaller infarcts (mean size 7% -vs- 17% of LV wall). The patients with and without clinically recognized AMI had similar numbers of the 4 major coronary arteries severely (76 to 100% reduction in cross-sectional area) narrowed (mean 2.8/4.0 -vs- 2.9/4.0 per patient), insignificant differences in frequency of severe narrowing for the LM coronary artery (18% -vs- 29%), similar overall percents of 5 mm segments of the 4 major coronary arteries severely narrowed (43% -vs- 42%), and similar percents of severely narrowed 5 mm segments of the right (46% -vs- 55%), LAD (39% -vs- 33%), and LC (41% -vs- 41%) coronary arteries.

DIAGNOSIS

A computer-derived protocol to aid in diagnosis of emergency room chest pain

Identification of patients whose chest pain represents AMI is often difficult. Because of fear of the consequences of missing patients at high risk, emergency room physicians are encouraged to admit patients to "rule out AMI" if the diagnosis is uncertain. Although this practice increases the number of admissions of patients who do have AMI, it has led to a situation in which as few as 30% of patients admitted to coronary care units are eventually diagnosed as having AMI. If the differentiation between AMI and other causes of chest pain could be made more accurately, the quantity of scarce resources spent on unnecessary admissions to the coronary care unit could be substantially reduced. To derive a protocol to identify AMI, Goldman and associates[4] from New Haven, Connecticut, and Boston, Massachusetts, derived a protocol to identify AMI in patients who went to 1 hospital emergency room with chest pain (Fig. 2-3). They then prospectively tested the protocol on 2 sets of patients at a second hospital. They analyzed 482 patients at 1 hospital. Using recursive partitioning analysis, they constructed a decision protocol in the format of a simple flow chart to identify AMI on the basis of 9 clinical factors. In prospective testing on 468

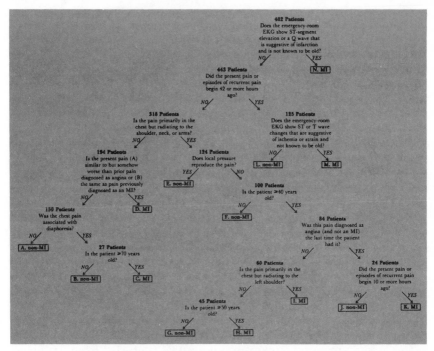

Fig. 2-3.   Computer-derived decision tree for classification of patients with acute chest pain. Each of the 14 letters (A through N) identifies terminal branch of tree. For any given patient, start with first question regarding ST-segment elevation and then trace patient through relevant subsequent questions until terminal branch is reached. In the Yale-New Haven Hospital sample, 7 terminal branches (C, D, H, I, K, M, and N) contained all 60 patients with AMI as well as 28 patients with unstable angina and 43 patients with other ultimate diagnoses. Reproduced with permission from Goldman et al.[4]

other patients at a second hospital, the protocol performed as well as the physicians. Moreover, an integration of the protocol with the physicians' judgments resulted in a classification system that preserved sensitivity for detecting AMI, significantly improved the specificity (from 67–77%) and positive predictive value (from 34–42%) of admission to an intensive care area. The protocol identified a subgroup of 107 patients among whom only 5% had AMI and for whom admission to nonintensive care areas might be appropriate. This decision protocol warrants further wide-scale prospective testing, but is not ready for routine clinical use.

Creatinine kinase—myocardial component in the absence of abnormally elevated total CK levels

Since the development of techniques to detect the isoenzymes of creatine kinase (CK) and lactic dehydrogenase (LDH), they have been used commonly to verify AMI. The presence of myocardial components (MB) of these enzymes is considered a highly specific and sensitive measure of myocardial cell death and has been especially helpful in the absence of diagnostic ECG changes. Of the 2 enzymes, CK and its myocardial isoenzyme MB are believed to have the greater predictive accuracy. Most reports confirming the accuracy of CK-MB in detecting AMI have found CK-MB in the presence of elevated total CK activity. A few reports have described the appearance of CK-MB in the absence of an abnormal elevation of total CK. Dillon and associates[5] from Durham, North Carolina, analyzed CK enzyme and isoenzyme patterns, LDH, and ECG changes in 724 consecutive patients admitted to their coronary care unit for chest pain. Of the 724, CK-MB was detected in 419 (58%). Of these, however, 69 (16%) had no abnormal elevation of total CK levels. The group with CK-MB but persistently normal total CK levels had fewer diagnostic QRS changes on ECG (17% -vs- 54%) and a lower frequency of LDH 1:2 inversion (28% -vs- 79%) than did the group with CK-MB and abnormally elevated CK levels. No specific level of either total CK or CK-MB, however, could segregate the patients with QRS or LDH level changes, suggesting that persistently normal levels of CK do not exclude the diagnosis of AMI.

Serum C-reactive protein

C-reactive protein (CRP) is the classic acute phase reactant, since serum CRP levels have long been known to increase after AMI. Earlier work using relatively insensitive and semiquantitative assays suggested that serial measurement of serum CRP levels may be useful in diagnosis and management of AMI. De Beer and associates[6] from London, England, investigated this possibility in a prospective study of well-characterized patients using a precise quantitative assay for CRP, together with measurements of creatine kinase (CK) MB, the specific myocardial isoenzyme. These authors measured CRP and CK-MB levels in patients with definite AMI, with spontaneous or exercise-induced angina pectoris, undergoing coronary angiography, and with noncardiac chest pain. All patients with AMI developed raised CRP levels and a significant correlation occurred between peak CRP and CK-MB values (Fig. 2-4). The CRP, however, peaked around 50 hours after the onset of pain at a time when the CK-MB, which peaked after about 15 hours, had already returned to normal. In 20 patients who recovered uneventfully, CRP levels fell, returning to normal about 7 days after AMI in 4 cases who were followed to that point. In 8 complicated AMI patients, including 4 who died within the first 10 days, the CRP level remained high. Angina alone or coronary arteriography did not cause a rise in the CRP or CK-MB concentrations.

Increased CRP production is a nonspecific response to tissue injury and raised CRP levels in cases of chest pain with a normal CK-MB indicates a process other than AMI. Regular monitoring of CRP levels also may assist in early recognition of intercurrent complications occurring after AMI.

Voulgari and associates[7] from Birmingham, England, studied serially by laser immunonephelometric assay in sera from 17 patients with AMI C-

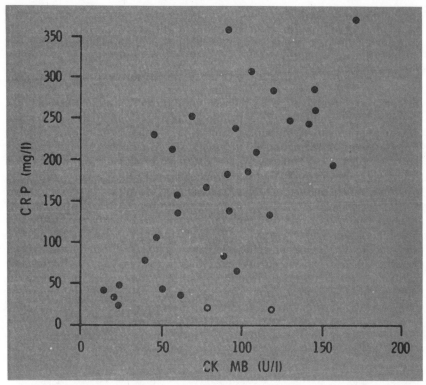

Fig. 2-4. Peak serum levels of CRP and CK MB in myocardial infarction. The 2 individuals with relatively poor CRP response are indicated (O). Reproduced with permission from DeBeer et al.[6]

reactive protein and 4 other acute phase reactant proteins of noncardiac origin. A similar comparison was made in 57 patients undergoing surgery and 72 with acute infections. C-reactive protein was consistently the most sensitive acute phase reactant in all 3 conditions. After AMI, a raised serum C-reactive protein level was found on admission in 4 patients before a rise in creatine kinase MB isoenzyme (CK-MB). The peak C-reactive protein level was reached by the third post-AMI day, and it then declined over 7 days with a half-life similar to myocardial tropomyosin. Serial monitoring of serum C-reactive protein, in parallel with cardiac proteins of short half-life (CK-MB) and long half-life (tropomyosin), provides maximal information for diagnosis and for detecting post-AMI complications.

Diagnosis by 2-D echo

To define the role of portable 2-D echo in the immediate diagnosis of acute chest pain syndrome, Horowitz and colleagues[8] from Philadelphia, Pennsylvania, studied 80 consecutive patients. Adequate 2-D echoes were obtained in 65 (81%). Thirty-three patients had clinical evidence of transmural and nontransmural AMI, 18 of whom had nondiagnostic initial ECG; 32 did not evolve a clinical AMI. Of the 33 patients,[31] 94% with clinical AMI had regional wall motion abnormalities on initial 2-D echo. The other 2 patients had uncomplicated nontransmural AMI diagnosed only by ECG in 1 and by ECG with moderate increase of cardiac enzymes in the other. Of the 32 patients without clinical AMI, 27 had normal regional wall motion on the initial 2-D echo and none had complications of arrhythmia, recurrent pain, CHF, or death in the hospital. Conversely, 10 of the 36 patients with initial 2-D echo regional wall motion abnormalities developed a complication. Thus, in patients with the acute chest pain syndrome, an initial 2-D echo that shows no regional wall motion abnormalities suggests that such patients will not develop an AMI or clinical complications during the hospital course. These investigators concluded that an initial 2-D echo with regional wall motion abnormalities identifies a high risk group of patients likely to evolve an acute infarction with important complications.

Quantification of size by 2-D echo

Visser and associates[9] from Amsterdam, The Netherlands, performed apex 2-D echo in 53 patients with AMI. All were studied within 12 hours of the onset of symptoms of their first AMI. Three apical long-axis views were obtained: the 2- and 4-chamber views and the right anterior oblique equivalent or 3-chamber view (Fig. 2-5). Satisfactory echos were obtained in 48 patients (91%). The individual apical views were divided into 3 segments and the area of asynergy was estimated in each view. Left ventricular asynergy was present in all 48 patients. In 46 patients, a positive correlation between the ECG and the echo was obtained as far as AMI localization was concerned. The estimated asynergic area correlated well with the peak value of the isoenzyme of creatine kinase (CK-MB) (Fig. 2-6). Thus, apex echo is a reliable alternative method of detecting and quantifying AMI soon after the onset of symptoms.

Thirty patients with chest pain syndromes were studied by Loh and colleagues[10] from Los Angeles, California, on admission by 2-D echo to confirm or exclude AMI. Twelve patients had nontransmural AMI and 18 patients had no AMI. There was no significant difference between these groups in background characteristics. Two-D echo studies were analyzed quantitatively and qualitatively. The most sensitive and specific technique for detecting AMI was qualitative analysis, using the presence of severe hypokinesis as the criterion for an abnormal study. Using this technique, 10 of 12 patients with AMI and all 18 patients without AMI were correctly identified. This analysis technique was highly reproducible. These data indicate that in patients with chest pain syndromes without diagnostic ECG findings of AMI, 2-D echo may provide a rapid, sensitive, specific tool to aid in the establishment of the correct diagnosis. In patients with nontransmural AMI, the presence of severe hypokinesis appears to be the best discriminator of AMI.

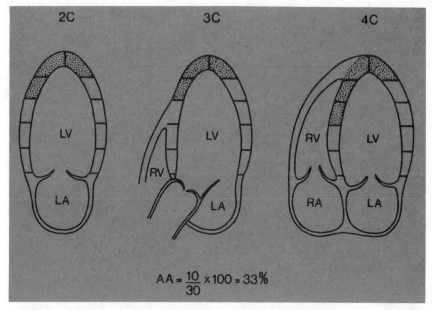

Fig. 2-5. Schematic diagram showing 3 apical long axis views. LV free wall and septum is divided into equal segments. Asynergic area (AA) of left ventricular wall (dotted segments) is expressed as percentage of total number of segments (30). In this example a total infarct size of 33% is obtained. Reproduced with permission from Visser et al.[9]

Relation of myocardial ischemia detected by stress perfusion scintigraphy and site of subsequent infarction

To determine the relation between scintigraphic regions of stress-induced ischemia and subsequent AMI, Frais and associates[11] from San Francisco, California, studied 21 patients who had previously undergone stress scintigraphy and who later had an AMI with scintigraphy on a second occasion soon afterward. After AMI, thallium-201 perfusion scintigraphy was performed in 16 patients (76%) and technetium-99m pyrophosphate in 14 patients (67%). All patients had at least 1 post-AMI scintigram and 9 (42%) had both perfusion scintigraphy and infarct imaging. Nineteen patients (90%) had scintigraphic evidence of stress-induced ischemia pre-AMI. Scintigraphic infarct regions were compared with regions of previously demonstrated stress-induced ischemia. In 11 patients (53%), the AMI was extensive; in 1, reimaged 1 week before AMI, and in 4 others (19%) there were matching defects; in 3 patients (14%) the AMI was less extensive, and in 2 patients (9%) the AMI was less extensive but also involved regions not previously shown to develop ischemia. In the final patient (5%) there was no match. AMI frequently involved regions previously shown to develop stress-induced

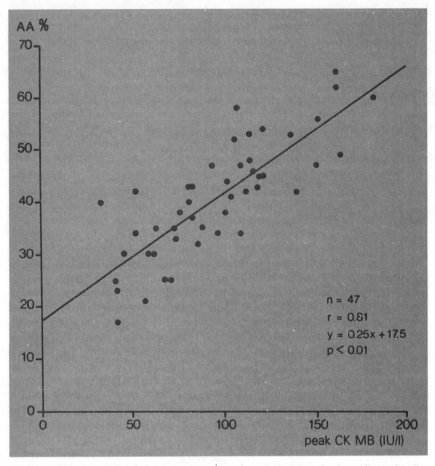

Fig. 2-6. Diagram of correlation between peak value of CK MB and echocardiographically estimated infarct size (AA). Reproduced with permission from Visser et al.[9]

ischemia, although these often underestimated the extent of myocardium at risk.

Characterization by positron emission tomography

Geltman and associates[12] from St. Louis, Missouri, assessed the sensitivity of positron emission tomography (PET) compared to thallium scintigraphy to characterize the value for delineating the extent, nature, and distribution of injury in patients with nontransmural and transmural AMI. Positron emission tomography was performed after the intravenous injection of carbon-11 palmitate in 10 normal subjects, 24 patients with initial nontransmural AMI defined by ECG, and 22 patients with transmural AMI. Depressed accumulation of carbon-11 palmitate was detected with sagittal, coronal, and transverse reconstructions and quantified based on 14 contiguous transaxial reconstructions. Defects with homogeneously intense depression of accumulation of tracer were detected in all 22 patients with transmural AMI. Abnormalities in the distribution of carbon-11 palmitate in the myocardium were detected in 23 patients with nontransmural AMI. Thallium-201 scinti-grams were abnormal in only 11 of 18 patients with nontransmural AMI. Estimated infarct size by tomography was greater among patients with transmural AMI compared with those with nontransmural AMI. Residual accumulation of carbon-11 palmitate within infarct regions was more intensely depressed among patients with transmural compared to nontrans-mural AMI. Thus, PET and metabolic imaging with carbon-11 palmitate is a sensitive means of detecting, quantifying, and characterizing nontransmural and transmural AMI.

DETERMINING INFARCTION SIZE

Effect of the haptoglobin phenotype

Haptoglobin (Hp) is a hemoglobin-binding serum α_2-globulin that is genetically determined by 2 autosomal codominant allelic genes, Hp 1 and Hp 2, which express themselves in 3 phenotypes designated as Hp 1-1, Hp 2-1, and Hp 2-2. Like other positive acute-phase reactants, serum Hp rises in infection and inflammation; the elevation is particularly marked after AMI and a relation between this increase and infarct size has been suggested by some authors. Chapelle and associates[13] from Liege, Belgium, and Bethesda, Maryland, investigated the relation between Hp phenotypes and serum levels of various biochemical markers after AMI in 496 patients. In 122 subjects selected on the basis of short delays until hospitalization, patients with Hp 2-2 had higher cumulated creatine kinase (CK) activity than did patients with Hp 1-1 or Hp 2-1 ($p < 0.05$), and higher myoglobin concentrations ($p < 0.02$) 12–28 hours after admission. Comparison of serum enzyme activities in the remaining 374 patients confirmed that Hp 2-2 patients had significantly higher total CK, CK isoenzyme MB fraction, aspartate aminotransferase and lactate dehydrogenase peak levels. Congestive heart failure also was more frequent in these patients ($p = 0.05$). These results suggest that Hp 2-2 patients have more severe AMI than Hp 1-1 and Hp 2-1 patients. No difference in the distribution of Hp phenotype was found between patients who had an AMI and healthy subjects, indicating that Hp 2-2 does not predispose to the occurrence of AMI.

By QRS scoring system

Although several clinical methods have been evaluated to estimate the size of an AMI, the 12-lead ECG remains the standard for recognizing the presence of and location of AMI. Wagner and associates (14) from Durham, North Carolina, and Downey, California, evaluated a simplified version of a previously developed QRS scoring system for estimating infarct size using observations of Q- and R-wave durations and R/Q and R/S amplitude duration ratios in the standard 12-lead ECG. Subjects with a minimal likelihood of having an AMI and minimal likelihood of having common non-AMI sources of QRS modification were studied to establish the specificity of each of the 37 criteria. Only 2 criteria required modification to achieve 95% specificity. These 37 criteria formed the basis of a 29-point QRS scoring system. A 98% specificity was achieved when a score >2 points was required to identify an AMI. Fifty patients were studied to determine the intra- and interobserver agreement with the scoring system and each criterion achieved at least 91% intra- and interobserver agreement. These investigators concluded that the standard ECG is inexpensive and can be obtained repetitively and noninvasively and that the QRS complex may be an important means of estimating the size, presence, and location of AMI.

Relation of size to performance at exercise soon after AMI

AMI size was estimated from serial serum creatine kinase (CK) MB measurements by Grande and Pedersen[15] from Copenhagen, Denmark, in 101 patients admitted <15 hours after their first AMI. A maximal symptom-limited exercise test comprising impedance measurements for the estimation of stroke volume at rest and at different levels of exercise was performed early after admission in 26 patients. A slight, but nonsignificant, negative correlation was observed between AMI size and physical capability as measured by the duration of work. The rise in systolic BP during exercise showed a significantly negative and the increase in heart rate a significantly positive correlation to AMI size. These findings suggest that the rise in BP, which is less in patients with larger AMI, is compensated for by an increase in heart rate, so that the maximum of cardiac performance and myocardial oxygen consumption is reached. The increase in cardiac stroke volume during exercise was negatively correlated with AMI size. Stroke volume only increased during lower levels of exercise. The increase in cardiac output at higher levels of exercise was achieved entirely by an increase in heart rate. The magnitude of ST-segment elevation during exercise showed a significantly positive correlation with AMI size, whereas the occurrence of arrhythmias during exercise was independent of it.

By single photon emission computed tomography and technetium-99m pyrophosphate

Holman and associates[16] from Boston, Massachusetts, determined the ability of single photon emission tomography with technetium-99m pyrophosphate to measure myocardial infarct size accurately in 20 patients with AMI. Imaging was performed with a standard gamma camera and with a multidetector transaxial emission computed tomographic body scanner 3 hours after the injection of technetium-99m stannous pyrophosphate. Pyrophosphate has been shown to localize in regions of AMI in previous studies performed by the nuclear cardiology group in Dallas, Texas. The location of increased technetium-99m pyrophosphate correlated well with the location of AMI by ECG. Measured from transaxial images, AMI size ranged from 14–117 g. There was a direct relation between AMI size and patient prognosis; in 13 patients with infarcts >40 g, 11 (85%) had complications, whereas only 2 of 7 patients with infarcts <40 g had complications during a follow-up period averaging 18 months (p < 0.05). These data suggest that pyrophosphate imaging may be used to detect and size AMI when single photon emission tomographic approaches are used. Furthermore, the data suggest that there is a relation between infarct size detected in this manner and subsequent complications of AMI.

LEFT VENTRICULAR FUNCTION AFTER AMI

Assessed by QRS scoring system

The value of the ECG in diagnosing and localizing an AMI is well established. Its use for measuring the size of an AMI or for assessing LV function has not been defined. Based on a QRS scoring system with computer simulation of the sequence of ventricular activation, Palmeri and associates[17] from Durham, North Carolina, evaluated the usefulness of the 12-lead ECG and a simplified version of this QRS scoring system for assessing LV function after AMI in 55 patients who did not have LV hypertrophy or conduction abnormalities. Serial 12-lead surface ECGs were scored according to a 29-point system based on the duration of Q and R waves and on the ratios of R-to-Q amplitude and R-to-S amplitude. The scores were proportional to the severity of wall-motion abnormalities, which were determined by radionuclide blood pool scanning and which correlated inversely with the radionuclide-determined LV EF. A score >3 was 93% sensitive and 88% specific for both severe regional dyssynergia and major depression of the global LV EF. The following equation was used to estimate the LV EF from the QRS score: LV EF (%) = 60− (3 × QRS score). After AMI, an ECG can provide important indirect quantitative information about LV function.

Assessed by 2-D echo

Gibson and associates[18] from Charlottesville, Virginia, studied 75 consecutive patients with AMI using 2-D echo 8 ± 3 hours after admission to determine if this procedure: 1) allows a recognition of regional LV asynergy, 2) identifies the relation of asynergy outside the ECG infarct zone to clinical events and coronary anatomic findings, and 3) identifies patients at high risk for cardiogenic shock before the onset of hemodynamic deterioration. The left ventricle was divided into 11 segments and individual segments were evaluated for systolic wall motion and thickening. Technically satisfactory 2-D echo studies were obtained in all 75 patients. Akinesia or dyskinesia was detected in at least 1 segment in all patients, including 15 (20%) who underwent imaging within 4 hours of the onset of symptoms and 19 (25%) with nontransmural AMI. Severe wall motion abnormalities outside the infarct zone were found in 47% of patients and correlated with a greater prevalence of death, cardiogenic shock, progression to a worse Killip class, reinfarction, and angina. Echo findings were related to coronary anatomic findings in 26 patients. In 66 patients initially assigned to Killip class I-II, the wall motion index was highly predictive with later hemodynamic deterioration. These data suggest that 2-D echo performed soon after admission to the coronary care unit provides useful and prognostic information concerning regional and global LV function during AMI.

Assessed by radionuclide ventriculography

Sanford and colleagues[19] from Dallas, Texas, evaluated 100 patients with AMI within 8 ± 3 hours (mean ± SD) after the onset of chest pain to evaluate the ability of admission radionuclide ventriculography to discriminate among various clinical subsets. Forty-one patients were in Killip functional class I, 52 in class II, and 7 in class III. The mean radionuclide LV EF was significantly lower in patients with higher Killip classification because of significant elevation of mean LV end-systolic volume rather than significantly altered end-diastolic volume. Killip classification frequently failed to correlate with EF in individual patients. Admission chest radiographic findings were categorized according to the presence of findings suggestive of impaired LV function. Mean LV EF was significantly lower in patients with abnormal than in patients with normal chest radiographs because of significant elevations in LV end-diastolic and end-systolic volumes. Chest radiographic findings frequently failed to correlate with the LV EF in individual patients. The most predictive variables in order of decreasing significance were anterior location of AMI, abnormal chest radiographic findings, rales to two-thirds of the posterior thorax, previous AMI, transmural AMI, and heart rate >100 beats/minute in the analysis of the ability of historical, physical, ECG, and chest radiographic findings to predict severity of ventricular dysfunction as established by radionuclide ventriculography. However, even these 6 optimal predictive variables explained only 42% of the observed variability in LV EF. Thus, the data obtained suggest that early radionuclide ventriculography adds significantly to the discriminant power of clinical and radiographic characterization of ventricular function in patients with AMI.

Nemerovski and colleagues[20] from Los Angeles, California, defined the sequential changes in LV and RV EF and regional LV wall motion following first transmural AMI. Fifty-four patients with either anterior (n, 28) or inferior (n, 26) AMI underwent RNA within 48 hours of onset of chest pain (study 1), between days 3 and 6 (study 2), and again between days 7 and 25 (study 3). Of the 28 patients with anterior AMI, 26 (93%) had initial LV EF <0.54, compared with 13 (50%) of 26 patients with inferior AMI. Eleven (42%) of 26 patients with inferior AMI had initial RV EF <0.39, compared with 8 (30%) of 27 patients with anterior AMI. There were no overall significant serial changes in mean LV EF or mean RV EF in patients with either anterior or inferior AMI. From study 1 to study 2, LV EF did not change in 24 patients (44%), improved in 13 (24%), and worsened in 17 (31%). From study 1 to study 3, LV EF remained unchanged in 15 patients (35%), improved in 17 (39%), and worsened in 11 (26%). From study 1 to study 2, RV EF did not change in 25 of 51 patients (49%), improved in 17 (31%), and worsened in 9 (17%). From study 1 to study 3, RV EF remained unchanged in 14 (38%), improved in 18 (48%), and worsened in 5 (14%). Changes in EF tended to occur early in the hospital course, with little subsequent changes. Serial changes in EF could not be predicted by clinical or demographic variables or by location of infarction. Significant changes in LV EF typically occurred without concurrent change in regional LV wall motion, suggesting alteration in ventricular loading rather than change in intrinsic myocardial performance. Initial depression of LV EF correlated with in-hospital mortality as well as with development of CHF and conduction defects. However, sequential changes in LV EF did not correlate with short-term prognosis. It is concluded that sequential changes in LV EF and RV EF occur frequently following AMI, appear to reflect ventricular loading conditions rather than intrinsic change in myocardial performance, and do not correlate well with short-term prognosis.

LV function was evaluated by Upton and colleagues[21] from Durham, North Carolina, by first-pass RNA in 42 patients at 3 and 8 weeks following AMI. The LV EF, diastolic volume, and wall motion were measured at rest and submaximal exercise at 3 weeks and at rest and submaximal and maximal exercise at 8 weeks. The mean EF, end-diastolic volume, and wall motion index did not change between 3 and 8 weeks in any group either at rest or during submaximal exercise. Ventricular function was decreased at rest in patients with previous anterior AMI, but not in patients with inferior and subendocardial AMI. During maximal exercise at 8 weeks, 9 patients (21%) had ST-segment depression, whereas 25 patients (60%) had a decrease in EF or a deterioration in wall motion. These abnormalities of ventricular function during exercise occurred equally among the infarct groups. RNA in patients with recent AMI demonstrated highly variable ventricular function at rest and/or during exercise in each infarct subgroup.

Buda and colleagues[22] from Toronto, Canada, examined regional myocardial perfusion after AMI in 26 patients with exercise ECG testing and thallium-201 perfusion imaging 3 weeks and 3 months after AMI. At 3 weeks, 9 (35%) of 26 patients had myocardial ischemia by exercise ECG testing, whereas 18 (69%) of 26 had ischemia by thallium-201 imaging. Three months after AMI, the extent of the thallium-201 perfusion defect was less and was associated with a loss of stress-induced ischemia in 8 patients. These data suggest that spontaneous improvement in thallium-201 myocardial perfusion imaging occurs in some patients after AMI.

Gibson and associates[23] from Charlottesville, Virginia, determined the clinical significance of increased lung thallium-201 uptake during submaximal exercise scintigraphy 2 weeks after AMI in 61 patients utilizing multigated blood pool imaging at rest and coronary angiography before hospital discharge. Thallium-201 uptake in the lung on the initial anterior projection image was graded qualitatively by comparing the intensity of thallium-201 activity in the lungs with that in the mediastinum. Thirty-nine patients had equal lung and mediastinal thallium-201 uptake and 22 had greater lung uptake. Patients with increased lung uptake had a greater prevalence of prior AMI (13% -vs- 36%, p < 0.05), less global cardiac reserve, more advanced Killip class in the coronary care unit (p < 0.05), a higher Norris coronary prognostic index, failure to achieve the target heart rate because of dyspnea, fatigue, or angina (36% -vs- 86%, p < 0.01), a greater incidence of exercise-induced ST-segment depression (18% -vs- 45%, p < 0.05), a greater number of anterior thallium-201 myocardial defects (p < 0.05); a lower LV EF at rest (50.4 ± 6.1% -vs- 39.6 ± 9.3%, p < 0.01), and a greater number of asynergic LV segments (p < 0.05). These data suggest that increased lung thallium-201 uptake during submaximal exercise scintigraphy in the early post-AMI period is frequent and is a marker of severe and functionally more important CAD associated with LV dysfunction.

When AMI occurs before age 36 years

Glover and associates[24] from San Diego, California, evaluated 120 consecutive patients ≤35 years of age who underwent coronary arteriography after AMI. Of the 120 patients, 92% were men. Four subgroups were identified: 1) 94 patients (78%) had significant CAD (>50% diameter narrowing of at least 1 major coronary artery); 2) 20 (17%) had normal coronary arteries; 3) 5 (4%) had major coronary arterial anomalies; and 4) 1 patient had coronary arteritis. Risk factors in these patients included cigarette smoking in 89%, positive family history of CAD in 48%, systemic hypertension in 21%, and a history of lipid abnormality in 20%. Risk factors were less frequent in the groups without coronary atherosclerosis. The data suggest that AMI before age 36 is a disease of men who smoke cigarettes and who often have a family history of premature CAD. Approximately 22% of such patients have normal coronary arteries, coronary arterial anomalies, or coronary vasculitis.

DETERMINING STATUS OF CORONARY ARTERIES AFTER AMI

Angiographic findings 1 month later

Since coronary arteriography is still not routinely performed after AMI, most retrospective studies deal with selective patients. Betriu and associates[25] from Barcelona, Spain, examined prospectively patients who survived AMI and related coronary anatomy to LV function. The study comprised 259 consecutive men ≤ age 60 years who underwent cardiac catherization 30 days after AMI. Coronary artery obtructive lesions >50% reduction in luminal diameter were found in 241 patients (93%), 118 (45%) of whom had total and 76 (29%) subtotal >90% stenotic occlusions of at least 1 coronary artery. Normal coronary arteries were seen in 8 patients and nonobstructive lesions in 10; 1-, 2-, and 3-vessel disease was present in 89, 86, and 66 patients, respectively. Patients with normal coronary arteries or nonobstructive lesions had higher EF than those with obstructive lesions in 1, 2, or 3 vessels. EF was lower and the percent of akinetic segments higher in patients with total or subtotal lesions and no collaterals. Adequate collaterals, seen in 29 patients, significantly improved regional wall motion and decreased the percent of akinetic segments. Thus, these investigators found that in a substantial percent of patients (32%), the infarcted area is spontaneously reperfused by collaterals or through the involved artery. Both of these mechanisms improve wall motion in the previously infarcted area.

Transaxial tomography and thallium -201

Ritchie and colleagues[26] from Seattle, Washington, determined whether transaxial tomographic imaging with thallium-201 is more sensitive in detecting significant CAD than standard planar imaging in 38 patients with remote AMI and in 15 normal individuals. Tomographic images were reconstructed from 64 views collected by a gamma camera rotated about the anterior circumference of the patient's chest. A series of consecutive transverse section images that encompassed the cardiac volume were reconstructed at a 6 mm plane spacing by filtered back projection. No correlation was made for attenuation. A set of transverse section images were reformatted by 3-D interpolation to obtain tomograms along the long and short axes of the myocardium. Tomographic and planar images were interpreted qualitatively. Tomography detected 33 (87%) of 38 patients with prior AMI, whereas planar imaging detected 24 (63%) of 38 (p = 0.01). The improvement in infarct detection occurred in the subset of patients with transmural inferior and subendocardial infarction, rather than in those with transmural anterior infarction. Peak increases in creatine kinase were smaller in patients detected only by tomography compared with those detected by both planar and tomographic images. Five patients (13%) with prior AMI were not detected by either approach. In 6 of the 9 patients detected by tomography alone, realignment of the image data along the short and long axes of the heart was essential for diagnosis. Fourteen of 15 patients without infarction were normal on both planar and tomographic images. A single normal patient had a defect detected by both techniques, thus providing a specificity of 93% for both techniques. Thus, transaxial tomography significantly improved the detection of thallium-201 myocardial perfusion defects in patients with prior AMI, especially in those with previous transmural inferior or nontransmural infarcts.

EARLY CHARACTERIZATION

Clinical signs -vs- hemodynamic state early after AMI

The initial pulmonary capillary wedge pressure, Killip-Scheidt classification, presence of third heart sound, and mortality were compared by Shell and colleagues[27] from Los Angeles, California, in 90 patients presenting with transmural AMI. Clinical and hemodynamic assessment was performed within 12 hours (time to clinical classification was 4.7 h and time to hemodynamic assessment was 5.8 h) of the AMI. A poor correlation was observed between early Killip-Scheidt clinical classification and early hemodynamic state when measured as percent correct classification (66%) or as a kappa probability statistic (36% for the total population, 9% for nonsurvivors). Increased initial LV filling pressure (>18 mmHg) was associated with increased mortality and early clinical classification was not. Addition of third heart sound information did not alter this observation. These data indicate that in the early hours of evolving AMI, the absence or presence of either pulmonary rales or third heart sounds is a poor guide to the hemodynamic state of the pulmonary circuit and to prognosis. Thus, during the initial stage of AMI, increases of LV filling pressure precede clinical manifestation of heart failure and this lag time, during which an increased LV filling pressure would not be detected by clinical examination, could delay the initiation of therapy designed to prevent pulmonary edema, resulting in increased morbidity and mortality.

Criteria for early discharge

As soon as AMI is suspected, hospitalization is advised to provide therapy for existing complications, to observe for subsequent complications, and to initiate a program of gradual rehabilitation that will minimize stress on the damaged myocardium. Some disagreement exists about the length of time patients in whom the diagnosis of AMI is established should be retained in the hospital. Severance and associates[28] from Durham, North Carolina, studied during an 18-month period all patients admitted to a community hospital coronary care unit to validate previously reported criteria for early hospital discharge after AMI (Fig. 2-7). Factors present during the first 4 hospital days, which predicted subsequent complications requiring urgent medical attention, were classified as either "urgent" or "prognostic" (Table 2-1, Fig. 2-8). Patients whose initial 4 days were marked by either no complications (81 patients) or prognostic complications (55 patients) were described. Only 1 of the 81 patients had a subsequent urgent complication and 4 of 55 patients had late urgent complications. Persistent sinus

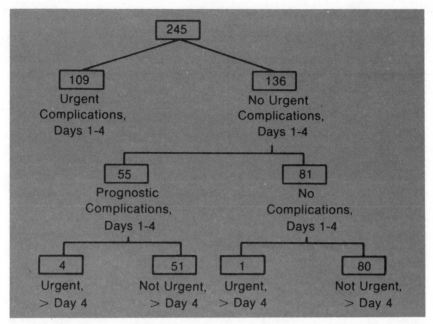

Fig. 2-7. Flow diagram of all patients with diagnosis of acute myocardial infarction; 109 patients with early urgent complications are not considered in this study. Reproduced with permission from Severance et al.[28]

tachycardia occurred during the first 4 days in 31 of the 55 patients. Early hospital discharge would be feasible in the group with neither urgent or prognostic complications. Further study of persistent sinus tachycardia, however, is required to improve its predictive ability.

TABLE 2-1. *Presence of early prognostic -vs- late urgent complications. Reproduced with permission from Severance et al.[28]*

COMPLICATION	# PATIENTS	# LATE URGENT COMPLICATIONS (%)
Neither prognostic complication	81	1 (1)
Persistent sinus tachycardia alone	31	2 (6)
Atrial arrhythmias alone	15	0
Both prognostic complications	9	2 (22)

Immediate detection of high risk patients by 2-D echo

Horowitz and Morganroth[29] from Philadelphia, Pennsylvania, studied 43 patients with AMI with serial 2-D echo to define a high risk subset for in-hospital cardiovascular complications, including pump failure, life-threatening arrhythmias, or death. A 2-D echo segment score was developed representing the extent of LV regional wall motion abnormality, which was correlated with peak total creatine kinase (CK) release. Patients with transmural AMI had a segment score of 7.2 ± 3.8, whereas those with nontransmural AMI had a segment score of 4.7 ± 3.4. Peak total serum CK enzyme level correlated statistically with segment score but with a low correlation coefficient. Thirteen (30%) of the 43 patients had an in-hospital complication and their segment score was 10.0 ± 3.4 compared to 4.6 ± 2.7 in those patients without a complication. A segment score ≥8 was found in 11 of 13 of those who had a cardiac complication and in only 5 (16%) of 30 patients without complication (sensitivity, 85%; specificity, 83%). Patient's initial clinical Killip classification was specific but very insensitive in predicting an early complicated course. Thus, 2-D echo study of LV regional wall motion can predict in the immediate post-AMI stage the in-hospital likelihood of such patients developing a cardiovascular complication during AMI.

Fig. 2-8. Incidences of both recurrent nonfatal infarcts and death are presented for period of hospitalization and for entire first 30 days and first year after acute infarct. Differences between groups with and without early prognostic complications are significant regarding death during all 3 time periods. Reproduced with permission from Severance et al.[28]

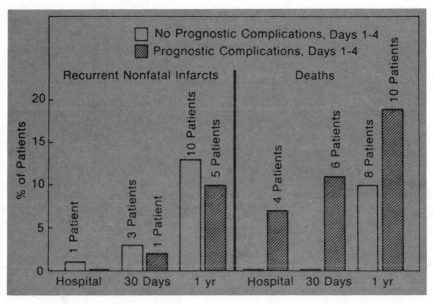

COMPLICATIONS

Angina pectoris

Koiwaya and colleagues[30] from Kitakyushu, Japan, repeated a recorded recurrent ST increase in leads where a new Q wave developed in 6 patients during the recovery phase of AMI. The ST increase was transient, occurred with or without chest pain, and returned to control levels. Enzymatic changes signifying recurrent myocardial necrosis were not observed after any episode. Coronary arteriography was performed in 1 patient and demonstrated a mild segmental stenosis in the artery perfusing the infarcted area. This artery became completely occluded after administration of ergonovine intravenously. The administration of calcium antagonists effectively reduced the frequency of postinfarction angina and ST increases in these patients. Therefore the clinical features suggested that post-AMI angina in these patients was produced by coronary artery spasm that could cause severe life-threatening arrhythmias.

Bundle branch block

Hauer and associates[31] from Utrecht, The Netherlands, followed 18 of 42 patients who survived >6 weeks after an anteroseptal AMI in which they acquired BBB. The remaining 24 patients had died primarily from cardiogenic shock or cardiac rupture. The remaining 18 (43%) patients were followed for an average of 13 months to assess long-term prognosis and evaluate whether the in-hospital monitoring period should be extended >6 weeks. Most of these 18 patients had bifasicular block develop during AMI, and in 3 it progressed to transient high degree AV block. Seven of the 18 survivors had potentially lethal complications during the first 6 weeks. Four of these 7 underwent aneurysmectomy between 10 and 20 weeks after AMI, and 1 died of a surgical complication. Major cardiac events occurred in 3 of 17 survivors. No patient died during the follow-up period. In 1 patient, complete AV block developed after aneurysm resection; this was the only patient treated with permanent pacing. Fifteen of the 17 patients were in functional class I or II. This study indicates that patients with BBB complicating anteroseptal AMI who survive the first 6 weeks after AMI have a relatively good prognosis during the first year. Prophylactic permanent pacing does not affect prognosis in these patients.

Dressler's syndrome

Lichstein and colleagues[32] from New York City examined the current incidence of postmyocardial infarction (Dressler's) syndrome. Of 282 patients with documented AMI evaluated during 1980, early postmyocardial infarction pericarditis was present in 18 (6.4%); 6 received corticosteroids and the remainder, salicylates or other anti-inflammatory agents. Information on the patient's status at 6 months was available in 229 patients who were discharged alive: 16 had died ≤6 months after discharge and 4 were lost to follow-up study. There were no documented cases of Dressler's syndrome. Thus, these data suggest that the frequency of Dressler's syndrome has decreased remarkably. This may be related to an increased use of medications to treat post-AMI pericarditis aggressively.

Left ventricular thrombus

Of 49 patients with acute MI studied by Friedman and associates[33] from Tuscon, Arizona, 11 had LV thrombus identified by 2-D echo. The patients with thrombi had a greater frequency of transmural AMI, high grade VPC on ambulatory monitoring, and lower radionuclide EF than the patients without thrombi. Most patients were receiving full dose heparin and/or warfarin from the time of admission to the hospital. Thus, the thrombi either developed before hospital admission or during anticoagulant therapy. Two patients with thrombi had peripheral emboli.

Right ventricular infarction

D'Arcy and Nanda[34] from Rochester, New York, performed real time 2-D echo studies in 10 patients with AMI who had clinical features suggestive of RV involvement. RV wall motion abnormalities were documented in all patients. In the 4-chamber views, 7 patients had akinesis of the entire RV diaphragmatic wall and 3 showed akinesis of segments of the diaphragmatic wall. Segmental dyskinetic areas that involved the RV free wall were found in 4 patients. One patient had a large RV aneurysm. Other echo features included RV enlargement in 8 cases, paradoxical ventricular septal motion in 7 cases, TR in 8 cases, gastric dilation in 4 cases, and localized pericardial effusion in 2. Supporting evidence for RV infarction was confirmed by radionuclide techniques in 7 patients, at surgery in 1 patient, and at autopsy in 2 patients.

Mitral regurgitation

Of 1,530 patients with CAD studied by Balu and associates[35] from Buffalo, New York, over a 5-year period, 104 had associated MR: 60 had no complications and 12 had CABG and both pre- and postoperative angiograms. In the 12, LV EF ranged from 34–75. The MR was considered severe (3+) in 3, moderate (2+) in 6, and trivial (1+) in 3. Following CABG, all except 2 patients were in class 1. (Preoperatively, all 12 were functionally class III or IV.) Of the 43 patients treated medically, 30 (72%) were in functional class III or IV. Angiographic results showed that 5 patients had 3+ MR, 14 had 2+ MR, and 24 had 1+ MR. The EF was <30 in 23 patients and ≥30 in 20 patients, and LV filling pressure was elevated. Twenty patients died, with a mean follow-up period of 11 months. Thus, their surgically treated patients with MR showed angiographic improvement in MR, improved functional status, and relief of symptoms compared with their medically treated patients.

Left ventricular aneurysm

Mason and associates[36] from Stanford, California, evaluated 127 patients treated by CABG and LV aneurysm resection for the control of refractory ventricular arrhythmias. Of the 127 patients, 82% survived surgery, and actuarial analysis of the results of conventional LV aneurysm resection in 32 patients with well-documented ventricular tachyarrhythmias demonstrated an arrhythmia recurrence rate of 50 ± 9% (SE) during the postoperative hospitalization. In contrast, after 10 months only 11 ± 9% of 18 patients who underwent myocardial resection guided by intraoperative electrical activation sequence mapping experienced arrhythmia recurrence. Thus, these data suggest that simple LV aneurysm resection is less effective in preventing venticular tachyarrhythmias than similar surgery guided by intraoperative mapping.

Faxon and colleagues[37] from Boston, Massachusetts, evaluated the prognosis of medically treated patients with angiographically defined LV aneurysm from data available from 1,136 patients with LV aneurysm. Prior AMI, reduced EF, absence of angina, and evidence of CHF were more commonly present in patients with LV aneurysm. Cumulative survival rates of medically treated patients at 1, 2, 3, and 4 years were 90, 84, 79, and 71%, respectively. A Cox analysis of survival indicated that age, residual LV function as assessed with angiography, LV end-diastolic pressure, functional impairment due to CHF, number of vessels narrowed, MR, and a third heart sound predicted outcome. When survival was stratified for similar degrees of LV dysfunction and functional impairment, there was no difference between the survival of patients with and without aneurysm. These data indicate that the survival of patients with LV aneurysm is better than previously recognized and that mortality is related primarily to age, LV function, and severity of CHF. The presence of a LV aneurysm does not independently alter survival.

To evaluate the complementary roles of 2-D echo and gated equilibrium RNA in the evaluation of patients with LV aneurysm, Sorensen and colleagues[38] from San Antonio, Texas, combined both techniques to evaluate wall motion, EF, and aneurysm detection in 35 patients undergoing cardiac catheterization who were suspected of having an LV aneurysm. Excellent agreement of qualitative wall motion analysis of 7 myocardial segments was obtained between RNA and contrast angiography (189 of 195 segments) and 2-D echo and contrast angiography (187 of 211 segments). The LV EF by both noninvasive techniques correlated with contrast angiography (RNA, r = 0.83; 2-D echo, r = 0.73). Both techniques tended to underestimate EF. Of 24 LV aneurysms identified by contrast angiography, RNA detected 21 and 2-D echo detected 22. RNA and 2-D echo combined detected all 24 contrast-defined aneurysms. Of 12 aneurysms confirmed at surgery, contrast angiography detected 11, 2-D echo detected 12, and RNA detected 10. Thus, RNA and 2-D echo are complementary noninvasive methods that accurately assess wall motion, estimate EF, and detect LV aneurysm.

PROGNOSTIC INDEXES

Mortality in survivors of AMI in the 1960s -vs- 1970s

Between 1968 and 1976, mortality from CAD declined in the USA by >20%. The exact reason for this decline is unclear. A conference sponsored by the National Heart, Lung, and Blood Institute (NHLBI) in 1978 concluded that both risk factor reduction and improved medical care contributed to the decline. The NHLBI is sponsoring pilot studies to evaluate the feasibility of determining if the incidence of nonfatal coronary events is changing. If the total incidence is decreasing, this fact implies that observed changes in coronary risk factors have been the cause of the decline in CAD mortality. If incidence is relatively unchanged, however, it suggests that survival secondary to improved health care is the more important cause for the decline. Two large studies of CAD patients served by the Health Insurance Plan of Greater New York (HIP) provided a unique opportunity to examine whether long-term prognosis of men who had survived AMI had improved during the decade from the mid-1960s to the mid-1970s. Weinblatt and associates[39] from New York City identified diagnostically comparable groups of patients from the 2 studies and performed new analyses to compare the risk of death during the 4.5 years after standard baseline examinations in the 2 different groups. They sought to identify any prognostic advantage for the patients studied in the 1970s over those studied in the 1960s. Although they compared 2 separate cohorts of patients with different characteristics, modern statistical methods were used in an attempt to correct for the measured discrepancies between the 2 populations. Even after statistical correction, there was no significant increase of survival in the latter cohort. Thus, this group concluded that improvements in long-term coronary care are unlikely to be major factors in explaining the decline in CAD mortality, although short-term benefits from acute care associated with the introduction of coronary care units could not be discounted.

Effect of AMI location

Thanavaro and associates[40] from St Louis, Missouri, studied the in-hospital prognosis of 1,105 patients who had their first transmural AMI; 611 patients had anterior AMI and 494 had inferior AMI. Patients with inferior AMI had a significantly lower in-hospital mortality rate (9% -vs- 16%) and significantly lower prevalences of CHF (39% -vs- 48%), cardiogenic shock (9% -vs- 13%), and conduction defects (left anterior hemiblock, right BBB, and intraventricular conduction defect). The patients with anterior AMI had significantly higher peak enzyme levels, and a greater percent of them (40% -vs- 26%) had SGOT values >240 IU/liter, whereas more patients with inferior AMI had SGOT values <120 IU/liter. When the parallel subgroups were compared according to the peak SGOT levels, the differences in the mortality and morbidity between the 2 infarct locations diminished. However, patients with anterior AMI still had a less favorable outcome. Logistic regression analysis demonstrated that both the peak enzyme level and the infarct location had an independent influence on the in-hospital prognosis of patients with first transmural AMI.

Two- -vs- 3-week hospitalization after AMI

Baughman and associates[41] from Boston, Massachusetts, obtained long-term follow-up in 138 patients who participated in a prospective, randomized study comparing 2 with 3 weeks of hospitalization following uncomplicated AMI. Follow-up information was available on 123 patients. The mean followup was 35 months for those patients who died and 99 months for those who survived. No differences were found between the 2 groups with respect to survival, cardiac-related deaths, frequency or severity of angina pectoris, subsequent AMI, incidence of CHF, number with LV aneurysms, or subsequent medical therapy. A significantly greater number of survivors in both groups stopped smoking and had a normal initial heart size than those who died. This long-term follow-up study further supports the conclusions of earlier short-term studies that 2 weeks of hospitalization is safe in patients with uncomplicated AMI.

Implications of diagnostic Q waves

Wasserman and colleagues[42] from Washington, DC, Richmond, Virginia, and Jackson, Mississippi, examined long-term prognostic implications of ECG location of AMI and the subsequent retention or disappearance of diagnostic Q waves in patients enrolled in the Aspirin AMI Study. In the 4,524 participants, aged 30–69 years, an AMI had occurred 8 weeks to 60 months before randomization to aspirin and placebo groups. The subjects were followed for ≥3 years (average, 38 months). Using the Minnesota Code, AMI was classified according to 3 ECG locations: lateral, inferior, and anterior, with further subdivision into major, moderate, and minor criteria based on Q-wave duration and Q/R ratios. Total mortality was not significantly different among patients with single infarct sites: lateral 12%, inferior 8%, and anterior 9%. Patients with multiple ECG infarct locations had a significantly higher mortality of 15%. Patients with Minnesota Code major criteria of AMI also had a significantly higher mortality (11%) than those with moderate (7%) or minor (7%) criteria. Loss of a previously documented diagnostic Q wave occurred in 14%. Mortality among patients who lost Q wave (7%) was not significantly different from that among those with persistent Q waves in a single infarct location (9%). No long-term prognostic significance could be attributed to the site of AMI or loss of Q wave on the resting ECG. Major Q-wave criteria and extent of AMI based on multiple coded sites were associated with a higher 3-year mortality.

Implications of ST-segment depression in posterior (inferior) AMI

Gelman and Saltups[43] from Melbourne, Australia, compared clinical features in hospital and posthospital course in patients with posterior (inferior) AMI by assessing prospectively precordial ST segment depression. They studied 110 consecutive patients without previous AMI and allocated them to 3 ECG groups. Group 1 consisted of 35 patients with posterior or posterolateral AMI without precordial ST depression. Group 2 consisted of 59 patients with ≥1 mm precordial ST depression subdivided into 36 patients with transient ST depression (2t) and 23 patients with ST depression persisting for ≥48 hours after admission ECG (2p). Group 3 had 16 patients with definite inferoposterior or inferoposterolateral AMI. Patients in group 2 were older than those in group 1, had higher peak creatine kinase (CK) levels, and had AF and AV block requiring treatment more frequently. These clinical differences were largely contributed by subgroup 2p. Compared with group 1, subgroup 2p contained relatively more women and there were more instances of VF and LV failure. The hospital stay was longer in this subgroup. Compared with group 3, patients in group 2p were older, had a greater proportion of women, and were more commonly previously hypertensive. Patients in subgroup 2t had higher CK levels and more frequent AV block than those in group 1. Differences in hospital mortality and in other clinical features were not significant among the groups. During follow-up of 12–32 months (mean, 17), LV failure was more common in subgroup 2p compared with groups 1 and 2t, and recurrent AMI occurred more often in subgroup 2p compared with group 1. No late deaths occurred in groups 1 and 3, but 3 (5%) patients in group 2 died. Thus, persistent precordial ST depression in patients with inferior AMI is a reliable marker of an adverse hospital and posthospital course.

Implication of QT > QS$_2$ syndrome

Boudoulas and colleagues[44] from Detroit, Michigan, determined whether the duration of electrical systole (QT) is more closely linked physiologically to the duration of electromechanical systole (QS$_2$) than to the heart rate and therefore might provide a more powerful prognostic indicator of sudden death than the relation of QT to heart rate. Of 100 stable patients studied 14 months after AMI and followed an average of 43 months, 20 had prolongation of their QT relative to QS$_2$ (QT > QS$_2$) and 13 patients had long QT intervals corrected for heart rate (QTc). Twenty died, 16 suddenly. Cumulative 5-year survival rate was 35% in patients with QT > QS$_2$ and 91% in patients with QT < QS$_2$ ($p < 0.001$). No significant difference in survival was observed in patients with long QTc compared with patients with a normal QTc. These data suggest that patients with CAD and a long QT interval (QT > QS$_2$) are at risk for sudden death.

Right atrial pacing early

Since patients recovering from AMI remain at risk for re-AMI and death during the first year after AMI, early identification of patients at risk could lead to a more intensive medical and surgical therapy. Tzivoni and colleagues[45] from Jerusalem, Israel, assessed the presence of residual myocardial ischemia and its prognostic significance soon after AMI with right atrial pacing (RAP) in 85 consecutive patients 1 day before hospital discharge. No patient was excluded from the study because of clinical condition. Their ages were 29–85 years (mean, 61). The study was performed at the bedside an average of 14 days after the AMI and no complications were noted during or after the test. The RAP was considered positive if ≥1 mm horizontal ST decrease developed. The mean maximal pacing rate achieved was 147 beats/minute. There were 46 patients (54%) with negative and 39 (46%) with positive RAP. In 30 patients with anterior AMI, 17% had RAP, which compared with 61% of the 23 patients with inferior AMI and 63% of the 32 patients with subendocardial AMI. Patients were followed for an average of 6 months. Among the 46 patients with negative pacing studies, there was 1 sudden death. No re-AMI occurred and 8 patients required hospitalization and 5 patients had chest pain. Among the 39 patients with a positive pacing study, 1 died suddenly and 2 after re-AMI. Four additional patients sustained reinfarction and survived. There were 20 hospitalizations in the group with positive RAP and 18 patients had chest pain. Treadmill exercise test was performed 6 months after AMI in 37 patients. Of the 21 patients with a negative RAP, 17 had a negative GETT; whereas 13 of the 16 patients with a positive RAP had a positive GETT 6 months later. Thus, RAP can be performed safely in patients with AMI. Of all postinfarction patients, 46% had residual areas of stress-induced myocardial ischemia. Thus, RAP was sensitive in predicting subsequent reinfarction, cardiac death, cardiac hospitalization, angina pectoris, and the response to GETT 6 months after AMI.

Prediction of sudden death by electrophysiologic studies

Hamer and associates[46] from Melbourne, Australia, studied 70 patients surviving an AMI complicated by CHF or arrhythmias or both 7–20 days after the AMI. The intent of this study was to develop the ability to predict sudden death in such high risk patients after AMI. Twenty-four hour ECG ambulatory monitoring and intracardiac electrophysiologic studies were performed in each patient. Electrophysiologic studies included an introduction of single RV stimuli during sinus rhythm, atrial pacing, or ventricular pacing and double RV premature stimuli in 33 patients and pacing at a second RV site in 50 patients. A repetitive ventricular response was defined as ≥2 spontaneous ventricular depolarizations in response to the premature stimulus with His bundle reentry and aberrant conduction of supraventricular impulses excluded by His bundle recording. Repetitive responses were found in 20 patients and 12 patients had responses that were either sustained VT or self-terminating VT of >5 complexes in duration. In 5 of 12 patients with sustained or self-terminating responses of >5 complexes, death occurred during a 12-month follow-up period; in 4 of these, death occurred suddenly and these responses were significantly associated with late sudden death because only 1 of 25 patients with responses of <5 complexes or no response to maximal provocation died suddenly. Therefore the data suggest that induced responses of >5 complexes in duration may be an important indicator of the risk of sudden death after AMI.

Relation of extension to survival

Myocardial infarct extension based either on specific enzyme changes or ECG changes had been reported to range from 9%–86%. Defined as reelevation or reappearance of creatine phosphokinase MB (CK-MB) 48 hours after the onset of symptoms, AMI extension was evaluated by Baker and associates[47] from Durham, North Carolina, prospectively in 56 consecutive patients with AMI. AMI extension occurred in 8 patients (14%). The sensitivity, specificity, and predictive accuracy in the diagnosis of AMI extension were 63, 85, 42%, respectively, for recurrent chest pain requiring morphine; 50, 65, and 19% for recurrent ST increase on routine 12-lead ECG; and 88, 63, and 28% for reelevation of total CK. Of the 8 episodes of extension, 3 were clinically silent. Four of 8 patients (50%) with extension expired, compared with 1 of 46 patients without extension. CK-MB persisted ≥72 hours in 16 patients and identified 7 of 8 who subsequently had AMI extension. Thus, myocardial infarct extension is an infrequent complication of AMI and is associated with a very high mortality rate. Persistence of CK-MB ≥72 hours identifies a subgroup of patients at high risk for subsequent AMI extension and death.

Determinants of prognosis

Sanz and associates[48] from Barcelona, Spain, studied 259 consecutive men (≤60 years of age) who survived AMI to identify predictors of late mortality. All patients underwent cardiac catheterization 1 month after onset of the AMI and were then followed for mean of 34 months. Nineteen patients (7%) died during the observation period. Of 79 baseline descriptors, 17 proved to be univariate predictors of survival. Cox regression analysis demonstrated that the EF ($p < 0.001$), the number of diseased vessels ($p < 0.005$), and the occurrence of CHF in the coronary unit ($p < 0.01$) were the only independent predictors of survival (Fig. 2-9). Risk stratification showed that the probability of survival at 4 years was highest in patients with normal EF (96–100%, depending on the number of diseased vessels) and lowest in those with EF <20% (30–75%). The prognosis in patients with EF from 21% to 49% was significantly worse (78%) than in those with normal EF only in the group with 3-vessel involvement ($p < 0.01$). Since most survivors of AMI who are likely to have their lives prolonged by CABG are in this group, it is reasonable to limit routine coronary angiography to the 56% of survivors who have EF between 21 and 49%.

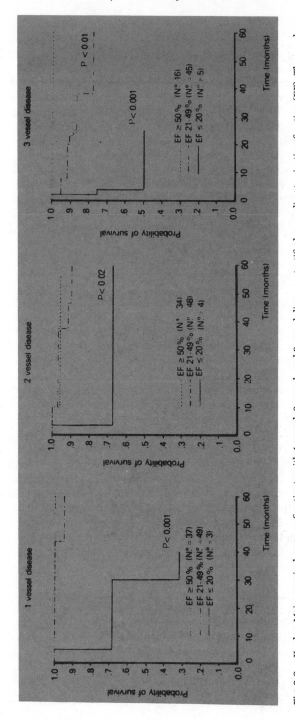

Fig. 2-9. Kaplan-Meier survival curves of patients with 1-vessel, 2-vessel, and 3-vessel disease, stratified according to ejection fraction (EF). The p values represent differences (log-rank test) between the group with ejection fraction of 50% and the other 2 groups. Reproduced with permission from Sanz et al.[48]

Implications of inotropic contractile reserve

Nesto and associates[49] from Boston, Massachusetts, related inotropic contractile reserve to 5-year prognosis in 54 patients receiving postextrasystolic potentiation or epinephrine infusion between 1971 and 1974. Recent LV function in surviving patients was assessed with radionuclide ventriculograms. Five-year survival was greater in patients with an initial change in EF >0.1 in both surgically treated (16 of 20 -vs- 5 of 15, p < 0.01), and medically treated groups (6 of 8 -vs- 1 of 11, p < 0.01). Among surviving patients in the surgical group, the most recent EF was significantly greater in patients demonstrating inotropic contractile reserve at their 1971–1974 contrast ventriculogram. These data support the notion that coronary revascularization enhances function of ischemic but viable myocardium and that the degree of postextrasystolic potentiation may be used to predict prognosis in patients with CAD undergoing either surgical or medical therapy.

Value of acute scintigraphic measurement of AMI size

Infarct, perfusion, and blood pool scintigraphy were performed by Perez-Gonzalez and colleagues[50] from San Francisco, California, in 62 patients during hospitalization for AMI. The largest measured infarct or perfusion image defect and LV EF were related to the late prognosis that was determined a mean of 16 months after the event. Breakpoint values for all scintigraphic variables could separate those who were asymptomatic on follow-up from those who died. The best indicators for selection of survivors and nonsurvivors were a scintigraphic infarct size ≥ 25 cm^2 and a perfusion abnormality $\geq 35\%$ of the projected LV area. Among patients with perfusion abnormalities above this limit, 61% died; 93% of those with small perfusion abnormalities survived. Scintigraphic measurements of relative myocardial perfusion and function best separate the patients asymptomatic on follow-up from those who develop heart failure and also best identify those with an unfavorable evolution who developed heart failure or died. Thus, early scintigraphic parameters appeared more accurate than other clinical laboratory indicators for determining late prognosis and could be important in planning treatment after AMI.

Implications of recurrent AMI

Marmor and associates[51] from St. Louis, Missouri, assessed the accuracy of multiple regression analysis as a prospective predictor of early recurrent AMI. From a new population of 150 patients admitted consecutively with AMI, regression coefficients derived by multiple logistic analysis were applied to the test set population and the presence or absence of recurrent AMI predicted correctly for 80% of the patients. Patients were followed for 9 months, ranging from 3–18 months and life table analysis was performed to assess the impact of recurrent AMI on short- and long-term survival. During the first 21 days after AMI, mortality was 23% for patients with transmural and 10% for nontransmural AMI. Among patients with nontransmural AMI, hospital mortality was 23% among those with early recurrent AMI and 8% for those without recurrence. At the conclusion of the follow-up, mortality was 34% among patients with nontransmural AMI recurrence, compared with 23% among patients with transmural AMI and no recurrence. Thus, this study demonstrates that early recurrent AMI has a distinct deleterious effect on survival and a subset of patients more likely to experience recurrent AMI can be prospectively identified.

Resting ECG -vs- predischarge exercise testing

Nikolic and associates[52] from Worcester, Massachusetts, investigated 50 consecutive patients aged 33–82 years (mean, 62) who underwent modified exercise ECG 8–18 days (mean, 13) after AMI. All were fit for discharge from the hospital on the day of testing. The outcome of the modified predischarge exercise test was predicted by 3 independent observers on the basis of ST-segment displacement in the resting pretest 12-lead ECG. The mean predictive accuracy for the 3 observers was 82% for a positive test defined as additional ST-segment depression or elevation ≥0.1 mV and rose to 94% for a positive test defined as additional ST-segment depression ≥0.1 mV alone. Thus, for most patients, the test result was already apparent in the resting 12-lead ECG. Only 3 of the 50 patients had chest pains associated with ST-segment depression during the exercise test. The others had negative, incomplete, or electrically positive tests. The authors believe that predischarge modified stress testing after AMI is unnecessary.

Early exercise testing

Miller and Borer[53] from New York City reviewed the potential risks and benefits of submaximal exercise testing in the early weeks after AMI. The potential benefits of such testing include: 1) promotion of patient self-confidence; 2) determination of posthospital exercise prescription; 3) detection of arrhythmias; and 4) determination of posthospital prognosis. However, the practical value of the apparent psychologic benefits and of the exercise prescription information in a patient not participating in formal exercise rehabilitation therapy is unclear. Detection of potentially important arrhythmias appears to be more adequately effected with 24-hour ambulatory ECG and detection of such arrhythmias appears to add relatively little prognostic information to that available from exercise ECG ST analysis or from resting radionuclide EF. Nonetheless, exercise-induced ST-segment depression can prove potentially useful prognostic information regarding morbid or fatal events during the year after AMI. Moreover, recent data suggest that exercise-induced angina and/or ST segment depression can aid importantly in the noninvasive determination of the anatomic extent of CAD. The additional benefit of RNA determination of LV function during exercise and of thallium-201 scintigraphic determination of myocardial perfusion during stress remain to be defined, although both approaches appear to provide important prognostic information. However, despite the potential benefits of exercise testing, in the absence of clinical trials of available therapy in the "high risk" patients defined by exercise testing, there remains an ill-defined relation between the information available from exercise testing and the results of management decisions based on this information.

Effects of exercise training on ventricular function

Cobb and associates[54] from Durham, North Carolina, and Ontario, Canada, evaluated the effects of 6 months of exercise training (bicycle ergometry, walking, and jogging) on exercise performance and ventricular function in patients with recent AMI. Fifteen patients were selected for study on the basis of AMI 1.5–6 months before study and age <65 years. The patients were evaluated by maximal treadmill exercise testing and RNA at rest and exercise before and after training. Before exercise training, maximal treadmill exercise time ranged from 1.5–11 minutes, EF at rest from 18%–67% and end-diastolic volume (EDV) from 108–208 ml. The mean EF 48% at rest did not change at maximal exercise. All 11 patients who completed the exercise training program achieved a significant training effect as defined by a reduction in heart rate at 50% maximal pretraining effect or an increase in maximal treadmill time. The mean EF and EDV and wall motion abnormalities at rest and at comparable pretraining exercise work loads and heart rates were not significantly different after training. Despite a wide range of rest and exercise ventricular function, patients with recent uncomplicated MI significantly increased their exercise performance. Because rest and exercise ventricular function were comparable before and after training, the improvement in exercise performance probably resulted from training effects on the peripheral vasculature.

Value of exercise testing, coronary angiography, and left ventriculography 6–8 weeks after myocardial infarction

deFeyter and associates[55] from Amsterdam, The Netherlands, examined the data on a consecutive series of 179 survivors of AMI who had symptom-limited treadmill exercise testing, coronary angiography, and left ventriculography within 6–8 weeks postinfarction. No patient in the series died and the prevalence of multivessel disease was higher in the symptomatic survivors. The prevalence of multivessel disease in inferior AMI was 63% and in anterior AMI, 42%. The LV impairment was more severe in anterior and preexisting AMI then in inferior and nontransmural AMI. During the mean follow-up period of 28 months, 11 cardiac deaths and 12 reinfarctions occurred. Total mortality was 22% in patients with EF <30% or 3-vessel disease and 1% in patients with an EF >30% and 1- or 2-vessel disease. A group at high risk of mortality is thus identified by angiography. The total reinfarction rate in this series was 9% in patients with an exercise tolerance of <10 minutes; 2% in patients with an exercise tolerance >10 minutes. The 58 patients who had an exercise tolerance of ≥10 minutes had very low risk for cardiac death or reinfarction. Thus, this investigation provides useful clinical information on mortality and recurrent coronary events based on early exercise testing, coronary angiography, and ventriculography following AMI.

TREATMENT

Intracoronary streptokinase

In an editorial, Sobel and Bergmann[56] from St. Louis, Missouri, discussed the basis of recent enthusiasm for intracoronary thrombolysis, unresolved issues, assessment of the success of intracoronary thrombolysis, and its long-term effects. Of these 4, of course, the most important is the long-term effects, and they have not been defined. Residual stenosis is unfortunately common. Recurrent thrombosis may ensue from a nidus of residual clot or atheroma. A CABG may be required even after successful intracoronary thrombolysis. Long-term effects on myocardium cannot be evaluated exclusively with indirect criteria. Unambiguous interpretation requires definitive characterization of effects of thrombolysis on the end points themselves. Long-term effects of intracoronary thrombolysis on symptoms of CAD, the incidence of AMI, quality of life, the risk of lethal arrhythmia, and overall survival remain speculative. Several issues require resolution, including 1) patient selection; 2) definition of intervals during which reperfusion may salvage myocardium (and those after which it may exacerbate injury); 3) identification of end points indicative of genuine benefits (and those indicative of potentially deleterious consequences); 4) elucidation of the persistence of restored angiographic patency; 5) selection of ancillary agents or regimens that may potentiate or sustain beneficial effects (e.g., anticoagulants or calcium antagonists). Clarification of these issues requires studies of at least 2 types: 1) those in which the response to thrombolysis of multiple end points can be rigorously compared so that appropriate end points for longitudinal studies can be identified; and 2) broadly based, longitudinal, rigorously controlled clinical trials employing the most suitable end points identified. Only when end points can be interpreted unambiguously and when criteria for patient selection and identification of intervals during which benefit may be achieved are available can we expect long-term clinical trials to elucidate definitively the efficacy of this intervention with so much promise alloyed with potential risk.

Rentrop and associates[57] from Gottingen, West Germany, assessed LV function sequentially with biplane cineventriculography in 18 patients with AMI in whom nonsurgical reperfusion was achieved with 8 ± 7 hours (mean ± SD) after the onset of chest pain utilizing intracoronary streptokinase. The

LV EF increased from 51 ± 10% before reperfusion to 56 ± 9% immediately after completion of streptokinase infusion (n, 13, p < 0.01). The length of the akinetic myocardial segment decreased from 10 ± 6–7 ± 5 cm (p < 0.025). These LV functional data were compared with data obtained in 2 medically treated groups that were matched retrospectively. Control group 1 included 9 patients with permanent obstruction of the infarcted vessel and control group 2, nine patients with spontaneous recanalization of the initially obstructed vessel. During AMI, EF and akinetic segment length were comparable in the 3 groups, but in the chronic stage EF was higher in the group receiving streptokinase than in control group 1 and the akinetic segment was shorter in length in the same group. Preservation of R waves was more extensive in the group receiving streptokinase. These data are compatible with the hypothesis that jeopardized myocardium is preserved by nonsurgical reperfusion during AMI.

Schwarz and associates[58] from Heidelberg, West Germany, evaluated the effects of early reperfusion after intracoronary infusion of streptokinase in patients with AMI. Serial analysis of serum creatine kinase (CK) activity, thallium-201 scintigraphy, and LV and coronary angiography were utilized in these assessments. Serial serum CK activity was measured at hourly intervals. Thallium-201 tomographic scintigrams were obtained before and 24 hours after recanalization. The size of the thallium-201 perfusion defect was measured from 8 scintigraphic LV cross sections. Regional EF was determined from the LV angiogram before and 4 weeks after recanalization. Three groups of patients were studied: group A, 10 patients with successful recanalization and a peak serum CK of <1,000 U/liter; group B, 9 patients with successful recanalization and a peak serum CK activity of >1,000 U/liter; and group C, 8 patients with unsuccessful recanalization. Patients in group A showed an increase in CK activity, a reduction in the thallium-201 perfusion defect, and an augmentation of regional EF with streptokinase therapy. Patients in group B had an increase in serum CK activity, only a moderate reduction in the thallium perfusion defect, and no change in regional EF. Patients in group C had an increase in serum CK activity, no change in thallium perfusion defect, and no change in regional EF. Patients in group A had a shorter duration of ischemia, (3.9 -vs- 4.8 hours), more frequently adequate collateral supply to the infarcting area before recanalization, and a smaller area supplied by the occluded vessel. Thus, conditions for tolerating myocardial ischemia did appear to be better in group A than in group B patients. These data show that early reperfusion may have a beneficial effect on the extent of myocardial necrosis as estimated from serum enzyme determinations, thallium-201 scintigraphy, and contrast ventriculography. The beneficial effect appears to depend upon the duration of myocardial ischemia and possibly on the blood flow to the ischemic area by collateral vessels.

Coronary arteriography and intracoronary streptokinase infusion were performed on 89 patients with evolving AMI by Smalling and colleagues[59] from Houston, Texas. Ventricular function was followed in these patients during hospitalization by gated RNA. In 35 patients, thallium imaging was performed on admission and 4 hours after reperfusion. An additional 30 patients with AMI who either met exclusion criteria for the streptokinase protocol or refused study served as controls. In patients admitted 0–6, 6–12, or 12–18 hours after onset of pain, there was no difference in change in LV EF from admission to discharge, in percent of patients with total occlusion demonstrating reperfusion, or in percent of patients demonstrating a significant increase in LV EF. The average increase in LV EF from admission to discharge in patients reperfused was 8% (40–48%). No change in LV EF was demonstrated in the controls or in patients in whom coronary reperfusion was unsuccessful. Reperfusion produced an increase in thallium uptake in the infarct-related myocardium that was accompanied by an improvement in regional function. Failure of reperfusion produced no change in either thallium uptake or regional function.

Efficacy and safety data from 209 USA cases in the Hoechst-Roussel intracoronary streptokinase registry were analyzed by Weinstein[60] from Sommerville, New Jersey. Successful recanalization was achieved in 76% of AMI-related occluded coronary arteries. Post-AMI complications (malignant arrhythmias, heart block, and pump failure) were substantially less frequent after successful recanalization compared with the recanalization failures. Cardiac in-hospital mortality was 2.5% in the recanalized group and 18% in the group in which recanalization failed. Severe hemorrhagic complications occurred in patients who were heparinized. These data suggest that myocardial reperfusion following streptokinase-coronary recanalization during evolving AMI may salvage myocardium. Except for excessive bleeding associated generally with heparinization, side effects and adverse reactions were readily controlled.

Thirty-four patients with AMI (mean age, 55 years) who received intracoronary streptokinase for coronary thrombosis were followed by Lee and associates[61] from Davis, California, up to 25 months (mean, 9.4) after the procedure of percutaneous transluminal coronary recanalization. Twelve patients had undergone CABG, 1 had PTCA, and 21 received medical therapy only. Among patients having CABG and PTCA, nearly 70% no longer had chest pain or reinfarction, and 62% were in New York Heart Association functional class I status; none died, 1 had another AMI but he had graft closure. In contrast, 43% of medically treated patients had chest pain or another AMI or had died on follow-up; only 32% of survivors were in class I functional status. Further, 71% of medically treated patients who were receiving warfarin had no chest pain and no reinfarction, whereas most (56%) patients who did not receive either warfarin or antiplatelet agents either had chest pain or reinfarction or died. The importance of CABG/PTCA and anticoagulant therapy is stressed to prevent recurrent ischemia, reinfarction, and reocclusion following successful reperfusion by means of percutaneous transluminal coronary recanalization in AMI.

Although intracoronary thrombolysis is potentially an exciting therapy for reducing the extent of AMI by lysing coronary clot, certain difficulties limit its widespread application. Since intravenous streptokinase could be widely applied if effective, Spann and colleagues[62] from Philadelphia and

Lancaster, Pennsylvania, as well as European investigators, evaluated whether high dose, brief duration intravenous streptokinase infusion given early in AMI would lyse coronary clots without bleeding. To date, these investigators treated 13 patients within 6 hours of onset of symptoms and with ECG and angiographic evidence of typical AMI caused by coronary clot. Clot lysis and angiographically proved coronary reperfusion were achieved in 6 patients within 1 hour of starting a systemic intravenous infusion of 850,000 IU of streptokinase. Schroeder and associates (Unstable Angina Pectoris, Georg Thieme-Verlag, 1981, p 167) from Berlin, West Germany, achieved angiographically proved coronary reperfusion in 11 of 21 patients with AMI following a 30-minute intravenous streptokinase infusion of 500,000 IU. Neuhaus and colleagues (Z Kardiol 70:791, 1981) from Gottingen, West Germany, achieved angiographically proved coronary reperfusion in 24 of 39 similar patients within 48 minutes by intravenous infusion of 1,700,000 IU of streptokinase. In these 3 studies, no serious bleeding occurred; LV function was improved in patients who achieved coronary reperfusion. Thus, rapid intracoronary clot lysis and coronary reperfusion can be achieved early in AMI by brief duration systemic intravenous infusion of high dose streptokinase without a high frequency of serious bleeding.

Schuler and colleagues[63] from Heidelberg, West Germany, studied 21 patients with AMI admitted to the hospital within 4 hours after onset of symptoms and obtained thallium scintigraphy before, 1 hour, and 24 hours after intracoronary fibrinolysis using streptokinase. The size of the thallium perfusion defect was assessed from myocardial cross-sections reconstructed from the original 7 pinhole data and expressed as a fraction of LV circumference. Recanalization was achieved in 16 patients within 4 hours after onset of symptoms. In these patients, the size of the perfusion defect had decreased from 36%–19% at 24 hours. No significant change was detected by redistribution at 1 hour after the intervention. In 5 patients, intracoronary fibrinolysis was unsuccessful and the vessels remained occluded. The thallium perfusion defect affected 40% of the LV circumference before the intervention; it remained virtually unchanged at 1 hour and at 24 hours after fibrinolysis. The perfusion defect was most reduced in patients with extensive collaterals supplying the ischemic area or a subtotal occlusion of the affected coronary artery. Thus, these investigators conclude that successful intracoronary fibrinolysis may reduce the size of the thallium perfusion defect in many patients with AMI. An important factor in the final result may be the presence of residual coronary flow supplied by extensive collaterals or by subtotal occlusion of the affected coronary artery when reperfusion is achieved within 4 hours after the onset of symptoms.

Schwarz and associates[64] from Heidelberg, West Germany, studied 39 patients treated with intracoronary infusion of streptokinase to define the effect of duration of myocardial ischemia on the late results after successful thrombolytic therapy in patients with transmural AMI. Patients with successful recanalization of the infarct-related vessel with a time lag between symptoms and reperfusion of <4 hours were included in 1 group (n, 15) and patients with successful recanalization with a time lag of >4 hours (n, 17) in another group. Coronary anatomy, LV volumes, LV EF and regional LV EF in the infarct area were determined before and 4 weeks after thrombolytic therapy with cineangiography. Before intervention, the groups were comparable with respect to age, Killip class, localization of AMI, frequency of previous AMI, extent of CAD, LV volume, LV EF, regional LV EF in the infarct area, and serum creatine kinase activity. Four weeks after thrombolytic therapy, patients in the group with symptoms for <4 hours before successful reperfusion had a higher LV EF and regional LV EF in the infarct area than patients with symptoms of >4 hours. Peak serum creatine kinase activity measured during the evaluation was lower in patients with a shorter duration of symptoms before thrombolytic therapy (764 U/liter) than in those patients with a longer duration of symptoms (1,580 U/liter, p < 0.05). These data are consistent with data obtained earlier in animal models that suggest infarct size is best contained and LV function best protected when thrombolytic therapy is applied early (within 4 hours) compared with late (>4 hours) in patients with AMI.

PTCA was performed in 21 patients with AMI treated by intracoronary infusion of streptokinase within 8 hours after the onset of symptoms by Meyer and colleagues[65] from Aachen, West Germany. Streptolysis therapy began a mean 3.6 hours after the onset of symptoms. The vessel was occluded in 14 patients and highly stenosed in 7. After the infusion of streptokinase over 26 minutes, patency of the occluded vessels was reached. A PTCA was performed 20–60 minutes after the end of the streptokinase treatment in 19 patients and 24 and 31 hours after treatment in 2 patients. The dilation was successful in 17 patients (81%). The degree of vessel obstruction was reduced from 90%–58%. No reocclusion was induced by PTCA and 20 patients were discharged. One patient died during hospitalization; at autopsy the treated vessel was still patent. During the follow-up period, 2 reinfarctions and 1 asymptomatic occlusion occurred. The clinical findings during the hospital course in the follow-up period were compared with those of a control group of 18 patients with AMI and comparable coronary stenoses who were treated only with streptokinase infusion. Four of these patients had a reinfarction during the hospital course and 3 died during the follow-up period. According to the present study, PTCA can be performed safely and successfully immediately after intracoronary infusion of streptokinase in patients with AMI. By reducing the subtotal stenosis, this treatment contributes to the reperfusion of ischemic myocardium, diminishes the risk of a reocclusion, and seems to improve the prognosis.

Mathey and associates[66] from Hamburg, West Germany, described observations in 6 patients with AMI whose coronary arteries were successfully recanalized but who died of cardiogenic shock 1–18 days after intracoronary thrombolysis. The 6 patients were among 101 with AMI treated by streptokinase. On admission, serum creatine kinase was still normal in all 6 patients but the ST segments were elevated without Q wave changes. The time between the onset of chest pain and coronary streptokinase infusion was approximately 2.9 hours. The total dose of intracoronary streptokinase averaged 200,000 units. Necropsy disclosed a patent coronary artery supplying the AMI in 5 patients and thrombotic reocclusion in 1 patient with a new AMI. All 6 patients had a transmural AMI. In 2 of the 6, the AMI was "anemic" and both had posterior wall AMI. In 3 patients with acute occlusion of the LAD coronary artery, the AMI was hemorrhagic and large. The hemorrhage was always confined to the area of necrosis. One other patient had both types of AMI, a large hemorrhagic one in the area of the recanalized LC coronary artery and an anemic one in the area supplied by a severely narrowed LAD coronary artery. Thus, despite coronary recanalization within 3.5 hours, reperfusion hemorrhage into the area of myocardial necrosis may occur. Whether or not the myocardial hemorrhage delays AMI healing is unclear.

Recent information suggests that 1 of the primary aims of the treatment of an evolving AMI should be to reestablish blood flow to the ischemic myocardium. Measures intended to reduce oxygen demand and enhance the development of collateral flow in patients with AMI fall far short of optimal survival rates and preservation of segmental wall function. Krebber and associates[67] from Hamburg, West Germany, reported 72 patients treated by intracoronary thrombolysis and in some instances subsequent CABG after AMI. All patients were admitted to the hospital within 4 hours after onset of symptoms. In each, there was significant ECG changes. All patients had intracoronary thrombolysis performed using streptokinase 2,000 U/minute as close as possible to the occluded coronary artery. In 78% (56 patients), the thrombus was successfully lysed. Patients in whom lysis was unsuccessful were treated in a standard fashion and were reevaluated for CABG 4–6 weeks after the acute episode. Patients in whom lysis was successful also were treated in a standard fashion if their clinical condition stabilized. A CABG was performed subsequently on an elective basis. Twenty patients required early surgical coronary revascularization because of persistent subtotal stenosis, intermittent severe coronary spasm, or unstable angina. Mean duration from onset of AMI to operation was 3.9 days. Six patients were operated on within 1–8 hours following intracoronary lysis and 14 patients, between the first and twelfth day after lysis. All 20 patients who underwent early CABG following intracoronary lysis survived and had uneventful postoperative courses. However, only 1 of these patients had a transmural AMI, and no patient was in cardiogenic shock. In the 17 patients studied 3–6 weeks postoperatively, the EF increased from 42% at the time of lysis to 55%. The overall mortality in the total group was 13% (9 of 72 patients), and all 9 were in cardiogenic shock.

No patient in the surgical group had cardiogenic shock. Furthermore, CABG was recommended electively to those patients. The authors suggested a 3-day waiting period for regeneration of high energy phosphates. The Hamburg group has demonstrated that in a selected group of patients after AMI, most of whom did not have evidence of transmural AMI, elective CABG can be done. They also have noted an improvement in global EF subsequent to CABG. Other groups should pursue and are pursuing an even more aggressive approach in which patients with AMI are immediately subjected to intracoronary streptokinase infusion followed, if necessary, by PTCA and, if appropriate, emergency CABG. The CABG could be delayed for 1 or 2 days in patients who are stable and who are not in cardiogenic shock. In patients with cardiogenic shock perhaps emergency CABG is indicated.

Nitroglycerin

Dunn and associates[68] from San Francisco, California, studied 18 patients an average of 36 hours after AMI and again at discharge to determine the ability of nitroglycerin to improve global and regional ventricular function after AMI. Equilibrium multigated blood pool scintigrams were performed at rest before and after the sublingual administration of nitroglycerin. Nitroglycerin increased both mean LV EF (0.51 ± 0.15–0.55 ± 0.15, $p < 0.02$) and mean RV EF (0.42 ± 0.14–0.47 ± 0.13, $p < 0.05$). In the early study, LV EF increased significantly in 5 of 18 patients. LV EF increased in the late study in 5 of 6 patients who had an increase early after nitroglycerin, but in only 2 of 12 patients who did not have an early increase ($p < 0.06$). Regional EF in the infarct zone increased late in 7 of 12 patients who had an early increase after nitroglycerin and in 0 of 6 who did not have an early increase ($p < 0.05$). Both RV and LV EF and regional EF showed little late responsiveness to nitroglycerin. These data suggest that in patients evaluated early after AMI, sublingual nitroglycerin improves LV, RV and regional EF in some patients. These nitroglycerin-induced changes appear to predict those patients in whom global ventricular function and regional LV function at the infarct site may improve late.

Kim and Williams[69] from Galveston, Texas, studied 30 patients with AMI 2.1 ± 1.1 (mean, $\pm$ SD) hours after the onset of pain and with ST-segment elevation in multiple leads. Either intravenous morphine (15 patients) or sublingual nitroglycerin (15 patients) was administered and the effect of each agent on pain and QRS changes observed. Nitroglycerin was administered repetitively in large doses while systolic BP was maintained >100 mmHg. Chest pain failed to respond within 30 minutes in 2 patients who received nitroglycerin; in the remaining 13 patients, nitroglycerin produced partial relief of pain in 17 ± 5 minutes and complete relief in 127 ± 605 minutes, requiring a cumulative dosage of 24 ± 39 mg in 16 ± 7 divided doses. An average of 15 ± 7 mg of morphine in 3.3 ± 1.5 divided doses produced complete relief of pain in a similar period (134 ± 77 minutes) (NS). In patients receiving morphine, Q waves developed at 24 and 48 hours, respectively, in 62 and 66 of a total of 86 sites with initial ST-segment elevation in the standard lead ECG. In nitroglycerin responders, Q waves developed in 24 and 48 hours, respectively, in only 21 (28%, $p > 0.001$) and 22 (29%, $p > 0.001$) of the 76 sites with initial ST-segment elevation. The percent R wave amplitude and relative changes in R and Q wave amplitude were significantly less in those patients receiving nitroglycerin. There was no in-hospital mortality. Thus, these data suggest that large and frequent doses of nitroglycerin when used in the hyperacute phase of AMI can effectively abolish chest pain and reduce later ECG indexes that might be indicative of the extent of myocardial necrosis.

Beta blockers

The Beta Blocker Heart Attack Trial (BHAT) sponsored by the National Heart, Lung, and Blood Institute, was a multicenter, randomized, double-blind, and placebo-controlled trial designed to test whether the regular administration of propranolol hydrochloride to men and women who had experienced at least 1 AMI would result in a significant reduction in total mortality during a 2- to 4-year period.[70] During a 27-month interval, 3,837 persons between the ages of 30 and 69 years were randomized to either propranolol (1,916) or placebo (1,921), 5–21 days after AMI. Depending on serum drug levels, the prescribed maintenance dose of propranolol hydrochloride was either 180 or 240 mg/day. The trial was stopped 9 months ahead of schedule. Total mortality during the average 25-month follow-up period was 7% in the propranolol group and 10% in the placebo group (Fig. 2-10). CAD mortality was 6.2% in the propranolol group and 8.5% in the placebo group. Sudden coronary death, a subset of CAD mortality, was 3.3% among the propranolol patients and 4.6% among the placebo patients. Serious side effects were uncommon. Hypotension, gastrointestinal problems, tiredness, bronchospasm, and cold hands and feet occurred more frequently in the propranolol group. In an editorial, Moser and Gorlin[71] had additional comments on the BHAT Trial.

Gundersen and colleagues[72] from Sandika, Norway, related long-term treatment with timolol in patients aged 65–75 years who survived AMI to a significant reduction, compared with placebo, in overall mortality, total cardiac death, sudden death, and reinfarction. The analyses were based on 732 patients (384 taking placebo, 348, timolol) from a cohort of 1,884 patients in a multicenter timolol study. The dosage of timolol was 10 mg twice daily, and the patients were followed for 12 to 33 months (average, 17). There were 83 deaths in the placebo group and 52 deaths in the timolol group, a reduction of 36%. There were 69 initial reinfarctions in the placebo group and 38 in the timolol group, a reduction of 40%. No difference was observed in the reduction of mortality and reinfarction between the ages 65 and 75 years and patients <65 years. The incidence of side effects, the number of withdrawals, and the reason for withdrawal were similar in older and younger patient groups. Thus, these investigators concluded that age should not be a decision-making factor concerning timolol therapy in post-AMI patients.

In AMI, beta adrenoceptor antagonists reduce heart rate, arterial pressure, and hence myocardial oxygen demand (MVO_2), and if given early in this condition may reduce AMI size. The relief of chest pain in AMI by beta blockers is thought to be due to reduction in MVO_2 following a fall in heart rate and BP. Ramsdale and colleagues[73] from Manchester and Oxford, England, demonstrated ischemic pain relief with the long-acting cardioselective beta blocker atenolol, in AMI by 3 separate studies. First, 18 patients were randomized to double-blind intravenous atenolol (5 mg) or saline immediately after admission, followed by oral atenolol (50 mg) or placebo 10 minutes later. In patients receiving atenolol, pain relief coincided with

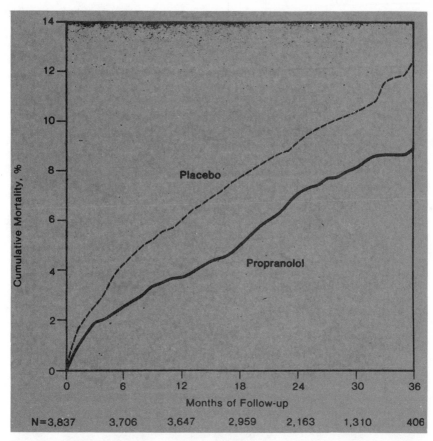

Fig. 2-10. Life-table cumulative mortality curves for groups receiving propranolol hydrochloride and placebo. N indicates total number of patients followed up through each time point. Reproduced with permission from Beta Blocker Heart Attack Trial Research Group.[70]

reduction in heart rate, systolic BP, and the heart rate times systolic BP product; however, pain and these parameters were unchanged by placebo. The degree of pain relief was related to the reduction in cardiac work achieved. A second open study involving 22 patients receiving intravenous atenolol (5–15 mg) early after AMI showed ischemic pain relief in 17 patients. They achieved a more significant reduction in the heart rate times systolic BP product than those whose pain remained unchanged. Finally, a retrospective study of 163 patients randomized to either atenolol or no beta blockade early after AMI revealed that patients receiving atenolol needed less opiate analgesia after admission. The safety of this therapy was illustrated by a decreased incidence of left heart failure and AF and no tendency to second and third degree heart block. It is concluded that early intravenous atenolol can safely play an important part in lessening ischemic chest pain and opiate requirements in AMI and that such success is usually related to the reduction in cardiac work achieved. These clinical benefits are in addition to that of potential infarct size limitation achieved by beta blockade.

For more than 10 years there has been interest in the long-term use of beta adrenoceptor blocking drugs to improve prognosis after recovery from AMI. Because earlier studies gave equivocal results, several further studies were begun in the late 1970s. In 1978, Julian and associates from Newcastle-upon-Tyne, England, started a multicenter trial with sotalol. This drug was selected because in addition to beta adrenoceptor blockade it had the advantage of a long half-life permitting once-daily dosage, and, uniquely for a beta blocking drug, class 3 antiarrhythmic action (prolongation of the action potential)., Julian and associates [74] in their present report of a double-blind randomized study, compared the effect of sotalol 320 mg once daily with that of a placebo in 1,456 patients surviving AMI. Treatment was started 5–14 days after AMI: 60% of the 1,456 patients were randomized to sotalol and 40% to placebo. Patients were followed for 12 months. The mortality rate was 7% (64 patients) in the sotalol group and 9% (52 patients) in the placebo group (Fig. 2-11). The mortality was 18% lower in the sotalol than in the placebo group, but this difference was not statistically significant. The rate of definite re-AMI was 41% lower in the sotalol group than in the placebo group (p < 0.05) (Fig. 2-12). Although the differences in mortality

Fig. 2-11. Cumulative mortality in 873 patients randomized to receive sotalol and 583 patients randomized to receive placebo, all followed-up for 1 year. Reproduced with permission from Julian et al.[74]

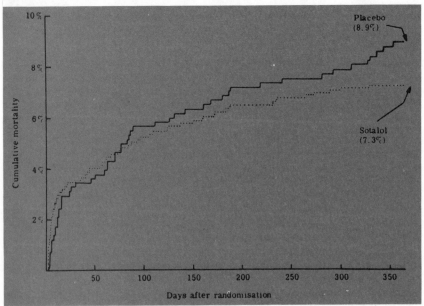

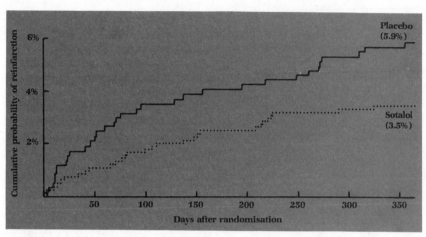

Fig. 2-12. Cumulative probability of reinfarction in 873 patients randomized to receive sotalol and 583 patients randomized to receive placebo. Reproduced with permission from Julian et al.[74]

were not significant, this trial supports the evidence that, in the year after AMI, beta adrenoceptor blocking drugs reduce mortality by 20%–25%. An unsigned editorial[75] discussed the article by Julian and associates and summarized observations in 11 trials of beta blockers after AMI in >13,000 patients.

Sulfinpyrazone

The Anturane Reinfarction Trial[76-78] was a randomized double-blind multicenter trial comparing the effects of sulfinpyrazone and a placebo on cardiac mortality after AMI. In this study, 1,558 eligible patients were followed for an average of 16 months, beginning 25–35 days after infarction. A reduction in overall cardiac mortality was observed, but this benefit occurred entirely during the first 6 months of treatment and appeared to be attributable to a decrease in the incidence of sudden death.

Subsequently, a critique of this study by the FDA was published.[79] The principal criticisms were that the criteria by which causes of death were classified were ambiguous and illogical and that there were inconsistencies in the application of these criteria; both faults were thought to be potential sources of bias. Furthermore, the practice of excluding from the primary analysis the patients determined to have been improperly enrolled (or "ineligible") and the practice of classifying certain deaths as "nonanalyzable," particularly after death, were also thought to be potential sources of bias.

To address these criticisms Sherry and associates[78] from several USA cities decided to check both the consistency and objectivity of the original classification by having the categorization of eligibility and analyzability, as well as the assignment of cause of death, repeated by external and independent reviewers. Accordingly, a committee was formed to review without knowledge as to treatment group the case report of each patient who died during the Anturane Reinfarction Trial and to classify the individual in regard to cause of death, eligibility, and analyzability according to the criteria provided by the Anturane Reinfarction Trial Policy Committee.

The result of that committee's work indicated that a fair agreement between the observed reductions in mortality based on the new committee classification and those based on the original classification was observed. Both analyses indicated a considerable lower incidence of both sudden deaths and total cardiac mortality in the sulfinpyrazone group during the initial 6 months. This, of course, was the benefit claimed in the original report. Thus, the reanalyses provided some renewed confidence about the original reports and answered at least in part the FDA's concerns about possible bias from misclassifications and exclusions. The concerns about study design persist, however. The FDA argues that the "intent-to-treat" approach—in which conclusions are based on outcome in all randomized patients, without exclusions—may be preferable. The Trial's policy committee argues that the "clinical efficacy" approach, which allows exclusions, may be superior when the objective is to determine the effect of an agent in the most appropriate treatment group. On reanalysis, the effects of sulfinpyrazone are, as expected, less impressive when the "intent-to-treat" principle is used.

The matter does not end here. Two recent events must be considered. The first is the report on the Italian trial of sulfinpyrazone in patients who had AMI[80]. This study involved 727 patients studied in a randomized double-blind trial of sulfinpyrazone and placebo. It was similar in overall design to the Anturane Reinfarction Trial, with the important exception that patients were withdrawn from the study if a "thromboembolic event" occurred, which was defined as an AMI, a stroke, or a transient ischemic attack. Treatment with sulfinpyrazone did not affect either the total mortality or the sudden death rate in this smaller series, but it did reduce the incidence of reinfarction and of all thromboembolic events over an average follow-up period of 19 months (Table 2-2). The effect was cumulative and did not show a plateau at 6 months.

The baseline characteristics of the Italian study population differed from those of the Anturane Reinfarction Trial in that the Italian group had a lower prevalence of prior AMI and fewer patients with CHF. The overall cardiac mortality in the first 6 months of study also was much lower in the Italian trial. These differences make a direct comparison difficult, but the finding of fewer nonfatal reinfarctions in the sulfinpyrazone-treated group in the Italian trial, even though nonfatal reinfarction is a relatively "soft" end point, reopens the question of whether sulfinpyrazone's action can be mediated by antithrombotic rather than antiarrhythmic action. The Anturane Reinfarction Trial also reported, without much elaboration, that fewer patients in the sulfinpyrazone-treated group had thromboembolic events.

The second development to consider is the advent of therapy with beta

TABLE 2-2. *Distribution of events during treatment period plus 7 days after stopping treatment. Reproduced with permission from the Anturan Reinfarction Italian Study.*[80]

EVENT	FULFILLING ENTRY CRITERIA		ALL RANDOMIZED	
	S (n = 346)	P (n = 348)	S (n = 365)	P (n = 362)
End-points				
Nonfatal reinfarction	10	25§	12	28¶
Nonfatal stroke	1	4	1	4
TIA	0	2	0	2
Fatal reinfarction	2	5	3	6
Sudden death	9	9	11	9
Other cardiac death	3	3	5	3
Fatal stroke	0	2	0	2
Total	25	50†	32	54*
Total events (see below)	26	50	33	55
Fatal and nonfatal reinfarction combined	12	30**	15	34**
Total thromboembolic end-points (fatal and nonfatal)	13	38‡	16	42‡
Average exposure to therapy (mo)	19.7	19.3	19.3	19.1

p values: Breslow and Mantel-Cox, * <0.025, † <0.005, ‡ <0.001; § Breslow <0.01, Mantel-Cox <0.025, ¶ Breslow <0.005, Mantel-Cox <0.025, ** Breslow <0.005, Mantel-Cox <0.01. "Total events" include 1 cancer death (S, fulfilling entry critiera) and 1 peritonitis death (P, all randomized).

adrenergic blocking agents to reduce mortality after AMI. Several large clinical trials of timolol, metoprolol, and propranolol have shown beneficial results. Treatment with these agents in patients lacking contraindications is rapidly becoming standard practice, and timolol has already been approved for this purpose by the FDA. Future trials of sulfinpyrazone, or, for that matter, of any other agent, will probably have to be conducted in patients with prior AMI who are being treated with beta blockers. Will sulfinpyrazone have an additive effect? In the Anturane Reinfarction Trial, 36% of the patients were taking beta blockers, and this therapy exerted an independent effect in reducing mortality. The numbers were too small to allow conclusions about an additive effect by sulfinpyrazone.

Where does this leave us? Numerous trials of beta blockers after AMI have been carried out over the past 15 years, with variable results. Only recently have adequate experimental design and sufficient numbers of patients finally allowed consistent findings and relatively clear-cut guidelines for therapy. Although sulfinpyrazone is an old agent and relatively free of side effects, it has no such body of accumulated knowledge. The 2 trials that have been published do show beneficial effects: in 1, an effect on the early incidence of sudden cardiac deaths, and, in the other, a sustained effect on reinfarction rate but not on sudden death. This is not a completely consistent picture. The mode of action of the agent is unknown. Only further trials will tell us whether sulfinpyrazone can add to the benefits of the beta blockers in the postinfarction patients. At this juncture it may be wise to wait for more information before adding this drug to the standard armamentarium for patients with prior AMI.

Aspirin or oral anticoagulant

A multicenter randomized clinical trial compared aspirin and oral anticoagulants in men and women who had had a documented AMI.[81] A firm conclusion about whether aspirin is effective in reducing mortality after AMI is still pending. Although not conclusive, the evidence is in favor of a beneficial effect of aspirin. Although the observed benefit varies from trial to trial and is on the average of minor importance (a 10–17% decrease in the death rate, compared with control), it is probably not attributable to chance. The results obtained with oral anticoagulants are similar. The main difference between these 2 antithrombotic therapies is that anticoagulants have been investigated in fewer controlled trials than has aspirin. As a result, there has been a long-standing and bitter controversy over the relative benefits and risks associated with these 2 agents. Review of previous publications leads to the conclusion that anticoagulants offer a possible reduction (10–20%) in the death rate after AMI. Despite the uncertainties, oral anticoagulants are still popular for this indication in some countries. French public health authorities decided to conduct a multicenter trial comparing aspirin and oral anticoagulants.[81] The primary end point was total mortality. Although causes of death and other events were less valuable end points, since the trial was not, and could not be, double blind, they also were assessed. The effects of aspirin (0.5 g given 3 times a day) and oral anticoagulant therapy were compared. Of 6,908 patients considered for entry, 1,303 were randomized to anticoagulant (652) (acenocoumarol, 422; fluindione, 140; ethylbiscoumacetate, 70; phenindione, 9; tioclomarol, 3) or aspirin (651) an average of 11.4 days after the onset of AMI and were followed 6–59 months (mean, 29). There were 65 deaths in the anticoagulant group and 72 in the aspirin group. The number of patients with reinfarction was higher in the aspirin group (33 -vs- 20). None of these differences was statistically significant. Almost twice as many patients were withdrawn from therapy in the aspirin group. There were 54% more patients with gastrointestinal events in the aspirin group and 4 times more patients with episodes of severe bleeding in the anticoagulant group. Thus, the aspirin in the dosage used (quite high) is probably not different from oral anticoagulants in affecting mortality and morbidity after AMI. This study, however, does not consider the effectiveness of either agent in comparison to no antithrombotic therapy, an issue that remains unsettled.

Nitroprusside

Durrer and associates[82] from Amsterdam, The Netherlands, gave sodium nitroprusside by intravenous infusion to 163 randomly selected patients during the first 24 hours after hospitalization for typical AMI and studied its effects on mortality at 1 week, on the frequency of cardiogenic shock, on clinical signs of LV failure, and on peak levels of creatine kinase (CK) isoenzyme MB. A control group of 165 patients received standard medical treatment and infusion of 5% glucose. The end point of the study was a significant reduction in mortality in the nitroprusside group; this was reached when 5 deaths had occurred in this group, compared with 18 among the controls (p < 0.05). The incidence of cardiogenic shock, clinical signs of LV failure, and mean peak levels of CK-MB were all reduced (p < 0.05). The results indicate that infusion of nitroprusside in the early phase of AMI limits complications, possibly by reducing infarct size. The drug was particularly effective in anterior wall AMI.

Cohn and associates[83] from Minneapolis, Minnesota and several other USA cities, summarized the results of a Veterans Administration Cooperative Study involving 812 men with presumed AMI and LV filling pressure ≥12 mmHg in a randomized double-blind placebo-controlled trial to assess the efficacy of a 48-hour infusion of sodium nitroprusside. The mortality rates at 21 days (10.4% in the placebo group and 11.5% in the nitroprusside group) and at 13 weeks (19% and 17%, respectively) were not significantly affected by treatment (Fig. 2-13). The efficacy of nitroprusside was related to the time of treatment: the drug had a deleterious effect in patients whose infusions were started within 9 hours of the onset of pain (mortality at 13 weeks, 24% - vs- 13%; p = 0.025) and a beneficial effect in those whose infusions were begun later (mortality at 13 weeks, 14% -vs- 22%; p = 0.04). Nitroprusside should probably not be used routinely in patients with high LV filling pressures after AMI. However, the results in the patients given late treatment suggest that those with persistent pump failure might receive sustained benefit from short-term nitroprusside therapy.

Although both of the previous trials[82 and 83] were prospective, randomized, and placebo controlled, included substantial numbers of patients, and used total mortality as the primary end point, the authors came to quite different conclusions. Durrer and colleagues[82] (whose study is here termed the European trial) report a treatment effect large enough to require cessation of the trial on ethical grounds: Patients assigned to nitroprusside therapy had a sufficient advantage in mortality over those given placebo to render further placebo assignments unethical. Cohn and colleagues[83] (in the Veterans Administration [VA] trial) report statistically indistinguishable mortality in the treatment and control groups and believe, moreover, that nitroprusside may be toxic in patients randomized within 9 hours of the onset of AMI. All patients admitted to the European trial were randomized

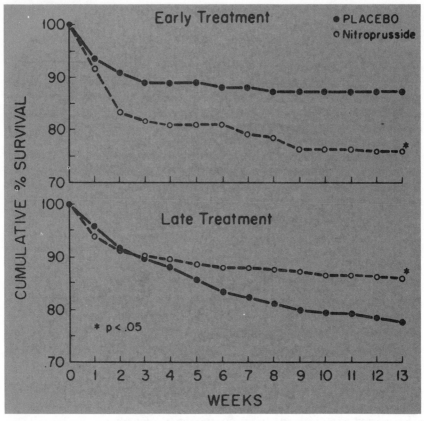

Fig. 2-13. Cumulative percentage of patients surviving after early treatment (within 9 hours of onset of AMI) and late treatment (later than 9 hours). Reproduced with permission from Cohn et al.[83]

within 12 hours of the onset of AMI, most within 9 hours. To confuse matters further, it is the large VA trial (812 subjects) that reports no difference and the smaller European trial (328 subjects) that reports a major therapeutic effect (72% reduction in 7-day mortality). Thus, the 2 trials seem contradictory. The VA trial included only men (mean age, 58 years), with clinical and ECG findings typical of AMI; all had elevated LV filling pressure, as determined by right-sided cardiac catheterization before randomization. The mean LV filling pressure was 19 mmHg. The interval between the onset of symptoms and randomization averaged 16 hours. Both trials excluded patients with shock and those with other illnesses likely to limit survival. The European trial included both men (78% of the sample) and women (mean age, 61). Clinical and ECG findings of AMI were similar to those in the VA trial. In contrast to the patients in the VA trial, most patients in the European trial (290 of 328) had no clinical evidence of elevated filling pressure on admission. Furthermore, the interval between the onset of symptoms and randomization was much shorter, averaging 5 hours. Thus, the patients involved in these trials were quite different: those in the European trial were largely without LV failure and were treated early, and the patients in the VA trial were treated later and had elevated LV filling pressures. Therefore the VA and European trials tested 2 different questions; congruent results are not necessarily expected.

Patients were randomly assigned to nitroprusside or placebo therapy in both trials. In addition, the VA investigators masked treatment assignment; this was not done (or at least not reported) by the European investigators, and it is a weakness in an otherwise well-designed and well-executed study. Were the treatment and control groups reasonably comparable with respect to prognostically important variables? The treatment and control groups in the VA trial were closely matched, particularly for variables used to stratify randomization (age, systolic pressure, and LV filling pressure). In a total of 29 reported baseline treatment-control comparisons, 4 were significantly different: Use of nitrates and prior angina, as well as baseline rales, were more common in the control group, and AV block was more common in the treatment group. In the European trial, randomization achieved well-matched treatment groups for age and systolic pressure. Six other baseline variables reported were evenly distributed, save for more common clinical CHF in the placebo group. Thus, randomization led to similar treatment groups in both trials, as judged by reported baseline variables. Baseline comparisons were more completely reported in the VA trial; particularly important is the assurance that baseline LV filling pressure was similar across treatment groups. This is unknown in the European trial, and the unequal proportions of patients with clinical CHF on admission (9% in the treatment group and 14% among the controls) imply that balance may not have been achieved with regard to this important variable.

The VA investigators stopped their trial after randomizing 812 of a planned 1,000 patients. It is quite unlikely that an additional 188 randomized patients would have materially affected their conclusions, given the contrast observed. The European trial included a sequential stopping rule within its design. The emergence of a large contrast in favor of the treatment group culminated with breach of the stopping rule boundary after 328 patients had been randomized, with 5 deaths in the treatment group and 18 deaths among the controls. The 7-day mortality in the nitroprusside group was 3% and 11% in the control group, a 72% reduction. This result is statistically significant and biologically extraordinary. Mortality was relatively low, however, in both groups, and this makes it possible for small changes in the difference between the groups to result in large swings in significance levels. Thus, the observed difference of 13 deaths is statistically significant, but significance would have been lost if the difference had been 9 deaths.

Nevertheless, the European trial has demonstrated that patients can be treated with nitroprusside in the early hours of AMI with minimal untoward effects, given careful monitoring. Furthermore, there appears to be a large difference in mortality in favor of the treated group. This promising result must be buttressed with further long-term follow-up and a more detailed analysis of the success of randomization in creating similar baseline groups. The conclusion would be strengthened if the significance level were unchanged after analysis with adjustment for baseline inequalities. The VA trial has established that the administration of nitroprusside to patients with suspected AMI and LV failure does not change the mortality rate at 13 weeks, although it does have a salutary effect on hemodynamics. The identification of a possibly harmful effect in patients randomized within 9 hours of onset in the VA trial was the result of extensive interrogation of the data set and thus could have arisen by chance. The possibility of a beneficial effect in those treated after 9 hours must be viewed with the same suspicion. Statistical techniques for judging the role of chance in the generation of a given treatment-control contrast are rendered impotent by extensive data exploration without prior statements of the hypothesis to be tested. Thus, the conclusion to be drawn from the VA trial is that the drug does not change 13-week mortality rates when compared with placebo. The subgroup findings are much less compelling, given the lack of prior stated hypotheses.

The major differences between the VA and European trials are the time from the onset of AMI to the initiation of therapy and the invariable presence of LV failure in patients in the VA trial. The drug probably does not affect mortality when given late to patients with CHF. This group of patients has an unfavorable outlook, and treatment many hours after the onset of AMI is unlikely to improve outcome. Nitroprusside may be effective in reducing mortality when given early to patients without CHF, but the jury is still out. Further analysis of the European trial and independent confirmation of its findings are needed before the use of nitroprusside even in selected patients with AMI can be recommended.

Methylprednisolone

The magnitude of damage in AMI remains a major determinant of long-term survival and various therapeutic interventions have been attempted in an effort to limit infarct size. Madias and Hood[84] from Boston, Massachusetts, compared 19 patients with transmural AMI treated with methylprednisolone within 4.5 hours after the onset of chest pain to 21 patients who received a placebo 4.5 hours after start of clinical symptoms. The study was a double-blinded, randomized protocol and the 2 groups were comparable with reference to sex, prevalence of risk factors, clinical status on admission, location of AMI, and magnitude of ischemic injury as assessed by standard ECG and precordial ST segment and QRS maps. Treated patients were older than patients who received placebo. Methylprednisolone in an intravenous dose of 2 g was administered on admission and a similar dose infused 3 hours later. Placebo administration followed an identical schedule. Mortality, cardiac rupture, incidence of ventricular arrhythmias, blocks, extension of AMI, pericarditis, post-AMI chest pain, persistent ST increase at discharge, and change in Killip classification during hospitalization were the same in both groups. Peak enzyme values and changes in ECG variables pertaining to resolution of ST increase and development of QRS evolutionary alterations were similar in both groups. Follow-up for 6 months did not reveal any differences in the clinical course of either of the 2 groups. Thus, these investigators have shown that methylprednisolone infused in a total dose of 4 g within 12 hours after the onset of chest pain in patients with transmural AMI does not produce any demonstrable beneficial or harmful effect.

Hyaluronidase preparation (GL enzyme)

Saltissi and associates[85] from London, England, assessed the effects of a highly purified hyaluronidase preparation (GL enzyme) on eventual AMI size as measured by ECG, enzymatic, and scintigraphic criteria in 79 patients with suspected AMI. Of the 71 patients with AMI, 35 received GL enzyme and 36 received placebo within 6 hours of the onset of chest pain. GL enzyme injected into a peripheral vein produced no adverse changes in the clinical, hemodynamic, biochemical, or hematologic variables studied. GL enzyme reduced precordial ECG indexes of infarct size as reflected by a diminution (p < 0.02) in the degree of both R-wave loss and Q-wave development. In addition, the number of leads developing pathologic Q waves (NAQ ⩾2), a sign of progression from ischemia to necrosis, was reduced (p < 0.05) after GL enzyme treatment. There were no significant differences in infarct size as measured by cumulative creatine kinase MB isoenzyme release or technetium-99m pyrophosphate scintigraphic infarct area, or in clinical outcome during the hospital stay. Interpretation of the enzymatic and scintigraphic data was complicated by chance bias in pretreatment randomization that resulted in more (p < 0.05) patients with severe hemodynamic impairment (and hence probably larger infarct sizes) entering the GL enzyme group. Nonetheless, a favorable effect of GL enzyme on infarct size was demonstrated by procordial ECG QRS mapping, where each patient acts as his own control.

Flint and associates[86] from Birmingham, England, assessed in a control trial among 483 patients presenting within 6 hours of onset of symptoms the influence of intravenous GL enzyme (hyaluronidase) on the outcome of AMI. A consistent trend toward reduced mortality was observed throughout the period of follow-up among GL enzyme-treated patients. When the fate of all patients entering the trial was considered, irrespective of final diagnosis, the reduction in mortality at 6 months (27 of 240 GL enzyme patients, 45 of 243 placebo) was statistically significant (p = 0.025).

GL enzyme was given in a double-blind placebo-controlled randomized study, by Henderson and associates[87] from New Castle upon Tyne, England, to 192 consecutive patients within 12 hours of suspected AMI. Compared with those receiving placebo, patients with definite AMI given GL enzyme had significantly less change in QRS complexes; in those with anterior AMI, the development of Q waves was less prominent. At 4 months, the overall mortality among those with definite and possible AMI receiving GL enzyme (6 of 83 patients, 7%) was lower than that in those receiving placebo (11 of 79, 14%). This difference was not significant. No adverse effects were observed.

Dopamine and/or dobutamine

The hemodynamic effects of dopamine and dobutamine were compared by Francis and associates[88] from Minneapolis, Minnesota, in 13 patients with acute cardiogenic circulatory collapse. All patients presented with acute pump failure and inadequate systemic perfusion, and most were hypotensive. Nine patients had an AMI; the other 4 patients had an acute decompensation of a previously stable ischemic cardiomyopathy and presented with low output syndrome in the absence of documented AMI. Patients were studied with a randomized single crossover design using each patient as his own control. Both drugs were given at doses of 2.5, 5, and 10 µg/kg/minute for periods of 10 minutes at each dose while hemodynamics were monitored. No other vasoactive drugs were used during the study. Because of advanced age or severe peripheral vascular disease, no patient was considered suitable for intraaortic balloon counterpulsation. There were no significant differences between the 2 drugs with regard to heart rate, mean arterial pressure, systemic vascular resistance, stroke work index, or mean RA pressure. Dobutamine improved stroke index and cardiac indexes significantly more than dopamine at doses of 5 µg/kg/minute. Dopamine increased LV filling pressure more than dobutamine at 5 and at 10 µg/kg/minute. Although both dopamine and dobutamine are useful in acute cardiogenic circulatory collapse, there appear to be important differences in their effect on LV filling pressure and in the mechanisms whereby they increase BP.

Coronary artery bypass grafting

CABG during AMI has been done in the USA primarily in 2 centers: Spokane, Washington, and Des Moines, Iowa. Both groups have reported initial results and the Des Moines, Iowa, group reported subsequent results in 1982. Phillips and associates[89] performed CABG in 156 patients during the early phases of evolving AMI. Six (4%) patients died in the hospital after CABG and 2 (1%) others later. Thrombectomy of the major coronary arteries supplying the area of myocardial necrosis was achieved in 79% of the patients and 17% of the patients showed no observable acute lesion in the major coronary artery supplying the area of myocardial necrosis. Graft patency was 99%. Late follow-up to 62 months disclosed 17 patients with residual limitations. The authors established some criteria for recognizing patients with early AMI who would benefit from CABG. Their criteria were derived by comparing preoperative and postoperative ventricular anatomy, creatine phosphokinase levels, and hemodynamics. All 156 patients were operated on from 1975–1981.

In a follow-up editorial, Gould[90] from Houston, Texas, pointed out the decision of the Phillips group for CABG depended on clinical evidence of ongoing ischemia that indicated remaining viable myocardium and not on a rigid time period based on the interval from onset of chest pain to the decision to perform CABG. EF increased to normal levels in hemodynamically stable patients and from very low to almost normal values in hemodynamically unstable patients. The dramatic increase in EF in the latter group and a hospital mortality of only 18% are promising, since higher mortality and severe LV impairment with pump failure have characterized such patients in the past. On the negative side, Gould pointed out that the patients studied by Phillips and colleagues were nonrandomized and this factor obviously may affect favorable outcome. Would comparable, medically treated patients at the same hospital have demonstrated similar or worse survival rates? In terms of ventricular function, the results of CABG were similar to those of medical reperfusion by intracoronary streptokinase therapy where EF rises an average of 10%–13% EF units in patients with initially reduced LV function. In the streptokinase studies, patients in whom reperfusion failed and also in untreated patients no improvement occurred in LV function. The selection of patients without an adequate control group treated medically makes the interpretation of the CABG results during AMI uncertain. If immediate CABG does improve EF, the question then still remains, is it worth it? Would medical reperfusion by intracoronary or intravenous thrombolysis followed by subsequent elective CABG accomplish the same end? The report of Phillips and associates raises important questions and in many respects is a step in the right direction. Better control groups and methods for assessing myocardial viability, however, will be necessary to define the future role of immediate CABG for AMI.

It is controversial whether CABG should be offered to patients in cardiogenic shock following AMI. Hines and Mohtashemi[91] from Mineola, New York, reviewed 45 patients who underwent intraaortic balloon counter-pulsation following an initial course of catecholamine infusion and afterload reduction. Intraaortic balloon insertion was then followed by coronary angiography. Surgical intervention was considered in 3 circumstances: the first group failed to respond to counterpulsation (1 patient); the second group of 7 patients, whose condition stabilized, could not be weaned from intraaortic balloon support; and the third group of 4 patients, who were successfully weaned, had significant CAD. Eighteen patients did not undergo angiography, only 4 of whom survived. Twenty-seven patients underwent coronary arteriography: 8 had 1-vessel disease and were not operated upon and are now alive 16–36 months after discharge; 7 patients had diffuse 3-vessel disease, global ventricular hypokinesis, and no bypassable distal vessels and were considered inoperable; 6 died in the hospital; the other patient survived, but is now New York Heart Association class IV. Of the remaining 12 patients, operation was considered. One patient died between the time of angiography and operation. The 1 patient in group 1 failed to respond to counterpulsation and underwent emergency operation and infarctectomy and is now class I, 4 years postoperatively. Of the remaining 11 patients, 7 could not be weaned from counterpulsation. Support was carried out from 7–16 days. One patient died before operation. Six others were operated upon. Five survived and are now alive 4–36 months postoperatively and are in class II and class III. Thus, 8 of 11 who underwent delayed CABG are long-term survivors.

In summary, in a small group of patients having cardiogenic shock after

AMI, intraaortic balloon counterpulsation was successful in stabilizing the hemodynamics, allowing coronary angiography, and finally leading to CABG. In this small group of patients operated upon, duration of survival ranged up to 4 years, and functional results were adequate. The present report details a selected group of patients culled from a larger group in cardiogenic shock where operation had a 67% long-term salvage.

Altering behavior

Friedman and colleagues[92] from San Francisco and Stanford, California, studied 1,035 consecutive post-AMI patients to determine the feasibility of altering type A behavior and the effects such alteration might have on subsequent rates of AMI and cardiovascular death. Approximately 300 subjects were enrolled in small groups and primarily received cardiologic counseling on the usually accepted coronary risk factors. In addition to cardiologic counseling, 600 subjects received advice and instructions designed to diminish the intensity of their type A behavior. The remaining subjects, who served as control, received no counseling but were examined and interviewed annually, as were those who dropped out of counseling groups. More than 98% of the 1,035 subjects exhibited moderate to severe type A behavior during a videotaped structured interview. After the first year of this 5-year study, the rates of infarction and cardiovascular death were lower statistically among subjects who received both cardiologic and behavioral counseling than among the control subjects. The rate of nonfatal AMI was lower among subjects who received behavioral counseling than among those who received only cardiologic counseling or those who dropped out of either counseling group. These investigators observed that the circumstances most often preceding recurrent AMI or cardiovascular death were emotional crises, excess physical activity, ingestion of a single fatty meal, or a combination of these.

Exercise

Ballantyne and associates[93] from Glasgow, Scotland, studied the effect of regular moderate exercise on the lipoprotein subfractions of male survivors of AMI. Nineteen men were randomly allocated to an incremental exercise program and 23 patients to a control group. Both groups were studied for 6 months. No change was recorded in any lipoprotein class in the control group. In the trained group, total triglyceride and LDL cholesterol concentration decreased significantly and HDL cholesterol and apolipoprotein rose. The concentration of the HDL subfraction increased with training, however; no relation was found between changes in lipoprotein and treadmill exercise test performance. Thus, in survivors of AMI, exercise may alter plasma lipoprotein values in a beneficial direction.

Walking is probably the most appropriate and widely applied initial mode of prescribed exercise for improving the functional capacity of CAD patients. Improvement in tolerance is indicated clinically by an increased external work load required to produce evidence of myocardial ischemia. Classic physiologic indicators of an aerobic training effect are increased maximal oxygen consumption ($\dot{V}O_2$ max) and reduced heart rate at submaximum work loads. Attenuation of heart rate and, to a lesser extent, the systolic BP responses to submaximal exercise reflects a reduction in myocardial oxygen demand ($M\dot{V}O_2$), which allows performance of higher work loads before reaching the ischemic threshold. According to current concepts, submaximal exercise heart rate is decreased after aerobic training, primarily due to peripheral mechanisms that increase $\dot{V}O_2$ max. Aerobic conditioning results in a lower heart rate at any given submaximal level of total somatic oxygen consumption ($\dot{V}O_2$). However, decreased heart rate might also occur if the trained patient became more mechanically efficient and performed external work with a lower $\dot{V}O_2$ requirement. To assess the effects of walk training on external work efficiency, and the determinants of $M\dot{V}O_2$, Dressendorfer and colleagues[94] from Davis, California, measured $\dot{V}O_2$, heart rate, and systolic BP in 8 male CAD patients during submaximal treadmill walking before and after at least 14 weeks of prescribed exercise. Each patient was tested before and after training at the individually determined horizontal treadmill speed that induced ischemic ST-segment depression in the pretraining test. Although $\dot{V}O_2$ max did not increase significantly with training, submaximal exercise heart rate and the product of heart rate and systolic BP were significantly reduced by 10% and 16%, respectively, and no patient had ischemic ECG changes after training. The reductions in the cardiac response to exercise were due primarily to a 10% decrease in $\dot{V}O_2$, indicating that the patients became more efficient walkers and reduced the $M\dot{V}O_2$ in proportion to the decreased total $\dot{V}O_2$. Thus, enhancement of external work efficiency, an extracardiac factor, can lessen $M\dot{V}O_2$ and thereby raise the exercise threshold for cardiac ischemia in CAD patients even when aerobic capacity, assessed by $\dot{V}O_2$ max, is not increased.

Reduction in heart rate during submaximal exercise is often used to judge the progress of patients with CAD in the course of a physical training program. Some patients, however, are treated with beta adrenergic blocking agents but it remains controversial if chronic beta blockade influences the effects of training and if heart rate remains a useful guide in the evaluation of the state of training in these patients. Vanhees and associates[95] from Leuven, Belgium, studied 30 men who recovered from an AMI: 15 were treated with beta blockers and 15 were not. All trained for 3 months 3 times a week. Cardiorespiratory results from uninterrupted incremental exercise tests before and after training were compared. In each subgroup, the heart rate and systolic BP were significantly reduced. For heart rate, the decrease after training became more pronounced with increasing work load and the overall reduction was significantly less in the beta blocker group compared with the patients not treated with beta blockers. For systolic BP the training-induced reductions were more pronounced in the patients on beta blockers. The increase of peak oxygen uptake was similar in the patients with and without beta blockers, namely, 36% and 35%. At submaximal exercise carbon dioxide output, pulmonary minute ventilation, and the respiratory exchange ratio were lower after training, and these effects of training were similar whether or not the patients were on beta blockers. The study showed that the usual effects of training were observed in patients on beta blockers and that heart rate remains a useful guide to their evaluation throughout a physical training program.

About 33% of patients who have severe LV dysfunction can achieve near normal levels of exercise. To elucidate the mechanisms, Litchfield and colleagues[96] from Iowa City, Iowa, studied 6 patients with severe LV dysfunction (average LV EF, 17%) who achieved near normal levels of exercise tolerance (>11 min treadmill exercise). All patients had normal pulmonary function at rest and during exercise. Hemodynamics were measured at rest and during supine and upright exercise. The major mechanism of the preserved exercise capacity in these patients were chronotropic competence, ability to tolerate elevated wedge pressures 33 mmHg without dyspnea, ventricular dilation, and increased levels of plasma norepinephrine at rest and during exercise. Also, whereas peripheral vascular resistance was unchanged during supine exercise, it decreased by 50% during similar levels of upright exercise. As a consequent, increases in cardiac output from rest to exercise were greater during upright than supine exercise, and pulmonary wedge pressures were lower during upright than supine exercise (21 -vs- 33 mmHg). Thus, multiple mechanisms permit some patients with severe LV dysfunction to achieve normal levels of exercise. These studies emphasize that LV function must be assessed by direct rather than indirect (exercise tolerance test) means.

For years, exercise, whether before or after AMI, has been considered a contributor to psychosocial improvement. Stern and Cleary[97] from Washington, DC, assigned 652 men who had at least 1 AMI 2–36 months earlier to participate ≥24 months as control subjects or subjects in a prescribed, supervised exercise training program. Psychosocial results at baseline and at follow-up of 6, 12, 24 months with minimal exception showed no differences between the control and exercise groups at any of the testing periods.

RELATED TOPICS

Management changes in past 10 years

Wenger and associates[98] from Atlanta, Georgia, examined changes in the patterns of care between 1970–1980 for patients with uncomplicated AMI. Questionnaires were sent to almost 6,000 physicians in 1979 and the responses compared with those of a similar survey taken in 1970. In 1979, almost all physicians reported the availability and use of intensive care unit facilities with continuous ECG monitoring. Also, becoming more widely available were progressive care facilities. The median length of hospitalization had decreased markedly and early ambulation with an earlier return to work were more common. Most physicians continued to recommend progressive physical activity after hospitalization. The routine use of anticoagulant therapy during hospitalization had declined. Prophylactic antiarrhythmic agents increased. Nitrate drugs and tranquilizers were more routinely prescribed by a large percentage of physicians for patients with uncomplicated AMI. Standard exercise test had increased from all physician specialties and the treadmill test was most often used typically 6 weeks post-AMI. Symptoms of new chest pain and palpitations were considered important enough to warrant the recommendation to report immediately to an emergency room. Also, the routine use of coronary arteriography by a large percent of physicians to evaluate the need for surgical intervention was noted and only a small percent of physicians recommended aspirin and nitrate drugs for patients with uncomplicated AMI.

Indications for cardiac catheterization and surgical therapy after AMI

An important question facing physicians is whether to recommend cardiac catheterization to a patient who has just had an AMI. To provide answers to this question, Epstein and associates[99] from Bethesda, Maryland, described their approach to selecting patients for coronary angiography after AMI and presented guidelines for identification and treatment of high risk patients after AMI. The authors recommended that after an AMI, patients with recurrent angina should undergo prompt catheterization, and those with evidence of severe LV dysfunction should be treated medically. Patients with adequate LV function and evidence of inducible ischemia provided by exercise stress testing should undergo cardiac catheterization (Fig. 2-14). Patients within this latter group who had subtotal occlusion of their LAD coronary artery should be considered candidates for PTCA and patients with LM or 3-vessel CAD should be considered for CABG. Until the results of prospective studies comparing mortality after medical and surgical therapy of high risk patients are available, however, these recommendations should serve only as guidelines. The authors recommended that the physicians' final diagnostic and therapeutic recommendations should continue to be individually tailored for each institute and each patient.

The authors suggested dividing patients by clinical criteria and noninvasive testing into subgroups whose members are at high and low risk of dying in the year after their hospital discharge. About 30% of patients will have clinical evidence of LV failure during their hospital course and about half of them will have a LV EF <30% (Fig. 2-15). Of the 70% without clinical CHF, <10% will have severe LV impairment. Thus, about 20% of patients surviving AMI will have severe LV dysfunction (EF <30%). Patients within this subgroup usually die of chronic CHF or refractory ventricular arrhythmias or both, with the first year mortality ranging from 25% to 45%. Death among this relatively small subset of the entire cohort of post-AMI patients constitutes most post-AMI deaths. Current surgical approaches with severe CHF patients who have no clinical evidence of reversible ischemia have not

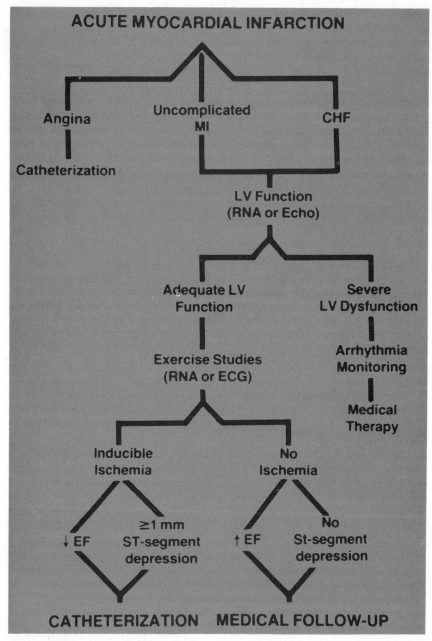

Fig. 2-14. Strategy for identifying patients who should undergo cardiac catheterization after AMI. The strategy is based on clinical assessment, evaluation of LV function by RNA or echo, arrhythmia analysis, and stress testing. Reproduced with permission from Epstein et al.[99]

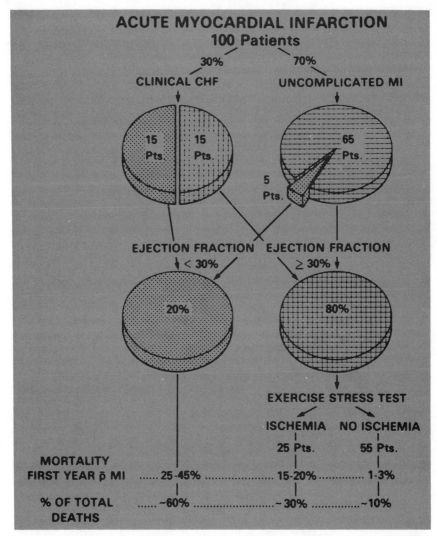

Fig. 2-15. First-year mortality rates for patients with AMI, according to subgroup. Hatched areas represent patients with ejection fractions of more than 30%; stippled areas represent patients with ejection fractions of less than 30%. (The percentages are necessarily rough approximations.) Reproduced with permission from Epstein et al.[90]

been shown to improve survival. Cardiac catheterization therefore is recommended only for patients in this poor prognosis subgroup who have recurrent angina or marked CHF symptoms refractory to medical therapy in association with noninvasive evidence of a discrete LV aneurysm or with physical findings consistent with a VSD of severe MR. Electrocardiographic monitoring (24 hours) was recommended to identify patients in this high risk subgroup who might benefit from antiarrhythmic therapy.

About 80% of patients who survive the in-hospital period after AMI will have resting LV EF ≥30%. Most patients will not have clinical evidence of LV failure or complex ventricular arrhythmias. The first year mortality for these patients with uncomplicated AMI is 5%–10%. Exercise stress testing conducted within 3 weeks of the AMI can be used to divide these patients into high risk "ischemic" and low risk "nonischemic" subgroups. Patients in whom angina develops or who have an ST-segment depression of ≥1 mm or whose LV EF decreases with exercise have a first year post-AMI mortality of 15%–20%. This subgroup of patients at high risk of dying represents a very different substrate than that of the high risk subgroup with severely impaired LV function. These patients not only have reasonably preserved LV function, but they have objective evidence of continuing ischemia, which is indicative of residual jeopardized myocardium, i.e., myocardium at risk of infarcting or of providing the focus for a potentially lethal arrhythmia. These patients, who constitute about one-third of all patients surviving an uncomplicated AMI, should undergo cardiac catheterization to determine whether they are candidates for either elective CABG or PTCA. Patients with negative exercise stress tests are in a very favorable prognostic subgroup, with an expected first year mortality of <3%. Since these patients would not be expected to benefit from CABG or PTCA, cardiac catheterization should be deferred in them.

Evidence that hospital care for AMI has not contributed to recent decline in coronary mortality

To investigate whether the reported 17% decline in the national rates of acute CAD mortality between 1973 and 1978 was attributable to a decreased in-hospital mortality for patients with AMI, Goldman and associates[100] from Boston, Massachusetts, surveyed all 63 acute care hospitals in the Boston area. Compared with 1973–1974, more 1978–1979 AMI patients were admitted to hospitals in metropolitan Boston, and especially to the 5 university teaching hospitals. Between 1973–1974 and 1978–1979, hospital admission rates decreased for younger patients and increased for older patients, but overall admission rates were almost identical. In-hospital mortality rates from AMI did not change significantly in any age group. Because overall AMI mortality declined while in-hospital mortality was unchanged, the proportion of AMI deaths that occurred inside the hospital increased from 30%–40%. Although recurrent hospital care undoubtedly benefits many individual patients, this study suggests improvements in the in-hospital care of AMI patients are not a major explanation for the nationwide mortality trends between 1973 and 1978.

AMI and angiographically normal coronary arteries

Legrand and associates[101] from Liege, Belgium, described 18 patients surviving an AMI and subsequently had a normal coronary arteriogram; 7 were < age 35 years; 11 were men and 6 were women; and the AMI was nontransmural in 11. The mean follow-up was 21 months. Eleven patients developed residual chest pain at rest early after AMI. One, treated by beta blockers, had a second AMI. Eight became asymptomatic, and 2 improved under antispastic therapy. Another patient developed severe variant angina 3 months after the AMI and died following plexectomy. Two patients had rare episodes of angina at rest. The stress ECG was negative in all 18 patients. Provocative test for spasm was positive in 3 of 9 patients. Diffuse narrowing associated with chest pain was demonstrated in 2 patients at angiography. Thus, of patients with an AMI and subsequent normal coronary arteries by angiogram, vasospastic phenomena and increased vasomotor tone are found in most patients. Whenever residual chest pain is controlled by antispastic therapy, the follow-up course seems benign.

References

1. CABIN HS, ROBERTS WC: Relation of healed transmural myocardial infarct size to length of survival after acute myocardial infarction, age at death, and amount and extent of coronary arterial narrowing by atherosclerotic plaques: analysis of 70 necropsy patients. Am Heart J 104:216–220, Aug 1982.

2. CABIN HS, ROBERTS WC: Comparison of amount and extent of coronary narrowing by atherosclerotic plaque and of myocardial scarring at necropsy in anterior and posterior healed transmural myocardial infarction. Circulation 66:93–99, July 1982.

3. CABIN HS, ROBERTS WC: Quantitative comparison of extent of coronary narrowing and size of healed myocardial infarct in 33 necropsy patients with clinically recognized and in 28 with clinically unrecognized ("silent") previous acute myocardial infarction. Am J Cardiol 50:677–681, Oct 1982.

4. GOLDMAN L, WEINBERG M, WEISBERG M, OLSHEN R, COOK EF, SARGENT K, LAMAS GA, DENNIS C, WILSON C, DECKELBAUM L, FINEBERG H, STIRATELLI R, MEDICAL HOUSE STAFFS YALE-NEW HAVEN HOSPITAL, BRIGHAM AND WOMEN'S HOSPITAL: A computer-derived protocol to aid in the diagnosis of emergency room patients with acute chest pain. N Engl J Med 307:588–596, Sept 2, 1982.

5. DILLON CM, CALBREATH DF, DIXON AM, RIVIN BE, ROARK SF, IDEKER RE, WAGNER GS: Diagnostic problem in acute myocardial infarction: CK-MB in the absence of abnormally elevated total creatine kinase levels. Arch Intern Med 142:33–38, Jan 1982.

6. DE BEER FC, HIND CRK, FOX KM, ALLAN RM, MASERI A, PEPYS MB: Measurement of serum C-reactive protein concentration in myocardial ischemia and infarction. Br Heart J 47:239–243, March 1982.

7. VOULGARI F, CUMMINS P, GARDECKI TIM, BEECHING NJ, STONE PCW, STUART J: Serum levels of acute phase and cardiac proteins after myocardial infarction, surgery, and infection. Br Heart J 48:352–356, Oct 1982.

8. Horowitz RS, Morganroth J, Parrotto C, Chen CC, Soffer J, Pauletto FJ: Immediate diagnosis of AMI by 2-D echo. Circulation 65:323–329, Feb 1982.

9. Visser CA, Kan G, Lie KI, Becker AE, Durrer D: Apex two dimensional echocardiography: alternative approach to quantification of acute myocardial infarction. Br Heart J 47:461–467, May 1982.

10. Loh IK, Charuzi Y, Beeder C, Marshall LA, Ginsburg JH: Early diagnosis of nontransmural myocardial infarction by two-dimensional echocardiography. Am Heart J 104:963–968, Nov 1982.

11. Frais M, Botvinick E, Shosa D, O'Connell W: Are regions of ischemia detected on stress perfusion scintigraphy predictive of sites of subsequent myocardial infarction? Br Heart J 47:357–364, Apr 1982.

12. Geltman EM, Biello D, Welch MJ, Ter-Pogossian MM, Roberts R, Sobel BE: Characterization of nontransmural MI by positron-emission tomo. Circulation 65:747–755, Apr 1982.

13. Chapelle J-P, Albert A, Smeets J-P, Heusghem C, Kulbertus HE: Effect of the haptoglobin phenotype on the size of a myocardial infarct. N Engl J Med 307:457–463, Aug 19, 1982.

14. Wagner GS, Freye CJ, Palmeri ST, Roark SF, Stack NC, Ideker RE, Harrell FE Jr, Selvester RH: Evaluation of a QRS scoring system for estimating myocardial infarct size. I. Specificity and observer agreement. Circulation 65:342–347, Feb 1982.

15. Grande P, Pedersen A: Myocardial infarct size and cardiac performance at exercise soon after myocardial infarction. Br Heart J 47:44–50, Jan 1982.

16. Holman BL, Goldhaber SZ, Kirsch C, Polak JF, Friedman BJ, English RJ, Wynne J: Measurement of infarct size using single photon emission computed tomography and technetium-99m pyrophosphate: a description of the method and comparison with patient prognosis. Am J Cardiol 50:503–511, Sept 1982.

17. Palmeri ST, Harrison DG, Cobb FR, Morris KG, Harrell FE, Ideker RE, Selvester RH, Wagner GS: A QRS scoring system for assessing left ventricular function after myocardial infarction. N Engl J Med 306:4–9, Jan 7, 1982.

18. Gibson RS, Bishop HL, Stamm RB, Crampton RS, Beller GA, Martin RP: Value of early two dimensional echocardiography in patients with acute myocardial infarction. Am J Cardiol 49:1110–1119, Apr 1982.

19. Sanford CF, Corbett J, Nicod P, Curry GL, Lewis SE, Dehmer GJ, Anderson A, Moses B, Willerson JT: Value of radionuclide ventriculography in the immediate characterization of patients with acute myocardial infarction. Am J Cardiol 49:637–644, March 1982.

20. Nemerovski M, Shah PK, Pichler M, Berman DS, Shellock F, Swan HJC: Radionuclide assessment of sequential changes in left and right ventricular function following first acute transmural myocardial infarction. Am Heart J 104:709–717, Oct 1982.

21. Upton MT, Palmeri ST, Jones RH, Coleman RE, Cobb FR: Assessment of left ventricular function by resting and exercise radionuclide angiocardiography following acute myocardial infarction. Am Heart J 104:1232–1343, Dec 1982.

22. Buda AJ, Dubbin JD, MacDonald IL, Strauss HD, Orr SA, Meindok H: Spontaneous changes in thallium-201 myocardial perfusion imaging after myocardial infarction. Am J Cardiol 50:1272–1278, Dec 1982.

23. Gibson RS, Watson DD, Carabello BA, Holt ND, Beller GA: Clinical implications of increased lung uptake of thallium-201 during exercise scintigraphy 2 weeks after myocardial infarction. Am J Cardiol 49:1586–1593, May 1982.

24. Glover MU, Kuber MT, Warren SE, Vieweg WVR: Myocardial infarction before age 36: risk factor and arteriographic analysis. Am J Cardiol 49:1600–1603, May 1982.

25. Betriu A, Castaner A, Sanz GA, Pare JC, Poig E, Coll S, Magrina J, Navarro-Lopez F: Angiographic findings 1 month after myocardial infarction: a prospective study of 259 Survivors. Circulation 65:1099–1105, June 1982.

26. RITCHIE JL, WILLIAMS DL, HARP G, STRATTON JL, CALDWELL JH: Transaxial tomography with thallium-201 for detecting remote myocardial infarction. Comparison with planar imaging. Am J Cardiol 50:1236–1241, Dec 1982.

27. SHELL WE, DeWOOD MA, PETER T, MICKLE D, PRAUSE JA, FORRESTER JS, SWAN HJC: Comparison of clinical signs and hemodynamic state in the early hours of transmural myocardial infarction. Am Heart J 104:521–528, Sept 1982.

28. SEVERANCE HW JR, MORRIS KG, WAGNER GS: Criteria for early discharge after acute myocardial infarction. Validation in a community hospital. Arch Intern Med 142:39–41, Jan 1982.

29. HOROWITZ RS, MORGANROTH J: Immediate detection of early high-risk patients with acute myocardial infarction using two-dimensional echocardiographic evaluation of left ventricular regional wall motion abnormalities. Am Heart J 103:814–822, May 1982.

30. KOIWAYA Y, TORII S, TAKESHITA A, NAKAGOKI O, NAKAMURA M: Postinfarction angina caused by coronary arterial spasm. Circulation 65:275–280, Feb 1982.

31. HAUER RNW, LIE KI, LIEM KL, DURRER D: Long-term prognosis in patients with bundle branch block complicating acute anteroseptal infarction. Am J Cardiol 49:1581–1585, May 1982.

32. LICHSTEIN E, ARSURA E, HOLLANDER G, GREENGART A, SANDERS M: Current incidence of postmyocardial infarction (Dressler's) syndrome. Am J Cardiol 50:1269–1271, Dec 1982.

33. FRIEDMAN MJ, CARLSON K, MARCUS FI, WOOLFENDEN JM: Clinical correlations in patients with acute myocardial infarction and left ventricular thrombus detected by two-dimensional echocardiography. Am J Med 72:894–898, June 1982.

34. D'ARCY B, NANDA NC: 2 dimensional echocardiographic features of right ventricular infarction. Circulation 65:167–173, Jan 1982.

35. BALU V, HERSHOWITZ S, MASUD ARZ, BHAYANA JN, DEAN DC: Mitral regurgitation in coronary artery disease. Chest 81:550–555, May 1982.

36. MASON JW, STINSON EB, WINKLE RA, OYER PE, GRIFFIN JC, ROSS DL: Relative efficacy of blind left ventricular aneurysm resection for the treatment of recurrent ventricular tachycardia. Am J Cardiol 49:241–248, Jan 1982.

37. FAXON DP, RYAN TJ, DAVIS KB, McCABE CH, MYERS W, LESPERANCE J, SHAW R, TONG TGL: Prognostic significance of angiographically documented left ventricular aneurysm from the Coronary Artery Surgery Study (CASS). Am J Cardiol 50:157–164, July 1982.

38. SORENSEN SG, CRAWFORD MH, RICHARD KL, CHAUDHURI TK, O'ROURKE R: Noninvasive detection of ventricular aneurysm by combined two-dimensional echocardiography and equilibrium radionuclide angiography. Am Heart J 104:145–152, July 1982.

39. WEINBLATT E, GOLDBERG JD, RUBERMAN W, FRANK CW, MONK MA, CHAUDHARY BS: Mortality after first myocardial infarction. Search for a secular trend. JAMA 247:1576–1581, March 19, 1982.

40. THANAVARO S, KLEIGER RE, PROVINCE MA, HUBERT JW, MILLER JP, KRONE RJ, OLIVER GC: Effect of infarct location on the in-hospital prognosis of patients with first transmural myocardial infarction. Circulation 66:742–747, Oct 1982.

41. BAUGHMAN KL, HUTTER AM, DeSANCTIS RW, KALLMAN CH: Early discharge following acute myocardial infarction. Long-term follow-up of randomized patients. Arch Intern Med 142:875–878, May 1982.

42. WASSERMAN AG, BREN GB, ROSS AM, RICHARDSON DW, HUTCHINSON RG, RIOS JC: Prognostic implications of diagnostic Q waves after myocardial infarction. Circulation 65:1451–1455, 1982.

43. GELMAN JS, SALTUPS A: Precordial ST segment depression in patients with inferior myocardial infarction: clinical implications. Br Heart J 48:560–565, Dec 1982.

44. BOUDOULAS H, SOHN YH, O'NEILL W, BROWN R, WEISSLER AM: The $QT > QS_2$ syndrome: a new

mortality risk indicator in coronary artery disease. Am J Cardiol 50:1229–1235, Dec 1982.

45. Tzivoni D, Kren A, Gottlieb A, Cranot C, Benhorin J, Gazala E, Golhman JO, Stern S: Right atrial pacing soon after MI. Circulation 65:330–335, Feb 1982.

46. Hamer A, Vohra J, Hunt D, Sloman G: Prediction of sudden death by electrophysiologic studies in high risk patients surviving acute myocardial infarction. Am J Cardiol 50:223–229, Aug 1982.

47. Baker JT, Bramlet DA, Lester RM, Harrison DG, Roe CR, Cobb FR: Myocardial infarct extension: incidence and relationship to survival. Circulation 65:918–923, May 1982.

48. Sanz G, Castañer A, Betriu A, Magriña J, Roig E, Coll S, Paré JC, Navarro-López F: Determinants of prognosis in survivors of myocardial infarction. A prospective clinical angiographic study. N Engl J Med 306:1066–1070, May 6, 1982.

49. Nesto RW, Cohn LH, Collins JJ, Wynne J, Holman L, Cohn PF: Inotropic contractile reserve: a useful predictor of increased 5 year survival and improved postoperative left ventricular function in patients with coronary artery disease and reduced ejection fraction. Am J Cardiol 50:39–44, July 1982.

50. Perez-Gonzalez J, Botvinick EH, Dunn R, Rahimtoola S, Ports T, Chatterjee K, Parmley WW: The late prognostic value of acute scintigraphic measurement of myocardial infarction size. Circulation 66:960–971, Nov 1982.

51. Marmor A, Geltman E, Schechtman K, Sobel BE, Roberts R: Recurrent myocardial infarction: clinical predictors and prognostic implications. Circulation 66:415–421, Aug 1982.

52. Nikolic G, Sugiura T, Spodick DH: Self-predicting stress tests: predischarge modified stress testing after acute myocardial infarction. Br Heart J 47:559–562, June 1982.

53. Miller DH, Borer JS: Exercise testing early after acute myocardial infarction: risks and benefits. Am J Med 72:427–438, March 1982.

54. Cobb FR, Williams RS, McEwan P, Jones RH, Coleman RE, Wallace AG: Effects of exercise training on ventricular function in patients with recent myocardial infarction. Circulation 66:100–107, July 1982.

55. deFeyter PJ, vanEenige MJ, Dighton DH, Visser FC, deJong J, Roos JP: Prognostic value of exercise testing, coronary angiography, and left ventriculography 6–8 weeks after myocardial infarction. Circulation 66:527–536, Sept 1982.

56. Sobel BE, Bergmann SR: Coronary thrombolysis—some unresolved issues. Am J Med 72:1–4, Jan 1982.

57. Rentrop KP, Blanke H, Karsch KR: Effects of nonsurgical coronary reperfusion on the left ventricle in human subjects compared with conventional treatment. Study of 18 patients with acute myocardial infarction treated with intracoronary infusion of streptokinase. Am J Cardiol 49:1–8, Jan 1982.

58. Schwarz F, Schuler G, Katus H, Mehmel HC, Olshausen K, Hofmann M, Herrmann HJ, Kubler W: Intracoronary thrombolysis in acute myocardial infarction: correlations among serum enzyme, scintigraphic and hemodynamic findings. Am J Cardiol 50:32–38, July 1982.

59. Smalling RW, Fuentes F, Freund GC, Reduto LA, Wanta-Matthews M, Gaeta JM, Walker W, Sterling R, Gould KL: Beneficial effects of intracoronary thrombolysis up to eighteen hours after onset of pain in evolving myocardial infarction. Am Heart J 104:912–920, Oct 1982.

60. Weinstein J: Treatment of myocardial infarction with intracoronary streptokinase: efficacy and safety data from 209 United States cases in the Hoechst-Roussel registry. Am Heart J 104:894–898, Oct 1982.

61. Lee G, Low RI, Takeda P, Joe P, DeMaria AN, Amsterdam EA, Lui H, Dietrich P, Lee K, Mason DT: Importance of follow-up medical and surgical approaches to prevent reinfarction, reocclusion, and recurrent angina following intracoronary thrombolysis with streptokinase in acute myocardial infarction. Am Heart J 104:921–924, Oct 1982.

62. Spann JF, Sherry S, Carabello BA, Mann RH, McCann WD, Gault JH, Gentzler RD, Rosenberg KM, Maurer AH, Denenberg BS, Warner HF, Rubin RN, Malmud LS, Comerota A: High-dose, brief intravenous streptokinase early in acute myocardial infarction. Am Heart J 104:939–945, Oct 1982.

63. Schuler G, Schwarz F, Hofmann M, Mehmel H, Manthey J, Maurer W, Rauch B, Herrmann HJ, Kubler W: Thrombolysis in AMI using intracoronary streptokinase: assessment by thallium-201 scintigraphy. Circulation 66:658–664, Sept 1982.

64. Schwarz F, Schuler G, Katus H, Hofmann M, Manthey J, Tillmanns H, Mehmel HC, Kübler W: Intracoronary thrombolysis in acute myocardial infarction: duration of ischemia as a major determinant of late results after recanalization. Am J Cardiol 50:933–937, Nov 1982.

65. Meyer J, Merx W, Schmitz H, Erbel R, Kiesslich T, Dorr R, Lambertz H, Bethge C, Krebs W, Bardos P, Minale C, Messmer BJ, Effert S: Percutaneous transluminal coronary angioplasty immediately after intracoronary streptolysis of transmural myocardial infarction. Circulation 66:905–913, Nov 1982.

66. Mathey DG, Schofer J, Kuck K-H, Beil U, Klöppel G: Transmural, hemorrhagic myocardial infarction after intracoronary streptokinase: clinical, angiographic, and necropsy findings. Br Heart J 48:546–551, Dec 1982.

67. Krebber HJ, Matheny D, Kuck KJ, Kalmar P, Rodewald G, Hill JD: Management of evolving myocardial infarction by intracoronary thrombolysis and subsequent aorta-coronary bypass. J Thorac Cardiovasc Surg 83:186–193, Feb 1982.

68. Dunn RF, Botvinick EH, Benge W, Chatterjee K, Parmley WW: The significance of nitroglycerin-induced changes in ventricular function after acute myocardial infarction. Am J Cardiol 49:1719–1727, May 1982.

69. Kim YI, Williams JF: Large dose sublingual nitroglycerin in acute myocardial infarction: relief of chest pain and reduction of Q wave evolution. Am J Cardiol 49:842–848, March 1982.

70. β-Blocker Heart Attack Trial Research Group: A randomized trial of propranolol in patients with acute myocardial infarction: I. mortality results. JAMA 247:1707–1714, March 26, 1982.

71. Moser M, Corlin R: Beta-blockers and myocardial infarction. Arch Intern Med 142:1618–1619, Sept 1982.

72. Gundersen T, Abrahamsen AM, Kjekshus J, Ronnevik PK: Timolol-related reduction in mortality and reinfarction in patients ages 65–75 years surviving AMI. Circulation 66:1179–1184, Dec 1982.

73. Ramsdale DR, Faragher EB, Bennett DH, Bray CL, Ward C, Cruickshank JM, Yusuf S, Sleight P: Ischemic pain relief in patients with acute myocardial infarction by intravenous atenolol. Am Heart J 103:459–467, Apr 1982.

74. Julian DG, Prescott RJ, Jackson FS, Szekely P: Controlled trial of sotalol for one year after myocardial infarction. Lancet 1:1142–1147, May 22, 1982.

75. Long-term and short-term beta blockade after myocardial infarction. Lancet 1:1159–1161, May 22, 1982.

76. The Anturane Reinfarction Trial Research Group: Sulfinpyrazone in the prevention of sudden death after myocardial infarction. N Engl J Med 306:250–256, April 22, 1982.

77. The Anturane Reinfarction Trial Research Group: Sulfinpyrazone in the prevention of cardiac death after myocardial infarction: the Anturane Reinfarction Trial. N Engl J Med 298:289–295, 1978.

78. Sherry S, Gent M, Lilienfeld A, McGregor M, Mustard JF, Yu P, Cartwright K, Ellis RA, Cohen MD: The anturane reinfarction trial: reevaluation of outcome. N Engl J Med 306:1005–1008, April 22, 1982.

79. Temple PR: The FDA's critique of the Anturane Reinfarction Trial. N Engl J Med 306:1488–1492, June 17, 1982.

80. Report From the Anturan Reinfarction Italian Study: Sulfinpyrazone in post-myocardial infarction. Lancet 1:237–242, Jan 30, 1982.

81. E.P.S.I.M. Research Group: A controlled comparison of aspirin and oral anticoagulants in prevention of death after myocardial infarction. N Engl J Med 307:701–708, Sept 16, 1982.

82. DURRER JD, LIE KI, VAN CAPELLE FJL, DURRER D: Effect of sodium nitroprusside on mortality in acute myocardial infarction. N Engl J Med 306:1121–1128, May 13, 1982.

83. COHN JN, FRANCIOSA JA, FRANCIS GS, ARCHIBALD D, TRISTANI F, FLETCHER R, MONTERO A, CINTRON G, CLARKE J, HAGER D, SAUNDERS R, COBB F, SMITH R, LOEB H, SETTLE H: Effect of short-term infusion of sodium nitroprusside on mortality rate in acute myocardial infarction complicated by left ventricular failure. Results of a veterans administration cooperative study. N Engl J Med 306:1129–1135, May 13, 1982.

84. MADIAS JE, HOOD JR WB: Effects of methylprednisolone on the ischemic damage in patients with AMI. Circulation 65:1106–1113, June 1982.

85. SALTISSI S, ROBINSON PS, COLTART DJ, WEBB-PEPLOE MM, CROFT DN: Effects of early administration of a highly purified hyaluronidase preparation (GL enzyme) on myocardial infarct size. Lancet 1:867–870, Apr 17, 1982.

86. FLINT EJ, DE GIOVANNI J, CADIGAN PJ, LAMB P, PENTECOST BL: Effect of GL enzyme (a highly purified form of hyaluronidase) on mortality after myocardial infarction. Lancet 1:871–874, Apr 17, 1982.

87. HENDERSON A, CAMPBELL RWF, JULIAN DG: Effect of a highly purified hyaluronidase preparation (GL enzyme) on electrocardiographic changes in acute myocardial infarction. Lancet 1:874–876, Apr 17, 1982.

88. FRANCIS GS, SHARMA B, HODGES M: Comparative hemodynamic effects of dopamine and dobutamine in patients with acute cardiogenic circulatory collapse. Am Heart J 103:995–1000, June 1982.

89. PHILLIPS SJ, ZEFF RH, KONGTAHWORN C, SKINNER JR, IANNONE L, BROWN TM, WICKEMEYER W, GORDON DF: Surgery for evolving myocardial infarction. JAMA 248:1325–1328, Sept 17, 1982.

90. GOULD KL: Coronary reperfusion: medical, surgical, or not at all? JAMA 248:1362–1363, Sept 17, 1982.

91. HINES G, MOHTASHEMI M: Delayed operative intervention in cardiogenic shock after myocardial infarction. Ann Thorac Surg 33:132–138, Feb 1982.

92. FRIEDMAN M, THORESEN CE, GILL JJ, ULMER D, THOMPSON L, POWELL L, PRICE V, ELEK SR, RABIN DD, BREALL WS, PIAGET G, DIXON T, BOURG E, LEVY RA, TASTO DL: Feasibility of altering type A behavior pattern after myocardial infarction. Recurrent coronary prevention project study: methods, baseline results, and preliminary findings. Circulation 66:83–92, July 1982.

93. BALLANTYNE FC, CLARK RS, SIMPSON HC, BALLANTYNE D: The effect of moderate physical exercise on the plasma lipoprotein subfractions of male survivors of MI. Circulation 65:913–917, May 1982.

94. DRESSENDORFER RH, SMITH JL, AMSTERDAM EA, MASON DT: Reduction of submaximal exercise myocardial oxygen demand post-walk training program in coronary patients due to improved physical work efficiency. Am Heart J 103:358–363, March 1982.

95. VANHEES L, FAGARD R, AMERY A: Influence of beta adrenergic blockade on effects of physical training in patients with ischemic heart disease. Br Heart J 48:33–38, July 1982.

96. LITCHFIELD RL, KERBER RE, BENGE JW, MARK AL, SOPKO J, BHATNAGAR RK, MARCUS ML: Normal exercise capacity in patients with severe LV dysfunction: compensatory mechanisms. Circulation 66:129–134, July 1982.

97. STERN MJ, CLEARY P: The national exercise and heart disease project: long-term psychosocial outcome. Arch Intern Med 142:1093–1097, June 1982.

98. WENGER NK, HELLERSTEIN HK, BLACKBURN H, CASTRANOVA SJ: Physician practice in the

management of patients with uncomplicated MI: changes in the past decade. Circulation 65:421–427, March 1982.

99. EPSTEIN SE, PALMERI ST, PATTERSON RE: Evaluation of patients after acute myocardial infarction: indications for cardiac catheterization and surgical intervention. N Engl J Med 307:1487–1492, Dec 9, 1982.

100. GOLDMAN L, COOK F, HASHIMOTO B, STONE P, MULLER J, LOSCALZO A: Evidence that hospital care for AMI has not contributed to the decline in coronary mortality bet. 1973–1974 and 1978–1979. Circulation 65:936–942, May 1982.

101. LEGRAND V, DELIEGE M, HENRARD L, BOLAND J, KULBERTUS H: Patients with myocardial infarction and normal coronary arteriogram. Chest 82:678–685, Dec 1982.

3

Arrhythmias, Conduction Disturbances, and Cardiac Arrest

ARRHYTHMIAS IN ATHLETES AND IN HEALTHY ELDERLY INDIVIDUALS

Viitasalo and associates[1] from Helsinki, Finland, recorded data from ambulatory ECG in 35 highly trained endurance athletes and in 35 nonathletic controls of similar age (Fig. 3-1.). The minimal, mean hourly, and maximal heart rates were significantly lower in athletes. Thirteen athletes (37%) and 2 controls (6%) had sinus pauses >2 seconds. Prolonged PR interval was observed in 13 athletes (37%) and in 5 controls (14%), second degree Wenckebach type block in 8 athletes (23%) and in 2 controls (6%) and second degree block with Mobitz II-like pattern in 3 athletes (9%) and in no controls. All athletes with Mobitz II-like pattern also had prolonged PR interval and Wenckebach-type second degree AV block. The behavior of sinus

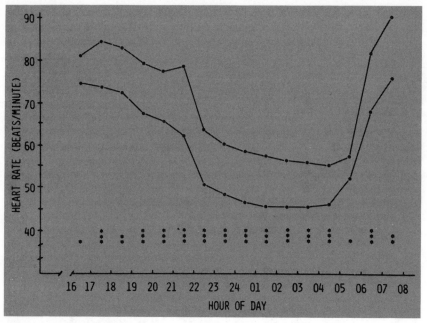

Fig. 3-1. Mean hourly heart rates in athletes (lower line) and controls (upper line). *p < 0.05, **p < 0.01, ***p < 0.001. Reproduced with permission from Viitasalo et al.[1]

rate on development of AV block varied, not only interindividually but also intraindividually, from absence of change to an increase or decrease in most subjects in both study groups. A decrease in sinus rate on appearance of AV block was found constantly in only 2 athletes and in 1 control, and AV dissociation with junctional rhythm occurred in 7 athletes (20%) and with ventricular rhythm in 1 athlete with neither phenomena occurring in a control. The athletes had slightly fewer VPC than controls and no athlete had VT, whereas 2 controls had VT.

Talan and associates[2] from Chicago, Illinois, made 24-hour ambulatory ECG recordings on 20 male long-distance runners, aged 19–28 years, during normal activities other than running. Average, maximum, and minimum waking heart rates, respectively, ranged from 58–108 (mean ± SD, 73 ± 15), 90–164 (120 ± 19), and 34–53 (43 ± 5) beats/minute. Longest waking sinus pauses ranged from 1.35–2.55 seconds (1.7 ± 0.3). Average, maximum, and minimum sleeping heart rates, respectively, ranged from 38–58 (47 ± 6), 69–114 (83 ± 14), and 31–43 (36 ± 3) beats/minute. Longest sleeping sinus pauses ranged from 1.60–2.81 (2.0 ± 0.3) seconds. All 20 runners had atrial premature beats, but only 1 (5%) had >100/24 hours. Fourteen runners (70%) had VPC, but only 2 (10%) had >50/24 hours, and none had ventricular couplets or VT. Eight runners (40%) had ≤1 episodes of type 1 second degree AV block. Compared with untrained men of similar age, the runners had slower heart rates (by approximately 10 beats/minute), longer sinus pauses, and a higher prevalence of AV block. Runners and untrained men did not differ with respect to prevalence of VPC, R-on-T phenomenon, ventricular couplets, or VT.

Twenty-four hour ambulatory ECG examination was performed in 98 healthy active subjects, aged 60–85 years, who were participants in a longitudinal study on aging by Fleg and Kennedy[3] from Baltimore, Maryland. Normal health was confirmed by noninvasive testing, including maximal treadmill exercise (98 of 98) and thallium scintigraphy (38 of 98). The studies indicated that a healthy population of elderly subjects shows a substantial prevalence of supaventricular ectopic beats and VPC, both isolated and complex. High degree AV block, profound sinus bradycardia, abnormal sinus pauses, and sinus arrest are rare in normal elderly subjects.

ATRIAL FIBRILLATION

Epidemiologic features

Kannel and associates[4] from Framingham, Massachusetts, described the frequency of AF in the Framingham population, which included 2,325 men and 2,866 women aged 30–62 years of age at entry. All were followed biennially >22 years and chronic AF developed in 49 men and 49 women. The frequency of AF rose sharply with age but did not differ significantly between the sexes. Overall, there was a 2% chance that AF would develop in 20 years. Atrial fibrillation usually followed the development of overt cardiovascular disease. Only 18 men and 12 women (31%) had chronic AF in the absence of cardiovascular disease. Rheumatic heart disease and CHF were the most powerful predictive precursors of AF, with relative risks in excess of 6-fold. Hypertensive cardiovascular disease was the most common antecedent cardiac abnormality. Among the risk factors for cardiovascular disease, diabetes mellitus and ECG evidence of LV hypertrophy were related to the occurrence of AF. The development of chronic AF was associated with a doubling of overall mortality and of mortality from cardiovascular disease.

A marker for abnormal left ventricular function in CAD

In a retrospective study of 1,176 patients with known CAD by cardiac catheterization, Kramer and associates[5] from Hyde Park and Stony Brook, New York, found 10 patients (0.8%) with AF. Comparison with 25 randomly selected patients with CAD in sinus rhythm showed that AF correlated significantly with impaired LV function, MR, and abnormalities of LV contraction. Thus, AF was considered a useful marker of extensive LV dysfunction.

Spontaneous conversion of long-standing AF

Spontaneous conversion to sinus rhythm after prolonged AF is uncommon, with only 11 recorded cases to the knowledge of Gardner and Dunn[6] from Kansas City, Kansas, in the English language "literature." Gardner and Dunn reported 4 cases of spontaneous conversion to an organized atrial rhythm (either sinus rhythm or atrial tachycardia with block) after 9–16 years of established AF. One case was due to a toxic reaction to digitalis. In the other 3 there was no apparent reason. M-mode and 2-D echo in 3 patients showed an akinetic and noncontractile left atrium in each. These observations lend support to an earlier hypothesis that "complete" fibrosis of the LA wall may be responsible for the conversion from AF.

In the post-thyrotoxic state

Nakazawa and associates[7] from Tokyo, Japan, designed a study to investigate the appropriate timing for cardioversion in patients with chronic AF who had been rendered euthyroid from a thyrotoxic state. They studied retrospectively 163 patients with thyrotoxic AF, with a mean follow-up of 34 months. With control of thyroid function alone, 101 patients has spontaneous reversion of AF to sinus rhythm and 62 patients had persistent AF. In those with spontaneous reversion, the longest duration of AF before the euthyroid state was 13 months. In those with persistent AF, the shortest duration of AF before the euthyroid state was 8 months. Almost 75% of those with spontaneous reversion had conversion to sinus rhythm within 3 weeks of becoming euthyroid. No spontaneous reversion occurred if AF was still present after the patient had been in a euthyroid state for 4 months. This study suggests that spontaneous reversion of AF to sinus rhythm is highly unlikely if the duration of AF before the euthyroid state exceeds 13 months or if it is still present after the patient has been in a euthyroid state for 4 months. Cardioversion should be performed at about the sixteenth week after the euthyroid state is achieved.

Verapamil treatment

Stern and associates[8] from Elmhurst, New York, evaluated the effectiveness of oral verapamil for control of ventricular rate in digitalized patients with AF with 3 clinical problems: chronic AF with rapid rate and rest (4 patients), chronic AF with accelerated rate during modest exercise (5 patients), and rapid rates during paroxysmal AF (4 patients). Patients in the first 2 categories were evaluated both by open label dosage titration and by a randomized, double-blind, crossover protocol. In chronic AF with rapid rate at rest, there was a significant reduction in resting heart rate (from 125 ± 7–87 ± 14 beats per minute, p < 0.01) and in peak exercise heart rate (from 162 ± 33–126 ± 25, p < 0.01). In chronic AF with rapid rate during exercise, there was also a significant decrease in resting heart rate (from 90 ± 7–66 ± 4, p < 0.01) and in peak exercise heart rate (from 126 ± 19–101 ± 15, p < 0.01). These effects continued during long-term follow-up of 1–12 months (mean, 7). In patients with paroxysmal AF, verapamil slowed the ventricular response (from 160 ± 24–72 ± 4, p < 0.01) with only some amelioration of symptoms. Therapy was well tolerated despite a high prevalence (7 of 13 patients) of radiographic cardiomegaly (cardiothoracic ratio >0.55). Thus, verapamil is a safe and useful drug for control of ventricular rate in digitalized patients with chronic and paroxysmal AF.

The elimination of verapamil and its n-demethylated metabolite, norverapamil, was studied by Schwartz and colleagues[9] from Stanford, California, in 9 patients with chronic AF after the first oral verapamil dose and during chronic oral verapamil administration. Significant increases were seen in the elimination half-lives of both verapamil (6.4 ± 3.5–12 ± 5 h) and norverapamil (10.3 ± 6–16.5 ± 7 h) during chronic oral verapamil administration. These pharmacokinetic observations have important clinical applications for the rational long-term administration of this agent. Once steady state serum concentrations have been achieved during chronic verapamil administration, verapamil doses should be given at less frequent intervals or in smaller doses to produce the desired serum concentration and therapeutic response and to minimize unwanted or toxic drug effects.

The safety, efficacy, and pharmacologic effect of combined verapamil and digoxin were studied in 10 patients with chronic AF by Schwartz and colleagues[10] from Stanford, California. Heart rate (HR) recordings, treadmill exercise test, physical examination, and serum digoxin concentration during chronic digoxin therapy were compared with those after the acute administration of verapamil and 1, 2, 4, 6, and 10 weeks after the addition of oral verapamil to digoxin therapy. After both intravenous and chronic oral verapamil administration, resting and exercise HR was significantly lower. Increasing serum concentrations of verapamil correlated with the increasing suppression of HR at rest and during exercise. The mean resting HR by 24-hour ambulatory ECG decreased from 87–72 beats/minute. The mean treadmill exercise HR decreased more markedly from a mean of 151–106 beats/minute. During chronic therapy, HR reductions were seen 1 week after the addition of verapamil and were maintained without change for the duration of the trial. The BP at rest and during exercise was unchanged. Cardiomegaly was present on the entry chest x ray in 6 patients. After verapamil, heart size decreased in 3 and was unchanged in 1, and 2 patients had transient CHF that responded to diuretics. Serum digoxin levels increased from a mean of 1.6–2.7 ng/ml during verapamil therapy. The increase was observed in 19 patients but was not related to clinical signs of digitalis excess and no episodes of asystole were seen on the serial 24-hour ECG. Chronic oral administration of verapamil 320 mg/day resulted in mean verapamil concentrations of 130–280 ng/ml with great intersubject and intrasubject variability. These investigators concluded that verapamil is effective in further suppressing the LV response rate in AF when given in combination with digitalis and can serve as an adjunct to digitalis therapy in the management of patients with chronic AF.

Transient AF and atrial flutter occur frequently in the early period following cardiac operation, even in patients with no preoperative rhythm disturbances. Plumb and colleagues[11] from Birmingham, Alabama, assess the efficacy and safety of using intravenous verapamil to treat these arrhythmias following cardiac operation. Twenty-eight patients with AF or atrial flutter received either low dose verapamil (0.075 mg/kg) or placebo using a randomized, double-blind crossover protocol. When low dose verapamil was given to 21 patients with AF, the ventricular rate fell from 150 ± 22–102 ± 14, and the rhythm in 1 patient converted to sinus. Eleven patients with AF in whom the response to low dose verapamil was either brief or incomplete later received standard dose verapamil (0.15 mg/kg), following which the ventricular rate fell from 139 ± 14–97 ± 13. The rhythm in 1 additional patient converted to sinus. The maximum decrease in ventricular rate occurred 1–3 minutes after verapamil infusion. A subset of 7 patients, 5 with AF and 2 with atrial flutter, who had rapid ventricular rates refractory to intravenous digoxin all showed good response to verapamil. There was a brief and clinically insignificant drop in systemic BP in most patients. No adverse effects were observed from verapamil administration.

The authors suggest that intravenous verapamil may be the most useful therapy available for AF, with rapid ventricular response occurring after cardiac operation. Whether subsequent therapy of AF is best accomplished with digoxin, repeated injections of verapamil, or oral verapamil is unknown. However, many patients probably would require no further therapy. Finally, the addition of verapamil therapy was very effective for patients in whom digoxin therapy suboptimally slowed ventricular rate.

SUPRAVENTRICULAR TACHYCARDIA WITH OR WITHOUT SHORT P-R INTERVAL SYNDROMES

Transplacental cardioversion of fetal tachycardia with procainamide

Persistent fetal tachycardia before and at the time of delivery may be associated with benign neonatal courses or result in severe CHF or in death. Intrauterine pharmacologic cardioversion with digoxin propranolol has been successful. Dumesic and associates[12] from San Francisco, California, described a newborn with fetal SVT complicated by intrauterine CHF that was diagnosed by 2-D and M-mode echo. The arrhythmia was temporarily cardioverted on several occasions by administering intravenous procainamide to the mother after digoxin and propranolol had failed to alter the fetal heart rate. The authors concluded that procainamide may be useful in the treatment of fetal SVT that is refractory to digoxin or propranolol.

In infants and children

Lundberg[13] from Stockholm, Sweden, reported a long-term follow-up study of 40 patients who had paroxysmal atrial tachycardia (PAT) in infancy. The follow-up period was 16–36 years (mean, 24); 86% males. Nine had AF or atrial flutter. There were 5 deaths in infancy, with 3 due to severe congenital heart disease. Males with preexcitation had by far the greatest frequency of recurrence, 60% in the long-term follow-up. Approximately 30% of subjects without preexcitation had recurrences in the third decade. Recurrences of AF/flutter were rare. Patients whose onset was at a mean age of 4 weeks had a greater tendency for recurrence than patients who had a mean age of onset at 10 weeks. Preexcitation was no longer observed in the ECG in 8 of 23 (35%) patients when their median age was 3 years, and 75% of those who lost preexcitation stopped having PAT. If preexcitation did not disappear, only 27% stopped having PAT. Three patients displayed apparent appearance or reappearance of preexcitation after 10 years of age.

This study is consistent with previous follow-up data regarding a higher incidence of recurrence of PAT in patients with preexcitation. In general, the long-term outlook is excellent for patients without complex heart disease. There was no late mortality except for a patient with a ruptured aortic aneurysm unrelated to the arrhythmia. These data are extremely useful in helping to counsel parents regarding long-term prognosis in this situation.

Greco and associates[14] from Napoli, Italy, compared the use of intravenous digitalis (lanatoside C), verapamil, and ATP for treatment of paroxysmal SVT in 62 children aged 4 days to 12 years (33 ≤ 1 yr). Twelve patients had heart disease and 17 had WPW. Patients who were in shock, who responded to vagal maneuvers, or who had AV dissociation before or after treatment were omitted from the study. Heart rates ranged from 180–320 beats per minute during SVT and ECG data suggested a reentry mechanism in most. Termination of SVT was successful in 21 of 32 (66%) with digitalis, 32 of 36 (89%) with adenosine triphosphate (ATP), and 36 of 39 (92%) with verapamil. The time from drug injection to termination of SVT was 75 ± 47 minutes with digitalis, 42 ± 6 seconds with ATP, and 128 ± 55 seconds with verapamil. Frequent transient gastrointestinal side effects and flushing occurred with ATP. Two patients had cardiac arrest with verapamil: 1 critically ill infant with low serum calcium and 1 6-month-old on a maintenance beta blocker. Both responded to catecholamine and calcium infusion.

These authors provide interesting comparative data regarding treatment of SVT. Since ATP is unavailable in the USA at present, the verapamil-digitalis question is more pertinent. First, it is clear that verapamil should not be used in a child who is in severe CHF, who has a low serum calcium, or who has received a beta blocker recently. Verapamil is an attractive drug, however, for the relatively stable patient with SVT because of its rapid onset of action, high success rate, and short half-life. It should be tried only with careful monitoring, intravenous access, and calcium drawn up ready to be used. In patients in whom it has been shown safe and effective, it could then be used to treat recurrent episodes of SVT in an expeditious manner.

Lidocaine for bidirectional tachycardia and for digitalis-induced tachycardia with block

Most recent studies discussing tachycardias with alternating QRS polarity have referred to them as *torsade de pointes*. In contrast, Castellanos and associates[15] from Miami, Florida, described 10 patients with bidirectional tachycardia and the effects of lidocaine on them. Three patients also had digitalis-induced atrial tachycardia with block. In 1 patient, a single bolus of lidocaine was followed 5 minutes later by VF, but the other 9 patients received 2 boluses of 75 mg followed by a drip infusion of 3 mg/minute. The drug terminated the episodes of atrial tachycardia with block and bidirectional tachycardia in all patients. Whereas the abolition of the bidirectional tachycardia was permanent in the 7 patients with digitalis intoxication, it recurred after stopping the drip infusion in the 2 patients without digitalis toxicity. Thus, lidocaine can be useful in the treatment of digitalis-induced bidirectional tachycardia and atrial tachycardia with block. From this study no conclusions can be drawn, however, as to whether lidocaine is superior to other class I or class IV agents.

Localization of site of ventricular preexcitation with body surface maps in WPW syndrome

Benson and associates[16] from Durham, North Carolina, studied 49 patients aged 7 weeks to 51 years with WPW syndrome by isopotential body surface maps during normal sinus rhythm, atrial pacing, or induced AF. The location of the accessory pathway was determined by multicatheter electrophysiologic studies or surgical ablation of the accessory pathway. When fusion was minimized and ventricular activation primarily controlled by a single accessory pathway, the distribution of positive and negative potentials on the anterior and posterior torso during QRS and the ST segment were an excellent index of the location of the site of the accessory pathway. The relation between a specific sequence of QRS-T wave body surface maps and a specific preexcitation site was similar from patient to patient in the presence of marked differences in age, size, and different cardiac status due to structural congenital cardiac defects. Localization of the site of the accessory pathway using distributions too early in QRS was unreliable because the early distributions varied from patient to patient for the same preexcitation site; however, the potential distributions during the ST segment were both stable and consistent from patient to patient for the same preexcitation site. The presence of significant fusion of ventricular activation initiated via a single accessory pathway and the normal conduction system or via multiple accessory pathways complicated the interpretation of body surface distributions. Thus, from this study the investigators predicted accurately at least 7 preexcitation sites by the combined use of QRS and ST-segment body surface maps.

Verapamil therapy

Klein and associates[17] from London, Canada, evaluated electrophysiologic effects of intravenous verapamil (bolus doses of 0.15 mg/kg body weight followed by infusion of 0.005 mg/kg/min) with those of oral verapamil (80 mg every 6 h for 48 h) in 8 patients with paroxysmal SVT. The mechanism of the SVT was AV nodal reentry in 4, and AV reentry utilizing an accessory pathway for retrograde conduction in 4. The electrophysiologic effects of oral and intravenous verapamil were similar. Both preparations prevented induced SVT in 6 patients, none of whom had recurrence of their arrhythmia while receiving long-term oral therapy during 5–10 months. Neither preparation had a significant effect in 2 patients acutely and this predicted failure of long-term oral therapy in 1 patient. Thus, the results of acute drug testing with intravenous verapamil can be utilized to predict electrophysiologic results and response to long-term therapy with oral verapamil.

Electrophysiologic drug testing of atrial fibrillation in preexcitation syndrome

Paroxysmal AF can be severely symptomatic when it complicates the preexcitation syndrome (WPW with short anomalous AV pathway refractoriness) or accelerated AV nodal conduction. In these conditions, paroxysmal AF is frequently sporadic, making it difficult to define effective prophylactic drug therapy using clinical trial and error. Thus, electrophysiologic drug testing was performed by Bauernfeind and colleagues[18] from Chicago, Illinois, in 9 patients with severely symptomatic and sporadic (2–13 attacks/24 months) paroxysmal AF. All patients had control inductions of sustained (>30 s) AF by high RA stimulation, and attempted inductions following serial administration of drugs. Drugs tested were intravenous procainamide (1.0–1.5 g, 5 patients); intravenous propranolol (0.1 mg/kg, 3 patients); oral quinidine (1.6–2.4 g/day, 6 patients); oral disopyramide (1.2–1.6 g/day, 4 patients), and oral aprindine (100–250 mg/day, 4 patients). In all patients, 1 or more drugs prevented induction of sustained AF: procainamide (1 patient), quinidine (5 patients), disopyramide (4 patients), and aprindine (4 patients). All patients were treated with drugs, which prevented induction of sustained AF, and were followed for 8–40 months (mean, 24). Seven patients tolerated the drugs: 6 had no AF and 1 had several short nonsustained attacks. Two patients did not tolerate the drugs: 1 had paroxysmal palpitation (on decreased aprindine dosage) and 1 had AF (while off of aprindine). Thus, electrophysiologic drug testing is feasible in patients with sporadic paroxysmal AF. Inability to induce sustained AF following drug administration suggests successful chronic prophylaxis of spontaneous paroxysmal AF with the same drug.

Ventricular response during atrial fibrillation in the WPW syndrome after verapamil

Gulamhusein and associates[19] from Ontario, Canada, examined the electrophysiologic effects of verapamil in 8 patients with WPW. In the present study, verapamil shortened the antegrade effective refractory period of the accessory pathway in 3 patients and abbreviated the shortest cycle length with 1-1 conduction over the accessory pathway in 2 patients. Verapamil also decreased the shortest R-R interval between preexcited ventricular complexes during AF. After verapamil, 2 patients required cardioversion for hemodynamic deterioration after acceleration of the ventricular response during AF. The ventricular rate accelerated after verapamil in 4 patients with predominately preexcited ventricular complexes during AF, whereas in patients with predominately normal ventricular complexes, the average ventricular rate decreased or did not change following the drug. Thus, verapamil may result in significant acceleration of ventricular response during AF in the the WPW syndrome and the investigators advise that the safety of verapamil in individual patients with this syndrome should be established by electrophysiologic testing before its use.

Effect of verapamil on accessory pathway in WPW syndrome

Harper and colleagues[20] from Melbourne, Australia, evaluated the effects of intravenous verapamil on the electrophysiologic properties of the accessory pathway in 12 patients with symptomatic WPW syndrome using intracardiac electrical recordings. Eleven of 12 patients had a reentrant supraventricular tachycardia produced with programmed AV pacing. After verapamil, it was still possible to induce supraventricular tachycardia in 6 of the 11 patients, but the mean cycle length of the tachycardia increased from a control value of 330 ± 20 ms (mean $\pm$ SE) to 369 ± 21 ms ($p < 0.05$). Verapamil had no significant effect on the antegrade refractory period or the accessory pathway as measured by the extrastimulus technique, but it did increase maximal AV conduction through the accessory pathway to incremental high rate atrial pacing in 10 of 12 patients. In 4 patients with AF verapamil decreased the average R-R interval from a control value of 327 ± 27 ms to 282 ± 28 ms ($p < 0.05$) and decreased the shortest R-R interval between preexcited beats from a control value of 237 ± 21 ms to 209 ± 18 ms ($p < 0.05$). These data suggest that in patients with symptomatic WPW syndrome, verapamil may increase the ventricular response through the accessory pathway if AF occurs.

Verapamil for tachyarrhythmias after cardiac operation

Although the antiarrhythmic effects of verapamil have been studied widely, its role in the treatment of atrial tachyarrhythmias after open heart surgery has not been defined. Accordingly, 22 patients were studied by Gray and colleagues[21] from Los Angeles, California, using a double-blind randomized crossover protocol 1–6 days after open heart surgery, except for 1 patient, who was studied 90 days after open heart surgery. AF was seen in 18 and atrial flutter was observed in 4 patients. Two doses were used, 0.075 and 0.15 mg/kg (not exceeding 10 mg/dose), depending on the response. A positive response consisted of: conversion to sinus rhythm or heart rate <100 beats/minutes. Eleven patients received verapamil as the first drug; the remaining 11 received placebo first. Digoxin had been given to 20 patients (0.5 mg, average dose) prior to inclusion in the study. Four patients converted to sinus rhythm within 30 minutes after verapamil and 1 additional patient did so within 10 seconds of placebo administration. The post-treatment heart rate combining both low and high dose response was 85 compared with 128 beats/minute for placebo. The heart rate remained lower than control 30 minutes after verapamil. Transient hypotension required intravenous fluid in 1 patient. Thus, verapamil safely and rapidly controls heart rate in supraventricular tachyarrhythmias, but is not likely to result in immediate conversion to sinus rhythm in patients following open heart surgery.

Procainamide in WPW syndrome

Wellens and associates[22] from Maastricht, The Netherlands, evaluated the influence of procainamide in identifying patients with the WPW syndrome with a short refractory period and an accessory pathway in an antegrade direction. Procainamide given intravenously in a maximal dose of 10 mg/kg body weight over a 5-minute period during sinus rhythm produced complete antegrade block in the accessory pathway in 20 of 39 patients with the WPW syndrome. An electrophysiologic investigation 24–48 hours later revealed that in 19 of the 20 patients, the effective refractory period of the accessory pathway was ≥270 ms. In 18 of the 19 patients not exhibiting antegrade block in the accessory pathway, the refractory period was <270 ms. Approximately the same effect occurred with 100 mg of procainamide as with 10 mg of ajmaline. These data suggest that intravenous procainamide is a reliable and rapid method of identifying patients with the WPW syndrome who may be at risk for circulatory insufficiency or sudden death with AF.

Disopyramide in WPW syndrome

Patients with the WPW syndrome may have 2 types of arrhythmias: a reciprocating tachycardia in which accessory pathway provides the retrograde limb of the reentrant circuit and atrial flutter/AF in which accessory pathway provides a route whereby a rapid ventricular response may be mediated. Kerr and associates[23] from Durham, North Carolina, evaluated the electrophysiologic effects of disopyramide phosphate in 12 patients with the WPW syndrome. The electrophysiologic studies were performed during a control period and after administering intravenous disopyramide (4 bolus doses of 0.5 mg/kg over 40 minutes superimposed on a continuous infusion of 1.0 mg/kg/h). All patients were then restudied after 3 days on oral medication in dosages of 800–1200 mg/day. In all patients, the investigators attempted to induce reciprocating tachycardia and AF. The cycle length during reciprocating tachycardia was not changed by intravenous disopyramide but increased after oral disopyramide from 331–370 ms. This increase occurred predominantly as the result of prolongation of retrograde conduction time in the accessory pathway. Despite prolonging cycle lengths during reciprocating tachycardia, disopyramide did not prevent its induction. The shortest and mean R-R interval during AF were used to assess antegrade refractoriness of the accessory pathway. Intravenous disopyramide prolonged the shortest R-R interval from 169–226 ms. Oral disopyramide prolonged the shortest R-R interval and the mean R-R interval significantly. After oral disopyramide, the episodes of AF were shorter and self-terminating. No acute hemodynamic side effects were observed but 5 patients had gastrointestinal or anticholinergic side effects on oral disopyramide. Seven patients elected to have surgical interruption of their accessory pathways and 5 were successfully treated with oral disopyramide for periods ranging from 14–33 months. Thus, disopyramide appears to have beneficial electrophysiologic effects in patients with WPW syndrome. Prolongation of refractoriness in the accessory pathway markedly slows the ventricular response during AF and therefore prevents the development of life-threatening arrhythmias.

Mechanisms responsible for spontaneous termination

Waxman and associates[24] from Toronto, Canada, studied 20 consecutive patients to determine possible mechanisms of early spontaneous termination of episodes of induced paroxysmal SVT that terminated spontaneously within 1 minute after initiation. Spontaneous conversion of SVT was associated with a reproducible course of hypotension at the onset of the arrhythmia followed by recovery of BP above control levels and termination. In the supine position, 9 (45%) patients had spontaneous termination in 35 (16%) of 219 episodes of SVT. In the head-down position, only 1 (8%) of 13 patients had spontaneous termination in 2 (4%) of 54 episodes. In the head-up position, only 1 (6%) of 18 patients had termination in 2 (2%) of 102 episodes. However, none of 5 patients demonstrated spontaneous termination of SVT in 25 episodes when pretreated with intravenous hyoscine butylbromide (cholinergic blocker) and none of 16 patients demonstrated spontaneous termination in 87 episodes of SVT after beta adrenergic blockade. The data suggest the initial hypotension during SVT causes a sympathetic response that increases BP resulting in a rise in vagal tone that terminates the SVT.

Isoproterenol in the WPW syndrome

Wellens and associates[25] from Maastricht, The Netherlands, evaluated the influence of beta adrenergic stimulation on the duration of the antegrade refractory period of the accessory pathway using isoproterenol infusions in 7 patients with the WPW syndrome. In 2 patients, the effect of isoproterenol was studied during long-term oral amiodarone administration. Isoproterenol shortened the antegrade refractory period of the accessory pathway in 6 of the 7 patients. In 2 of 3 patients with an initial antegrade refractory period in the accessory pathway of ≤290 ms, shortening measured 30 ms. In 3 patients having an antegrade refractory period of the accessory pathway of >290 ms, isoproterenol abbreviated these values by 30, 60, and 90 ms. The greatest amount of shortening was observed in patients with the longest initial values for their antegrade refractory period in their accessory pathway. In the 2 patients receiving amiodarone therapy, isoproterenol shortened the antegrade refractory period of the accessory pathway significantly, indicating that isoproterenol's effect cannot be prevented by long-term amiodarone administration. These data suggest that beta adrenergic stimulation induced by hypotension or anxiety may shorten the antegrade refractory period of the accessory pathway leading to rapid ventricular rates during AF in patients with the WPW syndrome.

Effect of sotalol on myocardial refractoriness

Bennett[26] from Manchester, England, gave sotalol intravenously to 15 patients with accessory AV pathways during intracardiac electrophysiologic studies. Eleven patients had the WPW syndrome and 4 had concealed left-sided accessory pathways. In contrast to the actions typical of beta blocking agents, intravenous sotalol prolonged the effective refractory periods of the ventricles and accessory pathways and reduced the ventricular response to AF in the patients with the WPW syndrome. Similar results were obtained with oral administration. These findings support the observation that sotalol, unlike other beta blocking agents, causes acute prolongation of the myocardial action potential and suggest that this action might be of therapeutic use.

Catheter technique for closed chest ablation of the atrioventricular conduction system for treatment of refractory supraventricular tachycardia

Patients with recurrent supraventricular tachyarrhythmias occasionally become disabled because available pharmacologic agents are ineffective or poorly tolerated, and pacemaker techniques fail to control recurrences. In the absence of an accessory AV pathway as the underlying cause of arrhythmia, surgical interruption of the AV conduction system with implantation of a permanent ventricular pacemaker has been shown to provide effective therapy. A variety of experimental techniques have been proposed to ablate the conduction system, but to date only open chest approaches have been used to accomplish interruption of the AV node and His bundle in human beings. Gallagher and associates[27] from Durham, North Carolina, described a catheter technique for ablating the His bundle and its application in 9 patients with recurrent SVT that was unresponsive to medical management. A tripolar electrode catheter was positioned in the region of the His bundle, and the electrode recording a large unipolar His bundle potential was identified. In the first patient, 2 shocks of 25 and 50 J, respectively, were delivered by a standard cardioversion unit to the catheter electrode, resulting in an intra-His bundle conduction defect. Subsequent delivery of 300 J resulted in complete heart block. In the next 8 patients, an initial shock of

200 J was used. The His bundle was ablated by this single shock of 6 of these patients and by an additional shock of 300 J in 1. In the remaining patient, conduction in the AV node was modified, resulting in alternating first and second degree AV block. A stable escape rhythm was preserved in all patients. The procedure was well tolerated, without complications, and all patients have remained free of arrhythmia, without medication, for follow-up periods of 2–6 months.

Anatomic effects of cryoablation of the atrioventricular conduction system

A cryosurgical technique for ablating the AV node-His bundle has been used by the medical and surgical group at Duke in patients with disabling supraventricular tachyarrhythmias unresponsive to medical management. Because of the value of cryoablation of the AV conduction system in the treatment of refractory cardiac rhythm disorders, the anatomic effects of cryoablation on the cardiac conduction system must be defined. Ohkawa and associates[28] from Durham, North Carolina, summarized studies on 4 patients who had intractable recurrent SVT or refractory AF or flutter. The patients were treated by cryoablation of the AV conduction system and died 8–360 days postoperatively. Serial sections of the AV conduction system were studied. Cryoablation produced lesions that completely destroyed most of the AV node in 3 cases, the penetrating portion of the His bundle in all 4 cases, and the branching portions of the His bundle in 2 cases. The right bundle branch was not involved markedly in any case. The lesions were discrete and sharply defined. The patient who died 8 days postoperatively had hemorrhage, necrosis, and slight inflammatory infiltrate. Patients who survived 49–360 days showed collagen deposition. The AV nodal artery and its branches showed slight to marked intimal thickening in 3 cases. Small, partly organized thrombi were present just behind the tricuspid in 2 patients. These investigators conclude that cryoablation of the AV system produced discrete cardiac lesions that did not markedly damage the tricuspid valve or aorta.

Electrophysiologic findings with accelerated atrioventricular nodal conduction

Certain clinical and electrophysiologic features of 42 patients with rapid AV nodal conduction during electrophysiologic study were described by Holmes and associates[29] from Rochester, Minnesota. The distinctive clinical feature of these patients was the high frequency of SVT, which was rapid and had been poorly responsive to conventional antiarrhythmic treatment. Abnormalities to both AV nodal conduction and AV nodal refractoriness were present. Medical management and late follow-up were characterized by inconsistent control of rhythm. In 4 patients, control of the SVT was finally achieved by successful ablation of an accessory extranodal pathway that participated in macroreentry paroxysmal SVT. In a fifth patient, the SVT was controlled with the use of a patient-activated radiofrequency atrial-stimulating pacemaker. Although the existence of shortened AV nodal conduction time and refractoriness may not cause supraventricular rhythm disturbances, symptoms are aggravated by resultant rapid ventricular rates. Treatment for patients with this anatomic and functional substrate must be highly individualized and based on electrophysiologic investigation.

Catheter-induced ablation of the atrioventricular junction for arrhythmias

In 5 patients with recurrent bouts of SVT resistant to, or intolerant of both conventional and experimental drugs, Scheinman and associates[30] from San Francisco, California, subjected them to a new procedure involving delivery of direct current shocks to an electrode catheter positioned adjacent to the bundle of His. Complete AV block was produced in all: 1 patient died suddenly 6 weeks after the shock therapy and the remainder had complete AV block with follow-up intervals ranging from 4–12 months. The shock therapy was associated with mild elevations of creatine phosphokinase MB (31 ± 18 units), but there was no hemodynamic evidence of TR. If this procedure proves safe and effective, it might supplant the need for open cardiac surgical procedures for His bundle ablation.

Antegrade and retrograde fast pathway properties with dual atrioventricular nodal pathways in the Lown-Ganong-Levine syndrome

Bauernfeind and colleagues[31] from Chicago, Illinois, analyzed antegrade dual AV nodal pathways, with or without AV nodal reentrant tachycardia, in 160 patients. A-H intervals reflecting antegrade fast pathway conduction ranged from 46–234 ms (mean, 91 ± 30, SD). The longest atrial paced cycle lengths at which block occurred in the antegrade fast pathway averaged 435 ± 112 ms. Retrograde fast pathway conduction was present at a ventricular paced cycle length slightly shorter than the sinus rhythm in 84 of 125 patients. Retrograde fast pathway conduction was intact at a cycle length of 375 ms in 41 of 124 patients. Eleven of 16 with an A-H inverval <60 ms, 22 of 57 with an interval 60–90 ms, 7 of 41 with an interval 91–130 ms, and 1 of 10 with an A-H interval >130 ms also had intact retrograde fast pathway conduction. Sustained AV nodal reentrant tachycardia could be induced in 51 of 160 patients. Seven of 17 patients with an A-H interval <60 ms, 27 of 72 with an interval 60–90 ms, 15 of 59 with an interval 91–130, and 2 of 10 with an interval >130 ms had sustained AV nodal reentrant tachycardia induced. Thus, in patients with dual AV nodal pathways, there are relations between the A-H interval and the ability of the fast pathway to sustain sequential antegrade conduction, and between the A-H interval and the ability of the fast pathway to sustain sequential retrograde conduction. Patients with a shorter A-H interval are more likely to have AV nodal reentrant tachycardia.

Surgery for WPW syndrome

Holmes and associates[32] from Rochester, Minnesota, described findings in 25 patients with the preexcitation syndrome who underwent operation for ablation of an accessory pathway. The mean age of the patients was 28 years and 20% had congenital heart disease. In 24, markedly symptomatic refractory SVT has been present for a mean of 13 years. The accessory pathway was RV or LV free wall in 22 patients and septal in 3 patients. Operation resulted in persistent ablation of the pathway in 80% of the patients. There was no perioperative mortality and no persistent complete heart block. During a mean follow-up of 16 months, 83% of patients with a preoperative history of SVT had no recurrence of the arrhythmia. Two patients (8%) had macroreentry paroxysmal SVT related to a persistently functioning bypass tract. The remaining 2 patients had SVT unrelated to a functioning accessory pathway. The authors concluded that the surgical treatment of patients with WPW syndrome is safe and effective. It should be considered in patients who are markedly symptomatic with refractory SVT, in those who have excessive potential for sudden cardiac death, in younger patients with symptomatic SVT in whom there is concern about the long-term effects of antiarrhythmic treatment, and in patients with SVT who are undergoing cardiac surgery for repair of associated conditions.

Burchell[33] from Minneapolis, Minnesota, wrote an accompanying editorial to the article by Holmes and associates to endorse the surgical approach to the arrhythmogenic preexcitation states; to underscore the complex nature of the arrhythmias with their exciting challenges for continued investigation; to suggest that while surgical therapy for paroxysmal tachycardia related to atavistic remnants of AV connections has now been established and is no longer experimental, it is not the proper province for the occasional procedure by a cardiac surgeon; and, as a corollary to these, to note that the patient for whom surgery for an arrhythmia is planned deserves study by clinicians, electrophysiologists, and surgeons who possess a dedication to and experience in this area.

VENTRICULAR ARRHYTHMIAS

Q-T prolongation and polymorphous ventricular arrhythmias with organophosphorus insecticide poisoning

Ludomirsky and associates[34] from Kfar-Saba, Tel-Aviv, Haifa, and Afula, Israel, evaluated 15 patients with organophosphorus poisoning and found Q-T prolongation in 14 and malignant ventricular tachyarrhythmias. Ventricular pacing was tried in 4 patients and successfully shortened the Q-T interval and eliminated the arrhythmias in all 4. Isoproterenol did the same in the fifth patient. The authors found that careful ECG monitoring was necessary until the Q-T interval returned to normal in such patients and that electrical pacing appeared to be an effective means for treating tachyarrhythmias arising as a complication of organophosphorus poisoning.

Treatment with acebutolol or quinidine

Shapiro and associates[35] from Dallas, Texas, studied 20 volunteers in a randomized double-blind crossover trial to evaluate the effects of acebutolol and sustained release quinidine sulfate. These patients had an average of ≥10/hour VPC on 2 24-hour ECG recordings, or ≥10/minute VPC during 2 cycle stress tests, or any number of complex forms of ventricular ectopic activity on either test. Acebutolol, 300 mg 3 times daily, produced effective beta receptor blockade and was better tolerated than sustained release quinidine sulfate in identical doses and had equal suppressant effects on ventricular ectopic activity.

Treatment with imipramine hydrochloride

Giardina and Bigger[36] from New York City studied 22 patients with ≥30 VPC without psychologic depression to determine the antiarrhythmic efficacy of imipramine and its half-life elimination and duration of action. Imipramine was given in a dosage of 1 mg/kg/day in 2 divided doses. Each day a 24-hour continuous ECG was recorded to determine the frequency of VPC and heart rate. During the acute dose-ranging period, 18 patients (82%) had an antiarrhythmic effect from imipramine. Two patients received 5 mg/kg/day without any decrease in frequency of VPC. The half-life of elimination of imipramine was 8.8 ± 3.72 hours but its duration of action was considerably longer. Four patients had treatment discontinued because of adverse side effects during a follow-up period of 19 ± 8.8 months. These data demonstrate that imipramine is a potent antiarrhythmic agent with a long duration of action and relatively few adverse side effects.

Treatment with mexiletine

Mehta and Conti[37] from Gainesville, Florida, studied 12 patients to determine the effectiveness of mexiletine, a new class 1 antiarrhythmic agent, in reducing VPC. Eleven patients completed 4 weeks of the trial with mexiletine and placebo with ambulatory Holter ECG recordings obtained at the end of each treatment period. Doses of mexiletine administered were designed to reduce the frequency of VPC ≥50% from baseline values. Mexiletine significantly reduced the rate of VPC by comparison with placebo (−66% -vs- 3%, p = 0.032). Mexiletine also reduced the median number/hour of ventricular couplets. Following 4 weeks of mexiletine therapy, 2, 2, 1, and 6 patients were taking 100, 200, 300, and 400 mg of mexiletine every 8 hours, respectively. Mexiletine produced no significant change in baseline values, including ECG intervals, BP, or heart rate. Mexiletine produced adverse side effects in 8 patients, including digestive difficulties and 7 other patients had central nervous system effects. These data demonstrate that mexiletine is efficacious and relatively safe for treatment of patients with VPC.

Implications during 24-hour ambulatory monitoring during catheterization

Califf and associates[38] in Durham, North Carolina, evaluated the prognostic importance of ventricular arrhythmias detected in 24-hour ambulatory monitoring in 395 patients with and 260 patients without significant CAD. Ventricular arrhythmias were found to be most strongly related to abnormal LV function, i.e., a LV EF of <40%. A modification of the Lown grading scheme was the most useful for classifying ventricular arrhythmias according to prognostic importance. When noninvasive characteristics were considered, the arrhythmia score contributed independent prognostic information, and the complexity of ventricular arrhythmias as measured by this score was related inversely to survival. When invasive measurements were used, however, the ventricular arrhythmia score did not contribute independent prognostic information. These data suggest that the LV EF is more useful than the ventricular arrhythmia score in identifying patients at high risk of sudden death.

Right ventricular dysplasia

Marcus and colleagues[39] from Paris, France, and Tucson, Arizona, reviewed patients with a RV dysplasia that is characterized by an abnormality in the development of part of the RV musculature. Patients with RV dysplasia may present with VT, supraventricular arrhythmias, right-sided CHF or asymptomatic cardiomegaly. Twenty-two adult patients with RV dysplasia who had recurrent VT were seen over a 7-year period. Males predominated over females by a ratio of 2.7:1, and the mean age at the time of hospitalization was 31 years. All except 1 patient had VT of a left BBB configuration. The heart was usually enlarged and the pulmonary vascularity appeared normal. Two-D echo in 6 patients showed increased RV diastolic dimension. All patients underwent RV angiography and the diagnosis of RV dysplasia was substantiated at surgery in 12 patients and at autopsy in another. This unique experience combined with a review of 34 previously reported adult cases provides a composite clinical profile of this condition in the adult.

Exercise provocable right ventricular outflow ventricular tachycardia

Palileo and colleagues[40] from Chicago, Illinois, identified 6 patients who met inclusion criteria of exertional palpitations, reproducible treadmill provocable VT, and performance of electrophysiologic studies, including isoproterenol infusion. There were 5 males and 1 female, aged 15–55 years.

Three patients were trained athletes, 2 had MVP, 3 had enlarged RV volumes (all trained athletes), and 2 had no evidence of organic heart disease. Treadmill exercise testing in all patients demonstrated reproducible exercise-provocable VT of at least 20 beats duration. Treadmill exercise VT was characterized by left BBB pattern QRS morphology and rates of 150–230 beats/minute. Electrophysiologic studies did not reproduce VT in 5 of 6 patients, whereas isoproterenol infusion at a dose of 2–4 μg/minute reproduced VT in all patients. Isoproterenol-induced VT was characterized by QRS morphology identical to treadmill exercise VT and rates of 165–230 beats/minute. Endocardial mapping of isoproterenol-induced VT revealed earliest activity in RV outflow tract. Serial treadmill exercise testing revealed suppression of exercise-VT in all 6 patients on propranolol therapy. Responses to class I drugs were variable and less successful. Thus, this subset of patients with common clinical, ECG, and electrophysiologic features share a common pathophysiology of VT.

Occult myocardial dysfunction with ventricular arrhythmias unassociated with clinically apparent heart disease

Kennedy and associates[41] from Baltimore, Maryland, studied 18 asymptomatic patients without apparent cardiac disease who were incidentally discovered to have frequent ventricular ectopic activity (mean, >100 beats/h during 24-h ambulatory ECG examination), and who were found by cardiac catheterization to have normal coronary arteriograms. Thirteen patients (72%) also demonstrated complex (multiform or repetitive patterns) of ventricular ectopic activity and 8 patients were found to have undiagnosed hypertension. The LV angiographic and hemodynamic data showed elevated LV end-systolic volume index in 10 patients (56%), elevated LV end-diastolic volume index in 12 (67%), and elevated LV end-diastolic pressure in 11 patients (61%). Although the EF of all but 3 patients was normal, impaired myocardial contractility, as measured by decreased mean velocity of circumferential fiber shortening (<1.0 circ/s), was found in 10 patients (56%). Abnormalities of LV function were more prevalent in patients with higher mean frequencies of ventricular ectopic activity (>300 beats/h), but did not seem related to the presence of complex types of ventricular ectopic activity. Etiologic mechanisms of the frequent and complex ventricular ectopic activity could not be defined. Thus, subclinical evidence of myocardial dysfunction is present in some persons without apparent cardiac disease who have frequent ventricular ectopic activity as evidenced by subtle abnormalities of increased LV volumes and end-diastolic pressure and decreased mean velocity of myocardial circumferential fiber shortening.

Sequential regional phase mapping or radionuclide-gated biventriculograms in sustained ventricular tachycardia

Mapping of VT has been employed as a guide to surgical therapy for this rhythm disturbance. Currently, mapping requires invasive techniques either in the electrophysiology laboratory or in the operating room. It has been recently reported that Fourier analysis and related techniques of gated RNA provide noninvasive data reflecting abnormalities of ventricular activation. Accordingly, RNA gated studies were performed by Swiryn and associates[42] from Chicago, Illinois, during sinus rhythm and during spontaneous or induced sustained VT in 6 patients with clinical VT. Fourier analysis of time-activity variation was used to calculate a RNA phase value for each pixel in the image. Color coding of each pixel according to the calculated phase resulted in a RNA phase map of the ventricle. The following results were considered to be consistent with the known electrophysiology of VT: 1) the phase map correlated with QRS morphology and axis in most but not all tachycardias; 2) earliest phase usually demonstrated the VT origin to be at the border of the ventricular wall motion abnormality; 3) endocardial mapping (available in 1 patient) showed close correlation with RNA phase mapping; 4) in 3 patients with CAD, VT with left BBB pattern had earliest LV phase along the septum; and 5) for 1 patient imaged during 2 different VT morphologies, the tachycardias had earliest phase at different borders of the same wall motion abnormality with differing progression of phase across the ventricles. Thus, RNA phase mapping of VT is feasible and appears to provide data consistent with the electrophysiology of this arrhythmia.

Multiformity of induced unifocal ventricular premature contractions

Booth and associates[43] from Chapel Hill, North Carolina, studied 30 patients undergoing cardiac catheterization to determine under what circumstances unifocal stimulated VPC could demonstrate multiformity of the QRS configuration. Multiformity was defined as unifocal response whose mean frontal axes differed by >15% with or without associated morphologic differences in the horizontal leads. Multiformity occurred in 12 (40%) of 30 patients. A statistically significant association was found between multiformity and LV wall motion abnormalities ($p < 0.01$), previous AMI ($p < 0.01$), and a LV EF of <60% ($p < 0.05$). Of the patients with multiformity 67% had CAD, but only 4 of these had a LV wall motion abnormality, prior AMI, or both. Multiformity was also dependent on the site of stimulation and on the degree of prematurity. These data demonstrate that the QRS configuration in early VPC cannot be used to indicate multifocal VPC nor to identify the site of origin of such beats.

Responses to programmed ventricular stimulation

Livelli and associates[44] from New York City studied 100 patients to determine the sensitivity and specificity of the repetitive ventricular response and VT induced by programmed electrical stimulation for identifying patients with spontaneous ventricular tachyarrhythmias. The authors found that the repetitive ventricular response was sensitive (92%) in the detection of patients with prior spontaneous ventricular tachyarrhythmias, but that it lacked specificity (57%). Indeed, the rate of false positive responses was 43%.

Inducible VT was less sensitive (65%) but more specific (98%); the rate of false positive responses was only 3%. In the 100 patients, 71 had heart disease and 29 did not. It was impossible to demonstrate that the presence of underlying heart disease had any significant effect on the sensitivity and specificity of repetitive ventricular responses or VT induced by programmed stimulation and it did not appear to increase the incidence of false positive responses. These data suggest that VT induced with programmed ventricular stimulation provides a good means for guiding the management of clinically significant ventricular tachyarrhythmias, irrespective of underlying heart disease, and that the repetitive ventricular response is not useful for this purpose because of its high rate of false positive responses among patients with or without significant heart disease.

Significance of repetitive ventricular response during programmed ventricular stimulation

Breithardt and associates[45] from Dusseldorf, West Germany, studied 65 patients to determine the incidence and prognostic significance of the repetitive ventricular response in predicting sudden death. Programmed RV stimulation was performed at a basic pacing rate of 120 beats/minute using 1 and 2 premature stimuli. Data were analyzed as to the presence or absence of a repetitive ventricular response and the patients' outcome subsequently determined. A repetitive ventricular response was observed in 23 (35%) of 65 patients after 1 and in 31 (48%) of 64 patients after 2 premature stimuli. It occurred in all 9 patients with VF and in 14 (82%) of 17 patients with VT. The mean follow-up period was 76 ± 39 weeks. Sixteen patients were classified as dying suddenly; the remaining patients survived or died nonsuddenly. After 1 premature stimulus, a repetitive ventricular response was observed in 33% of patients surviving or with nonsudden death and in 44% of patients with sudden death or malignant ventricular arrhythmias. After 2 premature stimuli, the incidence of a repetitive ventricular response increased from 41% in patients surviving or with nonsudden death to 69% in patients with sudden death. All nonsurviving patients who demonstrated a repetitive ventricular response had intraventricular reentry. Therefore the sensitivity of the test ranged between 37% and 88% and specificity between 45% and 92%, depending on the rigidity of the statistical criteria utilized. The proportion of false positive results was high (33–66%), but the proportion of false negative results was low (8–18%). Thus, these data show a correlation between sudden death and the incidence and number of repetitive ventricular responses, but there was a high incidence of false positive results.

Effect of encainide on programmed electrical stimulation and ventricular arrhythmia frequency

Duff and associates[46] from Nashville, Tennessee, studied the influence of encainide in the treatment of nonlife-threatening arrhythmias. Eight patients with chronic ventricular arrhythmias who had suppression of the ventricular ectopic activity by ambulatory monitoring during 6 months of outpatient treatment with encainide underwent programmed electrical stimulation testing in a drug-free state. Patients were assigned randomly to receive placebo or encainide. Thereafter, electrophysiologic testing was performed twice daily immediately before and 1 hour after administration of either placebo or encainide. In patients receiving encainide, the repetitive ventricular response was neither consistently absent during periods of arrhythmia suppression nor consistently present during periods of arrhythmia recurrence. Four patients showed increased ease of inducibility of the repetitive ventricular response during periods when encainide had suppressed the spontaneous ventricular arrhythmias. Three of 4 patients assigned randomly to placebo therapy initially manifested a repetitive ventricular response. Therefore time-dependent variations in cardiac electrophysiologic measurements should be taken into account when programmed electrical stimulation at a single electrode site is used to evaluate drug therapy. The presence or absence of the repetitive ventricular response bore no relation to arrhythmia frequency as encainide was administered or withdrawn.

Electrophysiologic testing for managing patients with ventricular tachycardia unrelated to CAD

Naccarelli and associates[47] from Indianapolis, Indiana, studied 83 patients with VT not due to CAD to establish the usefulness of programmed electrical stimulation in their management. In 39 patients with a history of sustained VT, programmed stimulation induced VT in 14 of 14 patients with MVP or primary electrical disease and in 13 of 25 with cardiomyopathy. Programmed stimulation induced nonsustained VT in 15 of 44 patients with a history of nonsustained VT. Of the 83 patients, 73 were treated with antiarrhythmic agents and followed for 14.4 ± 11.4 months. Drug therapy was determined with serial electrophysiologic testing in 31 patients. Twenty-four of these 31 patients had a history of sustained VT, and drugs prevented induction of VT in 9 but did not prevent it in 15. In 7 patients with a history of nonsustained VT, drugs prevented induction of VT in 5 and did not prevent it in 2. Forty-two patients were treated using the results of noninvasive testing. Drugs suppressed spontaneous VT in 15 of 15 patients with a history of sustained VT and in 26 of 27 with a history of nonsustained VT. Thus, in patients with VT unrelated to CAD, these data suggest the following: 1) programmed electrical stimulation induced VT less often than in patients whose VT was due to CAD; 2) programmed stimulation induced VT less often in patients with a history of nonsustained -vs- sustained VT; and 3) suppression of inducible VT appeared to predict effective drug therapy.

Importance of stimulation at more than 1 ventricular site during electrophysiologic drug testing in ventricular arrhythmias

Morady, and colleagues[48] from San Francisco, California, evaluated 64 patients with symptomatic VT or VF utilizing RV apical programmed stimulation to determine the efficacy of drug suppression of malignant ventricular arrhythmias. Thirty patients (group 1) did not undergo LV stimulation; LV stimulation in 38 drug trials induced no VT in 50% (group IIA), nonsustained VT in 26% (group IIB), and sustained VT in 24% (group IIC). Patients in groups I, IIA, and IIB received chronic antiarrhythmic drug therapy based on the results of electrophysiologic drug testing. Patients in group IIC underwent further drug testing until sustained VT was no longer inducible and were then entered in either group IIA or group IIB; 4 patients in whom the induction of sustained VT could not be suppressed by any drug regimen were excluded from long-term follow-up. The duration of follow-up was 15.8 ± 11.5 months in group I, 13.6 ± 3.7 months in group IIA, and 12.1 ± 4.9 months in group IIB. Recurrence rates of symptomatic VT or sudden death were 27% in group I, 0% in group IIA, and 20% in group IIB. These data suggest that approximately 50% of drug trials may be judged incorrectly as suppressing the induction of VT if only RV apical stimulation is performed during electrophysiologic drug testing in patients with malignant ventricular arrhythmias. Drug therapy that suppresses VT induction with both RV and LV programmed stimulation results in a significantly better clinical response than therapy based on the results of only RV apical stimulation.

Prediction of response to class 1 antiarrhythmic drugs during electrophysiologic testing

Swiryn and colleagues[49] from Chicago, Illinois, retrospectively examined data from 41 patients studied in their laboratory for symptomatic ventricular arrhythmias to test whether any clinical or electrophysiologic variables could be identified which would predict the patient's response to class I antiarrhythmic drugs. All patients had 1) clinically documented paraoxysmal sustained VT or VF remote from AMI, 2) inducible sustained VT during control electrophysiologic study, and 3) electrophysiologic study after ≥1 of the following class I antiarrhythmic drugs: intravenous procainamide (36 patients), oral quinidine (30 patients), and oral disopyramide (36 patients). Initially, patients were divided into those who had noninducible or only nonsustained VT after any 1 of the tested drugs (responders), and those who continued to have inducible sustained VT after all tested drugs (nonresponders). A logistic regression technique demonstrated no independent contribution to drug response by any of the following variables: sex, arteriosclerotic heart disease, cardiomegaly, age, time since the initial episode of VT, and cycle length of VT during control study. The number of antiarrhythmic drugs the patient had received before study was found to be a significant independent contributor, with responders having received an average of 2.5 drugs compared with 4.2 for nonresponders. In addition to the logistic regression, 12 other clinical and electrophysiologic variables were not predictors of drug response. It was also evaluated whether response or nonresponse to 1 class I drug predicts response or nonresponse to the other such drugs. Significant concordance of response and nonresponse was demonstrated for procainamide and quinidine, but not for either of these drugs and disopyramide. Thus, drug therapy for inducible sustained VT remains empiric.

Treatment with amiodarone

The antiarrhythmic efficacy and the electrophysiologic effects of amiodarone were determined by Nademanee and colleagues[50] from Los Angeles, California, in 13 consecutive patients with symptomatic life-threatening ventricular arrhythmias resistant to conventional agents. Amiodarone was initially given in high dosages (1,000–1,800 mg/daily); electrophysiologic effects, including induction of VT by programmed electrical stimulation, was undertaken before and after a mean period of 28 days of amiodarone therapy. Plasma drug levels determined by high pressure liquid chromatography were within the therapeutic range (0.92–11.99 mg/liter). Antiarrhythmic efficacy was determined on the basis of the quantitative analysis of 24-hour Holter recordings. Amiodarone reduced heart rate (−18%), lengthened P-R interval (+15%), A-H interval (+20%), and the Q-T_c by 13%, without effect on the QRS or H-V intervals. The atrial effective refractory period increased by 31% and the ventricular effective refractory period by 22%; effective refractory period of the AV node also increased, but could not be determined in all patients because of the longer refractory period of the atrium. Before amiodarone, AV Wenckebach during atrial pacing developed at a heart rate of 150 beats/minute and at 117 beats/minute during amiodarone therapy. In all 13 patients, amiodarone reduced the total counts of VPC by 95%–98% and eliminated complex ventricular ectopic activity and runs of VT. The effect has been sustained during a mean follow-up period of 12 months and there have been no symptoms. Before amiodarone was given, VT could be induced by programmed electrical stimulation in 12 of 13 patients (7 sustained, 5 nonsustained). On amiodarone, VT was provoked in 4 (3 sustained, 1 nonsustained). Side effects have included photosensitivity, proximal muscle weakness, elevation of hepatic enzymes, halo vision, and corneal deposits but without impaired vision; these could be reduced in severity or avoided by reduction in drug dosage. These data indicate that amiodarone is highly potent in suppressing symptomatic life-threatening VTs (VPC, ventricular ectopic activity, VT, and VF) without always being able to prevent the induction of VT by programmed electrical stimulation of the heart. The drug can be used in this context without the need for invasive electrophysiologic studies.

Waxman and associates[51] from Philadelphia, Pennsylvania, evaluated electrophysiologic effects of amiodarone and its ability to control ventricular arrhythmias in 51 patients with refractory sustained ventricular arrhythmia. Amiodarone was administered in doses of 400–800 mg/day and it prolonged refractoriness in the atria, AV junction, and ventricle and conduction through the AV node and His-Purkinje system. Clinical effectiveness was evaluated in 46 patients followed for 8.6 ± 6 months. It provided effective suppression of arrhythmias in 23 (50%); it was partly effective in 13 (28%) and ineffective in 10 (22%). Adverse effects occurred in 28 (55%) of 51 patients and in 11 (22%) patients the drug had to be discontinued because of adverse effects. These data suggest that amiodarone should be reserved for patients with life-threatening sustained ventricular arrhythmias because of the significant incidence of adverse effects. Good clinical effects and suppression of ventricular arrhythmias chronically can be observed in patients receiving amiodarone despite continued ability to induce these arrhythmias electrophysiologically.

Detailed electrophysiologic studies were performed by Finerman and colleagues[52] from Los Angeles, California, in 9 patients with chronic refractory ventricular arrhythmias before and after 7–20 weeks (mean, 11) of amiodarone therapy. The amiodarone dose at the time of the repeat study ranged from 400–800 mg/day. The drug reduced the sinus rate and prolonged the sinoatrial conduction time with some prolongation of the corrected sinus node recovery time. Intraatrial conduction was slightly prolonged both in sinus rhythm and during atrial pacing. Antegrade conduction through the AV node was significantly prolonged both in sinus rhythm and during atrial pacing, and Wenckebach AV block was seen at significantly lower atrial pacing rates after the drug. The H-V interval was prolonged both in sinus rhythm and during atrial pacing, and so was the QRS width during atrial pacing and the Q-T interval in sinus rhythm and during atrial pacing. Significant prolongation of the refractory periods in the atrium, AV node, and ventricular muscle, were also seen following the drug. Thus, significant electrophysiologic effects of this drug throughout the heart during chronic oral use attest to its clinical effectiveness in patients with atrial and ventricular arrhythmias. With appropriate care and despite its effects on the H-V interval and QRS width, amiodarone can be used in patients with intraventricular conduction defects complicating severe organic heart disease.

Treatment with mexiletine

Palileo and colleagues[53] from Chicago, Illinois, evaluated the efficacy of oral mexiletine in the therapy of recurrent VT in 17 patients (13 men and 4 women; mean age, 62 years) who had drug-refractory paroxysmal sustained VT associated with CAD in 14, valvular heart disease in 1, and primary myocardial disease in 1, and no heart disease in 1. All 17 patients had inducible sustained VT during the control electrophysiologic study and during serial electrophysiologic study on conventional drugs. Eleven patients tolerated a mean maximal daily dose of 1,073 ± 149 mg of mexiletine and underwent programmed ventricular stimulation; sustained VT was inducible in 10 patients and nonsustained VT in 1. In 10 patients with inducible sustained VT on mexiletine, the VT cycle length was longer during mexiletine therapy than during control. Programmed stimulation was not possible in 1 patient with severe neurologic side effects and in 5 patients with mexiletine-related worsening of ventricular arrhythmia. Seven patients had severe neurologic or gastrointestinal side effects, necessitating dose reduction in 5. The 47% incidence of noncardiovascular side effects is similar to that reported by others, but the 29% incidence of arrhythmia potentiation by mexiletine is higher than that noted by other investigators. Limited follow-up revealed recurrence of VT in 3 of 4 patients treated with oral mexiletine on a long-term basis. These data suggest that oral mexiletine may not be useful in the therapy of patients with drug-refractory, paroxysmal sustained VT. Its use is associated with a high incidence of adverse effects.

Treatment with bethanidine sulfate

Bacaner and Benditt[54] from Minneapolis, Minnesota, evaluated bethanidine sulfate, a chemical and pharmacologic analog of bretylium tosylate that has essentially identical antifibrillatory and inotropic actions in the heart. However, bethanidine sulfate is absorbed rapidly from the gastrointestinal tract in contrast to the poor absorption found with bretylium. Bethanidine was given to 23 patients with recurrent multiple drug refractory VT and VF. Eighteen patients (78%) had complete suppression of spontaneous and electrophysiologically inducible arrhythmias, 3 were improved, and 2 derived no benefit. In 6 of 9 patients in a small subgroup that was studied by programmed electrophysiologic drug testing, bethanidine completely prevented previously inducible ventricular tachyarrhythmias at the maximal stimulus tested. Bethanidine did not decrease cardiac output significantly. Ten patients on long-term therapy with bethanidine and protriptyline (to prevent orthostatic hypotension) were without detected arrhythmias for 2–26 (average, 13) months. The data suggest that bethanidine sulfate may be a useful addition to the armamentarium for the treatment of drug-resistant ventricular arrhythmias.

Acebutolol -vs- propanolol

Singh and colleagues[55] from Washington, DC, compared the effects on ventricular arrhythmia of acebutolol with those of propranolol in 31 patients who averaged more than 30 VPC per hour during 72 hours of ambulatory ECG monitoring. The treatment during the double-blind period was randomized to either oral acebutolol or propranolol given 3 times daily. Ambulatory ECG and maximal treadmill tests were performed after 1 and 5 weeks of therapy. Acebutolol and propranolol produced comparable levels of adrenergic blocade as reflected by significant reductions in mean heart rate during 24-hour ambulatory ECG and peak exercise compared with placebo. Acebutolol and propranolol produced comparable and significant reductions in VPC frequency during ambulatory ECG and exercise testing compared with placebo. Each agent produced similar and significant reductions in mean VPC grade compared with placebo during ambulatory ECG. No clinical or laboratory side effects of either agent necessitated drug discontinuance. These investigators concluded that acebutolol is a well tolerated beta blocking agent that compares favorably with propranolol in reducing the frequency and complexity of VPC at rest and during maximal exercise. Thus, acebutolol represents an important therapeutic addition to beta adrenergic blocking agents.

Various drug combinations

Combinations of antiarrhythmic drugs are frequently employed to treat refractory VT, but there are few data to support this form of therapy. Ross and colleagues[56] from Stanford, California, examined the efficacy and electrophysiology of 110 antiarrhythmic drug combination trials at electrophysiologic study in 74 patients with recurrent VT. Lidocaine was combined with quinidine in 33 trials, procainamide in 22 and encainide in 20. Propanolol was combined with quinidine in 17 trials, procainamide in 12, and encainide in 6. All individual drugs tested, except propranolol, which was usually not tested individually, had failed at electrophysiologic study or clinically in the presence of usually accepted plasma concentrations. Lidocaine in combination with quinidine was effective in 3% of the trials, with procainamide, in 5%, and with encainide in none of the trials. Propranolol in combination with quinidine was effective in 18% of the trials, with procainamide, in 17%, and with encainide in no trial. The electrophysiologic effects of the tested drug combinations were dominated by the individual effects of the type 1 antiarrhythmic agents. Thus, the tested antiarrhythmic drug combinations appear infrequently effective in preventing VT induction at electrophysiologic study when each agent has failed individually. The addition of lidocaine or propranolol to quinidine, procainamide, and encainide does not produce significant synergistic or new effects on the electrophysiologic variables analyzed.

Drug conversion of nonsustained to sustained ventricular tachycardia

Programmed electrical stimulation of the heart is a useful method to test drug effectiveness in recurrent VT, since patients who have inducible VT before but not after drug therapy usually do not have recurrence of VT while taking that drug. In addition, the demonstration is important of induction by programmed electrical stimulation of sustained VT during drug therapy in patients who only have nonsustained VT induced while receiving no drug therapy, since it is as necessary to avoid selecting a potentially harmful antiarrhythmic agent as it is to select an efficacious one. Rinkenberger and colleagues[57] from Indianapolis, Indiana, evaluated 11 of 83 patients who had VT and underwent serial electrophysiologic study with a more severe VT induced while receiving a particular antiarrhythmic drug compared with control study. For all patients, only nonsustained VT was initiated during control study, whereas sustained VT occurred during testing with disopyramide (2 patients), quinidine (2 patients), amiodarone (4 patients), and encainide (7 patients). Pacing techniques used to induce sustained VT were the same as those used in the control study in 8 patients and were less aggressive in 3 patients. Almost all episodes of sustained VT resulted in substantial hypotension, especially in patients who were taking encainide. Drugs associated with sustained VT increased the median tachycardia cycle length by 112 ms but increased the median ventricular effective refractory period by only 30 ms. Assuming reentry was responsible for VT, it is postulated that these drugs facilitated initiation of sustained VT by prolonging activation time while only minimally increasing refractoriness of the tachycardia circuit. Since induction of VT at programmed electrical stimulation appears to correlate with subsequent spontaneous recurrence of VT, this study shows that electrophysiologic study can be used to identify drugs that are potentially life-threatening to the patient.

Aggravation and provocation of ventricular arrhythmias by antiarrhythmic drugs

Antiarrhythmic drugs may aggravate or even induce ventricular arrhythmias. Velebit and associates[58] from Boston, Massachusetts, emphasized that this type of adverse reaction is becoming more prevalent as the use of antiarrhythmic agents become more widespread. In a retrospective analysis of antiarrhythmic drug action, these investigators documented a worsening of arrhythmias in 80 of 722 antiarrhythmic drug tests in 53 of 155 patients being treated for ventricular tachyarrhythmias. Aggravation of arrhythmias was defined as a 4-fold increase in the frequency of VPC, a 10-fold increase in repetitive forms, or the first emergence of sustained VT coincident with the time course of action of the particular drug under study. Such aggravation was observed with each of 9 drugs tested and included quinidine, procainamide, disopyramide, propranolol, metoprolol, aprindine, mexiletine, tocainide, and pindolol. The frequency of this complication for a specific drug ranged from 6%–16%. Drug blood concentrations were consistently in the therapeutic range. A study of the variability of ventricular arrhythmia during 48-hour Holter monitoring and exercise stress testing in no instance showed antiarrhythmic enhancement commensurate with that defining aggravation. Thus, these data suggest that this potentially serious complication is not readily predictable and requires a systematic approach to antiarrhythmic drug testing before a patient is prescribed a long-range maintenance program.

Prolonged survival with antiarrhythmic drugs

Graboys and associates[59] from Boston, Massachusetts, evaluated the protective effect of antiarrhythmic agents in 123 patients with malignant ventricular arrhythmias, including VF not caused by AMI or sustained VT causing hemodynamic deterioration. The studies were to determine survival dependent on the ability of antiarrhythmic drugs to prevent salvos of VT and R-on-T VPC. There were 35 deaths during an average follow-up of 30 months; in 23 patients death occurred suddenly, providing an 8.2 annual mortality rate. In 98 patients in whom antiarrhythmic drugs abolished the serious ventricular ectopic activity, only 6 sudden deaths occurred for a 2.3% annual mortality rate. In 25 patients in whom advanced VPC were not controlled, 17 died suddenly. In 44 patients with LV dysfunction (LV EF <50%), control of VPC was a critical element in predicting survival. The annual sudden death rate for the 12 noncontrolled patients with LV dysfunction was 41% compared with only 3.1% for the 32 patients with similar abnormalities in ventricular function in whom advanced VPC were abolished. Therefore, antiarrhythmic drugs can protect against the recurrence of life-threatening arrhythmias in patients who develop VF or VT.

Termination of ventricular tachycardia with ventricular stimulation by increased current strength

Waxman and associates[60] from Philadelphia, Pennsylvania, evaluated the effect of increased stimulus current strength on the RV effective refractory period (ERP) during sustained VT and on the ability of single premature RV stimuli to terminate VT. The studies were performed in 53 episodes of sustained VT in 25 patients. Of the 53 episodes, 44 were slowed by pharmacologic therapy. Current intensities of twice diastolic threshold, 5 mA and 10 mA, were employed. Increasing current from twice diastolic threshold to 5 mA shortened the mean ERP from 206–176 ms. There was a direct correlation between cycle length of VT and the ERP measured at twice diastolic threshold. The cycle length of VT and the amount of shortening of ERP as current was increased were not significantly correlated. Eleven episodes of VT that could not be terminated by ventricular stimulation at twice diastolic threshold were terminated when increased current strength was used. Thus, the ability to terminate VT was associated with a decrease in ERP and long tachycardia cycle length. The mean cycle length of the 11 episodes terminated was 455 ms compared with 381 ms in the 42 episodes not terminated at increased current.

Transvenous cardioversion via a catheter electrode

The study by Zipes and colleagues[61] from Indianapolis, Indiana, was to test the efficacy, safety, and patient tolerance of transvenous cardioversion and defibrillation in patients who had recurrent ventricular tachyarrhythmias. In 5 of 7 patients, a truncated exponential shock of 0.025–2.0 J synchronized to the QRS complex terminated 47 episodes of recurrent sustained VT. Cardioversion threshold was ≤0.25 J in 3 patients and 0.75–2.0 J in 2 patients. Shocks of 0.75 and 2.0 J failed to terminate VT in 1 patient each; higher energies were not tried because of hemodynamic decompensation. In 1 patient, a shock of 25 J terminated VF on 3 occasions, and in another patient a shock of 1.0 J terminated AF on 1 occasion. Shocks ≤0.5 J were well tolerated by the awake unsedated patient. Of 141 synchronized shocks (including subthreshold shocks), 140 produced no repetitive ventricular activity. In 1 seriously ill patient who had received multiple antiarrhythmic drugs and required balloon counterpulsation for hemodynamic support, on a single occasion each a synchronized transvenous shock and a synchronized conventional transthoracic shock produced ventricular flutter and VF, respectively. Thus, synchronized transvenous cardioversion by a catheter electrode offers promise as a new therapeutic approach for recurrent VT refractory to drug therapy, with eventual promise as a totally implanted system for chronic use.

Termination by a new pacing method

Gardner and associates[62] from Philadelphia, Pennsylvania, developed a new pacing technique for the determination of VT. Rapid ventricular pacing at cycle lengths 10–100 ms shorter than the VT cycle length and the introduction of 1 or 2 ventricular extrastimuli were assessed in 25 patients in whom ventricular extrastimuli and rapid ventricular pacing, delivered at cycle lengths and coupling intervals comparable to those used in the new method, had been unsuccessful. This combination method successfully terminated VT in 21 of 25 patients with cycle lengths of 230–400 ms. VT was terminated in 6 of 8 patients receiving drugs in whom VT could not be terminated by 1 or 2 ventricular extrastimuli or rapid ventricular pacing. This new technique was successful in 6 of 8 patients unresponsive to ventricular extrastimuli and in whom rapid ventricular pacing produced acceleration of VT, and in all 9 patients in whom antiarrhythmic agents made VT unresponsive to ventricular extrastimuli or rapid ventricular pacing. Thus, a combination of rapid pacing and extrastimuli can terminate VT unresponsive to ventricular extrastimuli or rapid pacing alone and may avoid acceleration of VT using rapid ventricular pacing at very short cycle lengths for termination.

SURGICAL TREATMENT OF VENTRICULAR TACHYCARDIA

To determine why some patients with a previous AMI develop serious or life-threatening ventricular arrhythmias, Klein and associates[63] from Birmingham, Alabama, performed electrophysiologic ventricular mapping during sinus rhythm in 38 patients during open heart surgery for CAD. Twenty-nine patients had a LV aneurysm or dyskinetic area, 8 had an akinetic area, and 1 had a severe hypokinetic area. Twenty-one had ventricular arrhythmias, 16 of whom had recurrent, sustained VT. Epicardial mapping was performed in all 38 patients. Endocardial mapping was done in 10 patients. In 20 patients with ventricular arrhythmias, an area of delayed activation (>100 ms after onset of QRS complex) was found (Fig. 3-2). This type of delay was present in 2 of 17 patients without arrhythmias. Of the 21 patients with arrhythmias, 20 had fractionated electrograms (3 exclusively with endocardial mapping) and 13 patients had double potentials. Fractionation and double potentials were found in only 1 of the 17 patients without arrhythmias. Thus, in patients with previous AMI and serious ventricular arrhythmias, areas of significantly delayed epicardial

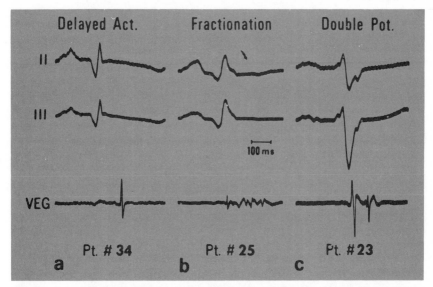

Fig. 3-2. ECG leads II and III recorded simultaneously with bipolar ventricular electrogram (VEG) in 3 patients recorded with exploring electrode. (A) Delayed activation in which ventricular electrogram occurs 145 ms after onset of QRS complex. (B) Fractionation of ventricular electrogram. (C) A double potential in which the second deflection is separated from the initial deflection by 75 ms and occurs 140 ms after the onset of the QRS complex and 12 ms after end of QRS complex. Reproduced with permission from Klein et al.[63]

activation, fractionation, and double potentials are characteristic findings of ventricular mapping during sinus rhythm, and presumably constitute the substrate for development of these arrhythmias.

To determine the correlation of regional contraction abnormalities with ventricular activation in patients with CAD, Wiener and colleagues[64] from New York City performed intraoperative epicardial mapping in 24 patients who underwent surgery for CAD. Nine patients had normally contracting ventricles, 5 had areas of hypokinesis and 10 had areas of akinesis or dyskinesis. Four patients with asynergy had VT or VF. The earliest epicardial activation occurred in the anterior right ventricle in patients with and without asynergy. Each patient with normal contraction or areas of hypokinesis had 2 LV epicardial breakthrough sites. The breakthrough site was defined as emergence of a radially propagating wave front at the epicardial surface, providing an island of early activation that was completely surrounded by points of later activation. The patients with areas of akinesis or dyskinesis had an average of 1.2 ventricular epicardial breakthrough sites. Breakthrough did not occur in areas of akinesis or dyskinesis. The latest epicardial activation occurred at the base of either ventricle in all patients with normal ventricle or areas of hypokinesis but in only 4 of 10 patients with akinesis or dyskinesis. In 6 of 10 patients with akinesis or dyskinesis, the latest activation was over an abnormally contracting segment. Regional activation time in hypokinetic zones was not significantly different from that in normal zones, but was significantly delayed in akinetic and dyskinetic zones. Among patients with asynergy, there was no difference in epicardial activation pattern between those with and those without malignant arrhythmias. Thus, akinesis and dyskinesis but not hypokinesis appear to be associated with marked changes in epicardial activation patterns.

In 7 patients with documented VT and prior AMI, late potentials (LP) were recorded by Breithardt and colleagues[65] from Düsseldorf, West Germany, at the end of or after the QRS complex from the body surface using high gain amplification and the signal averaging technique. In 6 of 7 patients, VT could be initiated by programmed RV stimulation; in 1 patient VT was inducible only from the left ventricle during surgery. Surgery was guided by epicardial and endocardial mapping. In most cases besides resection of scar tissue, a partial or complete subendocardial encircling ventriculotomy was performed. Postoperatively, LP were abolished in 5 patients, VT being no longer inducible. In the remaining 2 patients, LP were still present. VT was still inducible in 1 of these 2 patients, whereas in the other patient no programmed testing was done postoperatively. These data suggest that the abolition of LP by surgery is closely related to the disappearance of the propensity to stimulus-induced VT. Thus, the averaging technique represents a new approach to the noninvasive control of the efficacy of surgery in patients with VT and prior AMI.

Fontaine and colleagues[66] from Ivry and Paris, France, evaluated 24 patients with VT unrelated to myocardial ischemia and resistant to antiarrhythmic therapy. Surgery was performed utilizing epicardial mapping during sinus rhythm and during VT and various surgical techniques were employed, including simple ventriculotomy, encircling endocardial ventriculotomy, and cryosurgery. Aneurysmectomy associated with encircling endocardial ventriculotomy was successful in all 3 cases of idiopathic LV aneurysm during a mean follow-up of 14 months. In 12 patients with arrhythmogenic RV dysplasia, simple ventriculotomy alone or combined with small excision (4 cases) were able to prevent sustained VT in all patients except 2 whose arrhythmia was controlled subsequently by long-term antiarrhythmic therapy. Two patients died of nonarrhythmic causes 30 and 58 months after operation. One patient with Uhl's anomaly died of CHF in the postoperative period. In the 5 patients with idiopathic VT 1 was cured and 4 had recurrent postoperative episodes of VT similar to those present before operation. However, 2 of these patients had good clinical results; the arrhythmia was controlled by drugs in 1, and the other patient had only nonsymptomatic short-lasting episodes. Two patients died in the postoperative period. The mean follow-up period in these patients was 36 months. In 2 patients with nonobstructive cardiomyopathy, ventriculotomy prevented recurrences in 1 patient who died of CHF 6 months postoperatively and the other had immediate lethal recurrences. One patient had a fibroma in the ventricular septum and did not survive operation. The data suggest that surgery can either prevent or make VT simpler to control with antiarrhythmic therapy. However, the results of surgery are not perfect and some failures occur. Nevertheless, this type of surgery is relatively early in its evolution and further developments can be expected.

Ventricular arrhythmias remain a potentially lethal complication of CAD and appear related to areas of abnormal contraction, particularly LV aneurysm. Weiner and associates[67] from New York City performed epicardial and endocardial mapping in 11 patients with LV aneurysm. Six patients had chronic recurrent VT and 5 had ventricular arrhythmias no more severe than isolated VPC. Endocardial points were recorded during stable sinus rhythm in each patient and local electrograms were evaluated as to timing and presence of fragmentation. Activation of the epicardial surface of the aneurysm was abnormal in all patients and extended beyond completion of the QRS in 3 patients in the arrhythmia group and 2 in the nonarrhythmia group. Activation of the epicardial border zone was normal in all patients. Electrograms from the endocardial surface of the aneurysms were abnormally fragmented in all patients and the mean duration of activation was not different between patients with and without arrhythmias. In patients with VT, electrograms of the endocardial border zone showed fragmentation compared with a much smaller area of the endocardial border zone in patients without arrhythmias. Fragmentation was always recorded along the septal border of the aneurysm. In VT patients 5 of 6 had electrical activity in the endocardial border zone extending beyond the end of the QRS compared with only 1 of 5 patients without VT. These investigators concluded that fragmented electrical activity is present in all patients with LV aneurysm but the extent and severity of fragmentation in the endocardial border zone is greatest in patients with recurrent VT.

Of 65 patients having surgery for recurrent ventricular tachyarrhythmias and reported by Mason and colleagues[68] from Stanford, California, intraoperative electrophysiologic-directed LV surgery frequently eliminated ventricular tachyarrhythmias and probably was more effective than blind resection of LV aneurysm. Thirty-two patients (group I) underwent simple LV aneurysm resection. Thirty-three patients (group II) underwent myocardial resection or incision guided by intraoperative mapping and the electrical activation sequence. The clinical hemodynamic and angiographic characteristics of the 2 groups were similar; however, this was not a randomized study. Actuarial survival in the 2 groups was similar through 24 months; however, late attrition in group I patients left only 21 ± 13% alive by life table analysis at 94 months (Fig. 3-3). Arrhythmia occurrence was greater in group I than in group II. Death was caused by ventricular tachyarrhythmias in 12 of the 17 patients (71%) who died in group I, but arrhythmia was causal in only 3 of 12 who died in group II. However, 67% of the deaths in group II were due to CHF, and this may have been the result of myocardial injury by the map directed surgery. Thus, routine LV aneurysm resection in patients with VT is unsatisfactory. They suggest either encircling endocardial myotomy or extended endocardial resection in addition to aneurysm resection. Compared with patients without preoperative ventricular tachyarrhythmias having CABG, the survival of the patients (as reported in this and other

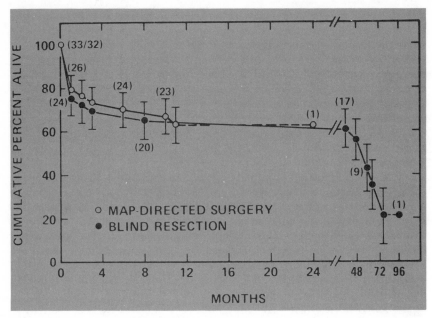

Fig. 3-3. Postoperative survival. The cumulative proportion of patients surviving in 2 groups after surgery is plotted against time. These actuarial curves show no significant difference in survival in the 2 groups through 24 months of follow-up. The subsequent decrease in survival in the blind aneurysm resection group is shown on a compressed time scale. Standard errors of the means are indicated by vertical bars. Numbers in parentheses indicate number of patients remaining in follow-up at beginning of given interval. Reproduced with permission from Mason et al.[68]

studies of patients with ventricular tachyarrhythmias) is appreciably less satisfactory.

The surgical treatment of various cardiac arrhythmias has received increased attention in the last few years. Ungerleider and colleagues[69] and Cox and associates[70] from Durham, North Carolina, discussed electrophysiologic effects, regional myocardial blood flow effects, regional LV functional effects, and finally the clinical indication, surgical technique, mechanism of action, and results of the encircling endocardial ventriculotomy (EEV) for refractory ischemic VT. Before the description by Guiraudon (*Ann Thorac Surg* 26:438, 1978) of an encircling endocardial myotomy and by Harken and colleagues (*Ann Surg* 190:456, 1979) of endocardial resection, most surgical attempts to eradicate intractable ischemic VT could be classified as indirect. Ungerleider and colleagues[69] collected reports of 179 patients treated either by sympathectomy, CABG alone, resection of LV aneurysm, or combined CABG and aneurysmal resection and termed these "indirect" procedures. The operative mortality was 26% and only 58% of patients were "cured" of their arrhythmia.

These investigators found EEV in the absence of induced myocardial

TABLE 3-1. *Results of indirect and direct surgical procedures for treatment of refractory ischemic ventricular tachycardia. Reproduced with permission from Cox et al.*[70]

PROCEDURE	# PATIENTS	OPERATIVE DEATHS		LATE DEATHS		POSTOP RECURRENCE WITHOUT DRUG THERAPY		REFRACTORY POSTOP WITH DRUG THERAPY		OVERALL SUCCESS RATE*	
		#	%	#	%	#	%	#	%	#	%
Indirect	179	47	26	?	?	29	16	29	16	103	58
EEV	47	8	17	4†	9	3	7	1	0	37	79
ERP	76	7	9	10‡	13	4	5	1	1	68	89

Legend: EEV, Encircling endocardial ventriculotomy. ERP, Endocardial resection procedure. * Overall success rate includes total number of patient (column 1) minus operative deaths (column 2), late deaths related to operation or recurrent ventricular tachycardia, and postoperative recurrences on medical therapy (column 5). † Two late deaths related to EEV. ‡ No late deaths related to ERP.

ischemia caused an epicardial conduction delay of 23 ± 3 ms (Fig. 3-4). When the myocardium was made ischemic by coronary artery ligation, the EEV was capable, in certain instances, of isolating spontaneous ventricular electrical activity to the myocardium encompassed by the incision. Surprisingly, the EEV resulted in total ablation of all fast electrical activity at 20 of 48 (42%) subendocardial electrode sites and at 12 of 44 (27%) subepicardial sites monitored within the encompassed myocardium. Thus, although some tachyarrhythmias might be encompassed by the EEV, the procedure most commonly ablated the electrical activity within the EEV and thus might modify the anatomic electrophysiologic substrate necessary for the genesis and perpetuation of these arrhythmias. Some investigators have found that in patients treated with EEV there was a deterioration of LV function. Ungerleider and associates studied the effect of EEV on local myocardial blood flow in 10 dog hearts using the radioactive tracer microsphere technique. They demonstrated that following EEV, blood flow in all regions and layers of the encompassed myocardium was less than that in the uninvolved normal myocardium. This relative decrease in flow was most marked in the central portion of the encompassed myocardium. Subsequent occlusion of the distal LAD coronary artery resulted in a further decrease in relative flow to the encompassed myocardium. The authors noted that when done in the clinical setting EEV was performed only around the border of a previous AMI, but that is the very place where coronary collateral vessels are likely to be present. Although the dogs did not mimic exactly the clinical situation, the implication of performing an EEV would appear to be the same, that is, that myotomy reduced blood flow to the encompassed myocardium. This might explain the higher operative mortality with this

Fig. 3-4. Concurrent electrograms from 2 regions of the left ventricle obtained after an EEV-encompassed region was made ischemic by occlusion of the distal LAD coronary artery. The heart was in a normal sinus rhythm. Activation within EEV myocardium appears fragmented. Spontaneous impulse initiation occurs within EEV (arrow) and is not reflected outside its boundaries, demonstrating that the EEV isolates this arrhythmia from the remainder of the heart. Reproduced with permission from Ungerleider et al.[69]

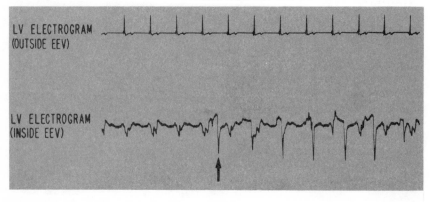

procedure and the decrement in LV function. In a subsequent article, the authors demonstrated that the EEV procedure resulted in significant stiffening of a LV portion encompassed by the EEV. Furthermore, there was an increase in resting end-diastolic length within the EEV. In addition to the demonstration of a change in regional diastolic compliance within the EEV, the authors also showed that normalized systolic excursion (percent delta L) during the ejection phase of systole was diminished within the EEV region after myotomy was done. These experiments were done in canine hearts with normal myocardium, as opposed to the clinical situation in which EEVs are placed around fibrotic myocardium. Nevertheless, the authors demonstrated both diminished blood flow and decrements of systolic and diastolic function within the encircled myocardium. They suggested that this functional impairment may translate to decrements in LV function in patients undergoing this procedure. With EEV, there was an overall success rate of 79%, and with endocardial resection, there was an overall success rate of 89%. The authors employed both EEV and ERP for medically refractory ischemic VT arising in the left ventricle. They suggest that a localized region of myocardial abnormality be documented either by ECG or by LV angiography before operation, since the effectiveness of both procedures depends upon identification of an abnormal anatomic substrate intraoperatively. The EEV, as described by Guiraudon and associates, involved opening the left ventricle through the previously healed AMI or aneurysm. If an aneurysm was present, an aneurysmectomy was performed. The border between the endocardial fibrosis at the base of the aneurysm and surrounding normal myocardium was identified. An incision perpendicular to the plane of the LV wall was placed just outside the border of the endocardial fibrosis, and continued around the entire base of the fibrotic endocardium. The depth of the incision on the LV free wall was such that only a narrow bridge of subepicardium, epicardium, and overlying vessels were spared. Incision was made approximately 1 cm deep on the septal side of the aneurysm. This incision was then closed with nonabsorbable suture and buttressed with felt pledgets. For posterior scars or aneurysms, the incision was started as near the LV base as possible and parallel to and within 1 cm of the posterior portion of ventricular septum to avoid the posterior papillary muscle.

Ungerleider, Cox and colleagues have contributed new knowledge on the electrophysiology and decrement of ventricular function associated with the Guiraudon (EEV) procedure. They have brought together reports from several institutions to document an improved success rate for EEV or endocardial resection over indirect procedures. In summary, the success rate for an indirect procedure is 58% (70% confidence limits, 53–62%) and the overall success rate for direct procedures is 85% (70% confidence limits, 81–89%). Thus, there is a statistical superiority of the direct over the indirect procedure.

Josephson and colleagues[71] from Philadelphia, Pennsylvania, evaluated 60 patients with recurrent sustained VT refractory to medical therapy who underwent subendocardial resection. There were 52 men and 8 women, aged 39–74 years, all with CAD. Each had had an AMI 1 week to 11 years before surgery and 52 had LV aneurysms. The mean EF was 27%. All 60 patients underwent endocardial resection with or without aneurysmectomy guided by intraoperative and/or catheter endocardial mapping. Thirty-seven endocardial resections were from the ventricular septum, 14 from the interoposterior free wall, and 16 were from the anteroapical or anterolateral free wall. There were 5 (8%) surgical deaths. The 55 survivors underwent programmed stimulation in the control state 28 days following the operation. In 42 patients (group A) VT was not inducible but was inducible in 13 patients (group B). Group B patients underwent drug testing and were discharged on the antiarrhythmic agent that made the VT noninducible or more difficult to induce. There have been only 4 recurrences of sustained VT with an average follow-up time of 19 months. There have also been 9 late nonarrhythmic deaths. The actuarial survival curve predicted 62% survival at 40 months. It is concluded that activation-guided endocardial resection provides long-term effective therapy for drug-resistant VT.

Martin and associates[72] from Philadelphia, Pennsylvania, evaluated 62 patients who underwent aneurysmectomy and endocardial resection for control of recurrent sustained VT. Forty patients also had CABG (1.5 grafts per patient). The mean preoperative LV end-diastolic pressure was 18 mmHg, cardiac index was 2.7 liters/min/m^2, and EF was 28%. In a subset of 32 patients with clearly demarcated aneurysmal and contracting ventricular sections, the mean EF of the residual contracting section was 35% and 26 of these patients had a contracting section EF <45%. There were 5 operative deaths (8%). No hemodynamic findings distinguished the patients who died during surgery. Patients with an LV end-diastolic pressure above the group mean or an overall EF below the group mean had an operative mortality of 10% and 7%, respectively. In the subgroup of 26 patients with a contracting segment EF <45%, the operative mortality was 12%. In the surgical survivors as a whole, the LV end-diastolic pressure decreased from 17–14 mmHg, and the overall EF increased from 28–39%, whereas the cardiac index did not change. Linear regression analysis revealed that patients with the highest preoperative LV end-diastolic pressures and the lowest overall EF were most likely to have improvement in these parameters postoperatively. Patients with a preoperative contrasting segment EF <45% had similar postoperative changes in the LV end-diastolic pressure and overall EF. In addition, the incidence of inducible VT postoperatively was similar in patients with a preoperative contracting segment EF <45% (4 of 23), and in the rest of the group (8 of 34). It is concluded that: 1) patients with LV aneurysm and medically refractory VT often have marked dysfunction of the residual contracting LV section; 2) aneurysmectomy and endocardial resection is an effective mode of therapy for VT and can be performed with a low operative mortality; and 3) postoperatively, the angiographic EF usually increases and the LV end-diastolic pressure often decreases, especially in patients with the most marked preoperative LV dysfunction.

Moran and colleagues[73] from Chicago, Illinois, have published their results using extended endocardial resection for the treatment of VT and VF. They reported 40 patients with drug-refractory, life-threatening cardiac rhythm disturbances. These patients had extended endocardial resection of scar tissue due to healing of AMI in 38 patients, to previous congenital heart operation in 1 patient, and to cardiac sarcoidosis in 1. The endocardial resection was, in some cases, directed by epicardial and endocardial mapping during VT, occasionally induced by low dose isoproterenol during normothermic cardiopulmonary bypass. Epicardial mapping most often revealed a breakthrough of the VT morphology on either the right or left side of the ventricular septum, usually anteriorly if the infarct was anterior, and inferiorly if the infarct was inferior. Endocardially the septum was commonly documented as the earliest site of activation, nearly always at the margin of dense white scar with normal-appearing septal endocardium. The operative mortality was 10%. Of 36 survivors, 33 (92%) are free of arrhythmia at follow-up periods ranging from 3–36 months (mean, 12.5). The arrhythmia in the remaining 3 patients is now drug controlled. Thirty-three patients had postoperative electrophysiologic studies, and in 30 (91%) the arrhythmia was no longer inducible. The authors present excellent results in a difficult group of patients. They emphasize that although operation was at times guided by endocardial mapping, all visible endocardial scar tissue was removed, as opposed to resection of simply those areas with abnormal mapping findings.

CARDIAC ARREST

Most patients with cardiac arrest outside the hospital have VF by the time personnel from a mobile coronary care team arrives. Adgey and associates[74] from Belfast, Northern Ireland, assessed 48 consecutive patients who had sudden cardiac problems outside the hospital but neither VF nor VT were present on arrival of the mobile coronary care team. Before the initiation of VF, which occurred after arrival of the coronary care team in all 48 patients, late cycle VPC were recorded in 38 patients (79%) and R-on-T VPC in 27 patients (56%). R-on-T VPC were relatively infrequent, an average of 3 occurring during a mean monitoring time of 27 minutes. Multifocal VPC occurred in only 3 patients (6%), consecutive VPC in 14 (29%), and self-terminating VT in 3 (6%); VPC occurring at >5 a minute were uncommon during this phase. The time from "warning arrhythmias" to the development of VF in many patients was short, thus limiting the administration of antiarrhythmic agents. A significant increase in the heart rates recorded immediately before VF when compared with those documented initially was observed. Thus, an increase in cardiac rate appeared to be a predisposing factor in the initiation of VF. An R-on-T VPC was the most important factor in the initiation of VF. It occurred in 33 patients (69%). In 9 (19%) VT and in 6 (12%) a late cycle VPC or idioventricular rhythm initiated VF.

To explore the relation between vigorous physical activity and primary cardiac arrest, Siscovick and associates[75] from Seattle, Washington, identified through emergency service incident reports, 163 patients aged 25–75 years with primary cardiac arrest. Control subjects matched for age, sex, residence, and the absence of prior clinical heart disease were identified from the community. Spouses of subjects were interviewed to quantify leisure time activity during the previous year. Energy expended in high intensity leisure time activity, requiring 60% of maximum oxygen intake, was determined. The risk of primary cardiac arrest was 60% lower in patients in the 2 upper quartiles of high intensity leisure time activity than in persons without high intensity leisure time activity. Because this association was demonstrated in a clinically healthy population without prior morbidity, the data support the hypothesis that high intensity leisure time activity protects against primary cardiac arrest. An extensive review of the relation between exercise and sudden death appeared recently.[76]

Thompson and associates[77] from Providence and Pawtucket, Rhode Island, determined the cause of death in 12 men who died while jogging in the state of Rhode Island in the 6 years from 1975–1980. The cause of death in 11 was CAD and in 1, acute gastrointestinal hemorrhage. The prevalence of jogging in the Rhode Island population was determined using a random-digit telephone survey. Among men aged 30–64 years, 7% reported jogging at least twice a week. The incidence of death during jogging for men of this age group was 1 death per year for every 7,620 joggers, or approximately 1 death per 396,000 man-hours of jogging. This rate is 7 times the estimated death rate from CAD during more sedentary activities in Rhode Island and suggests that jogging contributes to sudden death in susceptible persons. The occurrence, however, of only 1 death per 7,620 joggers per year demonstrates that the risk of exercise is small and suggests that the routine exercise testing of healthy subjects before exercise training is not justified. Of the 11 CAD deaths, at least 4 had preexisting symptomatic CAD apparently before they became joggers; total cholesterol values were available in 9 and in 6 of them the value was >200 mg/dl; in the other 3, the values were 185, 190, and 195 mg/dl.

Virmani and associates[78] from Washington, DC, studied at necropsy 30 men who were joggers. Information on their jogging habits was available, however, for only 18, who ran 7–105 miles/week, from 1–28 years. Three of the 30 patients were "marathon runners." Sixteen (53%) had histories of systemic hypertension, hypercholesterolemia, and/or family histories of premature CAD. Eight patients had previous clinical evidence of CAD. Two had transient ischemic attacks. Nineteen of the 30 patients died suddenly while jogging, 6 died suddenly shortly after jogging, 3 had chest pains soon after jogging, and 2 were found dead in bed. The heart was increased in weight in 16 (53%). Severe coronary artery atherosclerosis was present in 22 patients (73%), and 6 of them had coronary arterial thrombi. Acute or healed myocardial infarction was present in 14 (47%). One patient had MVP. In 7 patients no cause of death could be established: 3 of them had cardiomegaly and 6 had myocytolysis. Myocytolysis also was present in 11 patients with severe CAD. Although this is the largest series of runners studied at necropsy, it is diluted by the fact that 8 of the 30 patients had previous clinical evidence of CAD and information regarding running habits was available for only 18 patients. Another interesting feature of this study is the absence of a discernible cause of death in 7 of the 30 patients. One would have to wonder if the authors had access to the hearts in these patients or was their information entirely derived from autopsy protocols.

Rabkin and associates[79] from Winnipeg, Canada, determined whether ECG abnormalities detected on routine examination in men without clinical evidence of heart disease predicted sudden death in the absence of preexisting clinical manifestations of heart disease. The Manitoba study consisted of a cohort of 3,983 men with a mean age at entry of 31 years who had been followed with regular examination, including ECG, since 1948. During the 30-year observation period, 70 men without previous clinical manifestations of heart disease died suddenly (Fig. 3-5). The prevalence of ECG abnormalities before sudden death was 71% (50 of 70). The frequency of ECG abnormalities were as follows: major ST-segment and T-wave abnormalities (22 patients, 31%); VPC (11 patients, 16%); voltage criteria for LV hypertrophy (9 patients, 13%); complete left BBB (5 patients, 7%); and pronounced left axis deviation (4 patients, 6%). When these ECG findings in men without clinical manifestations of heart disease were related prospectively to the

Fig. 3-5. The age adjusted sudden death incidence for those with and without each of the following ECG abnormalities: pronounced left axis deviation (LAD), ventricular extrasystoles (VE), left ventricular hypertrophy (LVH), major ST-segment or T-wave abnormalities (Maj ST-T), and complete left bundle branch block (LBBB). The number of sudden death cases observed (OBS) in each subgroup with each ECG abnormality and the relative risk for sudden death are also shown. Reproduced with permission from Rabkin et al.[79]

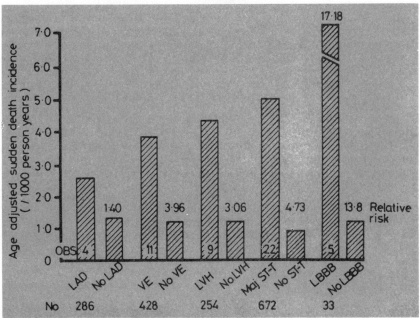

frequency of sudden death, each, except pronounced left axis deviation, was a significant predictor of sudden death. Two variables were examined in more detail. Increased severity of primary T-wave abnormalities and the association of ST-segment and T-wave abnormalities with increased QRS voltage further increased sudden death risk. The combination of VPC with either ST-T abnormalities or LV hypertrophy much increased the risk of sudden death. Thus, these data indicate that ECG abnormalities detected on routine examination in men without clinical evidence of heart disease are significantly related to the occurrence of sudden cardiac death.

Weaver and associates[80] from Seattle, Washington, evaluated 90 ambulatory patients previously resuscitated from out of hospital VF an average of 11.5 months after the episode. Physical activity immediately before cardiac arrest was known in 86 patients; in 23 (27%), VF occurred with exertion and in 63 (73%), while performing very low level activity. Chest pain and AMI occurred with equal frequency with both levels of activity. The subsequent exercise test results showed few differences between the 2 groups. Angina occurred in only 11 patients, and exercise-provoked ST changes suggestive of myocardial ischemia occurred in less than half of the patients in each group. More patients who had collapsed during nonexertional activities had exercise-produced complex ventricular arrhythmias than did patients who had collapsed during exertion (52% -vs- 26%, respectively; p < 0.05).

The patients were followed ≥2 years; at 24 months of follow-up, there were 27 deaths, of which 19 were the result of sudden cardiac arrest. In retrospect, only 2 of the exercise test findings were associated with subsequent fatal events. Seven of 11 patients with angina during testing had cardiac arrest or died later compared with 20 patients (25%) who had stopped exercising for other reasons (p > 0.01). In addition, the failure of systolic arterial pressure to increase ≥10 mmHg during the test also was associated with poor survival, i.e., respective mortalities at 2 and 4 years were 54% and 69% in those with this response compared with 26% and 42% in those whose pressure increased normally (p < 0.004). These data suggest that most patients developing VF do so at low activity levels. Routine exercise testing later is of limited value in the assessment of these patients except that angina and systolic hypotension developing during exercise appear predictive of a risk of future cardiac arrests.

Weaver and associates[81] from Seattle, Washington, described 144 patients with CAD previously resuscitated from out of hospital VF who underwent 24-hour ambulatory ECG monitoring 5 months after cardiac arrest. Patients were then followed for an average of 32 months. Fifty-one patients died, 32 from subsequent unexpected cardiac arrest. One hundred twenty-nine patients (90%) had uniform ventricular ectopy, two-thirds had complex ventricular ectopy, consisting of bigeminy, trigeminy, repetitive forms, or frequent multiforms. Complex ectopy present in 20% or more of the 30-minute recording intervals occurred in 18 of the patients who developed subsequent cardiac arrest compared with 26 of 92 (28%) who survived. Other forms of ectopy, uniform, multiform, and repetitive beats, were more sensitive but less specific predictors of death or recurrent VF. Complex ventricular arrhythmia was associated with certain clinical histories. It occurred in 95% of patients with a history of CHF and in 79% with remote AMI compared with 59% and 56% without these histories. As expected, mortality also was greater in patients who had these clinical characteristics. Thus, complex ectopy was related to mortality regardless of clinical history.

Nikolic and colleagues[82] from Worcester, Massachusetts, reported 6 instances of sudden death recorded by Holter monitoring that showed VF in 5 and a bradyarrhythmia in 1. Complex ventricular ectopic activity preceded cardiac arrest in 5 patients, including the 1 with the bradyarrhythmic arrest. Two patients with chronic bifascicular block arrested as a result of VF. Fifteen previously reported cases were reviewed. The composite profile included advanced myocardial disease, complex ventricular ectopic activity, R-on-T initiation of the terminal rhythm except in patients with prolonged Q-T interval, and variations in cycle length preceding the onset of VT or VF.

Utilizing incidence cases of CAD occurring in Rochester, Minnesota, during the years 1950–1975, Beard and associates[83] studied the distribution of sudden cardiac death (1,054 cases) by day of the week and season of the year. Overall, sudden cardiac death, defined as that occurring within 24 hours of onset of symptoms, occurred with greater frequency on Saturdays than on other days of the week. The frequency of occurrence of sudden death by season varied somewhat, the highest being in winter and the lowest in summer, but no more than expected by chance. Among men, there was a decreasing trend by day of the week from Saturday to Friday, and this was so for those with and those without a history of CAD.

Although most patients dying suddenly in the Western world do so because of severe narrowing of the coronary arteries from atherosclerosis, the final event in virtually all of them is a ventricular arrhythmia. What actually is the final stimulus producing the ventricular arrhythmia is unclear. Lown[84] from Boston, Massachusetts, for many years has studied the neural and psychologic mechanisms related to sudden coronary death, and in an editorial summarized his and others' views on the relation between mental stress, arrhythmias, and sudden coronary death. He concludes that higher nervous system inputs to the heart clearly constitute transient risk factors for sudden coronary death. Whereas data from animal studies are direct and persuasive, findings in humans are as yet incomplete and at best circumstantial. The neuroeffector sequence impinging on the myocardium is a summated expression emanating from complex interactions, including immediate sensory perception, recall of past emotional events, established conditioned reflex pathways, concentrations of neurotransmitters and their precursors at various brain sites, and a host of other factors. The very complexity of the matrix to be unraveled will no doubt slow acquisition of decisive insights, especially since biobehavioral and psychologic tools are still primitive. But substantial progress is now possible utilizing the prodigious recent advances in neurochemistry and psychopharmacology. Brain neurotransmitter synthesis, for example, can be modified by dietary manipulation of their precursors. The neutral amino acids L-tryptophan and tyrosine, precursors for serotonin and norepinephrine, respectively, when administered to animals protect against VF. Lown's final statement, although it is a little too optimistic and ignores the problem of atherosclerosis, is, "appreciation of the role of the central nervous system in modulating cardiac electro-physiologic properties will hasten the day when sudden cardiac death will no longer be the leading cause of fatality in the industrially developed world." If the coronary arteries stay wide open, sudden death may not be eliminated, but its cause will not be the heart in most instances.

Mittleman and Wetli[85] from Miami, Florida, analyzed the demographic features and predisposing factors to fatal food asphyxiation (café coronary) in 141 such fatalities over a 20-year period. Old age, poor dentition, and alcohol consumption were expected findings. Other predisposing factors included institutionalization in long-term medical care facilities, sedative drugs, and natural diseases, most notably parkinsonism. Since institutionalized patients tended to asphyxiate on soft, friable, or snacklike foods, future improvements in rescue techniques should take this into consideration. The incidence of 0.66/100,000 population has remained unchanged over the 2 decades studied. Observers were present at the time of the fatal incident in 85% of the cases. In only a third, the food was lodged in a supraglottic location. These data indicate that continued efforts toward greater awareness of the café coronary syndrome still are needed. Special attention should be directed to the predisposing role of institutionalization, sedative drugs, and natural diseases.

Since cardiopulmonary resuscitation (CPR) was introduced nearly 30 years ago, its use has spread from specialized units to all areas of the hospital and into the community. Now any person seems to be a candidate for CPR regardless of underlying condition, prognosis, and age. Despite a relatively low overall success rate, CPR has saved the lives of many persons. A patient's response to CPR varies with the area of the hospital in which it is done, cause of arrest, and underlying disease. Hershey and Fisher[86] from Cleveland, Ohio, compared the success rate of CPR with the outlook in terms of a return to semi-independent existence, and with the suitability of CPR as practiced in one hospital. They evaluated the records of all patients who had CPR in their hospital during the 6 months from July–December 1980. They chose to analyze primarily the patients resuscitated on the general floors of the hospital rather than those in an intensive care unit (ICU). Of 88 CPRs done on 79 patients during the 6-month period, 28 (32%) were performed in the emergency department (ED), 22 (25%) in ICU, 36 (41%) in the general wards, and 2 in miscellaneous areas. The success rate, as measured by the patient's response to CPR (return of vital signs), did not vary significantly with the area of the hospital and was 60% overall. The success rate, as measured by discharge from the hospital, was much less and varied (with borderline significance) by area of the hospital. Of the 35 patients who underwent 36 CPRs in the general hospital floors, there were only 2 long-time survivors. For each of the 35 patients, their most serious condition was put into 1 of 4 categories: acute disease, neoplasm, end-stage disease, and neurologic disease. In general, the patients in the acute illness group had other severe underlying disease. Before admission to the hospital 13 of the 35 patients were living independently in the community, 10 were living at home, and 10 had to be cared for by relatives. Only 4 of the 35 patients, appeared to the authors to be "viable." Of the first resuscitations received by these 35 patients, the authors judged 8 to be reasonable, 5 indeterminate, and 22 not reasonable. Of the 20 patients responding to their initial CPR, 4 died subsequently after a second CPR, 5 were receiving intensive care but did not receive CPR at the time of death, 9 were allowed to die without aggressive management, and 2 were still alive. This experience reemphasizes the low success rate of CPR in certain types of patients. The acute cases in the ED or ICU have a statistically much better chance of a long-term successful outcome than do patients in a general ward. Patients who are deteriorating have a very poor survival rate. Those who do respond to CPR usually die fairly soon afterward while still in intensive care and having used up much of the hospital's resources. The suitability of patients for CPR should be considered and a decision should be made beforehand as to whether CPR is to be instituted when a cardiorespiratory arrest occurs.

Bjork and associates[87] from Minneapolis and St. Paul, Minnesota, reviewed the clinical courses of 63 survivors of cardiopulmonary arrest to determine the frequency and temporal occurrence of noncardiac complications and their relation to mortality. Complications were grouped as occurring ≤48 hours, 48–96 hours, or >96 hours after arrest. Acute pneumonia, electrolyte level disturbances, and gastrointestinal hemorrhage each occurred in 28 (45%) of the 63 patients. Resuscitation-related injuries, seizures, and hepatic function test abnormalities each occurred in at least 18 (28%) of the 63 patients. Pneumonia and hepatic function test abnormalities were each significantly correlated with increased mortality. Septicemia, acute renal failure, and acute respiratory distress syndrome each occurred in 3 (5%) or 4 (7%) of the 63 patients and were always associated with death.

SYNCOPE

Controversy has concerned the need to treat patients with a hypersensitive carotid sinus reflex since this was first recognized as a cause of syncope. Evidence exists that syncopal patients with a hypersensitive carotid sinus reflex will continue to have disabling symptoms unless treated. Pacing is now accepted as a treatment of first choice for syncopal patients with a pure or predominant cardioinhibitory response to carotid sinus massage. A predominant cardioinhibitory response is found in up to 80% of patients with carotid sinus syndrome. A pure vasodepressor response is rare, occurring in only about 8% of patients, but a mixed vasodepressor or cardioinhibitory response is common. Patients with such a mixed type of response pose a therapeutic problem, since ventricular pacing does not correct their vasodepressor response and symptoms may persist. Morley and associates[88] from London and Sussex, England, described observations in 70 patients who had been paced for carotid sinus syndrome for 4 years. Of the 70 patients, 12 had persistent symptoms despite adequate ventricular pacing. These 12 were found to have a significant vasodepressor response, a significant hypotensive response to ventricular pacing (pacemaker effect), and a severe hypotensive response to carotid sinus massage with introduction of ventricular pacing, which reproduced symptoms in all patients. A group of 14 asymptomatic paced carotid sinus patients was found to have a significantly lower vasodepressor response, pacemaker effect, and combined vasodepressor response plus pacemaker effect than the group with persistent symptoms. Thus, AV sequential pacing eliminated the hypotensive effect of ventricular pacing and is considered the treatment of choice for patients with carotid sinus syndrome who have both cardioinhibitory and significant vasodepressor responses.

Silverstein and associates[89] from Boston, Massachusetts, reviewed the records of 108 patients admitted to a medical intensive care unit (ICU) for syncope during a 2-year period. Explicit criteria were used to classify patients by presumed etiologic diagnosis. Of the cases of syncope, 36% were due to cardiovascular disease, 17% to noncardiovascular disease, and 47% were unexplained at hospital discharge (Table 3-2). Of presumed etiologic diag-

Table 3-2. *Syncope diagnoses. Reproduced with permission from Silverstein et al.*[89]

	#	%
Cardiovascular		
Myocardial infarction	6	
Ventricular arrhythmia	13	
Arterial fibrillation	6	
Sick sinus syndrome	4	
Conduction disease	2	
Pacemaker failure	4	
Aortic stenosis	4	
	39	36
Noncardiovascular		
Neurological disease	5	
Pulmonary embolus	3	
Vasovagal syncope	1	
Posttussive syncope	1	
Drug toxicity	4	
Orthostatic hypotension	4	
	18	17
Unexplained	51	47
Total	108	100

noses, 72% were based on information available at the time of patient admission; the remainder were based on ICU monitoring and additional diagnostic tests. Patients were prospectively studied after hospital discharge. The 1-year mortality was 19% in the cardiovascular group, 6% in the noncardiovascular group, and 6% among patients whose syncope remained unexplained. Age-standardized comparisons between the unexplained syncope group, the USA population, and other ICU patients suggest that patients with syncope unexplained at hospital discharge do not have an increased risk of death during the subsequent year.

Gulamhusein and associates[90] from London, Canada, and Indianapolis, Indiana, assessed the value of clinical electrophysiologic study using intracardiac recording and programmed electrical stimulation in 34 patients who had unexplained syncope and/or presyncope. All patients had a normal ECG, and no abnormality was detected by clinical examination, ambulatory ECG recording, or treadmill testing. The electrophysiologic results were diagnostic in 4 patients (12%) and led to appropriate therapy that totally relieved symptoms. The results were abnormal but not diagnostic in 2 patients (6%) and normal in the remaining 28 patients (82%). The patients were followed 2–44 months (mean, 15) after electrophysiologic testing: 16 patients (47%) had no further episodes in the absence of any intervention; in 4 patients (12%), a definitive diagnosis was made during follow-up; in 7, permanent pacing was instituted empirically with relief of syncope, and 2 patients continued to have syncope. Thus, the diagnostic yield of electrophysiologic testing is low in patients having no ECG abnormality or evidence of cardiac disease. Empirical permanent pacing in patients with symptoms continuing after study appears beneficial, but this result was difficult to evaluate because of the high frequency of spontaneous remission in that group. The ECG documentation of abnormalities during syncope is the only definitive way to confirm or exclude an arrhythmic cause of the symptoms.

Hess and colleagues[91] from San Francisco, California, studied 32 patients with syncope of undetermined cause using conventional neurologic and cardiovascular testing. All patients underwent invasive electrophysiologic studies to assess sinus nodal function, AV conduction, and the inducibility of supraventricular and VT. Eleven patients (34%) had laboratory-induced VT, 5 (15%) had sinus node dysfunction, 1 (3%) had infra-His AV block during atrial pacing, and 1 (3%) probably had quinidine-related VT. In the remaining 14 patients, no detectable abnormalities were found during electrophysiologic studies. After a mean follow-up period of 21 ± 1 months, 10 of the 11 patients with inducible VT were asymptomatic while receiving laboratory-directed antiarrhythmic therapy. One patient died from VF after discontinuing the chosen antiarrhythmic regimen. Five of the remaining 7 patients with an electrophysiologic abnormality were asymptomatic after implantation of a permanent pacemaker or alteration of previous drug therapy or both. In 14 patients with a normal electrophysiologic study, empiric treatment was used with recurrent syncope occurring in 4 patients during follow-up. These data indicate that invasive electrophysiologic studies provide a presumptive diagnosis in 56% of patients with syncope of undetermined etiology. Therapy specific for the electrophysiologic abnormality was usually successful in preventing recurrent syncope.

PACEMAKERS

Pacemaker malfunction (such as lead-related, unit malfunction, insertion site problems) can still occur despite the availability of lithium batteries. Reinhart and associates[92] from Portland, Oregon, observed pacemaker failure, i.e. repeat surgical procedure required, after initial implantation in 22 of 115 (19%) patients. Failure occurred within the first month in 12, with 10 being lead related. Insertion site problems did not occur. Although most endocardial pacemaker complications occur early, patients are at risk as long as the units are in place. Despite improvements in the batteries, there continue to be sufficient problems with pacemakers to emphasize the need for selectivity in determining which patients receive permanent units.

Bergfeldt and associates[93] from Stockholm, Sweden, by radiographic screening for sacroiliitis in a population of 223 men who had permanently implanted pacemakers found sacroiliitis in 19 men (8.5%), 15 of whom fulfilled diagnostic criteria for ankylosing spondylitis. In 6 patients, sacroiliitis was asymptomatic and 2 patients were completely free of symptoms other than those originating from their heart manifestations. In 7 of the 15 patients with ankylosing spondylitis and the 4 patients with sacroiliitis without clinical criteria of ankylosing spondylitis, the diagnosis was previously unknown. Uveitis and AR occurred in 5 patients each, whereas peripheral arthritis was twice as common. The prevalence of sacroiliitis and ankylosing spondylitis of 8.5% and 6.7%, respectively, differ significantly (p < 0.01) from the frequencies found in general Caucasian populations of 1%–2% and 0.1%–0.5%, respectively. HLA B27 was present in >80% of the patients with sacroiliitis and/or ankylosing spondylitis, compared with 10% in the general population. This strong association is in accordance with previous studies of patients with symptomatic sacroiliitis and/or ankylosing spondylitis. Thus, sacroiliitis, diagnosed by x ray, can be considered a marker for this relatively common cause of severe disturbances of the cardiac conduction system.

Sixty-nine patients receiving AV sequential (DVI) pacemakers were compared by Stone and colleagues[94] from Detroit, Michigan, and Minneapolis, Minnesota, with 67 patients receiving ventricular demand (VVI) pacemakers for control of the symptoms of sinus node dysfunction. The populations were similar with comparable prepacing incidences of each assayed symptom and number of symptoms per patient (symptom density). Syncope was well controlled by both DVI and VVI pacing. DVI pacing was better than VVI pacing for control of all other symptoms. Symptom density responses were: DVI pre, 3.3 ± 0.95, post, 0.43 ± 0.63; VVI pre, 3.2 ± 0.97, post, 1.75 ± 1.44. Atrial electrode problems were encountered in 5 (7%) of the DVI patients and 1 (0.74%) ventricular electrode required repositioning.

SICK SINUS SYNDROME

The effects of therapeutic doses of orally administered quinidine sulfate on sinus rhythmicity and automaticity were observed in 11 patients with sick sinus syndrome (SSS) by Vera and colleagues[95] from Davis, California. Evaluation of sinus node function was undertaken by assessing sinus nodal recovery time (SNRT), treadmill exercise testing, and 24-hour ambulatory ECG monitoring before and after quinidine administration (25 mg/kg; range, 800–1,600 mg daily). Corrected SNRT ranged from 100–1,320 ms (average, 551) before quinidine and was not significantly altered after quinidine to 346–660 ms (average, 481). Further, quinidine did not induce accelerated infrasinus pacemaker activity. Spontaneous sinus rate evaluated with ambulatory monitoring revealed average rate of 57 beats/minute (range, 53–63) before quinidine without significant increase to average 59 beats/minute (range, 52–80) after quinidine therapy. Similarly, the maximal sinus node response to exercise was not significantly affected by quinidine (average, 129 beats/minute before and after drug therapy). Thus, therapeutic doses of quinidine do not exert adverse effects on sinus node function in SSS patients. Chronic oral quinidine therapy therefore can be used safely in patients with chronic sinus node disease when indicated for control of tachyarrhythmias.

The SSS has become the most common indication for permanent pacemaker insertion. Patients who require pacemakers for SSS are generally elderly, with a mean age in most series of >60 years. There have been no previous series of symptomatic SSS in younger patients who have not had cardiac surgery. To determine the characteristics of SSS, and the role of permanent pacemaker therapy in younger patients, Kay and associates[96] from New York City reviewed their experience over 10 years with such patients. Of 1,484 pacemakers placed at their institution between 1970 and 1980, there were 18 patients aged 20–40 years who were not postoperative congenital heart disease patients. Twelve patients had primary SSS as the indication for pacing. Eleven of them were markedly symptomatic with syncope, near syncope, or lightheadedness. Ambulatory monitoring revealed evidence of sinus node disease in all patients. Electrophysiologic studies were falsely negative in the 5 patients in whom they were performed. The patients tolerated pacemaker therapy well and became asymptomatic with pacing. Thus, SSS in young adults is uncommon, but still represents the most common indication for permanent pacemaker therapy in this age group. The decision for pacemaker therapy should depend on symptoms and results of ambulatory monitoring. In young adult patients with troubling symptoms and evidence for SSS, pacemaker therapy can be expected to alleviate symptoms and is well tolerated.

Depressed conduction in the sinoatrial junction, common in the SSS, should decrease the maximum pacing rate at which 1:1 capture of the sinoatrial node occurs. This may result in shorter than expected sinus node recovery time (SNRT) and maximal prolongation of SNRT at relatively slow pacing rates. To test this hypothesis, Reiffel and colleagues[97] from New York City evaluated the range of pacing rates necessary to demonstrate maximal SNRT in 34 patients with and 20 patients without sinus node dysfunction. Atrial pacing was performed at multiple paced cycle lengths (PCL) between 400 and ≥1,000 ms, 4 times at each. A mean corrected SNRT (CSRT) was determined at each PCL, and the PCL of the longest CSRT was determined (PCL_p). The PCL_p varied linearly with sinus cycle length, was dependent on sinoatrial conduction time, and was longer in patients with SSS than in normal persons. Only 2 of 20 normal persons, but 21 of 34 patients with SSS, had a PCL_p > 600 ms. A long PCL_p (>600 ms) suggests the possibility of recovery times that have been limited by atrial-sinus node entrance block and appears to be indicative of sinus node dysfunction.

SUPRAVENTRICULAR PARASYSTOLE

Kinoshita and associates[98] in Sapporo, Japan, have previously shown that in most patients with ventricular parasystole, Mobitz type I second degree entrance block is present. The investigators presented electrophysiologic studies in 2 patients with supraventricular parasystole (1 AV and 1 atrial). In both patients, reentrant VPC appeared to occur as the results of Mobitz type I second degree entrance block. The authors believe that when a sinus impulse fell soon after the absolute refractory period of the pathway containing the parasystolic focus, it reached and discharged a focus after marked delay and thereafter became a reentrant VPC. In enter ectopic intervals containing more than 1 sinus beat, the number of intervening sinus beats was always even, suggesting the presence of concealed reentrant extrasystolic bigeminy. The authors concluded from the observations in the present report and in previous patients with ventricular parasystole that most cases of parasystole, whether ventricular or supraventricular or whether intermittent or continuous, may be governed by second degree entrance block.

BUNDLE BRANCH BLOCK

To assess whether gross pathologic differences exist between hearts with left BBB and left axis deviation (LAD) than those with left BBB and a normal frontal plane axis, Havelda and colleagues[99] from Louisville, Kentucky, examined 70 hearts with left BBB in a series of 1,410 sequential dissections. The incidence of left BBB was 5%. Thirty-two hearts had LAD and 34 had normal axes on the correlative ECG. Left ventricular enlargment occurred frequently (90%). No significant differences were found in age distribution, LV weight, coronary anatomy, or infarct location. Quantitative analysis revealed larger inferoposterolateral and apical infarcts in hearts with left BBB and LAD. The accuracy of various ECG signs of LV enlargement and AMI in the presence of left BBB was assessed and voltage criteria and QRS duration poorly defined anatomic chamber enlargement. Anterior infarction was suggested by a Q or a pathologic Q wave in lead I, a Q wave in leads I, V_5, V_6, or notched S waves in V_3 or V_4. Pathologic Q waves or ST shifts in the inferior leads had high diagnostic specificity but low sensitivity for an inferior infarction.

A triad of exertional chest discomfort, transient rate-dependent left BBB and normal coronary arteries was presented by Virtanen and associates[100] from Helsinki, Finland, in 7 patients. Although the clinical symptoms resembled effort angina, qualities atypical of classic angina pectoris were common: 1) the onset was always abrupt; and 2) the pain was local never radiating; 3) palpitations were frequent; and 4) "walk through" phenomenon often was present. The abrupt pain took place simultaneously with the appearance of left BBB induced by physical exercise in all 7 patients. Atrial pacing or spontaneous resting heart rate changes produced similar sensations and left BBB in 4 of the 5 patients examined. Similary, in the same 4 patients kinetocardiographic recordings disclosed a sudden occurrence of paradoxical cardiac movement at the moment LBBB and chest pain appeared. The paradoxical systolic motion disappeared at reversion to normal conduction.

Peters and colleagues[101] from San Francisco, California, Chicago, Illinois, and Portland, Oregon, in a collaborative study obtained serial His bundle recordings during 1-1 AV conduction in 90 patients with chronic BBB over a mean interval of 30 months. The AV conduction time increased (A-H), infranodal conduction time (H-V) similarly increased in 29 patients, but only 10 patients had parallel increases in A-H and H-V intervals. Increases in conduction times were independent of age, time interval between studies, cause of heart disease, or initial A-H or H-V intervals. Women were significantly more likely than men to show an increase in H-V interval and spontaneous trifascicular block. Spontaneous progression to second or third degree AV block occurred at the AV node in 7 patients and below the node in 12 patients. The initial A-H interval was prolonged in 5 of 7 patients with AV nodal block and increased further in only 2 at restudy. The initial H-V interval was abnormal in 8 of 12 patients who progressed to infranodal block and was prolonged further in 8 at restudy. The investigators conclude that in patients with chronic BBB, 1) approximately 33% show progressive AV conduction system disease and AV nodal and infranodal disease progress independently; 2) progression of infranodal disease is more common in women: 3) AV nodal disease is a common cause of AV block and can occur without further prolongation of the A-H interval once a critical level of disease is attained, whereas infranodal block is usually accompanied by progressive lengthening of the H-V interval; and 4) progression of AV conduction disease is not readily predictable from clinical and electrophysiologic variables.

McAnulty and associates[102] from Portland, Oregon, conducted a prospective study in which 554 patients with chronic bifascicular and trifascicular conduction abnormalities were followed for an average of 42 ± 8 months.

Complete heart block occurred in 19 patients, and 17 were successfully treated (Fig. 3-6). The actuarial 5-year mortality from an event that could conceivably have been a bradyarrhythmia was 6% (35% from all causes) (Fig. 3-7, Table 3-3). Of the 160 deaths, 67 (42%) were sudden; most of these were not ascribable to bradyarrhythmia but to tachyarrhythmia and AMI (Table 3-3). Mortality was higher in patients with CAD ($p < 0.01$) and CHF ($p < 0.05$). Patients in whom syncope developed before or after entry into the study had a 17% incidence of heart block (2% in those without syncope) ($p < 0.05$); however, no single variable was predictive of which patients were at high risk of death from a bradyarrhythmia. The predictors of death were increasing age, CHF, and CAD; the predictors of sudden death were CAD and increasing age. The risks of heart block and of death from a bradyarrhythmia were low; in most patients, heart block was recognized and successfully

Fig. 3-6. Cumulative incidence (mean ± S.E.) of complete heart block. Reproduced with permission from McAnulty et al.[102]

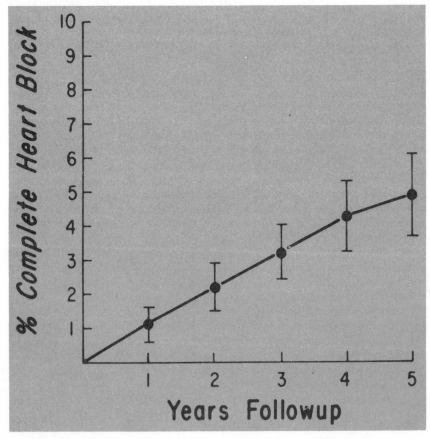

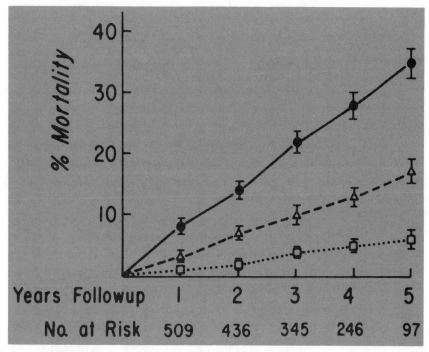

Fig. 3-7. Actuarially determined cumulative incidence (mean ± S.E.) of all deaths (circles), sudden deaths (triangles), and "special events" (squares). Number at risk refers to number of patients who were followed for designated period of time (for example, 509 patients who completed 1 year of follow-up). Reproduced with permission from McAnulty et al.[102]

treated with a pacemaker. The authors suggested the following guidelines: Patients who are asymptomatic require no special evaluation or treatment for BBB. Since most of these patients have serious heart disease and a high 5-year mortality, particularly if they have CAD or CHF or both, appropriate investigation and treatment of their underlying heart disease is advisable. In addition, patients with BBB and symptoms suggestive of a bradyarrhythmia should be evaluated to determine the cause of the symptoms and should undergo intensive efforts to document bradyarrhythmia. If a bradyarrhythmia is documented, permanent pacemaker implantation is indicated. If a bradyarrhythmia is not documented, pacemaker insertion is not recommended. If symptoms are recurrent, extensive investigations are indicated. There may be individual exceptions to the application of these guidelines.

M-mode echoes were obtained by Strasberg and colleagues[103] from Chicago, Illinois, in 48 patients with complete left BBB. Of these 48 patients, 28 had left BBB with normal frontal plane QRS axis ($-20°$ to $+90°$) and 20 had left BBB with left axis deviation ($-30°$ to $-60°$). In the group with left BBB and normal axis, 25 patients had typical early systolic posterior septal

TABLE 3-3. *Events in all 554 patients. Reproduced with permission from McAnulty et al.*[102]

	# PATIENTS
Death	160
Nonsudden	86
Sudden	67
Secondary to bradyarrhythmias	(2)
Secondary to other cause	(49)
Unknown cause	(16)
Unknown	7
Complete heart block	19
Permanent	17
Transient	2
Permanent pacemaker implantation	30
Syncope (after entry into study)	47
Secondary to bradyarrhythmia	19
Recurrent	12

motion characteristic of left BBB. Septal motion following early posterior septal motion (through the ejection period) was posterior in 24 patients (86%), anterior (paradoxical) in 2 (7%), and flat in 2 (7%). In the group with left BBB and left axis deviation, 16 patients had the typical early systolic posterior septal motion; subsequent septal motion was posterior in 3 (15%), anterior (paradoxical) in 13 (65%), and flat in 4 (20%). Patients with left BBB and normal axis had a higher frequency of posterior septal motion, and patients with left axis deviation had a higher frequency of anterior septal motion. The correlation of abnormal axis and paradoxical septal motion may be explained by the activation pattern producing left axis deviation or by a septal disease process producing both abnormalities of axis and abnormal septal motion.

Dancy and associates[104] from London, England, studied 27 patients with complete right BBB as the only abnormal finding via high speed M-mode echo to determine the effect of electrical delay on the mechanical events of RV systole. Pulmonic valve opening (PVO) was delayed in all cases. In some, the delay was mainly between mitral valve closure (MVC) and tricuspid valve closure (TVC), and this was designated "proximal block." In the others, the main delay was between TVC and PVO and this was designated "distal block." The patients were divided into those with proximal and those with distal block by calculating the ratio TVC-PVO/MVC-TVC. Twelve of 13 with distal delay but only 1 of 14 with proximal delay had episodes of syncope or near syncope. These results are consistent with previous theories about the pathophysiology of right BBB. Echo may offer a noninvasive method to estimate the prognosis in isolated right BBB.

CONGENITAL COMPLETE HEART BLOCK

Pinsky and associates[105] from Houston Texas, reported 65 patients with congenital complete heart block seen between 1955 and 1979. The median age at diagnosis was 7 months, with 26 (40%) diagnosed before 1 month of age. Anatomic defects were present in 25 (39%) with ventricular inversion/L-TGA present in 20 of 25 (80%). Permanent pacing was performed in 17 (26%) for bradycardia, CHF, or syncope; 6 of 17 (35%) had anatomic defects. There were 10 deaths in the 65 patients (15%) and 7 of the 10 had complex cardiac defects. These authors report a much more favorable outcome for the child without anatomic heart disease than has been noted previously: 95% survival in the child without heart disease and only 68% survival during the study in the child with heart disease. A strong case is made for permanent pacing based on bradycardia alone (resting ventricular rate <40/minute in a child). The neonate is more difficult to assess in regard to need for permanent pacing based on rate only; Pinsky and associates suggest that rates consistently <55/minute in a symptomatic neonate indicate the need for pacing. In this group, observation and even temporary pacing may obviate the need for permanent pacing, particularly in the neonate with no heart disease or only a PDA.

Reid and associates[106] from Glasgow, Scotland, reported their 18-year experience with 35 patients with congenital complete heart block. The age at presentation ranged from 12 days to 85 years, with 14 (40%) presenting by 10 years and 27 (77%) by 20 years. Cardiac defects were present in 6 (17%). Permanent pacing was required in 21 (60%) patients because of syncope or CHF with no deaths in the paced group 1–12 years after implantation. Age at pacing ranged from 12 days to >50 years with 10 of 21 (48%) paced by 30 years of age. Only 2 patients survived beyond their 50th birthday without permanent pacing. In the 14 patients without pacing, 1 died suddenly at age 5 years. The question of long-term prognosis for the child with congenital complete heart block remains incompletely answered. For the child without complex heart disease, the prognosis is good. It appears, however, that many if not most patients eventually will need permanent pacing. How does one predict when to intervene to prevent the rare occurrence of Stokes-Adams attacks or sudden death? QRS duration, resting ventricular rate (except when extremely low, probably <40/min), exercise ventricular rate, and atrial rates do not appear to hold up as markers for the need to intervene prophylactically. More investigations regarding exercise response and continuous ambulatory ECG monitoring over extended periods are needed.

Young adults with nonsurgically induced heart block do not necessarily have a benign prognosis and pacemaker implantation may be necessary. There have been no previous reports of long-term pacemaker follow-up in young adults with nonsurgically induced (congenital) complete heart block. Besley and colleagues[107] from Cleveland, Ohio, studied 13 patients aged 15–37 years (mean, 24) at pacemaker implantation. There were 9 females and 4 males. All were functional class II or III (New York Heart Association) before pacemaker implantation. Syncope, dizziness, fatigue, shortness of breath, and dyspnea on exertion were the most common symptoms. Cardiac catheterization findings (11 patients) were normal in 5, and additional cardiac anomalies were present in 6. His bundle studies (9 patients) showed absent A-H intervals in all patients, with H-V intervals not identified in 2, 20–30 ms in 1, and 30–50 ms in 6 patients. Holter monitor recordings (8 patients) demonstrated complete heart block in all 8 with intermittent second to third degree block in 2. Two patients had occasional PVC. Stress exercise tests (9 patients) demonstrated increased ventricular rate response (although subnormal in some patients); symptoms developed in 7. All 13 patients were contacted 3 months to 7 years (mean, 4 years) after pacemaker implantation. Two patients had died, but the deaths were not related to pacemaker dysfunction. All patients who are currently alive had marked improvement in functional symptomatology and all are currently functional class I. Congenital complete heart block is not a benign condition in young adults and may require pacemaker implantation, which improves symptoms and allows the patient to lead a normal life.

RELATED TOPICS

Ventricular arrhythmias during bedside pulmonary arterial catheterization

The flow-directed, balloon-tiped catheter is commonly used in intensive care units for hemodynamic monitoring of critically ill patients. One of the originally described advantages of this type of catheter over conventional stiff catheters was its failure to induce significant ventricular arrhythmias in patients undergoing PA catheterization. More recent studies have shown a frequency of ventricular arrhythmias up to 50%, including episodes of VT and VF. Spring and associates[108] from Miami, Florida, determined the frequency of advanced arrhythmias and acute right BBB during bedside PA catheterization in 119 critically ill patients undergoing 150 PA catheterizations. All were studied prospectively using continuous ECG monitoring with permanent recordings. Ventricular arrhythmias other than VPC occurred during 80 of the 150 catheterizations (53%). These included ventricular salvos (3–5 consecutive VPC) in 30%, nonsustained VT (5–30 VPC in 20%) and sustained VT (>30 consecutive VPC) in 3%. In 2 patients, VF developed. In another 3 patients, lidocaine or a precordial thump was required to terminate the episode of VT. A new right BBB developed in 7 patients (5%) and persisted for a mean of 10 hours. The frequency of advanced ventricular arrhythmias was statistically correlated with either the presence of predisposing risk factors for ventricular ectopic beats or prolonged catheterization time.

Esophageal pacing

The proximity of the esophagus to the atria is the anatomic basis for using esophageal electrodes to record electrical activity from the atria and several investigators have suggested this route to deliver electrical stimulation to the atria or ventricles for diagnostic and therapeutic purposes. Gallagher and associates[109] in Durham, North Carolina, developed guidelines for reproducible esophageal pacing of the atria and determined the incidence of successful initiation and termination of tachycardia using this technique. In 39 patients with a history of spontaneous SVT, strength-duration curves were performed in 39 patients using a bipolar esophageal lead with a 2.9 cm interelectrode distance. The esophageal current threshold decreased progressively as pulse duration was increased to the limit of the stimulator (9.9 s). At pulse durations of 8–9.9 ms, atrial capture was achieved in all patients. Shorter pulse durations resulted in capture in progressively fewer patients despite stronger current. In 38 patients with documented SVT overdrive pacing from the esophagus was performed at cycle lengths of 240–400 ms using a pulse duration of 7–9.9 ms. Reciprocating tachycardia was induced in 35 of 38 patients and was terminated by overdrive pacing in 33 of 38 patients. AF was induced incidently in 4 patients: sinus rhythm returned spontaneously. Other effects included ventricular pacing in 2, unmasking of latent preexcitation in 3, induction of VT by atrial pacing in 2 patients with a history of VT, and phrenic nerve pacing in 1 patient. All patients experienced discomfort, usually described as a mild burning sensation or chest pain similar to indigestion. No patient had discomfort sufficiently severe to force discontinuation of the study. Thus, atrial pacing can be achieved from the esophagus with minimal discomfort in most patients. Rapid atrial pacing from the esophagus can be used to induce and terminate SVT for diagnostic or therapeutic purposes and esophageal pacing provides a convenient way to assess repeatedly the efficacy of long-term drug therapy and screen patients for preaccess excitation syndromes.

Arrhythmias and conduction disturbances in the sleep apnea syndrome

Miller[110] from Hershey, Pennsylvania, evaluated the prevalence of cardiac arrhythmias and conduction disturbances by 24-hour continuous ECG monitoring in 23 patients with the sleep apnea syndrome. During sleep, marked sinus arrhythmia (>30 beats/min variation) occurred in 18 patients. Extreme sinus bradycardia (heart rate < 30 beats/min) and sinus pauses(>1.8 s) occurred in 2 patients. First degree and type I second degree AV block occurred in another patient. A decrease in the number of VPC occurred from wakefulness to sleep. These data suggest that the prevalence of serious arrhythmias and conduction disturbances during sleep in patients with the sleep apnea syndrome is relatively low.

Comparison of ventricular inhibited and atrial synchronous ventricular inhibited pacing

Kruse and associates[111] from Skovde, Sweden, examined 16 patients treated with a noninvasive programmable pacemaker after a prolonged period of ventricular inhibited (VVI) and atrial synchronous ventricular inhibited (VDD) pacing. Maximal work capacity was determined by bicycle ergometry. Atrial and ventricular rates, brachial artery cuff pressure, and breathing rate were measured at rest and during exercise. There was a mean increase in working capacity of 24% with VDD compared with VVI pacing. Thirteen patients underwent cardiac catheterization. During VDD pacing, cardiac output was significantly higher, particularly during exercise, due to the capability of heart rate increase and despite a substantial compensatory stroke volume increase during VVI pacing. Arterial venous oxygen difference was much higher during VVI pacing during the highest work load, whereas the corresponding level during VDD pacing was significantly lower. During exercise, arterial blood lactate was significantly higher during VVI than during VDD pacing. Heart size was also significantly smaller during VDD pacing. According to a questionnaire completed by the patient, to evaluate subjective symptoms and pacemaker preference, the VDD mode of pacing was favored. This study concluded that VDD pacing is superior to VVI pacing.

Effects of flecainide acetate on cardiac conduction and refractoriness

Hellestrand and associates[112] from London, England, assessed in 47 patients the electrophysiologic effects of flecainide acetate (2 mg/kg as an intravenous infusion over 5 min). Seven patients had normal electrophysiology, 16 had a direct accessory AV pathway, 12 had dual AV nodal (A-H) pathways, 5 had VT, 6 had conduction system disease, and 1 patient had a LA tachycardia. No significant change occurred in sinus cycle length. The PA, A-H and H-V intervals were all significantly prolonged. The QRS complex duration increased significantly. The Q-T interval was slightly prolonged due to the increase in QRS duration. Refractoriness of the atrial and ventricular myocardium was slightly prolonged, but was significant only at the ventricular level. No significant change occurred in refractoriness of the normal AV node. Pronounced prolongation of retrograde "fast" A-H pathway refractoriness was observed in those patients with dual A-H pathways. Antegrade and retrograde accessory pathway refractoriness were both greatly increased. These electrophysiologic properties strongly suggest that flecainide will be useful in the management of a wide variety of cardiac arrhythmias. It should be administered, however, with caution to patients with preexisting conduction system disease. Because repolarization is not delayed, flecainide is unlikely to induce ventricular arrhythmias related to prolongation of the Q-T interval.

Effects of sotalol

Nathan and associates[113] from London, England, assessed the electro-physiologic effects of intravenous sotalol hydrochloride (0.4 mg/kg) in 24 patients, including 13 with the WPW syndrome, undergoing routine electro-physiologic study. Fifteen to 30 minutes after sotalol administration, there was a significant increase in sinus cycle length and in sinus node recovery time. There was a small increase in the A-H interval, but the H-V interval was unchanged. The Q-T and J-T intervals, measured during sinus rhythm, were both increased. The atrial, ventricular, and AV nodal effective refractory periods were all prolonged, as was the AV nodal functional refractory period. In 13 patients with ventricular preexcitation there was an increase of the accessory pathway antegrade and retrograde effective refractory periods. In 12 of these 13 sotalol was given during AV reentrant tachycardia, resulting in termination in 5. Tachycardia cycle length increased in all patients, with the major effect being in the AV direction. Although some effects seen in these patients are consistent with the beta adrenergic antagonist properties of sotalol, the effect on atrial, ventricular, and accessory pathway effective refractory periods and on ventricular repolarization is not typical of that observed with other beta blockers but may be the result of lengthening of the action potential duration. These findings suggest that sotalol may be a more versatile antiarrhythmic agent than other beta receptor antagonists.

Pneumonitis with fibrosis from amiodarone

Introduced in Europe in 1961 as an antianginal agent, amiodarone hydrochloride is a benzofuran derivative subsequently found to have impor-tant antiarrhythmic properties. Sobel and Rakita[114] from Cleveland, Ohio, described 6 patients who developed pulmonary infiltrates of undetermined origin while being treated for severe ventricular arrhythmias with amiodar-one hydrochloride. Biopsy material was available in 4 patients and revealed interstitial or alveolar fibrosis and pneumonitis. Four patients recovered and 2 died of severe cardiopulmonary decompensation. All patients who recov-ered received corticosteriod therapy. Thus, pulmonary fibrosis is a previously unreported complication of amiodarone therapy.

Low energy countershock using an intravascular catheter

Yee and associates[115] from London, Canada, evaluated 8 patients with recurrent ventricular arrhythmias to determine the feasibility, effectiveness, and safety of using an intravascular catheter positioned in the RV apex for countershock in a coronary care unit (CCU). Countershock using 2.5–40 J stored energy was attempted 115 times to terminate 100 episodes of VT. Eight-six (87%) of 99 countershock attempts for VT, 3 of 5 for ventricular flutter, and 4 of 11 for VF were successful using this technique. The catheters remained in stable position for 1–16 days without dislodgment and most countershocks were delivered by the regular nursing staff in the CCU. These data suggest that low energy countershock through an intravascular catheter system is feasible, safe, and often effective in a CCU setting. This catheter lead system also may prove useful in managing VT that occur during electrophysiologic studies.

Accurate rapid compact analog method for quantification of frequency and duration of myocardial ischemia by semiautomated analysis of 24-hour Holter ECG recordings

Although the semiautomated analysis of 24-hour Holter recordings is now widely used in the detection and quantitation of disorders of cardiac rhythm and conduction, there are still no comparable methods for routine clinical use for the detection of the frequency and duration of myocardial ischemic episodes in patients with CAD. Research methods available to detect ischemic ST-T wave changes depend on sophisticated computer systems, are ill-suited for clinical use, and are not readily validated. However, Nademanee and colleagues[116] from Los Angeles, California, showed that when Holter tape is replayed at 60 times real time on heat-sensitive paper recorder at slow speeds (3.3–10 cm/min) rapid compact analog representation of 24-hour recording can be compressed into 480–1440 cm of paper. By this method, close juxtaposition of QRST complexes produces distinctive patterns; from these the frequency and duration of myocardial ischemic episodes can be identified promptly, accurately, and reproducibly. When combined with conventional Holter scanning assembly, the accuracy of detection can be validated continuously by intermittent printout of the abnormality and ventricular ectopy can be quantitated simultaneously. The analysis of a technically acceptable 24-hour recording can be accomplished in 24–40 minutes (at 60 times real time playback) by an experienced operator. The fast compact analog representation of 2-channel 24-hour recordings permitted the reliable detection of ST segment elevation and depression, pseudonormalization of ST-T wave abnormality, T-wave augmentation, AV block, VT, and intermittent BBB. The technique also allowed the relation of chest pain to the onset of ischemia to be established. Holter recordings from 22 CAD patients known to have myocardial ischemic episodes were examined; 275 episodes with ST segment deviations were identified, 92 (33%) being associated with angina that developed 2–8 minutes after the onset of ischemia. The method of compact analog ECG signal recording proved considerably superior to ST segment trend plotting; when combined with intermittent printout of observed abnormalities, the technique is simple, rapid, and extremely accurate in identifying the frequency and duration of myocardial ischemia from 2-channel 24-hour Holter recordings. This system permits the use of Holter monitoring for the noninvasive detection of myocardial ischemic episodes in a manner analogous to the quantitation of drug-induced suppression of ventricular ectopy from continuous ECG recordings.

Cardiac conduction abnormalities in the Reiter syndrome

Cardiac involvement in the Reiter syndrome is considered uncommon. The cardiac involvement usually consists of an aortitis similar to that observed in syphilis and in ankylosing spondylitis. The urethritis, arthritis, ocular, and dermal manifestations need not be present at the onset of cardiac symptoms and a long latent period may exist between the active Reiter syndrome and the appearance of cardiac symptoms. Ruppert and associates[117] from Washington, DC, reviewed retrospectively 22 patients with the Reiter syndrome who had been hospitalized. Of the 22, 8 had 1 or more conduction disturbances, and the conduction disturbance was the initial manifestation of the Reiter syndrome in 3 of the 8 patients. Of the 8 with conduction disturbances, prolongation of the PR interval occurred in 5, left BBB in 2, right BBB in 1, and complete heart block in 1. Testing for the B27 antigen gave positive results in all patients with conduction disturbances. The B27 antigen also occurs in patients with ankylosing spondylitis. The heart, like the joints and iris, appears to be a target organ for B27-associated disease by an undefined mechanism.

Ventricular defibrillation using 175 J -vs- 320 J shocks

Patients treated for cardiac arrest due to VF commonly receive shocks from defibrillators set to deliver the highest available level of energy. The reason for using maximum energy is not clear, but probably reflects an intuitive sense that the maximum available energy should be most effective. Cardiac damage, both transient and irreversible, may follow high energy shocks, and such damage may attenuate resuscitation and lower the survival rates. When shocks are delivered with minimum delay to patients with AMI, energy levels of 100–200 J are successful in most. Accordingly, Weaver and associates[118] from Seattle, Washington, compared the effects of initial electric shocks using 175 and 320 J in 249 patients with VF (Figs. 3-8 and 3-9). Survival was unrelated to the energy level used for defibrillation. Reversion to an organized rhythm occurred in a similar proportion of both treatment groups after 1 or 2 shocks. The rhythm identified after the first shock was related to outcome (the survival rate was 42% in patients with supraventricular rhythm, 30% in persistent VF, 26% in idioventricular rhythm, and 14% in asystole, $p < 0.02$). Ventricular fibrillation recurred in 68% of patients who had been initially defibrillated to an organized rhythm. Repeated shocks at the higher energy level resulted in a higher incidence of AV block after defibrillation (24% of patients receiving 320 J and 9% of those receiving

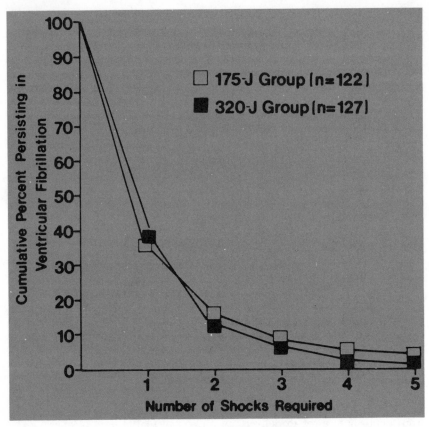

Fig. 3-8. Effectiveness of 175-J and 320-J shocks in treating defibrillation. Ventricular fibrillation was removed at least transiently in over 60% of patients with 1 shock and in more than 85% after 2 shocks. Defibrillation rates were virtually the same in the 2 treatment groups. Defibrillation occurred in all patients. Shocks of 320 J were delivered to both treatment groups when 3 or more shocks were required. Reproduced with permission from Weaver et al.[118]

shocks of lower energy, $p < 0.005$). Patients who survived required fewer shocks than patients who later died in the hospital (2.6 shocks compared with 3.6, $p < 0.005$). Thus, initial defibrillatory shocks using 175 J are as safe and effective as shocks of nearly twice that energy level.

Response to exercise after taking psychotropic drugs

Psychotropic drugs may prolong the Q-T interval and therefore potentially predispose to ventricular arrhythmias and/or sudden cardiac death. Exercise prescribed as therapy for depression also may prolong the Q-T

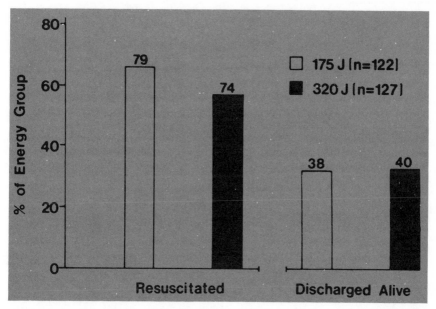

Fig. 3-9. Resuscitation and survival rates in patients initially treated with 175-J and 320-J defibrillatory shocks. Approximately 60% of both groups were resuscitated and admitted to hospital; 31% were resuscitated and later discharged alive from hospital. Figures above bars refer to numbers of patients. Reproduced with permission from Weaver et al.[118]

interval and augment arrhythmia risk. To determine Q-T interval (Q-T wave peak, or QTPK) response to exercise in patients receiving psychotropic drugs, Johnson and associates[119] from Atlanta, Georgia, performed treadmill exercise tests on 20 mentally competent psychiatric inpatients clinically free of heart disease. Twenty-four hour ambulatory ECG was performed within 1 day of exercise testing. Exercise test results for psychiatric patients were compared with those of normal subjects receiving no medication. Separate regression lines relating heart rate to QTPK interval, calculated for each group, showed no significant difference. No serious arrhythmias occurred during routine daily activities or exercise. Patients without heart disease taking psychotropic drugs have appropriate QTPK interval shortening with exercise.

References

1. VIITASALO MT, KALA R, EISALO A: Ambulatory electrocardiographic recording in endurance athletes. Br Heart J 47:213–220, March 1982.
2. TALAN DA, BAUERNFEIND RA, ASHLEY WW, KANAKIS C JR, ROSEN KM: Twenty-four hour continuous ECG recordings in long-distance runners. Chest 82:19–24, July 1982.

3. FLEG JL, KENNEDY HL: Cardiac arrhythmias in a healthy elderly population. Chest 81:302–307, March 1982.

4. KANNEL WB, ABBOT RD, SAVAGE DD, McNAMARA PM: Epidemiologic features of chronic atrial fibrillation: the Framingham study. N Engl J Med 306:1018–1022, Apr 29, 1982.

5. KRAMER RJ, ZELDIS SM, HAMBY RI: Atrial fibrillation—a marker for abnormal left ventricular function in coronary heart disease. Br Heart J 47:606–608, June 1982.

6. GARDNER JD, DUNN M: Spontaneous conversion of long-standing atrial fibrillation. Chest 81:429–432, Apr 1982.

7. NAKAZAWA HK, SAKURAI K, HAMADA N, MOMOTANI N, ITO K: Management of atrial fibrillation in the post-thyrotoxic state. Am J Med 72:903–906, June 1982.

8. STERN EH, PITCHON R, KING BD, GUERRERO J, SCHNEIDER RR, WIENER I: Clinical use of oral verapamil in chronic and paroxysmal atrial fibrillation. Chest 81:308–311, March 1982.

9. SCHWARTZ JB, KEEFE DL, KIRSTEN E, KATES RE, HARRISON DC: Prolongation of verapamil elimination kinetics during chronic oral administration. Am Heart J 104:198–203, Aug 1982.

10. SCHWARTZ JB, KEEFE D, KATES RE, KIRSTEN E, HARRISON DC: Acute and chronic pharmacodynamic interaction of verapamil and digoxin in AF. Circulation 65:1163–1170, June 1982.

11. PLUMB VJ, KARP RB, KOUCHOUKOS NT, ZORN GL, JAMES TN, WALDO AL: Verapamil therapy of atrial fibrillation and atrial flutter following cardiac operation. J Thorac Cardiovasc Surg 83:590–596, Apr 1982.

12. DUMESTIC DA, SILVERMAN NH, TOBIAS S, GOLBUS MS: Transplacental cardioversion of fetal supraventricular tachycardia with procainamide. N Engl J Med 307:1128–1131, Oct 28, 1982.

13. LUNDBERG A: Paroxysmal atrial tachycardia in infancy: long-term follow-up study of 49 Subjects. Pediatrics 70:638–642, Oct 1982.

14. GRECO R, MUSTO B, ARIENZO V, ALBORINO A, GAROFALO S, MARSICO F: Treatment of paroxysmal supraventricular tachycardia in Infancy with digitalis, adenosine-5'-triphosphate, and verapamil: a comparative study. Circulation 66:504–508, Sept 1982.

15. CASTELLANOS A, FERREIRO J, PEFKAROS K, ROZANSKI JJ, MOLEIRO F, MYERBURG RJ: Effects of lignocaine on bidirectional tachycardia and on digitalis-induced atrial tachycardia with block. Br Heart J 48:27–32, July 1982.

16. BENSON DW JR, STERBA R, GALLAGHER JJ, WALSTON A II, SPACH MS: Localization of the site of ventricular preexcitation with body surface maps in patients with WPW syndrome. Circulation 65:1259–1268, June 1982.

17. KLEIN GJ, GULAMHUSEIN S, PRYSTOWSKY EN, CARRUTHERS SG, DONNER AP, KO PT: Comparison of the electrophysiologic effects of intravenous and oral verapamil in patients with paroxysmal supraventricular tachycardia. Am J Cardiol 49:117–124, Jan 1982.

18. BAUERNFEIND RA, SWIRYN SP, STRASBERG B, PALILEO E, SCAGLIOTTI D, ROSEN KM: Electrophysiologic drug testing in prophylaxis of sporadic paroxysmal atrial fibrillation: technique, application, and efficacy in severely symptomatic preexcitation patients. Am Heart J 103:941–949, June 1982.

19. GULAMHUSEIN S, KO P, CARRUTHERS SG, KLEIN GJ: Acceleration of the ventricular response during AF in the WPW after verapamil. Circulation 65:348–354, Feb 1982.

20. HARPER RW, WHITFORD E, MIDDLEBROOK K, FEDERMAN J, ANDERSON S, PITT A: Effects of verapamil on the electrophysiologic properties of the accessory pathway in patients with the Wolff-Parkinson-White Syndrome. Am J Cardiol 50:1323–1330, Dec 1982.

21. GRAY RJ, CONKLIN CM, SETHNA DH, MANDEL WJ, MATLOFF JM: Role of intravenous verapamil in supraventricular tachyarrhythmias after open-heart surgery. Am Heart J 104:799–802, Oct 1982.

22. WELLENS HJJ, BRAAT S, BRUGADA P, GORGELS APM, BÄR FW: Use of procainamide in patients with the Wolff-Parkinson-White syndrome to disclose a short refractory period of the accessory pathway. Am J Cardiol 50:1087–1089, Nov 1982.

23. KERR CR, PRYSTOWSKI EN, SMITH WM, COOK L, GALLAGHER JJ: Electrophysiologic effects of disopyramide phosphate in patients with WPW syndrome. Circulation 65:869–878, May 1982.

24. WAXMAN MB, SHARMA AD, CAMERON DA, HUERTA F, WALD RW: Reflex mechanisms responsible for early spontaneous termination of paroxysmal supraventricular tachycardia. Am J Cardiol 49:259–272, Feb 1982.

25. WELLENS HJJ, BRUGADA P, ROY D, WEISS J, BÄR FW: Effect of isoproterenol on the anterograde refractory period of the accessory pathway in patients with the Wolff-Parkinson-White syndrome. Am J Cardiol 50:180–184, July 1982.

26. BENNETT DH: Acute prolongation of myocardial refractoriness by sotalol. Br Heart J 47:521–526, June 1982.

27. GALLAGHER JJ, SVENSON RH, KASELL JH, GERMAN LD, BARDY GH, BROUGHTON A, CRITELLI G: Catheter technique for closed-chest ablation of the atrioventricular conduction system. A therapeutic alternative for the treatment of refractory supraventricular tachycardia. N Engl J Med 306:194–200, Jan 28, 1982.

28. OHKAWA S-I, HACKEL DB, MIKAT EM, GALLAGHER JJ, COX JL, SEALY WC: Anatomic effects of cryoablation of the AV conduction system. Circulation 65:1155–1162, June 1982.

29. HOLMES DR JR, HARTZLER GO, MERIDETH J: The clinical and electrophysiologic characteristics of patients with accelerated atrioventricular nodal conduction. Mayo Clin Proc 57:339–344, June 1982.

30. SCHEINMAN MM, MORADY F, HESS DS, GONZALEZ R: Catheter-induced ablation of the atrioventricular junction to control refractory supraventricular arrhythmias. JAMA 248:851–855, Aug 20, 1982.

31. BAUERNFEIND RA, SWIRYN S, STRASBERG B, PALILEO E, WYNDHAM C, DUFFY CE, ROSEN KM: Analysis of anterograde and retrograde fast pathway properties in patients with dual atrioventricular nodal pathways. Observations regarding the pathophysiology of the Lown-Ganong-Levine syndrome. Am J Cardiol 49:283–290, Feb 1982.

32. HOLMES DR JR, OSBORN MJ, GERSH B, MALONEY JD, DANIELSON GK: The Wolff-Parkinson-White syndrome: a surgical approach. Mayo Clin Proc 57:345–350, June 1982.

33. BURCHELL HB: The surgical treatment of reentrant atrioventricular tachycardia (Wolff-Parkinson-White Syndrome). Mayo Clin Proc 57:387–393, June 1982.

34. LUDOMIRSKY A, KLEIN HO, SARELLI P, BECKER B, HOFFMAN S, TAITELMAN U, BARZILAI J, LANG R, DAVID D, DISEGNI E, KAPLINSKY E: Q-T prolongation and polymorphous ("torsade de pointes") ventricular arrhythmias associated with organophosphorus insecticide poisoning. Am J Cardiol 49:1654–1658, May 1982.

35. SHAPIRO W, PARK J, KOCH GG: Variability of spontaneous and exercise-induced ventricular arrhythmias in the absence and presence of treatment with acebutolol or quinidine. Am J Cardiol 49:445–454, Feb 1982.

36. GIARDINA EV, BIGGER JT: Antiarrhythmic effect of imipramine hydrochloride in patients with ventricular premature complexes without psychological depression. Am J Cardiol 50:172–179, July 1982.

37. MEHTA J, CONTI CR: Mexiletine, a new antiarrhythmic agent, for treatment of premature ventricular complexes. Am J Cardiol 49:455–460, Feb 1982.

38. CALIFF RM, MCKINNIS RA, BURKS J, LEE KL, HARRELL FE, BEHAR VS, PRYOR DB, WAGNER GS, ROSATI RA: Prognostic implications of ventricular arrhythmias during 24 hour ambulatory monitoring in patients undergoing cardiac catheterization for coronary artery disease. Am J Cardiol 50:23–31, July 1982.

39. MARCUS FI, FONTAINE GH, GUIRAUDON G, FRANK R, LAURENCEAU JL, MALERGUE C, GROSGOGEAT Y: RV dysplasia: a report of 24 adult cases. Circulation 65:384–398, Feb 1982.

40. PALILEO EV, ASHLEY WW, SWIRYN S, BAUERNFEIND RA, STRASBERG B, PETROPOULOS AT, ROSEN KM: Exercise provocable right ventricular outflow tract tachycardia. Am Heart J 104:135–193, Aug 1982.

41. KENNEDY HL, PESCARMONA JE, BOUCHARD RJ, GOLDBERG RJ, CARALIS DG: Objective evidence of occult myocardial dysfunction in patients with frequent ventricular ectopy without clinically apparent heart disease. Am Heart J 104:57–65, July 1982.

42. SWIRYN S, PAVEL D, BYROM E, BAUERNFEIND RA, STRASBERG B, PALILEO E, LAM W, WYNDHAM CRC, ROSEN KM: Sequential regional phase mapping of radionuclide gated biventriculograms in patients with sustained ventricular tachycardia: close correlation with electrophysiologic characteristics. Am Heart J 103:319–332, March 1982.

43. BOOTH DC, POPIO KA, GETTES LS: Multiformity of induced unifocal ventricular premature beats in human subjects: electrocardiographic and angiographic correlations. Am J Cardiol 49:1643–1653, May 1982.

44. LIVELLI FD, BIGGER JT, REIFFEL JA, GANG ES, PATTON JN, NOETHLING PM, ROLNITZKY LM, GLIKLICH JI: Response to programmed ventricular stimulation: sensitivity, specificity and relation to heart disease. Am J Cardiol 50:452–458, Sept 1982.

45. BREITHARDT G, SEIPEL L, MEYER T, ABENDROTH RR: Prognostic significance of repetitive ventricular response during programmed ventricular stimulation. Am J Cardiol 49:693–698, March 1982.

46. DUFF HJ, RODEN DM, DAWSON AK, OATES JA, SMITH RF, WOOSLEY RL: Comparison of the effects of placebo and encainide on programmed electrical stimulation and ventricular arrhythmia frequency. Am J Cardiol 50:305–312, Aug 1982.

47. NACCARELLI GV, PRYSTOWSKY EN, JACKMAN WM, HEGER JJ, RAHILLY GT, ZIPES DP: Role of electrophysiologic testing in managing patients who have ventricular tachycardia unrelated to coronary artery disease. Am J Cardiol 50:165–171, 1982.

48. MORADY F, HESS D, SCHEINMAN MM: Electrophysiologic drug testing in patients with malignant ventricular arrhythmias: importance of stimulation at more than one ventricular site. Am J Cardiol 50:1045–1060, Nov 1982.

49. SWIRYN S, BAUERNFEIND RA, STRASBERG B, PALILEO E, IVERSON N, LEVY PS, ROSEN KM: Prediction of response to class I antiarrhythmic drugs during electrophysiologic study of ventricular tachycardia. Am Heart J 104:43–50, July 1982.

50. NADEMANEE K, HENDRICKSON J, KANNAN R, SINGH BN: Antiarrhythmic efficacy and electrophysiologic actions of amiodarone in patients with life-threatening ventricular arrhythmias: potent suppression of spontaneously occurring tachyarrhythmias versus inconsistent abolition of induced ventricular tachycardia. Am Heart J 103:950–959, June 1982.

51. WAXMAN HL, GROH WC, MARCHLINSKI FE, BUXTON AE, SADOWSKI LM, HOROWITZ LN, JOSEPHSON ME, KASTOR JA: Amiodarone for control of sustained ventricular tachyarrhythmia: clinical and electrophysiologic effects in 51 patients. Am J Cardiol 50:1066–1074, Nov 1982.

52. FINERMAN WB JR, HAMER A, PETER T, WEISS D, MANDEL WJ: Electrophysiologic effects of chronic amiodarone therapy in patients with ventricular arrhythmias. Am Heart J 104:987–995, Nov 1982.

53. PALILEO EV, WELCH W, HOFF J, STRASBERG B, BAUERNFEIND RA, SWIRYN S, COELHO A, ROGEN KM: Lack of effectiveness of oral mexiletine in patients with drug-refractory paroxysmal sustained ventricular tachycardia. A study utilizing programmed stimulation. Am J Cardiol 50:1075–1081, Nov 1982.

54. BACANER MB, BENDITT DG: Antiarrhythmic, antifibrillatory, and hemodynamic actions of bethanidine sulfate: an orally effective analog of bretylium for suppression of ventricular tachyarrhythmias. Am J Cardiol 50:728–734, Oct 1982.

55. SINGH SN, DIBIANCO R, DAVIDOV ME, GOTTDIENER JS, JOHNSON WL, LADDU AR, FLETCHER RD: Comparison of acebutolol and propranolol for treatment of chronic ventricular arrhythmia: a placebo-controlled, double-blind, randomized crossover study. Circulation 65:1356–1364, June 1982.

56. ROSS DL, SZE DY, KEEFE DL, SWERDLOW CD, ECHT DS, GRIFFIN JC, WINKLE RA, MASON JW:

Antiarrhythmic drug combinations in the treatment of VT. Circulation 66:1205–1210, Dec 1982.

57. RINKENBERGER RL, PRYSTOWSKY EN, JACKMAN WM, NACCARELLI GV, HEGER JJ, ZIPES DP: Drug conversion of nonsustained ventricular tachycardia during serial electrophysiologic studies: identification of drugs that exacerbate tachycardia and potential mechanisms. Am Heart J 103:177–184, Feb 1982.

58. VELEBIT V, PODRID P, LOWN B, COHEN BH, GRABOYS TB: Aggravation and provocation of ventricular arrhythmias by antiarrhythmic drugs. Circulation 65:886–893, May 1982.

59. GRABOYS RB, LOWN B, PODRID PJ, DESILVA R: Long-term survival of patients with malignant ventricular arrhythmia treated with antiarrhythmic drugs. Am J Cardiol 50:437–443, Sept 1982.

60. WAXMAN HL, CAIN ME, GREENSPAN AM, JOSEPHSON ME: Termination of VT with ventricular stimulation: salutary effect of increased current strength. Circulation. 65:800–804, Apr 1982.

61. ZIPES DP, JACKMAN WM, HEGER JJ, CHILSON DA, BROWNE KF, NACCARELLI GV, RAHILLY GT JR, PRYSTOWSKY EN: Clinical transvenous cardioversion of recurrent life-threatening ventricular tachyarrhythmias; low energy synchronized cardioversion of ventricular tachycardia and termination of ventricular fibrillation in patients using a catheter electrode. Am Heart J 103:789–794, May 1982.

62. GARDNER MJ, WAXMAN HL, BUXTON AE, CAIN ME, JOSEPHSON ME: Termination of ventricular tachycardia. Evaluation of a new pacing method. Am J Cardiol 50:1338–1345, Dec 1982.

63. KLEIN H, KARP RB, KOUCHOUKOS NT, ZORN GL, JAMES TN, WALDO AL: Intraoperative electrophysiologic mapping of the ventricles during sinus rhythm in patients with a previous myocardial infarction: identification of the electrophysiologic substrate of ventricular arrhythmias. Circulation 66:847–853, Oct 1982.

64. WIENER I, MINDICH B, PITCHON R, PICHARD A, KUPERSMITH J, ESTIOKO M, JURADO R, CAMUNAS J, LITWAK R: Epicardial activation in patients with coronary artery disease: effects of regional contraction abnormalities. Circulation 65:154–160, Jan 1982.

65. BREITHARDT G, SEIPEL L, OSTERMEYER J, KARBENN U, ABENDROTH RR, BORGGREFE M, YEH HL, BIRCKS W: Effects of antiarrhythmic surgery on late ventricular potentials recorded by precordial signal averaging in patients with ventricular tachycardia. Am Heart J 104:996–1003, Nov 1982.

66. FONTAINE G, GUIRAUDON G, FRANK R, FILLETTE F, CABROL C, GROSGOGEAT Y: Surgical management of ventricular tachycardia unrelated to myocardial ischemia or infarction. Am J Cardiol 49:397–410, Feb 1982.

67. WEINER I, MINDICH B, PITCHON R: Determinants of VT in patients with ventricular aneurysms: results of intraoperative epicardial and endocardial mapping. Circulation 65:856–861, May 1982.

68. MASON JW, STINSON EB, WINKLE RA, GRIFFIN JC, OYER PE, ROSS DL, DERBY G: Surgery for ventricular tachycardia: efficacy of left ventricular aneurysm resection compared with operation guided by electrical activation mapping. Circulation 65:1148–1155, June 1982.

69. UNGERLEIDER RM, HOLMAN WL, STANLEY TE, LOFLAND GK, WILLIAMS JM, IDEKER RE, SMITH PK, QUICK G, COX JL: Encircling endocardial ventriculotomy for refractory ischemic ventricular tachycardia. J Thorac Cardiovasc Surg 83:840–864, June 1982.

70. COX JL, GALLAGHER JJ, UNGERLEIDER RM: Encircling endocardial ventriculotomy for refractory ischemic ventricular tachycardia. J Thorac Cardiovasc Surg 83:865–872, June 1982.

71. JOSEPHSON ME, HARKEN AH, HOROWITZ LN: Long-term results of endocardial resection for sustained ventricular tachycardia in coronary disease patients. Am Heart J 104:51–57, July 1982.

72. MARTIN JL, UNTEREKER WJ, HARDEN AH, HOROWITZ LN, JOSEPHSON ME: Aneurysmectomy and endocardial resection for ventricular tachycardia: Favorable hemodynamic and antiar-

rhythmic results in patients with global left ventricular dysfunction. Am Heart J 103:960–965, June 1982.

73. MORAN JM, KEHOE RF, LOEB JM, LICHTENTHAL PR, SANDERS JH, MICHAELIS LL: Extended endocardial resection for the treatment of ventricular tachycardia and ventricular fibrillation. Ann Thorac Surg 34:538–552, Nov 1982.

74. ADGEY AAJ, DEVLIN JE, WEBB SW, MULHOLLAND HC: Initiation of ventricular fibrillation outside hospital in patients with acute ischaemic heart disease. Br Heart J 47:55–61, Jan 1982.

75. SISCOVICK DS, WEISS NS, HALLSTROM AP, INUI TS, PETERSON DR: Physical activity and primary cardiac arrest. JAMA 248:3113–3117, Dec 17, 1982.

76. McMANUS BM, WALLER BF, GRAYBOYS TB, MITCHELL JH, SIEGEL RJ, MILLER HS JR, FROELICHER VF, ROBERTS WC: Exercise and sudden death. Parts I and II. Current Problems Cardiol 6:1–89, Dec 1981, 7:1–57, Jan 1982.

77. THOMPSON PD, FUNK EJ, CARLETON RA, STURNER WQ: Incidence of death during jogging in Rhode Island from 1975 through 1980. JAMA 247:2535–2538, May 14, 1982.

78. VIRMANI R, ROBINOWITZ M, McALLISTER HA JR: Nontraumatic death in joggers: a series of 30 patients at autopsy. Am J Med 72:874–881, June 1982.

79. RABKIN SW, MATHEWSON FAL, TATE RB: The electrocardiogram in apparently healthy men and the risk of sudden death. Br Heart J 47:546–552, June 1982.

80. WEAVER WD, COBB LA, HALLSTROM AP: Characteristics of survivors of exertion- and nonexertion-related cardiac arrest: value of subsequent exercise testing. Am J Cardiol 50:671–676, Oct 1982.

81. WEAVER WD, COBB LA, HALLSTROM AP: Ambulatory arrhythmias in resuscitated victims of cardiac arrest. Circulation 66:212–217, July 1982.

82. NIKOLIC G, BISHOP RL, SINGH JB: Sudden death recorded during Holter monitoring. Circulation 66:218–225, July 1982.

83. BEARD CM, FUSTER V, ELVEBACK LR: Daily and seasonal variation in sudden cardiac death, Rochester, Minnesota, 1950–1975. Mayo Clin Proc 57:704–706, Nov 1982.

84. LOWN B: Mental stress, arrhythmias and sudden death. Am J Med 72:177–180, Feb 1982

85. MITTLEMAN RE, WETLI CV: The fatal cafe coronary. Foreign-body airway obstruction. JAMA 247:1285–1288, March 5, 1982.

86. HERSHEY CO, FISHER L: Why outcome of cardiopulmonary resuscitation in general wards is poor. Lancet 1:31–34, Jan 2, 1982.

87. BJORK RJ, SNYDER BD, CAMPION BC, LOEWENSON RB: Medical complications of cardiopulmonary arrest. Arch Intern Med 142:500–503, March 1982.

88. MORLEY CA, PERRINS EJ, GRANT P, CHAN SL, McBRIEN DJ, SUTTON R: Carotid sinus syncope treated by pacing: analysis of persistent symptoms and role of atrioventricular sequential pacing. Br Heart J 47:411–418, May 1982.

89. SILVERSTEIN MD, SINGER DE, MULLEY AG, THIBAULT GE, BARNETT GO: Patients with syncope admitted to medical intensive care units. JAMA 248:1185–1189, Sept 10, 1982.

90. GULAMHUSEIN S, NACCARELLI GV, KO PT, PRYSTOWSKY EN, ZIPES DP, BARNETT HJM, HEGER JJ, KLEIN GJ: Value and limitations of clinical electrophysiologic study in assessment of patients with unexplained syncope. Am J Med 73:700–705, Nov 1982.

91. HESS DS, MORADY F, SCHEINMAN MM: Electrophysiologic testing in the evaluation of patients with syncope of undetermined origin. Am J Cardiol 50:1308–1315, Dec 1982.

92. REINHART S, McANULTY JH, DOBBS J: Type and timing of permanent pacemaker failure. Chest 81:433–435, Apr 1982.

93. BERGFELDT L, EDHAG O, VEDIN L, VALLIN H: Ankylosing spondylitis: an important cause of severe disturbances of the cardiac conduction system: prevalence among 223 pacemaker-treated men. Am J Med 73:187–191, Aug 1982.

94. STONE JM, BHAKTA RD, LUTGEN J: Dual chamber sequential pacing management of sinus

node dysfunction: advantages over single-chamber pacing. Am Heart J 104:1319–1327, Dec 1982.

95. VERA Z, AWAN NA, MASON DT: Assessment of oral quinidine effects on sinus node function in sick sinus syndrome patients. Am Heart J 103:80–84, Jan 1982.

96. KAY R, ESTIOKO M, WIENER I: Primary sick sinus syndrome as an indication for chronic pacemaker therapy in young adults; incidence, clinical features, and long-term evaluation. Am Heart J 103:338–342, March 1982.

97. REIFFEL JA, GANG E, BIGGER JT JR, LIVELLI F JR, ROLNITZKY L, CRAMER M: Sinus node recovery time related to paced cycle length in normals and patients with sinoatrial dysfunction. Am Heart J 104:746–752, Oct 1982.

98. KINOSHITA S, NAKAGAWA K, KATO N, NISHINO T, TANABE Y: Mechanism of supraventricular parasystole. Circulation 65:208–212, Jan 1982.

99. HAVELDA CJ, SOHI GS, FLOWERS NC, HORAN LG: The pathologic correlates of the ECG: complete LBBB. Circulation 65:445–451, March 1982.

100. VIRTANEN KS, HEIKKILA J, KALA R, SILTANEN P: Chest pain and rate-dependent left bundle branch block in patients with normal coronary arteriograms. Chest 81:326–331, March 1982.

101. PETERS RW, SCHEINMAN MM, DHINGRA R, ROSEN K, McANULTY J, RAHIMTOOLA SH, MODIN G: Serial electrophysiologic studies in patients with chronic BBB. Circulation 65:1480–1485, June 1982.

102. McANULTY JH, RAHIMTOOLA SH, MURPHY E, DEMOTS H, RITZMANN L, KANAREK PE, KAUFFMAN S: Natural history of "high-risk" bundle-branch block: Final report of a prospective study. N Engl J Med 307:137–143, July 15, 1982.

103. STRASBERG B, RICH S, LAM W, SWIRYN S, BAUERNFEIND R, ROSEN KM: M-mode echocardiography in left bundle branch block: significance of frontal plane QRS axis. Am Heart J 104:775–779, Oct 1982.

104. DANCY M, LEECH G, LEATHAM A: Significance of complete right bundle-branch block when an isolated finding. An echocardiographic study. Br Heart J 48:217–221, Sept 1982.

105. PINSKY WW, GILLETTE PC, GARSON A, McNAMARA DG: Diagnosis, management, and long-term results of patients with congenital complete atrioventricular block. Pediatrics 69:728–733, June 1982.

106. REID JM, COLEMAN EN, DOIG W: Complete congenital heart block: report of 35 cases. Br Heart J 48:236–239, Sept 1982.

107. BESLEY DC, McWILLIAMS GJ, MOODIE DS, CASTLE LW: Long-term follow-up of young adults following permanent pacemaker placement for complete heart block. Am Heart J 103:332–337, March 1982.

108. SPRUNG CL, POZEN RG, ROZANSKI JJ, PINERO JR, EISLER BR, CASTELLANOS A: Advanced ventricular arrhythmias during bedside pulmonary artery catheterization. Am J Med 72:203–208, Feb 1982.

109. GALLAGHER JJ, SMITH WM, KERR CR, KASELL J, COOK L, REITER M, STERBA R, HARIE M: Esophageal pacing: a diagnostic and therapeutic tool. Circulation 65:336–341, Feb 1982.

110. MILLER WP: Cardiac arrhythmias and conduction disturbances in the sleep apnea syndrome: prevalence and significance. Am J Med 73:317–321, Sept 1982.

111. KRUSE I, ARNMAN K, CONRADSON TB, RYDEN L: A comparison of the acute and long-term hemodynamic effects of ventricular inhibited and atrial synchronous ventricular inhibited pacing. Circulation 65:846–855, May 1982.

112. HELLESTRAND KJ, BEXTON RS, NATHAN AW, SPURRELL RAJ, CAMM AJ: Acute electrophysiologic effects of *flecainide acetate* on cardiac conduction and refractoriness in man. Br Heart J 48:140–148, Aug 1982.

113. NATHAN AW, HELLESTRAND KJ, BEXTON RS, WARD DE, SPURRELL RAJ, CAMM AJ: Electrophysiologic effects of sotalol—just another beta blocker? Br Heart J 47:515–520, June 1982.

114. SOBEL SM, RAKITA L: Pneumonitis and pulmonary fibrosis associated with amiodarone treatment: a possible complication of a new antiarrhythmic drug. Circulation 65:819–824, Apr 1982.

115. YEE R, ZIPES DP, GULAMHUSEIN S, KALLOK MJ, KLEIN GF: Low energy countershock using an intravascular catheter in an acute cardiac care setting. Am J Cardiol 50:1124–1129, Nov 1982.

116. NADEMANEE K, SINGH BN, GUERRERO J, HENDRICKSON J, INTARACHOT V, BAKY S: Accurate rapid compact analog method for the quantification of frequency and duration of myocardial ischemia by semiautomated analysis of 24-hour Holter ECG recordings. Am Heart J 103:802–813, May 1982.

117. RUPPERT GB, LINDSAY J, BARTH WF: Cardiac conduction abnormalities in Reiter's syndrome. Am J Med 73:335–340, Sept 1982.

118. WEAVER WD, COBB LA, COPASS MK, HALLSTROM AP: Ventricular defibrillation—a comparative trial using 175-J and 320-J shocks. N Engl J Med 307:1101–1106, Oct 28, 1982.

119. JOHNSON RE, WARE JD, MOFFITT S, ARENSBERG D, WENGER NK: Response to exercise in patients taking psychotropic drugs: arrhythmias and the QT interval (QT wave peak). Arch Intern Med 142:755–759, Apr 1982.

Systemic Hypertension

DETECTION, EFFECTS OF VARIOUS NATURAL STATES AND SUBSTANCES, AND CONSEQUENCES

BP during normal daily activities, sleep, and exercise

Pickering and associates[1] from New York City recorded BP every 15 minutes using a noninvasive ambulatory BP recorder during 24 hours in 25 subjects with normal BP, 25 with borderline systemic hypertension, and 25 with established essential hypertension. Readings were analyzed for 4 situations: 1) physician's office, 2) work, 3) home, and 4) asleep. Treadmill exercise tests also were performed on a separate occasion with the Bruce protocol. The 24-hour recording in all 3 groups showed the highest BPs during work and the lowest during sleep. The situational BP changes were generally similar, but both hypertensive groups differed from normal subjects in that they showed consistently higher BPs in the physician's office than at home, whereas normal subjects showed little difference. During exercise, the hypertensive groups showed a similar rise of systolic pressure to that of normal subjects. Pressures recorded in the physician's office gave good predictions of the average 24-hour pressure in normal and established hypertensive subjects, but not in the borderline group; in such patients, 24-

hour monitoring may be of particular value in establishing the need for treatment.

Circadian BP patterns

Noninvasive ambulatory circadian BP monitoring was recently introduced as a technique to define BP better in patients with borderline systemic hypertension. This technique also has been used to quantify variability of BP and to assess the effects of hypertensive therapy. Early experiences using BP monitoring during the day or at night have shown that the variability of BP increases with the height of the BP but not with the patient's age. Other studies, however, using circadian ambulatory BP monitoring equipment failed to agree whether variability of BP is related to age. Drayer and associates[2] from Long Beach and Irvine, California, performed circadian BP monitoring in 50 untreated ambulatory patients with systemic hypertension to study the effects of age on the pattern and variability of BP and heart rate. Casual BP, measured in the morning, was greater than the average of the BPs measured at 7.5-minute intervals for 24 hours ($148 \pm 2/95 \pm 2$ and $137 \pm 2/88 \pm 2$ mmHg, $p < 0.001$) (Table 4–1). The correlation between casual systolic pressure and the 24-hour average was stronger ($p < 0.05$) in younger (<55 years of age) patients ($r = 0.69$, n, 24, $p < 0.001$) than in older patients ($r = 0.42$, n, 26, $p < 0.1$). Similarly, diastolic pressures correlated more strongly ($p < 0.05$) in younger patients ($r = 0.71$, $p < 0.001$) than in older patients ($r = 0.43$, $p < 0.05$). Variability of systolic pressure, defined as the standard deviation of all readings obtained during 24 hours, was greater than that of diastolic pressure (17 and 13 mmHg, respectively, $p < 0.001$). Moreover, the variability of systolic pressure was greater in older than in younger patients (18 and 15 mmHg, respectively, $p < 0.01$) (Table 4-2). The variability of diastolic pressure was slightly but not significantly greater in older patients (14 and 13 mmHg, NS). The circadian pattern of BP expressed as averages of readings obtained during consecutive 2-hour intervals was similar in the 2 age groups. However, the level of systolic pressure was consistently higher ($p < 0.01$) and that of both diastolic pressure and heart rate consistently lower ($p < 0.01$) in older patients. Thus, ambulatory circadian BP monitoring reveals significant changes in BP levels and its variability with age; the casual BP does not accurately reflect these changes. Longer periods of BP monitoring are required for accurate assessment of the characteristics of hypertension in the aged.

A representative value for whole day BP

Weber and associates[3] from Long Beach, and Irvine, California, analyzed shorter-term alternatives to 24-hour monitoring of BP in 6 patients with systemic hypertension. Average BP during the 24-hour period was lower than averages during a 2-hour morning period or those based on either 3 readings or a single reading taken at 8 a.m. The systolic and diastolic BP 2-hour averages correlated more strongly with the 24-hour averages than did the 3-

TABLE 4-1. *Comparison of casual blood pressure and heart rate with parameters obtained during 24-hour monitoring in 50 patients with hypertension.*

	CASUAL*	P	24H AVERAGE	VARIABILITY†	HIGHEST 2H AVERAGE	LOWEST 2H AVERAGE
Systolic blood pressure (mmHg)	148 ± 2	<0.001	137 ± 2	16.7 ± 0.6	155 ± 2	116 ± 2
Diastolic blood pressure (mmHg)	95 ± 2	<0.001	88 ± 2	13.1 ± 0.4	104 ± 2	74 ± 2
Pulse pressure (mmHg)	53 ± 2	<0.001	48 ± 2	14.3 ± 0.5	51 ± 2	35 ± 2
Heart rate (beats/min)	74 ± 2	ns	75 ± 2	11.8 ± 0.5	89 ± 2	62 ± 1

* n = 44. † Variability is defined as the standard deviation of all readings obtained during 24 h. ns = not significant.

TABLE 4-2. *Comparison of different variables of blood pressure and heart rate between younger (55 years of age or less, n = 24) and older (over 55 years of age, n = 26) patients with hypertension.*

	YOUNGER PATIENTS	P	OLDER PATIENTS
Casual systolic pressure (mmHg)	143 ± 3	<0.1	153 ± 3
Average 24 h systolic pressure (mmHg)	135 ± 3		136 ± 3
Variability of systolic pressure (mmHg)*	15.2 ± 0.7	<0.01	18.1 ± 0.8
Casual diastolic pressure (mmHg)	96 ± 3		94 ± 2
Average 24 h diastolic pressure (mmHg)	89 ± 2		87 ± 2
Variability of diastolic pressure (mmHg)*	12.5 ± 0.5		13.7 ± 0.6
Casual pulse pressure† (mmHg)	47 ± 2	<0.01	59 ± 3
Average 24 h pulse pressure (mmHg)	46 ± 2		49 ± 3
Variability of pulse pressure (mmHg)*	13.4 ± 0.6	<0.1	15.2 ± 0.7
Casual heart rate† (beats/min)	74 ± 2		74 ± 3
Average 24 h heart rate (beats/min)	76 ± 2		74 ± 2
Variability of heart rate (beats/min)*	12.6 ± 0.6	<0.01	11.0 ± 0.7

* Variability is defined as standard deviation of all readings obtained during 24 h. † n = 22 in each subgroup.

reading or single-reading alternatives. Thus, the average of serial BP readings obtained during a 2-hour morning period is a consistent predictor of the whole day BP and represents it more closely than the conventionally used single reading.

BP in teenagers

It has been suggested that a hyperkinetic circulatory state with high cardiac output causes high BP in childhood and secondarily in adulthood. Hofman and associates (4) from Boston, Massachusetts, studied BP and cardiac output in 319 subjects aged 15–19 years. The BP was measured with an automated device; cardiac output was estimated by M-mode echo and indexed by body surface area. The distribution of cardiac output was stratified using quartiles. Mean arterial pressure was virtually constant over these strata, with boys and girls showing essentially the same pattern. Linear regression of mean arterial pressure on cardiac output yielded a coefficient that was not significantly different from 0. A history of high BP in the parents was positively associated with mean arterial pressure, but unrelated to cardiac output, in the offspring. These data do not support the hypothesis that the hyperkinetic circulatory state causes high BP in childhood; rather, raised BP in adolescents appears to relate to increased peripheral vascular resistance. Therefore these findings lend support to the view that change in BP over time is caused by a gradual increase in peripheral resistance beginning early in life.

Relation of BP at ages 20–39 to subsequent BP

Since identification of persons at risk developing systemic hypertension may permit earlier detection and perhaps prevention of this condition, Rabkin and colleagues[5] from Winnipeg, Canada, investigated the relation of BP in men aged 20–39 years to their subsequent BP from the perspective of BP tracking, position in BP distribution, and later evidence of hypertensive BP values. The group followed 3,983 men since 1948, and 90% were 20–39 years of age at entry. The BP in individuals not treated with antihypertensive medication was examined at 5-year intervals to 1978. To adjust for age, BP was examined within 5-year age groups at entry. The correlations between entry and subsequent BP at the same length of follow-up were greater for systolic than for diastolic BP. Men whose BP was below the mean at entry were less likely to have a BP > 1 standard deviation (SD) above the mean at any of the examinations. Men with an entry BP > 1 SD above the mean were more likely to have BP above the mean at later follow-up. The relation decreased considerably after 20 years, espeically in the 20–24 year age groups. The results were similar for the probability of hypertensive values (systolic BP > 141–150 mmHg and a diastolic BP > 90–95 mmHg) at later examination. Thus, these investigators concluded from a 30-year follow-up, that BP in later life can be predicted from BP at ages 20–39 years and can identify groups at higher or low risk for hypertension.

Isolated systolic hypertension in elderly

Since 1980, both the National Coordinating Committee of the High Blood Pressure Education Program and the Joint National Committee on Detection, Evaluation, and Treatment of High Blood Pressure have addressed the problem of isolated systolic systemic hypertension in the elderly. This issue is important because there are now 25 million Americans aged ≥ 65 years and it is estimated that by 1990 there will be nearly 30 million such Americans. Gifford[6] from Cleveland, Ohio, reviewed this subject. He defined isolated or pure systolic systemic hypertension as an elevation of systolic BP ≥160 mmHg and a diastolic BP of <90 mmHg. Although there are no control prospective trials confirming a reduction in morbidity and mortality with treatment, Gifford believes that a reduction in the systolic BP will clearly reduce LV work load and if systolic hypertension is clearly established by

TABLE 4-3. *Doses of some antihypertensive drugs recommended for elderly patients with isolated systolic hypertension. Reproduced with permission from Gifford.[6]*

DRUG	INITIAL DOSAGE, MG	USUAL MAXIMAL DOSAGE, MG
Diuretics		
Hydrochlorothiazide	25 qd	50 qd
Chlorthalidone	25 qd or qod	50 qd
Metolazone	2.5 qd or qod	5 qd
Sympathetic depressants		
Methyldopa	250 qd	500 qd
Clonidine hydrochloride	0.1 qd	0.6 bid
Vasodilator		
Hydralazine hydrochloride	25 qd	100 bid

multiple determinations he believes that therapy for these individuals is appropriate. He recommends administering any hypertensive agents cautiously and in low doses initially with slow, incremental increases (Table 4-3).

Usefulness of home BP determinations

The results of the Hypertension Detection Follow-up Program (HDFP) group study substantially lowered the BP levels at which any hypertensive therapy should be started. Attention is now focusing on treatment of patients with borderline systemic hypertension, those whose readings oscillate above and below 150 mmHg systolic and 90 mmHg diastolic. The major clinical problem in the treatment of patients with borderline hypertension is the variability of clinic BP readings. The problem of separating spontaneous BP variability from the effects of treatment are so large that 3 recent studies of mild hypertension found it necessary to remove from the trial those patients with occasionally normal readings. Cottier and associates[7] from Ann Arbor, Michigan, designed a study to investigate the sensitivity of home BP measurements in detecting minor changes induced by any hypertensive therapy. Sixteen untreated patients underwent a double-blind trial of propranolol hydrochloride (average dose, 105 mg), clonidine hydrochloride (0.24 mg), and placebo. Home BP readings decreased with both active compounds (-8/-5 with propranolol and -11/-7 with clonidine) (Fig. 4-1). During placebo, the readings increased to levels identical to untreated values. This study demonstrates that patients with borderline hypertension are consistently capable of detecting small average changes in home BP. It is also shown that sympatholytic monotherapy can be effectively used to lower the BP in such patients.

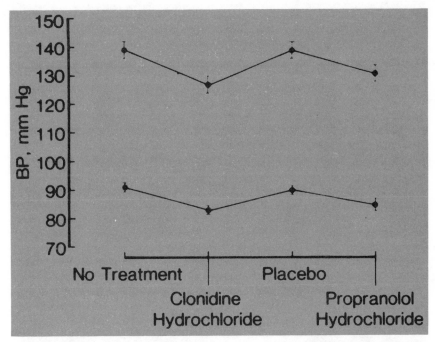

Fig. 4-1. Systolic and diastolic BP ± SEM throughout trial. Analysis of variance to test significance of difference was used. With clonidine hydrochloride -vs- placebo and clonidine -vs-baseline, untreated BPs were significantly different ($p < .01$). Similarly, propranolol hydrochloride -vs- placebo and propranolol -vs- baseline were significantly different ($p < .01$). There was no significant difference between baseline and placebo periods. Systolic BP with clonidine was lower than with propranolol ($p < .01$). Reproduced with permission from Cottier et al.[7]

Coital BP in hypertensives

In the investigation of patients with systemic hypertension, Mann and associates[8] from Harrow, England, performed a large number of ambulatory recordings of intraarterial BP. Subjects were encouraged to behave as normally as possible, being little encumbered by the monitoring apparatus, and several had sexual intercourse during the recording period. Technically satisfactory recordings of coital BP were made on 18 occasions in 11 hypertensive subjects. Their ages were 29–56 years (mean, 42) and 3 were women. Peak BP values up to 300/175 mmHg were observed during coitus, the mean for men being 237/138 and for women 216/127 mmHg (Fig. 4-2). The recordings, however, showed that both heart rate and BP fluctuated widely during sexual activity, occasionally reaching very high levels. Though patterns varied greatly, the highest peak of heart rate and BP (presumably

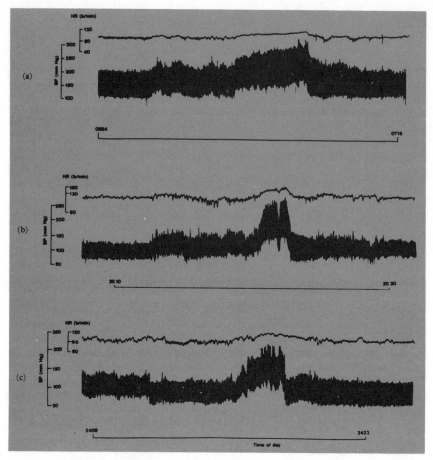

Fig. 4-2. Examples of coital blood pressure recordings in 3 hypertensive men: (a) case 2; (b) case 6; (c) case 8. Note the widely fluctuating pattern and simultaneous peaks in heart rate and blood pressure at time of presumed orgasm. Reproduced with permission from Mann et al.[8]

associated with orgasm) were generally simultaneous and were followed by a rapid fall to precoital levels or below. The peak levels of both BP and heart rate were sustained in each case for only a few seconds. Peak heart rates were 131 beats/minute for men and 96 beats/minute for women.

Cardiovascular effects of obesity and hypertension

Messerli[9] from New Orleans, Louisiana, reviewed the association between obesity and systemic hypertension. The evidence linking high BP and obesity is based on 3 basic observations: 1) hypertensive patients tend to become obese; 2) obese patients are at higher risk of hypertension than

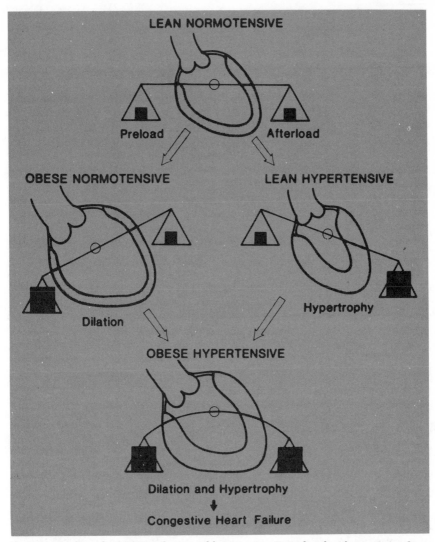

Fig. 4-3. Cardiac adaptation to obesity and hypertension. Reproduced with permission from Messerli et al.[9]

nonobese subjects, and weight gain might indicate whether or not borderline hypertension evolves into established hypertension; 3) caloric restriction leading to weight loss is commonly associated with fall in arterial BP irrespective of whether the patient restricts his salt intake. Despite the clinical and epidemiologic evidence, pathogenetic mechanisms of the relation between high BP and obesity remain poorly understood, and whether or not this relation is causal has not been firmly established. Messerli presents

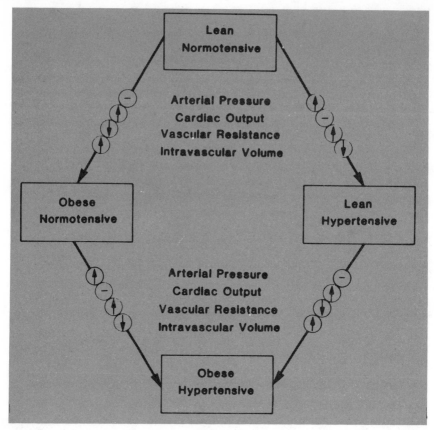

Fig. 4-4. Cardiovascular effects of obesity and hypertension. Reproduced with permission from Messerli et al.[9]

the following hypotheses in this respect: 1) high BP or the drugs used in its treatment stimulate a patient to increase caloric intake inappropriately; 2) obesity and its metabolic changes or a high caloric (and salt) intake with lack of exercise predispose a subject to high BP; 3) both hypertension and obesity are influenced by a common, yet unknown, pathophysiologic factor; 4) the common denominator of high BP and obesity could be the factitious phenomenon of inaccurate BP recording due to increased arm girth. Messerli reviewed some cardiovascular findings that are induced by obesity and high BP or the combination of these disorders.

Although often coexisting in the same patient, obesity and essential hypertension exert disparate cardiovascular effects. An excess of adipose tissue augments cardiac output, stroke volume, and LV filling pressure, expands intravascular volume, and lowers total peripheral resistance. (Figs. 4-3 and 4-4). In contrast, essential hypertension in a nonobese patient is associated with a contracted intravascular volume, high total peripheral resistance, and normal cardiac output, but with increased LV stroke work due to high afterload. Left ventricular adaptation will consist of eccentric hypertrophy in the obese (irrespective of arterial pressure) and concentric hypertrophy in the nonobese hypertensive patient. The combination of obesity and hypertension burdens the heart with high preload and high afterload, thereby greatly enhancing the risk of CHF. Peripheral resistance and intravascular volume may be normal in mildly hypertensive obese patients because of the mutually antagonizing effects of the increase in arterial BP and the increase in body weight. The fall in arterial pressure associated with weight loss seems to be caused by a decrease in adrenergic activity, which leads to a fall in cardiac output without change in vascular resistance. Obesity hypertension may be the result of an inappropriately raised cardiac output in the presence of a relatively restricted arterial capacity due to the low vascularity of adipose tissue. In morbid obesity increased blood viscosity may contribute to the raised arterial pressure.

Error in BP measurement due to incorrect cuff size in obesity

A cuff of inappropriate size in relation to the patient's arm circumference can cause considerable bias in BP measurement. Since the standard 12 cm wide cuff is the only one generally used, the expected error in BP measurements would be greatest in obese subjects, who make up at least 25% of the adult population in the west. Studies to determine the error in BP determination attributable to inappropriate cuff size have been conducted almost exclusively in nonobese subjects. Maxwell and associates[10] from Los Angeles, California, analyzed 84,000 serial BP measurements made with cuffs of 3 different sizes by trained nurse specialists in 1,240 obese subjects during a program of rapid weight reduction. The differences in readings between the 3 cuffs were smallest in nonobese subjects and became progressively greater with increasing arm circumference in the obese patients. The regular cuff (12 × 23 cm) showed the greatest bias in relation to arm circumference. Formulae and a table were derived to correct the measurement error caused by cuffs of inappropriate size at various arm circumferences. (Table 4-4). The reported high prevalence of systemic hypertension in obese subjects may be greatly overestimated according to these authors.

Habitual excessive dietary salt intake and BP levels in renal transplant recipients

Kalbfleisch and associates[11], from Columbus, Ohio, and Milwaukee, Wisconsin, observed that renal transplant recipients with good graft function (mean serum creatinine level 1.5 mg/dl ± 0.5 SK, n, 68) had dietary salt intakes (estimated from serial measurements of 24-hour sodium excretion rate) that averaged 43% higher than that of a comparable group of healthy subjects. There was no correlation between BP levels and salt intake and, despite the high dietary salt intake, systemic hypertension was present in

TABLE 4-4. *Correction of systolic and diastolic BP readings obtained with cuffs of different sizes at various ACs. Reproduced with permission from Maxwell.*[10]

	CORRECTION (mmHg)					
	LARGE CUFF		REGULAR CUFF		THIGH CUFF	
AC (cm)	S	D	S	D	S	D
20	+11	+7	+11	+7	+11	+7
22	+9	+6	+9	+6	+11	+6
24	+8	+5	+7	+4	+10	+6
26	+7	+5	+5	+3	+9	+5
28	+5	+4	+3	+2	+8	+5
30	+4	+3	0	0	+7	+4
32	+3	+2	−2	−1	+6	+4
34	+2	+1	−4	−3	+5	+3
36	0	+1	−6	−4	+5	+3
38	−1	0	−8	−6	+4	+2
40	−2	−1	−10	−7	+3	+1
42	−4	−2	−12	−9	+2	+1
44	−5	−3	−14	−10	+1	0
46	−6	−3	−16	−11	0	0
48	−7	−4	−18	−13	−1	−1
50	−9	−5	−21	−14	−1	−1
52	−10	−6	−23	−16	−2	−2
54	−11	−7	−25	−17	−3	−2
56	−13	−7	−27	−19	−4	−3

For correction of BP readings in individual patients, positive numbers should be added to and negative numbers subtracted from the reading obtained. S = systolic correction; D = diastolic correction.

only 29 patients and was usually mild; mean systolic and diastolic BP was 132 ± 10 and 89 ± 7 mmHg, respectively, while the patients were receiving antihypertensive medication (median number of standard doses of antihypertensive medication was 1.0 doses/patient/day). These observations suggest that high dietary salt intake does not exert a powerful BP elevating effect, since any effect of high dietary salt intake to raise BP should have been magnified in the renal transplant recipients because of their reduced renal mass and their chronic glucocorticoid therapy.

Pressor effect of alcohol

Arkwright and colleagues[12] in Perth, Australia, examined 30 pairs of drinking and nondrinking men matched for age and weight from a working population in which a close relation between alcohol consumption and BP had been demonstrated. Men who drank an average of 408 ml of ethanol/

week had a higher supine and standing systolic and supine diastolic BP than nondrinkers. Resting plasma concentrations of free and sulfonated norepinephrine and epinephrine renin activity, angiotensin II, aldosterone, and cortisol were similar in drinkers and nondrinkers. To investigate differences that may arise when sympathoadrenal activity was stimulated, the subjects underwent a series of standardized physiologic stresses: isometric handgrip, mental arithmetic, cold pressor testing, standing and bicycle exercise. Heart rate and BP responses were similar in drinkers and nondrinkers, although the differences in BP between the 2 tended to become smaller after certain stresses. No differences in the plasma levels of free or conjugated catecholamines were apparent after these stresses. The plasma renin activity increased only after bicycle exercise and this appeared similar in both groups. The plasma cortisol levels did not increase. Thus, the higher BP in drinkers cannot be explained by increased activity of the sympathoadrenal and renal pressor mechanisms.

The relation between alcohol consumption and BP was studied in 491 males aged 20–45 by Arkwright and associates[13] in Perth, Australia. The subjects volunteered to complete a health questionnaire and submit to standardized measurements of BP, heart rate, and body size. Average weekly alcohol consumption correlated with systolic pressure but not diastolic pressure. Systolic pressure increased progressively with increasing alcohol consumption, with no obvious threshold effect. In moderate and heavy drinkers, the prevalence of systolic hypertension >140 mmHg was 4 times that of teetotalers. The effect of alcohol on systolic BP was independent of the effects of age, obesity, cigarette smoking, and physical activity. The exheavy drinkers had BP similar to those of teetotalers, suggesting that the effect of alcohol is reversible. Cigarette smokers had lower diastolic pressures than nonsmokers, an effect independent of obesity. The linear correlation between alcohol consumption and systolic BP and the lower BP in exdrinkers suggest a cause and effect relation. These results indicate that alcohol ranks close to obesity as a potentially preventable cause of hypertension.

Effect of coffee drinking and cigarette smoking on BP in hypertension

Freestone and Ramsay[14] from Sheffield, UK, examined 16 patients with mild systemic hypertension who habitually smoked cigarettes and consumed caffeine after they had abstained from both overnight. Their mean BP (147/89 mmHg) was substantially lower than values recorded in the clinic (164/102 mmHg) and remained so when they continued to abstain (149/94 mmHg at 2 hours). Smoking 2 cigarettes (3.4 mg nicotine) elevated BP by 10/8 mmHg, but for only 15 minutes. Drinking coffee (200 mg caffeine) elevated BP by up to 10/7 mmHg between 1 and 2 hours. Combined coffee ingestion and cigarette smoking caused a substantial rise in BP from 5–120 minutes to levels similar to those measured in the clinic (162/102 mmHg at 2 hours). Similar results were obtained in thiazide-treated patients. The interaction of coffee and cigarettes on BP, but not on pulse rate, was significant. The pressor effect of cigarette smoking and caffeine ingestion in combination may be important in the evaluation of patients with mild hypertension.

Thus, the authors have shown that patients with mild systemic hypertension had BPs substantially lower than clinic values when they abstained from caffeine and nicotine overnight, but the BP did not rise when they continued to abstain, and that it rose promptly and persistently to clinic values when they smoked 2 cigarettes and drank coffee. The circumstances of the experiment were relevant to the ordinary habits, and the observations should not be discounted because epidemiologic data are at variance. The combination of caffeine consumption and cigarette smoking may be important as a cause of elevated clinic BP readings in some patients. Although the magnitude of the effect, averaging 11/8 mmHg over ≥ 2 hours, may not impress the clinician dealing with individual patients, it must be remembered that an upward shift of BP of this degree in the population, whatever the cause, would have a large effect on the prevalence of hypertension.

Effect of calcium on BP

In some theories concerning the pathogenesis of systemic hypertension, intracellular calcium plays an important part. In an epidemiologic survey focusing on the relation between sodium consumption and BP, Kesteloot and Geboers[15] from Leuven and Brussels, Belgium, also measured serum calcium concentration and in a subsample, 24-hour urinary calcium excretion. In this epidemiologic survey of BP in 9,321 men, an independent and highly significant positive correlation was found between serum calcium and both systolic and diastolic BP. A significant but weaker correlation also was found between 24-hour urinary calcium excretion and BP. In the same study, neither a positive correlation between 24-hour sodium excretion and BP nor a negative one between 24-hour potassium excretion and BP could be demonstrated.

Relation between lithium efflux and sodium content of erythrocytes and a family history of systemic hypertension

Essential hypertension has long been attributed to some change in the balance or distribution of sodium. The sodium content of erhthrocytes, lymphocytes, and leukocytes is increased, owing to inhibition of the sodium pumps. This inhibition disappears from leukocytes when the BP is lowered with diuretics and is probably due to a circulating inhibitor of sodium transport. Sodium ions leave erythrocytes through pathways other than the sodium pump but these are exchange pathways and changes in them have little effect on the sodium content of the cells. Two pathways are the furosemide-sensitive sodium-potassium cotransport system and the sodium-sodium exchange mechanism that can be measured as a sodium-dependent lithium efflux. Abnormalities in these 2 sodium pathways have been reported in patients with essential hypertension. Clegg and associates[16] from Leeds and Rochdale, England, measured the lithium efflux and sodium content of erythrocytes in 75 patients with untreated essential hypertension. The average values of both were higher than those of normotensive control subjects. Values above the range in the controls were found only in patients with a family history of systemic hypertension and in those the frequency of raised lithium efflux was 76% and of raised sodium content was 36%. Measurement of lithium efflux and sodium content, together with the family history, allows patients with essential hypertension to be categorized into 4 groups.

Absenteeism and labeling in hypertensives

In a specific work-site population (the Massachusetts Mutual Life Insurance Company in Springfield, Massachusetts) the illness absenteeism of 259 persons with systemic hypertension was studied by Charlson and associates[17] from New York City in the year after they were screened and labeled. Absenteeism due to illness increased more in 48 patients who were unaware of their hypertension (newly labeled) than in the 211 subjects who were aware that they were hypertensive. Among the newly labeled subjects, only the young subjects and those with pure systolic hypertension experienced increased absenteeism. The newly labeled subjects who received active follow-up and treatment with antihypertensive medication had only minimal increases in absenteeism. In contrast, those who received active follow-up without medication and those who received only episodic follow-up had significantly greater increases. Vigorous efforts are warranted to ensure active follow-up and treatment for hypertensive subjects after their condition has been labeled. Caution should be exercised in labeling, however, if no antihypertensive treatment is initiated.

Adrenal and renal abnormalities in essential hypertension

To determine whether the previously described abnormalities in adrenal secretion and renal blood flow in essential systemic hypertension are associated, Williams and associates[18] from Boston, Massachusetts, examined the responses to the relevant systems in 18 patients with essential hypertension. Patients <30 years of age were studied to minimize the likelihood that the phenomena were secondary to long-standing hypertension. To achieve a wide span of sodium balance, studies were performed during a high (200 mEq) sodium intake, a restricted (10 mEq) sodium intake, and a restricted sodium intake supplemented by a further short-term diuretic-induced volume deficit (furosemide, 180–300 mg, to reduce body weight by 1–1.5 kg). The indexes measured included cardiac output (indocyanine green indicator dilution), plasma volume (^{125}I albumin space), renal blood flow (radioxenon transit), plasma renin activity and aldosterone levels and aldosterone secretory rate. All of these variables, with the exception of BP and total peripheral resistance, were within the normal range during the 2 diets. The aldosterone secretory response to diuretic-induced volume depletion on a low-sodium diet was clearly blunted in 9 subjects. These 9 subjects (abnormal responders) had a virtually absent aldosterone increment (23 ± 34 μg/24 hours) compared with the normal responders (502 ± 70 μg/24 hours). In addition, renal blood flow was significantly higher in these 9 subjects during both a high sodium intake (434 ± 19 -vs- 342 ± 26 ml/100 g/min) and a restricted sodium intake (446 ± 11 -vs- 285 ± 39 ml/100 g/min). Yet, there were no significant differences between these 2 groups in sodium or potassium balance, BP, plasma volume, cardiac index, or plasma renin activity during a high or low sodium intake. Normally, control of both aldosterone release by the adrenal and renal perfusion is dominated by angiotensin; an apparently blunted response of both systems suggests that there may be a generalized abnormality in the way angiotensin interacts with its target tissues in many young patients with essential hypertension.

Saralasin test

Recently, saralasin acetate was approved by the Food and Drug Administration for use as a diagnostic agent for the detection of angiotensin II dependent (renin-mediated) systemic hypertension. A committee,[19] composed of clinical investigators with extensive experience with saralasin, outlined the present and potential uses of this agent in the diagnosis and treatment of various forms of systemic hypertension (Fig. 4-5); Frohlich and associates from New Orleans, Louisiana, summarized the consensus of the committee.

Saralasin is an angiotensin II analogue that differs from the natural agent in that the terminal amino acids (in the 1 and 8 positions) are substituted. As a result, it binds to angiotensin II tissue receptors, but as a much weaker vasoconstrictor agonist than angiotensin II. It therefore may have dual action, depending on the circulating levels of the natural pressor substance, angiotensin II. At high levels of circulating angiotensin II, saralasin competitively inhibits binding of angiotensin II to the receptor sites of the vasculature, diminishing vasoconstriction and reducing arterial pressure. At low levels of circulating angiotensin II, saralasin may act as an agonist, raising the pressure. Therefore its depressor action is mediated by reducing total peripheral resistance; but this is unassociated with a compensatory increase in heart rate, cardiac output, or myocardial contractility.

The saralasin test consists of an intravenous (IV) infusion of saralasin at a constant rate for 20–30 minutes or an infusion at increasing rates up to 45 minutes while BP is constantly monitored. To facilitate responsiveness, mild sodium depletion is achieved by a single dose (40 or 80 mg) or oral furosemide 12–14 hours before the test or by 3–5 days of a low sodium (10 mEq) diet. Antihypertensive medications, except diuretics, are withheld for at least 1 week before testing.

The IV infusion of saralasin almost always is associated with an initial immediate transient elevation of arterial pressure lasting 2–4 minutes. Test results are judged only by the subsequent pressure response, commencing 6 minutes after the start of the infusion. Control pressure is the average of the last 4 diastolic pressure readings obtained just before the saralasin infusion;

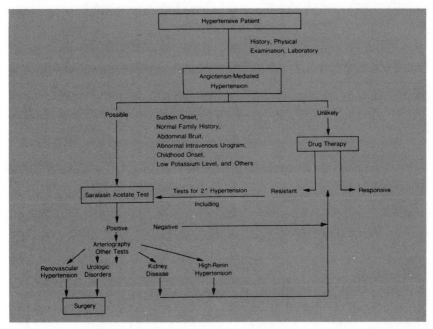

Fig. 4-5. Conceptual schema presenting evaluation of patient with renin-dependent hypertension and role of saralasin acetate test in algorithm. Reproduced with permission from Report of a Consensus Committee.[19]

saralasin pressure is the average of the 4 consecutive diastolic pressures that differ most from control pressure. A positive saralasin test is defined as a sustained decrease in diastolic pressure of at least 7 mmHg, indicating renin-mediated hypertension.

A positive saralasin test when performed after modest sodium depletion is an indication that angiotensin II is contributing to the hypertension. The drug is more specific than a converting enzyme inhibitor (e.g., captopril), which may affect pressure through other mechanisms. Renin-mediated forms of hypertension include the following: 1) Renovascular hypertension and experimental (2-kidney model) and clinical arterial disease are generally acknowledged to be angiotensin mediated, despite normal plasma renin activity. 2) High-renin essential hypertension comprises 5%–15% of the hypertensive population. 3) Hypertension in coarctation of the aorta, renin-secreting renal tumors, segmental renal infarction, renal parenchymal disease, and renal transplant hypertension is often, but not always, angiotensin mediated.

Although saralasin is primarily a diagnostic agent, it has proved useful for short-term (hours to days) emergency treatment of malignant hypertension, severe CHF, and in reducing BP during and after renal arteriography.

Stroke incidence in the hypertension detection and follow-up program

The Hypertension Detection and Follow-up Program (HDFP) previously reported a 17% reduction in all-cause mortality among its stepped care (SC) group relative to the community-treated referred care (RC) group. The current report[20] compares cerebrovascular disease morbidity and mortality in the SC and RC populations. The SC 5-year stroke incidence (2%/100 persons) was significantly lower than that found among the RC (3%/100 persons). Reduction in stroke rates among SC were experienced for all race and sex groups, all diastolic BP strata, all ages, and among those with or without evidence of long-standing systemic hypertension. Comparisons of the cardiovascular death rates for SC (1.06/1,000 persons) and RC (1.91/1,000 persons) with those obtained for the general USA population (0.83/1,000 persons) indicate that the cardiovascular death rate decreased in the SC hypertensive population to a level approaching that of the general USA population.

MANAGEMENT OF *MILD* HYPERTENSION

In 1975, while several major trials of the treatment of mild systemic hypertension were under way, a joint World Health Organisation/International Society of Hypertension committee was formed to establish liaison between the trials, to facilitate an exchange of opinions among the investigators, and to promote common approaches to the analyses of future results. Since that time, the results of 4 important mild hypertension trials have been reported; the U.S. Public Health Service Study (USPHS), the Australian National Blood Pressure Study (ANBPS), the U.S. Hypertension Detection and Follow-up Program (HDFP), and the Oslo Study. The ANBPS and HDFP studies concluded that mortality of mild hypertensives was reduced by active treatment. The USPHS and the Oslo Study, which were smaller trials, were unable to demonstrate any overall reduction in mortality. The Medical Research Council (MRC) trial in Britain is still in progress, and the European Working Party on High Blood Pressure in the Elderly (EWPHE) is also continuing its trial in hypertensives >60 years of age. Each of the 4 major studies are summarized here and in the accompanying tables[21] (Tables 4-5–4-12).

Can authoritative recommendations for treatment of mild hypertension be based on the results of these 4 trials? In some respects, between trial agreement is good; all 4 are consistent in showing benefit, conferred by treatment, in terms of cerebrovascular complications. These results confirm, and extend to a lower BP range, the earlier results published by the Veterans Administration trials. The 2 larger studies, ANBPS and USPHS, and the Oslo Study are consistent in showing no benefit in terms of nonfatal AMI among treated subjects compared with controls. The 3 trials that have published

TABLE 4-5. *Design characteristics of the 5 trials. Reproduced from WHO/ISH Mild Hypertension Liaison Committee.*[21]

TRIAL	DESIGNED TO DETECT	BLINDNESS	α-FACTOR*	β-FACTOR*	DURATION FOR EACH PARTICIPANT
U.S.P.H.S.	Reduction in overall mortality to that of U.S. male population not dying of cardiovascular diseases	Double-blind, placebo-controlled	0.05	0.95	7 yr
A.N.B.P.S.	30% reduction in all-causes mortality and morbidity from cardiovascular complications	Single-blind, placebo-controlled	0.05	0.90	5 yr
H.D.F.P.	40% reduction in all-causes mortality	Open—comparison of two methods of antihypertensive care	0.05	0.90	5 yr
Oslo	Significant reduction in cardiovascular complications	Open—observation of untreated control group	Not stated	Not stated	5½ yr
M.R.C.	40% reduction in mortality from stroke and hypertensive heart disease and in morbidity from stroke	Single-blind, placebo-controlled	0.01	0.95	5 yr

* β is the probability of detecting as significant (at level α) a true reduction of a specified amount.

TABLE 4-6. *Trial participants in the 5 trials. Reproduced from the WHO/ISH Mild Hypertension Liaison Committee.*[21]

TRIAL	POPULATION SAMPLE	#	% MALE	% WHITE	AGE RANGE (yr)
U.S.P.H.S.	Merchant seamen, active and retired servicemen and their dependants, hospital and social-security employees	389	80	72	21–55
A.N.B.P.S.	General population; screened volunteers from 4 areas in Australia	3427	63	100	30–69
H.D.F.P.	General population; screened samples from 14 areas in U.S.A.	10 940	54	56	30–69
Oslo	Screened population of all men aged 40–49 living in Oslo	785	100	Not stated	40–49
M.R.C.	General population; screened total populations on lists at 176 general practices and 14 industrial clinics or screening organizations	17 290	52	99	35–64

analyses of ECGs show a reduced incidence of ECG evidence of LV hypertrophy in the actively treated groups.

Given that despite minor discrepancies all the trials show some benefits from drug treatment, can we proceed to recommend this form of management for all persons with mild hypertension? Neither ANBPS nor HDFP showed significant benefit in terms of mortality for subjects <50 years old,

TABLE 4-7. *Drug regimens in the actively treated groups* in the 5 trials. Reproduced from the WHO/ISH Mild Hypertension Liaison Committee.*[21]

TRIAL	DRUG REGIMEN
U.S.P.H.S.	Chlorothiazide and rauwolfia
A.N.B.P.S.	Chlorothiazide (first order); plus beta blocker or methyldopa (second order); plus hydralazine or clonidine (third order)
H.D.F.P.	Chlorthalidone; triamterene or spironolactone as supplements or alternatives (step 1); plus reserpine or methyldopa (step 2); plus hydralazine (step 3); plus guanethidine (step 4); other drugs added or substituted (step 5)
Oslo	Hydrochlorothiazide (first order); plus methyldopa or propranolol (second order)
M.R.C.	Bendrofluazide (first order) supplemented by methyldopa or guanethidine (second order); or propranolol (first order) supplemented by methyldopa or guanethidine

* Stepped care in H.D.F.P.

TABLE 4-8. *Comparability of blood pressure measurements in men aged 45–54 with entry diastolic (V) pressures 90–109 mmHg: from entry to 3 yr. Reproduced from the WHO/ISH Mild Hypertension Liaison Committee.*[21]

BLOOD PRESSURE MEASUREMENTS AT	U.S.P.H.S.*		A.N.B.P.S.*		H.D.F.P.*		OSLO†		M.R.C.*	
	TREATED	CONTROL	TREATED	CONTROL	STEPPED CARE	REFERRED CARE	TREATED	CONTROL	TREATED	CONTROL
Mean of pre-entry visits	147/98	146/96	154/100	155/100	152/100	151/101	156/97	155/96	155/98	155/98
Entry	145/97	144/97	152/99	153/99	153/98	153/99	151/92	149/92	158/98	156/98
3 or 4 mo	132/88	144/96	137/90	145/94	133/87	...	...	...	132/86	142/92
1 yr	133/88	143/95	135/90	147/95	131/88	143/93	131/84	150/93	137/87	147/93
2 yr	129/85	150/96	134/88	145/94	129/86	141/92	129/84	149/93	135/86	149/93
3 yr	131/84	146/96	132/87	143/90	...	...	128/84	148/93	135/85	152/94
4 yr	126/83	146/95	137/87	146/91	...	...	132/85	151/94	136/85	155/94

* Data provided to the W.H.O./I.S.H. Liaison Committee. † Data for men aged 40–49, from Oslo study publication.[4]

TABLE 4-9. Crude mortality rates (per 1000 person years) in treated subjects and controls* in A.N.B.P.S., H.D.F.P. (stratum I), and the Oslo trial, and in controls in the M.R.C. trial. Reproduced with permission from the WHO/ISH Mild Hypertension Liaison Committee.[21]

								MORTALITY					
TRIAL	DIASTOLIC BLOOD-PRESSURE (mmHg)	AGE RANGE (yr)	PERSON YEARS	ALL CAUSES		ALL CARDI-OVASCULAR		ALL CEREBRO-VASCULAR		CORONARY HEART DISEASE		NON-CARDIO-VASCULAR	
				#	RATE	#	RATE	#	RATE	#	RATE	#	RATE
A.N.B.P.S.													
Treated	95–109	30–69	6991	25	3.6	8	1.1	3	0.4	5	0.7	17	2.4
Controls			6868	35	5.1	18	2.6	6	0.9	11	1.6	17	2.5
H.D.F.P.													
Stepped care	90–104	30–69	19 115	231	12.1	122	6.4	17	0.9	86	4.5	109	5.7
Referred care			19 063	291	15.3	165	8.7	31	1.6	107	5.6	126	6.6
Oslo													
Treated	<110	40–49	2233	10	4.5	7	3.1	0	0.0	6	2.7	3	1.3
Controls			2088	9	4.3	6	2.9	2	1.0	2	1.0	3	1.4
M.R.C.													
Controls	90–109	35–64	16 415	83	5.1	46	2.8	7	0.4	35	2.1	37	2.3

* Stepped care and referred care for H.D.F.P.

TABLE 4-10. *Australian national blood pressure study. Numbers of trial endpoints by diagnostic categories. Reproduced with permission from WHO/ISH Mild Hypertension Liaison Committee.*[21]

END-POINT EVENTS	INTENTION-TO-TREAT ANALYSIS				ON-TREATMENT ANALYSIS			
	ACTIVE (6991 person-years)	PLACEBO (6868 person-years)	TOTAL	%	ACTIVE (5294 person-years)	PLACEBO (5184 person-years)	TOTAL	%
Fatal:								
MI	5	11	16		2	8	10	
Stroke	3	6	9	19.6	2	4	6	12.8
Other cardiovascular	0	1	1		0	1	1	
Noncardiovascular	17	17	34		5	6	11	
Nonfatal:								
MI	28	22	50		18	17	35	
Other coronary heart disease	65	76	141		50	63	113	
Stroke	10	16	26	80.4	7	13	20	87.2
TIA	4	9	13		3	8	11	
Retinopathy	2	5	7		1	4	5	
Congestive heart failure	3	3	6		2	1	3	
Renal failure	1	2	3		1	2	3	
Total	138	168	306	100.0	91	127	218	100.0

TABLE 4-11. *Hypertension detection and follow-up program. Percentage reduction in cardiovascular and non cardiovascular mortality in stepped-care subjects, according to diastolic pressure on entry. Reproduced with permission from WHO/ISH Mild Hypertension Liaison Committee.*[21]

	STEPPED CARE		REFERRED CARE		
PARTICIPANTS	# DEATHS	RATE/1000 PATIENT YEARS	# DEATHS	RATE/1000 PATIENT YEARS	REDUCTION IN MORTALITY (%)
All participants:					
Cardiovascular	195	7.3	240	9.1	18.8
Noncardiovascular	154	5.7	179	6.8	14.0
Total	349	13.0	419	15.8	16.7
Strata II and III (105 mmHg+):					
Cardiovascular	73	9.5	75	10.1	5.9
Noncardiovascular	45	5.8	53	7.1	15.1
Total	118	15.3	128	17.3	7.8
Stratum I (90–104 mmHg):					
Cardiovascular	122	6.4	165	8.7	26.0
Noncardiovascular	109	5.7	126	6.6	13.5
Total	231	12.1	291	15.3	20.6

although USPHS demonstrated a 57% reduction in the lesser complications of hypertension in those <55 years. The risks in younger and less hypertensive subjects are, of course, lower and the chances of demonstrating benefit correspondingly reduced. The HDFP study has shown that once target organ damage has occurred, the risks of hypertension cannot be lowered, with good care, to the level of risk experienced by those without target organ damage. Is it justifiable to wait and observe? Mild hypertension, because it is so common, is perhaps the most important risk factor underlying cardiovascular morbidity and mortality in industrialized countries; more cardiovascular events occur against a background of mild than severe hypertension. Millions of persons would be affected by widespread acceptance of a recommendation that a diastolic pressure sustained at 90 mmHg necessitated life-long therapy. The social and economic consequences would be considerable both for the individual and for the community. Costs in terms of adverse reactions to drugs are not negligible, and some attempt to show the balance between enhanced survival and adverse reactions seems necessary, even though these cannot be measured on the same scale. The reports published to date do not provide adequate information on adverse drug reactions. Unless it can be determined which persons with mild hypertension will benefit most from therapy (and those who will come to no harm if left untreated), the community benefit would be bought at the expense of many previously symptom-free individuals who would experience drug side effects and derive

TABLE 4-12. *Hypertension detection and follow-up program. Percentage reduction in all-causes mortality in stratum-I stepped-care subjects, according to entry characteristics. Reproduced with permission from WHO/ISH Mild Hypertension Liaison Committee.*[21]

ENTRY CHARACTERISTICS	STEPPED CARE		REFERRED CARE		REDUCTION IN MORTALITY (%)
	# DEATHS	RATE/1000 PATIENT YEARS	# DEATHS	RATE/1000 PATIENT YEARS	
Not on antihypertensive treatment and without target-organ damage* at entry:					
Entry diastolic pressure					
90–94 mmHg	36	7.0	54	10.6	34.0
95–99 mmHg	39	8.4	53	11.6	27.6
100–104 mmHg	31	9.3	44	11.6	19.8
On antihypertensive treatment or with target-organ damage* at entry:					
Entry diastolic pressure					
90–104 mmHg	125	20.8	140	25.0	16.8

* Target-organ damage included "hard" left-ventricular hypertrophy on ECG, history of MI, history of stroke, history of intermittent claudication, serum-creatinine >1.7 mg/dl.

no benefit. These studies, in other words, suggest that the first line of treatment for persons with mild hypertension should be observation, perhaps combined with general health measures, such as weight reduction and restriction of salt intake. Any reduction in underlying vascular damage, morbid events, and mortality as a result of drug treatment must, of course, be balanced against any harmful consequences: although HDFP and ANBPS seem to have demonstrated the benefits of drug treatment in subjects with sustained diastolic pressures >90 mmHg, the decision to prescribe antihypertensive drugs for any individual should not be automatic.

Subsequent to this review, the full report of the HDFP and the ANBPS trials were reported,[22, 23] and they were analyzed and compared with the other reports by Freis.[24]

In view of the uncertainties, Freis suggested that we may be doing more harm than good by giving life-long drug treatment to patients with borderline or mild hypertension. However, because of the possibility of benefit, even though it is unproved, a compromise position, as suggested by others, including Freis, may be most appropriate. Patients with diastolic BP of 90–99 mmHg (average of ≥3 visits) are treated or not, according to the number of risk factors present. Patients with few other risk factors are given low sodium diets but not drugs. The Australian study found a gradual fall in BP in many of their placebo control patients. By the third year of follow-up 48% of the patients who began with diastolic pressures ≥95 mmHg had pressures below this level, 12% had progressed to a more severe stage, and only 32% remained in their initial range of 95–109 mmHg. This experience demonstrates the wisdom of waiting for an extended period before initiating antihypertensive drug treatment in mild hypertension. Patients with many risk factors may have their BP reduced with drugs if necessary. If drugs are used, they should be given by the step care method, beginning with a diuretic alone and avoiding complicated multiple drug regimens. All patients with elevated BP should be followed periodically to detect any evidences of progression to a more severe stage of hypertension. By such a discriminative approach, many millions of people could be spared needless life-long exposure to drugs.

An alternative to medication for systemic hypertension is to avoid excess dietary sodium. The treatment effect of such diet had been known for nearly 80 years but regarded as inconvenient and unpalatable, especially since the advent of diuretics that remove excess sodium. Beard and associates[25] from Canberra, Australia, randomly allocated 90 patients on medication for mild hypertension to diet and control groups and kept them under surveillance by their own doctors every 2 weeks for 12 weeks to test the short-term effectiveness of a diet free from sodium additives as an alternative to medication. Mean urinary sodium excretion was reduced to 37 mmol/24 hours in the diet group and 161 mmol/24 hours in the control group, with average K/Na ratio of 3.9/0.50. Both groups had a fall in mean systolic and diastolic BP, but the diet group finished on half of the initial amount of medication, with 1 patient in 3 off medication and 4 of 5 having either stopped or reduced the dose. The control group remained on almost the full amount of medication, with 2 of 3 patients having made no reduction. The diet group had a mean weight loss of 2.1 kg, a rise in serum potassium, and a fall in serum bicarbonate. There was no increase in overall frequency of muscle cramp, and the diet group reported feeling happier, less depressed, and less dependent on analgesics. Two-thirds of the diet group intend to continue to diet indefinitely. Reduction of sodium intake permitted drug treatment to be substantially reduced without side effects or loss of BP control.

Levinson and associates[26] from Washington, DC, discontinued antihypertensive therapy in 24 patients with mild systemic hypertension whose BP had been well controlled with diuretics alone. Eleven patients (46%) maintained normal diastolic BP (90 mmHg) for 6 months after stopping treatment and 5 patients (21%) for 12 months. All patients who remained normotensive 6–12 months had mean diastolic BP ≤82 mmHg during treatment. There was no significant correlation between maintenance of normotension and any of the following: pretreatment BP, presence of target organ damage, duration of known hypertension, family history of hypertension, heart rate, body weight, weight gain after stopping diuretic therapy, 24-hour urinary sodium and potassium excretion, serum electrolyte values, or renin profile. This study demonstrates that hypertension may be favorably modified, sometimes for many months, by effective antihypertensive treatment.

TREATMENT

Effects on offspring of treatment during pregnancy

Systemic hypertension in pregnancy is associated with an increased perinatal mortality and more preterm deliveries. A higher proportion of small-for-date babies and a higher incidence of subsequent neurologic impairment also have been reported. It is agreed that maternal systemic hypertension should be treated to prevent maternal complications, and methyldopa is the most widely used agent. Methyldopa, however, is known to cross the placenta, and the systolic BP of full-term infants born to mothers treated with the drug was shown to be lower than that of randomly selected control infants during the first 2 days after delivery. In 2 randomly controlled trials of methyldopa treatment in systemic hypertension during pregnancy, fetal survival was significantly greater in the treated group. The children born to mothers in the second and larger trial have been followed up regularly since birth to assess growth and development. Cockburn and associates[27] from Oxford, England, followed 195 children from birth who were born to hypertensive women treated with methyldopa during pregnancy. The children were extensively examined at the age of 7½ years. The frequency of problems with health, physical or mental handicap, sight, hearing, and behavior was the same in children of treated and untreated women. Sons of the untreated women were heavier and taller than those of treated women, as were their mothers. Among children of women who entered the trial between 16 and 20 weeks' gestation, sons of untreated women had larger heads than sons of treated women, but there was no difference in mean intelligence quotients. There were no significant differences between the children in the treated and untreated groups in standing and supine BP or 14 tests of ability. Methyldopa therefore seems safe to use in pregnancy and is probably preferable to other drugs from the point of view of the neonate.

In a private practice

Systemic hypertension is one of the most common conditions seen by the practicing physician. Yet, because of noncompliance, conditions of many hypertensive patients are not effectively controlled by treatment. Zismer and associates[28] from Minneapolis, Minnesota, and Los Angeles, California, tested the efficacy of a patient education program in reducing the BP of hypertensive patients in a private solo medical practice. The intervention program focused on 3 behavioral objectives: pill taking, appointment keeping, and dietary sodium reduction. It was hypothesized that patients receiving this treatment approach would have a substantial reduction in BP compared with patients receiving usual medical care. Of 39 hypertensive patients receiving drug therapy randomized into a treatment group and a control group and followed for 6 months, the BP fell in the treatment group (−13 mmHg systolic, −8 mmHg diastolic) and rose in the control group (+3 mmHg systolic, +1 mmHg diastolic). Both differences are significant.

Natriuretic hormone

De Wardener and MacGregor[29] from London, England, reviewed the evidence for the hypothesis that the rise in peripheral resistance in inherited systemic hypertension is due largely to the observed rise in the circulating level of a sodium-transport inhibitor. A sequence of events was proposed to link a postulated genetic defect in the kidney's ability to excrete sodium, salt intake, the rise in the circulating concentration of a sodium-transport inhibitor, and the rise in peripheral resistance in essential hypertension (Fig. 4-6).

Improving adherence to dietary sodium restriction

To improve adherence to dietary sodium restriction, Kaplan and associates[30] from Dallas, Texas, validated 2 simple techniques for providing rapid and accurate estimates of urinary content: overnight urine collections and an immediate analysis of urine sodium content. These techniques were then applied in a trial with a group of patients with systemic hypertension who were considered to be resistant to the adoption of dietary changes. After 6 months, 68% of the patients on the lower sodium diet reduced their urine

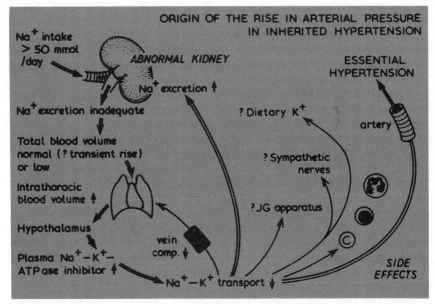

Fig. 4-6. Sequence of events to explain a postulated inherited defect in kidney's ability to excrete sodium, observed rise in concentration of circulating sodium-transport inhibitor, salt intake, and rise in peripheral resistance in essential hypertension. JG = juxtaglomerular; vein comp. = venous compliance. Reproduced with permission from DeWardener and MacGregor.[29]

sodium content by ≥33%. They had an 11 mmHg fall in mean BP compared with a 3 mmHg rise in the control group, who were not on a lower sodium diet, and a lesser fall in plasma potassium levels.

Moderate sodium restriction

Nearly 80 years ago it was demonstrated that salt restriction lowered BP. Very low levels of sodium intake, around 10 mmol/per day, greatly reduced BP, and, in patients with severe hypertension, an increase in sodium intake raised BP. A 10 mmol/day sodium diet in the Western World requires special foods and is extremely difficult even for the most compliant patient. A more modest reduction of sodium intake, achieved by not adding salt and avoiding foods loaded with sodium, has been claimed to lower BP in patients with mild to moderate essential systemic hypertension, but the studies that yielded this finding have been criticized for their lack of adequate controls, their open nature, and the methodology of BP measurement. MacGregor and associates[31] from London, England, conducted a double-blind randomized crossover study of the effect a modest restriction of dietary sodium intake on 19 unselected patients with mild to moderate essential hypertension whose average supine BP after 2 months' observation on no treatment was 156/98 mmHg. They were advised not to add salt to food and to avoid sodium-laden foods. After 2 weeks of sodium restriction, patients were entered into an 8-week double-blind randomized crossover study of "slow sodium" versus "slow sodium placebo." The mean supine BP was 7 mmHg (6%) lower in the fourth week of placebo than that in the fourth week of slow sodium (p < 0.001). Urinary sodium excretion in the fourth week of slow sodium was 162 ± 9 mmol/24 hours (p < 0.001). There was no difference in potassium excretion. These results suggest that moderate sodium restriction achieved by not adding salt and avoiding sodium-laden foods should, if not already, become part of the management of patients with essential hypertension.

Potassium

Khaw and Thom[32] from London, England, conducted in 20 young healthy men on normal sodium unrestricted diet a randomized double-blind crossover study of increased oral potassium 64 mmol a day versus placebo. A significantly greater proportion had lower systolic and diastolic BP on potassium than on placebo. The mean diastolic BP was significantly lowered by 2.4 mmHg during potassium supplementation. Change in diastolic BP correlated negatively with change in 24-hour urinary potassium and positively with change in 24-hour urinary sodium/potassium ratio in individual subjects. These results indicate that in healthy young volunteers on a normal unrestricted Western diet, added potassium can lower mean diastolic BP. Although the change was small, this effect may be important for several reasons. 1) The group consisted of healthy young normotensive persons who might perhaps be thought not susceptible to the changes in dietary electrolytes that may affect a hypertensive patient. A reduction of their BP therefore was evidence for an etiologic role of potassium in determining the mean BP levels in the population as a whole rather than just in hypertensive patients. 2) This effect was shown after just 2 weeks of intervention, suggesting that BP is a dynamic reflection of current electrolyte status. 3) This effect was shown on a group with unrestricted salt intake. If dietary potassium affects BP, either independently or through lowering the overall sodium/potassium ratio, individuals wanting to lower their BP might find it easier to increase their potassium intake in the form of fruit and vegetables than to decrease their sodium intake. The evidence suggests that the 2 work synergistically.

It was suggested >50 years ago that potassium supplementation might lower BP in man. There is only 1 randomized study of potassium supplementation alone in patients with essential hypertension, and, although a fall in BP was seen, this was a short inpatient study for only 10 days on each diet and involved a very high sodium intake and a large increase in potassium. MacGregor and associates[33] from London, England, in 23 unselected patients with mild to moderate essential hypertension whose average supine BP after 2 months' observation on no treatment was 154/99 mmHg randomized them into an 8-week double-blind crossover study of 1 month's treatment with slow release potassium tablets (60 mmol/day) -vs- placebo without alteration of dietary sodium or potassium intake. By the fourth week, mean supine BP had fallen by 4% on potassium supplementation compared with placebo (Fig. 4-7). Urinary potassium excretion increased from 62 ± 5 mmol/24 hours on placebo to 118 ± 7 mmol/24 hours on potassium. The fall in BP was not related to urinary sodium excretion before entry to the trial or while on placebo. Moderate potassium supplementation caused a small but significant fall in BP in patients with mild to moderate essential hypertension and could be additive to the effects of moderate sodium restriction. This increase

Fig. 4-7. Average systolic and diastolic blood pressures and urinary potassium excretion before and during treatment with potassium and placebo. *p < 0.05; **p < 0.025; ***p < 0.001. Reproduced with permission from MacGregor et al.[33]

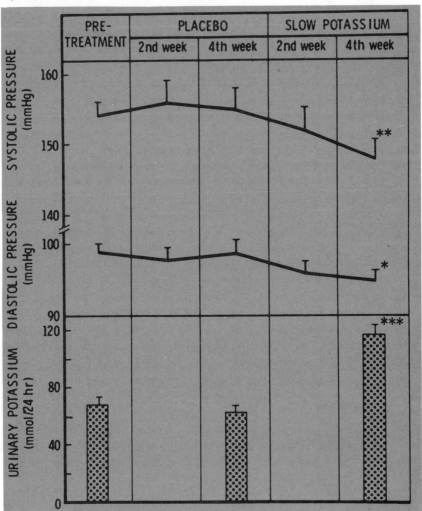

in potassium intake could be achieved with a potassium-based salt substitute and a moderate increase in vegetable and fruit consumption. Moderate dietary sodium restriction with dietary potassium supplementation may obviate or reduce the need for drug treatment in some patients with mild to moderate hypertension.

Harrington and associates[34] from Boston, Massachusetts, in an editorial discussed with considerable logic the contention that the popular practice of prescribing either oral potassium supplements or potassium-sparing agents routinely to patients being treated with diuretics for systemic hypertension is one based largely on tradition and erroneous premises, and not on a careful consideration of benefits and risks. They ask 3 questions: How did the national obsession with potassium come about? Do existing data justify the current widespread prescribing practices? If not, what kinds of data are needed to clarify an issue that affects millions of people and costs hundreds of millions of dollars? They concluded that until more data are available potassium salts or potassium-sparing diuretics should not be prescribed routinely for diuretic-treated hypertensive patients unless they are also receiving digitalis. Furthermore, in their view, such treatment is warranted only for severe potassium depletion or for manifestations that clearly can be related to a potassium deficit.

Verapamil

Since an increase in peripheral resistance is a consistent hemodynamic finding in a hypertensive patient, Gould and colleagues[35] from Middlesex, England, reasoned that it might be logical to counteract the vasoconstriction by using drugs that would produce direct vasodilation. These investigators performed a controlled study to monitor the reduction of BP over a 24-hour period with verapamil in patients with essential hypertension using a system for continuous recording of intraarterial BP during a series of exercises and observation during daily activities. Sixteen patients underwent continuous monitoring over a 48-hour period before and after at least 6 weeks of therapy with a dose range from 120–160 mg of verapamil 3 times daily. Each monitoring period included physiologic tests, such as the tilt table, maximal handgrip, and riding a bicycle. Mean standing BP in the clinic before therapy was 130/110 and after therapy 145/86 mmHg. Verapamil produced a consistent reduction in BP over 24 hours, but particularly during the day. Heart rate was similarly reduced. There was no evidence of postural hypotension and the absolute responses to the dynamic and isometric exercises were reduced. The degree of reduction of the BP was consistent and suggested that slow-channel inhibitors may be appropriate for antihypertensive therapy.

Atenolol

Hemodynamic, metabolic, and cardiovascular reflexive variables were measured before and after 4 weeks of beta blockage with atenolol in 10 patients with mild essential hypertension by Dreslinski and associates[36] in New Orleans, Louisiana. Atenolol reduced mean arterial pressure, heart rate, cardiac index, and renal vascular resistance and increased total peripheral resistance. Glomerular filtration rate and renal blood flow were unchanged; plasma renin activity fell 43%. Reflexive cardioacceleration during the Valsalva maneuver and upright passive tilt was blunted. No changes were observed in circulating fluid volumes. In 6 patients followed for 1 year, BP and heart rate were maintained at levels similar to those during the first 4 weeks. Thus, this study showed that atenolol is an effective oral antihypertensive that has no apparent deleterious hemodynamic effects on the renal and splanchnic circulations.

Nadolol

Although it has been demonstrated repeatedly that propranolol and other beta blocking agents diminish heart rate and cardiac output, their role in determining regional perfusion under clinical conditions is not clear. Several studies have indicated that these agents may decrease renal plasma flow and adversely affect glomerular filtration rate. Rarely have both systemic and renal hemodynamic changes been evaluated together, leaving open the question of whether changes in renal blood flow passively follow the fall in cardiac output or reflect other mechanisms. In contrast, early studies using intravenous injections of nadolol in sodium-restricted hypertensive subjects demonstrated a rise in renal blood flow measured by xenon washout, whereas a decrease was observed during propranolol administration. Textor and associates[37] from Cleveland, Ohio, undertook to define the changes in both systemic and renal hemodynamics before and during oral nadolol therapy (80 mg in the first phase of the study and 160 mg in the second) in patients with systemic hypertension. As anticipated, BP and cardiac index fell, whereas peripheral resistance rose. Renal blood flow, however, was well preserved, indicating a redistribution of cardiac output to the kidneys. The results suggest that a direct renal vasodilator effect of nadolol allows independent regulation of the renal circulation.

Pindolol

The antihypertensive effect of pindolol, a beta receptor blocking agent with intrinsic sympathomimetic activity (ISA, or partial agonist activity), has been demonstrated in several hundred clinical trials performed in many countries. The results representative of such trials are reviewed by Fanchamps[38] from Basle, Switzerland. In a cooperative study of pindolol by Swiss internists, BP normalization was achieved in 76% of patients. In a French trial, BP reduction correlated with the initial pressure level. Pindolol also was found effective in treating renal hypertension (West Germany) and was considered particularly useful in hypertensive patients with coexistent angina pectoris (South Africa). A favorable effect on the BP profile registered during the whole day was demonstrated by means of BP telemetry (West

Germany). A Swedish long-term study showed pindolol to have a sustained antihypertensive effect over 16 months associated with a progressive decrease in systemic vascular resistance. In a study conducted in New Zealand, pindolol compared favorably with drugs previously used for hypertension (methyldopa, diuretics, rauwolfia, guanethidine). Pindolol proved slightly less effective than methyldopa in a Canadian trial, but significantly more effective than this drug in a South African study. Danish investigators found pindolol equivalent to chlorthalidone in lowering the resting BP but more effective than the diuretic in reducing the BP and pulse response to exercise. Of particular interest are comparisons of pindolol with other beta blockers performed in West Germany, Sweden, Australia, and New Zealand. The BP reductions obtained with pindolol did not differ significantly from those obtained with the other beta blockers, whether they were cardioselective (metoprolol, atenolol) or not (propranolol, timolol, nadolol); however, pindolol produced less slowing of resting heart rate than these 5 other drugs, which are devoid of ISA. Pindolol proved somewhat more effective than other nonselective beta blockers with ISA (oxprenolol), although both produced less bradycardia than propranolol (New Zealand). In resistant cases, the combination of pindolol with diuretics, methyldopa, or hydralazine was found to increase the responder rate significantly (Australia, Denmark, England, Italy).

Nifedipine plus atenolol

The calcium channel blocker, nifedipine, was used by Opie and colleagues[39] from Cape Town, South Africa, as additional oral therapy to beta adrenergic receptor blockade by the cardioselective agent atenolol in the therapy of 31 patients with systemic hypertension. Initial studies were directed toward control of associated angina pectoris in 15 of the patients, but no effects were found on angina except in 2 patients. However, arterial BP was consistently reduced in all patients. Further studies by Opie and colleagues on 16 patients were directed toward the use of nifedipine as an antihypertensive agent in addition to atenolol and a thiazide diuretic. Nifedipine (10 mg sublingually) acutely dropped systolic/diastolic BP by about 30/20 mmHg within 20 minutes. Follow-up studies made after 4–8 weeks showed that the initial acute response to nifedipine predicted the long-term response to oral nifedipine, 10 mg twice daily. Of 31 hypertensive patients tested, only 1 failed to respond to nifedipine.

Captopril

The BP lowering effect of the orally active angiotensin-converting enzyme inhibitor captopril was studied by Waeber and associates[40] from Boston, Massachusetts, and Lausanne, Switzerland, in 59 hypertensive patients maintained on a constant sodium intake. Within 2 hours of the first dose of captopril, BP fell from 171/107 to a low of 142/92 mmHg, and after 4–8 days of treatment, BP averaged 145/94 mmHg. The magnitude of BP drop induced by captopril was significantly correlated to baseline plasma renin activity (PRA) both during the acute phase and after the 4–8 day interval. Because of considerable scatter in individual data, renin profiling was not precisely predictive of the immediate or delayed BP response of individual patients. However, the BP levels achieved following the initial dose of captopril closely correlated with BP measured after 4–8 days of therapy and appeared to have greater predictive value than control PRA of the long-term efficacy of chronic captopril therapy despite marked BP changes occurring in some patients during the intermediate period. Further, because of these intermediate BP changes, addition of a diuretic to enhance antihypertensive effectiveness of angiotensin blockade should be restrained for several days after initiation of captopril therapy.

In a study to assess the effects of the angiotensin-converting enzyme inhibitor captopril on patients with systemic hypertension, nephrotic syndrome developed in 1 patient and a serum sicknesslike condition in another. Because of the possibility of subclinical glomerular lesions developing in this population, renal biopsy specimens from hypertensive, nonproteinuric patients were studied. Electron microscopy revealed dense spherical deposits along the epithelial side of the glomerular capillary basement membrane. Because of these observations, the Captopril Collaborative Study Group,[41] which included several centers in the USA, set up a study. Renal biopsy material was studied from 38 hypertensive patients, 19 of whom had received captopril for ≥6 months. Comparable immunofluorescence findings and prominent arteriolar and mesangial deposits of C3 and IgM were noted equally in all patients. Within the noncaptopril group, 1 biopsy showed mesangial IgA glomerulonephritis, and, in another, microscopy revealed typical membranous glomerulonephritis. The biopsy specimens from 4 patients in the captopril group showed evidence of glomerular deposits and 2 had typical membranous glomerulonephritis. Small, spherical electron-dense deposits were seen with equal frequency along the outer aspect of the glomerular basement membrane in both groups, but were not thought to be immune deposits. Renal biopsy material from hypertensive patients may have ultrastructural and immunohistologic abnormalities that cannot be ascribed to captopril. Subclinical glomerulonephritis appears to exist in the hypertensive population. The membranous glomerulonephritis could be drug related, but this cannot be determined with certainty from the small sample studied. Caution must be shown in attributing glomerulonephritis to any drug without information about the kidneys before treatment.

Aldigier and associates[42] from Paris, France, administered captopril to 17 patients with essential hypertension and 9 with renovascular hypertension for 6–26 days. All patients were on a low sodium diet and were treated after the third day in the hospital with progressively increasing doses of captopril (75–450 mg/day). Mean systolic BP decreased from 142 ± 20–117 ± 18 mmHg in essential hypertension and from 136 ± 11–106 ± 10 mmHg in those with renovascular hypertension. Plasma renin activity, plasma aldosterone, urinary aldosterone, and vasopressin were higher in renovascular hypertension than in essential hypertension. Captopril decreased plasma aldosterone and urinary aldosterone and vasopressin and increased plasma renin activity in patients in both groups. These data indicate that captopril decreases the activity of the renin-angiotensin-aldosterone-vasopressin system in patients with essential and renovascular hypertension, although its renal effects are different. Marked increases in plasma creatinine were observed among patients with renal artery stenosis. These data suggest caution in the use of converting enzyme inhibitors in patients with renovascular hypertension, especially those on a low sodium diet, but they emphasize the efficacy of captopril in treating systemic arterial hypertension.

To evaluate the therapeutic efficacy of oral angiotensin-converting enzyme inhibition with low dose (average 30 mg/day) captopril in diuretic-resistant systemic hypertension, Fujita and associates[43] from Ibaraki, Japan, determined its long-term circulatory action by a dye dilution method and venous occlusion forearm plethysmography in 11 uncontrolled patients taking a thiazide diuretic. Significant declines in mean BP (average $12 \pm 4\%$) and systemic vascular resistance ($29 \pm 3\%$) were accompanied by an increase in cardiac output ($25 \pm 4\%$). Forearm vascular resistance ($16 \pm 3\%$) decreased considerably, but the decrease in limb vascular resistance did not parallel the fall in systemic vascular resistance in magnitude ($p < 0.01$), indicating that arteriolar dilation occurred on a selective basis. Plasma renin activity (PRA) increased after therapy as plasma aldosterone levels consistently fell, whereas plasma norepinephrine concentrations were not changed. There was a direct correlation between pretreatment PRA and the magnitude of the decline in systemic vascular resistance ($p < 0.05$). These findings suggest that the inhibition of angiotensin-converting enzyme with captopril in diuretic-resistant hypertensive patients improves cardiocirculatory function through selective dilation. The reordering of regional blood flow, which appears to result from release of angiotensin-mediated vasoconstriction as well as the suppression of aldosterone, may underlie the prolonged observed benefit. This oral vasodilator in very low doses appears to represent an effective adjunct for the treatment of hypertension refractory to diuretics.

Since the hypotensive effects of angiotensin antagonists and converting enzyme inhibitors have been shown to result from a decrease of systemic vascular resistance and sometimes accompanied by an increase in cardiac output, Fagard and associates[44] from London, England, examined the hemodynamic effects of captopril at rest and during exercise in hypotensive patients. The study was restricted to sodium-replete patients because a single dose of captopril had been reported to produce adverse hypotension after sodium depletion. Twenty patients were allocated either to a placebo or a captopril treatment group. The studies were performed in the laboratory and measurements obtained from a brachial artery puncture for intraarterial pressure recording and a Swan-Ganz catheter introduced in antecubital vein and positioned in the PA. After a period of rest, the patients were seated on a bicycle and graded exercise performed with continuous measurement of oxygen and carbon dioxide output. Each patient was investigated in rest recumbent (RR) and rest sitting (RS) positions and during an uninterrupted graded submaximal exercise test to the anaerobic threshold for treatment and with a similar protocol, 75 minutes after treatment with captopril or placebo. Captopril decreased brachial intraarterial pressure by 7/4 mmHg at RR, by 16/10 mmHg at RS, and by 19/10 mmHg during exercise. Slight increases of cardiac output and of HR were noted at rest. Cardiac output was not significantly affected during exercise but the increase of heart rate of 2.4 beats/minute was significant. Captopril decreased PA and capillary wedge pressures with unchanged pulmonary vascular resistance. These data indicate that the action of captopril in hypertensive patients is characterized by arteriolar and possibly venous dilation at rest and during exercise but no effect was observed on pulmonary vascular resistance.

The effect of low dose (25 mg 3 times a day) captopril was evaluated by Vlasses and associates[45] from Philadelphia, Pennsylvania, in 16 patients with mild to moderate essential systemic hypertension, previously uncontrolled by hydrochlorothiazide. After a no-treatment period, mean 8-hour seated diastolic BP was 103 ± 5 mmHg on placebo, 95 ± 8 after single dose of captopril, 96 ± 4 after 2 weeks of captopril alone, and 90 ± 6 mmHg after its combination with hydrochlorothiazide. Although 9 patients had ≥ 10% fall in seating diastolic BP after the initial dose of captopril, only 3 had a comparable fall after 2 weeks; after captopril and hydrochlorothiazide, however, 12 patients had such a response. Captopril decreased mean angiotensin-converting enzyme activity and plasma aldosterone, although to a lesser extent with continued therapy. Because its side effects appear dose related, low doses of captopril combined with a diuretic are effective and may be well tolerated.

Diazoxide

Diazoxide, as usually given in a single bolus, may cause precipitous falls in BP with resultant tissue hypoperfusion. To examine the efficacy and safety of slow infusion, Garrett and Kaplan[46] from Dallas, Texas, treated 18 patients with mean initial BP of 220/143 mmHg by 2 regimens: group A (9 patients) received 15 mg/minute; group B (9 patients) received 30 mg/minute. The goal of therapy, diastolic BP 100–105 mmHg, was reached in 16 of the 18 with no immediate drug-related side effects. Infusion time was 38 minutes in group A and 21 minutes in group B. Slow intravenous infusion of diazoxide appears to be safe and effective treatment for severe hypertension and should replace the rapid bolus technique.

Diazoxide plus beta blocker

Huysmans and associates[47] from Nijmegen, The Netherlands, evaluated the effects of beta adrenoreceptor blocking agents administered intravenously either immediately before or after diazoxide infusion, in the acute management of severe hypertension or hypertensive crises. Twenty-nine patients with severe hypertension (n, 14) or hypertensive crisis (n, 15) were treated with diazoxide infusion and intravenous injection of a beta blocker. In 13 patients, diazoxide was administered first. It gradually reduced mean arterial BP by 16%, and increased heart rate by 27%, and plasma renin activity (PRA) by 49%. Beta blockade thereafter lowered mean arterial BP by only 1% despite reductions of heart rate by 36% and of PRA by 17%. In 16 other patients, a beta blocker when given first reduced mean arterial BP by 3%, heart rate by 9% and PRA by 24%. Diazoxide infusion thereafter gradually reduced mean arterial BP further by 22% and raised heart rate and PRA to pretreatment levels. No complications were observed. Beta blockade before diazoxide infusion effectively prevents a rise in heart rate above control levels, whereas its acute effect on BP is negligible. It is advisable to use this combined regimen in all situations in which the occurrence of tachycardia might be dangerous.

Minoxidil

Alpert and Bauer[48] from Columbia, Missouri, studied 9 symptomatic patients whose diastolic BP > 120 mmHg 2 hours after receiving a combination of 40 mg of oral propranolol hydrochloride and 40 mg of oral furosemide. Systemic and pulmonary hemodynamics were measured before and after a 20 mg loading dose of oral minoxidil. A booster dosage of 5–20 mg of minoxidil was given at 4 hours if the diastolic BP > 100 mmHg. There was a progressive and significant reduction of systemic vascular resistance and systolic diastolic BP during hemodynamic monitoring. The decrease in systemic vascular resistance occurred without notable change in cardiac output or pulmonary wedge pressure. These results indicate that an orally administered regimen of propranolol, furosemide, and loading-booster doses of minoxidil produces prompt, progressive, and sustained BP reduction due to vasodilation in patients with severe hypertension who require prompt (but not immediate) BP control.

Multiple agents

The risks of systemic hypertension are correlated with the degree of BP elevation, and patients with untreated malignant hypertension can be expected to die within months. Severe hypertension, of course, is more difficult to control than mild or moderate hypertension, mainly because a greater fall in BP is needed. Other factors, however, probably add to the difficulty of treatment, since some patients show no significant response to potent antihypertensive drugs even when compliance is believed to be adequate. The term "drug-resistant hypertension" is often used, but since the patients may in some circumstances respond to medication, the term "refractory hypertension" may be preferred. Swales and associates[49] from Leicester, England, reviewed their experience with 126 patients with BP that was unacceptably high despite a conventional stepped care regimen (diuretic, beta blocker, and vasodilator). A comparative assessment of different approaches to the treatment of refractory hypertension was performed. One of 4 regimens was used: oral diazoxide, minoxidil, captopril, or quadruple therapy (diuretic plus beta adrenoceptor blocker plus hydralazine plus prazosin). Despite the severity of hypertension, BP could be controlled in almost all these patients, and no patient died from cerebrovascular disease while on treatment. Two patients died of renal failure and 5 patients required long-term hemodialysis. However, CAD remained a problem and caused death in 10 patients. Diazoxide was the most effective treatment but was the most difficult and unpleasant to use. Captopril was the best tolerated but failed to control BP in 6 of 15 patients. This experience indicates that there are now sufficient therapeutic alternatives to achieve acceptable BP control in almost all patients with "refractory" hypertension, although no treatment is ideal.

Nyberg and associates[50] from Goteborg, Vasteras, Torshalla, and Malmo, Sweden, gave a beta blocker (pindolol) and a diuretic (clopamide) in different dosages, singly and in 2 different combinations, to 71 patients with mild essential hypertension. The trial design was such that patients took both drugs singly and in combination, and in different doses, according to a set plan. The best regimen for each patient was determined by taking into account not only BP but also resting heart rate, body weight, serum potassium, and serum urate. For 19 patients (27%), monotherapy was best— pindolol for 16 and clopamide for 3. For the remaining patients, a combination of pindolol 10 mg and clopamide 5 mg was best for 39, and in 35 of these 1 tablet daily was sufficient. All patients reached the preset target BP. The differences in proportions responding best to the following pairs of regimens compared—monotherapy -vs- combination, and combination of clopamide 5 mg and pindolol 5 mg -vs- combination of clopamide 5 mg and pindolol 10 mg—were significant ($2p < 0.01$). The process by which the best treatment is chosen according to this study design resembles much more closely that followed in general medical practice than does the process in the conventional hypertension trial, in which only average effects are reported and compared.

Glucose tolerance, glycohemoglobin and serum lipids after discontinuing antihypertensive drugs

Diuretic-based antihypertensive drug therapy causes a disturbance in glucose tolerance and in serum lipid and lipoprotein concentrations. To evaluate the reversibility of the glucose intolerance and to identify mechanisms of the metabolic alterations, Ames and Hill[51] in New York City examined a short glucose tolerance test insulin glycohemoglobin and lipid concentrations during the supervised withdrawal of long-term therapy in 35 patients with primary hypertension. An average of 7 weeks after stopping drugs, glucose tolerance and glycohemoglobin improved, total cholesterol decreased 18 mg/dl, triglyceride decreased 27 mg/dl and the ratio of total to HDL cholesterol significantly decreased. The changes in lipid concentration from the treated to untreated state correlated with the changes in glycohemoglobin and indexes of glucose metabolism. These findings suggest that insulin resistance develops during drug therapy and disturbs both glucose and lipid metabolism. Attention to these alterations could provide directions for further control of atherosclerotic complication during the drug treatment of hypertension.

Transluminal dilation of atherosclerotic and nonatherosclerotic renal artery stenosis

Although percutaneous transluminal dilation was initially employed in peripheral and subsequently in coronary arteries, a recent application of this method has been in patients with renal vascular hypertension. Mahler and associates[52] from Bern, Switzerland, treated 16 consecutive patients with renovascular hypertension by transluminal dilation and observed them for 6–39 months. Poststenotic renal artery pressure increased and the renal arteries were patent on angiogram taken immediately after dilation. In 13 patients, angiogram was repeated 2–9 months later. At that time, the selective renal vein renin ratio had decreased significantly. At the end of the follow-up period, BP was improved or normal in 14 patients. One of the 8 patients with atherosclerosis was normotensive without treatment compared with 5 or 6 patients with fibromuscular dysplasia (FMD). The results in 2 patients with vasculitis remained uncertain. The 4 patients with relapses, 1 after intimal catheter dissection, were treated successfully by redilation. Thus, these investigators found that renovascular hypertension can be improved by transluminal dilation in patients with atherosclerosis and in patients with FMD with lasting success and a low morbidity rate.

Response of left ventricular mass to antihypertensive therapy

Rowlands and associates[53] from Birmingham, England, monitored continuously intraarterial ambulatory BP and did M-mode echo in 50 patients with mild to moderate essential hypertension. All patients had outpatient casual measurements of BP > 140/90 mmHg on 3 separate occasions; the mean casual BP of the group was 162 ± 14. There was no clinical evidence in any patient of target organ damage or of LV hypertrophy as assessed by standard ECG and x ray criteria. Indexes of LV mass were derived from echo data by standard formulae. Of the 50 patients, 43 were followed for 12 ± 7 months with repeat M-mode echo and casual BP measurements. Of them, 25 received antihypertensive therapy and 18 were untreated. Mean 24 hour systolic BP correlated significantly with echo LV mass; mean 24 hour diastolic BP also correlated but the relation was weaker. In the treated group there was a significantly greater fall in BP and LV mass index than in the untreated group, and there was a significant correlation between the fall in systolic BP and the fall in LV mass index in the treated group. Systolic BP appears to be an important factor in the pathogenesis of LV hypertrophy, and in hypertensive patients changes in LV mass assessed by echo correlate with changes in BP.

References

1. PICKERING TG, HARSHFIELD GA, KLEINERT HD, BLANK S, LARAGH JH: Blood pressure during normal daily activities, sleep and exercise. Comparison of values in normal and hypertensive subjects. JAMA 247:992–996, Feb 19, 1982.

2. DRAYER JIM, WEBER MA, DEYOUND JL, WYLE FA: Circadian blood pressure patterns in systemic hypertension. Am J Med 73:493–499, Oct 1982.

3. WEBER MA, DRAYER JIM, WYLE FA, BREWER DD: A representative value for whole-day blood pressure monitoring. JAMA 248:1626–1628, Oct 1, 1982.

4. HOFMAN A, ELLISON RC, NEWBURGER J, MIETTINEN OS: Blood pressure and hemodynamics in teenagers. Br Heart J 48:377–380, Oct 1982.

5. RABKIN SW, MATHEWSON FAL, TATE RB: Relationship of BP in 20–39 y.o. men to subsequent BP and incidence of HT over a 30 year observation period. Circulation 65:291–299, Feb 1982.

6. GIFFORD RW: Isolated systolic hypertension in the elderly: some controversial issues. JAMA 247:781–785, Feb 12, 1982.

7. COTTIER C, JULIUS S, GAJENDRAGADKAR SV, SCHORK A: Usefulness of home blood pressure determination in treating borderline systemic hypertension. JAMA 248:555–558, Aug 6, 1982.

8. MANN S, CRAIG MWM, GOULD BA, MELVILLE DI, RAFTERY EB: Coital blood pressure in hypertensives: cephalgia, syncope, and the effects of beta-blockade. Br. Heart J 47:84–89, Jan 1982.

9. MESSERLI FH: Cardiovascular effects of obesity and hypertension. Lancet 1:1165–1168, May 22, 1982.

10. MAXWELL MH, WAKS AU, SCHROTH PC, KARAM M, DORNFELD LP: Error in blood-pressure measurement due to incorrect cuff size in obese patients. Lancet 2:33–35, July 3, 1982.

11. KALBFLEISCH JH, HEBERT LA, LEMANN J, PIERING WF, BERES JA: Habitual excessive dietary salt intake and blood pressure levels in renal transplant recipients. Am J Med 73:205–210, Aug 1982.

12. ARKWRIGHT PD, BEILIN LJ, VANDONGEN R, ROUSE IA, LALOR C: The pressor effect of moderate alcohol consumption in man: a search for mechanisms. Circulation 66:515–518, Sept 1982.

13. ARKWRIGHT PD, BEILIN LJ, ROUSE I, ARMSTRONG BK, VANDONGEN R: Effects of alcohol use and other aspects of lifestyle on BP levels and prevalence of hypertension in a working population. Circulation 66:60–66, July 1982.

14. FREESTONE S, RAMSAY LE: Effect of coffee drinking and cigarette smoking on the blood pressure of untreated and diuretic-treated hypertensive patients. Am J Med 73:348–353, Sept 1982.

15. KESTELOOT H, GEBOERS J: Calcium and blood pressure. Lancet 1:813–815, Apr 10, 1982.

16. CLEGG G, MORGAN DB, DAVIDSON C: The heterogenicity of essential hypertension. Relation between lithium efflux and sodium content of erythrocytes and a family history of hypertension. Lancet 2:891–894, Oct 23, 1982.

17. CHARLSON ME, ALDERMAN M, MELCHER L: Absenteeism and labelling in hypertensive subjects: prevention of an adverse impact in those at high risk. Am J Med 73:165–170, Aug 1982.

18. WILLIAMS GH, TUCK ML, SULLIVAN JM, DLUHY RG, HOLLENBERG NK: Parallel adrenal and renal abnormalities in young patients with essential hypertension. Am J Med 72:907–914, June 1982.

19. Report of a Consensus Committee: Use of saralasin as a diagnostic test in hypertension. Arch Intern Med 142:1437–1440, Aug 1982.

20. Hypertension Detection and Follow-up Program Cooperative Group: Five-year findings of the hypertension detection and follow-up program. III. Reduction in stroke incidence among persons with high blood pressure. JAMA 247:633–638, Feb 5, 1982.

21. W.H.O./I.S.H. Mild Hypertension Liaison Committee: Trials of the treatment of mild hypertension. An interim analysis. Lancet 1:149–156, Jan 16, 1982.

22. Untreated mild hypertension. A report by the Management Committee of the Australian Therapeutic Trial in mild hypertension. Lancet 2:185–191, Jan 23, 1982.

23. Hypertension Detection and Follow-Up Program Cooperative Group: The effect of treatment on mortality in "mild" hypertension: results of the hypertension detection and follow-up program. N Engl J Med 307:976–980, Oct 14, 1982.

24. FREIS ED: Should mild systemic hypertension be treated? N Engl J Med 307:306–309, July 29, 1982.

25. BEARD TC, COOKE HM, GRAY WR, BARGE R: Randomized controlled trial of a no-added-sodium diet for mild systemic hypertension. Lancet 2:455–458, Aug 28, 1982.

26. LEVINSON PD, KHATRI IM, FREIS ED: Persistence of normal BP after withdrawal of drug treatment in mild systemic hypertension. Arch Intern Med 142:2265–2268, Dec 1982.

27. COCKBURN J, MOAR VA, OUNSTED M, REDMAN CWG: Final report of study on hypertension during pregnancy: the effects of specific treatment on the growth and development of the children. Lancet 1:647–649, March 20, 1982.

28. ZISMER DK, GILLUM RF, JOHNSON A, BECERRA J, JOHNSON TH: Improving hypertension control in a private medical practice. Arch Intern Med 142:297–299, Feb 1982.

29. DE WARDENER HE, MACGREGOR GA: The natriuretic hormone and essential hypertension. Lancet 1:1450–1453, June 26, 1982.

30. KAPLAN NM, SIMMONS M, MCPHEE C, CARNEGIE A, STEFANU C, CADE S: Two techniques to improve adherence to dietary sodium restriction in the treatment of hypertension. Arch Intern Med 142:1638–1641, Sept 1982.

31. MACGREGOR GA, MARKANDU ND, BEST FE, ELDER DM, CAM JM, SAGNELLA GA, SQUIRES M: Double-blind randomised cross-over trial of moderate sodium restriction in essential hypertension. Lancet 1:351–354, Feb 13, 1982.

32. KHAW KT, THOM S: Randomised double-blind cross-over trial of potassium on blood-pressure in normal subjects. Lancet 2:1127–1129, Nov 20, 1982.

33. MACGREGOR GA, SMITH SJ, MARKANDU ND, BANKS RA, SAGNELLA GA: Moderate potassium supplementation in essential hypertension. Lancet 2:567–570, Sept 11, 1982.

34. HARRINGTON JT, ISNER JM, KASSIRER JP: Our national obsession with potassium. Am J Med 73:155–159, Aug 1982.

35. GOULD BA, MANN S, KIESO H, SUBRAMANIAN B, RAFTERY B: The 24 hr ambulatory blood pressure profile with verapamil. Circulation 65:22–27, Jan 1982.

36. DRESLINSKI GR, MESSERLI FH, DUNN FG, SUAREZ DH, REISIN E, FROHLICH ED: Hemodynamic, biochemical and reflexive changes produced by atenolol in hypertension. Circulation 65:1365–1368, June 1982.

37. TEXTOR SC, FOUAD FM, BRAVO EL, TARAZI RC, VIDT DG, GIFFORD RW JR: Redistribution of cardiac output to the kidneys during oral nadolol administration. N Engl J Med 307:601–605, Sept 2, 1982.

38. FANCHAMPS A: Therapeutic trials of pindolol in hypertension: comparison and combination with other drugs. Am Heart J 104:388–406, Aug 1982.

39. OPIE LH, JEE L, WHITE D: Antihypertensive effects of nifedipine combined with cardioselective beta-adrenergic receptor antagonism by atenolol. Am Heart J 104:606–612, Sept 1982.

40. WAEBER B, GAVRAS I, BRUNNER HR, COOK CA, CHAROCOPOS F, GAVRAS HP: Prediction of sustained antihypertensive efficacy of chronic captopril therapy: relationships to immediate blood pressure response and control plasma renin activity. Am Heart J 103: 384–390, March 1982.

41. Does captopril cause renal damage in hypertensive patients? Report from the Captopril Collaborative Study Group. Lancet 1:988–990, May 1, 1982.

42. ALDIGIÉR J, PLOUIN P, GUYENE TT, THIBONNIER M, CORVOL P, MENARD J: Comparison of the hormonal and renal effects of captopril in severe essential and renovascular hypertension. Am J Cardiol 49:1447–1452, Apr 1982.

43. FUJITA T, ANDO K, NODA H, SATO Y, YAMASHITA N, YAMASHITA K: Hemodynamic and endocrine changes associated with captopril in diuretic-resistant hypertensive patients. Am J Med 73:341–347, Sept 1982.

44. FAGARD R, BULPITT C, LIJNEN P, AMERY A: Response of the systemic and pulmonary circulation to converting-enzyme inhibition (captopril) at rest and during exercise in hypertensive patients. Circulation 65:33–39, Jan 1982.

45. VLASSES PH, ROTMENSCH HH, SWANSON BN, MOJAVERIAN P, FERGUSON RK: Low-dose captopril: its use in mild to moderate hypertension unresponsive to diuretic treatment. Arch Intern Med 142:1098–1101, June 1982.

46. GARRETT BN, KAPLAN NM: Efficacy of slow infusion of diazoxide in the treatment of severe hypertension without organ hypoperfusion. Am Heart J 103:390–394, March 1982.

47. HUYSMANS FThM, THIEN TA, KOENE RAP: Combined intravenous administration of diazoxide and beta-blocking agent in acute treatment of severe hypertension or hypertensive crisis. Am Heart J 103:395–400, March 1982.

48. ALPERT M, BAUER JH: Rapid control of severe hypertension with *Minoxidil*. Arch Intern Med 142:2099–2104, Nov 1982.

49. SWALES JD, BING RF, HEAGERTY A, POHL JEF, RUSSELL GI, THURSTON H: Treatment of refractory hypertension. Lancet 1:894–896, Apr 17, 1982.

50. NYBERG G, ANAGREUS N, LEPPERT J, OVERMO J, ASPLUND J, ASTROM B, BERGSTROM R, KULLMAN S: New design for clinical trial of antihypertensive drugs applied to pindolol, clopamide, and combinations thereof. Lancet 1:355–358, Feb 13, 1982.

51. AMES RP, HILL P: Improvement of glucose tolerance and lowering of glycohemoglobin and serum lipid concentrations after discontinuation of antihypertensive drug therapy. Circulation 65:899–904, May 1982.

52. MAHLER F, PROBST P, HAERTEL M, WEIDMANN P, KRNETA A: Lasting improvement of renovascular hypertension by transluminal dilatation of atherosclerotic and nonatherosclerotic renal artery stenosis. A follow up study. Circulation 65:611–644, March 1982.

53. ROWLANDS DB, GLOVER DR, IRELAND MA, McLEAY RAB, STALLARD TJ, WATSON RDS, LITTLER WA: Assessment of left-ventricular mass and its response to antihypertensive treatment. Lancet 1:467–470, Feb 27, 1982.

5

Valvular Heart Disease

MITRAL REGURGITATION

Etiology of clinically isolated, severe, chronic, pure MR severe enough to warrant valve replacement

The etiology of clinically isolated, severe, pure MR was determined by Waller and colleagues[1] from Bethesda, Maryland and Washington, DC, in 97 patients older than 30 years of age utilizing examination of the operatively excised mitral valves. None had any degree of MS or a dysfunctioning aortic valve as determined by preoperative catheterization. The etiology of MR was leaflet prolapse in 60 patients (62%), papillary muscle dysfunction from coronary heart disease in 29 (30%), infective endocarditis on previously normally functioning valves in 5 (5%), and rheumatic heart disease in 3 (3%) (Figs. 5-1 and 5-2). Thus, nonrheumatic conditions caused the MR in 94 (97%) of the 97 patients. The history alone (previous AMI, rheumatic fever, active infective endocarditis) usually provided adequate information in the patients with coronary, infective endocarditis, and rheumatic etiologies to predict accurately the cause of the MR preoperatively; conversely, the lack of a history of 1 of these other 3 conditions strongly suggested MVP as the cause of the MR preoperatively. All 60 patients with MVP had increased mitral valve circumferences, leaflet areas, and/or products of the circumference

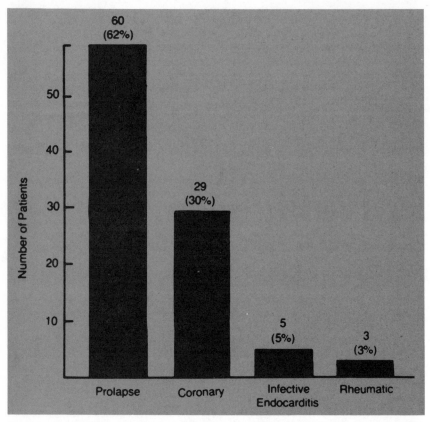

Fig. 5-1. Bar graph showing the 4 conditions causing chronic, isolated, pure, mitral regurgitation in 97 patients with operatively excised valves. Reproduced with permission from Waller et al.[1]

times the area (Fig. 5-3). In contrast, only 1 of the 37 patients in whom the MR was due to another cause had increased mitral circumference, increased area, or the product of the 2. A systolic click was not heard preoperatively in any of the 97 patients, including the 60 with MVP.

Left atrial volume overload

Gehl and associates[2] from Philadelphia, Pennsylvania, measured LA volume by 2-D echo in 36 patients undergoing cardiac catheterization, including 9 subjects with normal findings, 5 with severe MR and sinus rhythm, 5 with severe MR and AF, 6 with mild MR and sinus rhythm, 3 with mild MR and AF, 6 with severe MS, and 2 with severe MS and moderate MR. The LA dimension was measured by planimetry of the LA area and assuming

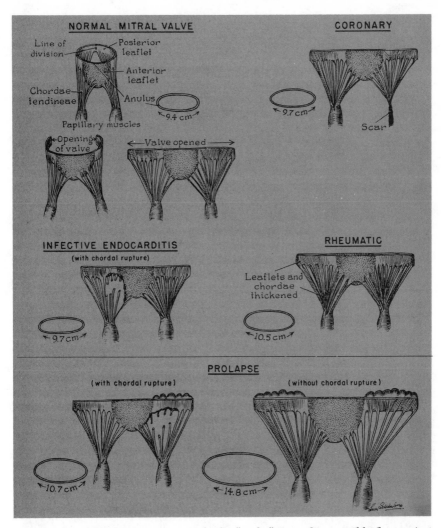

Fig. 5-2. Morphologic variations in mitral valve "anular" circumference and leaflet area in 4 conditions causing isolated, pure mitral regurgitation. Reproduced with permission from Waller et al.[1]

spherical geometry, LA volume was calculated. Patients with severe MR had marked LA systolic expansion with large phasic changes in the LA cubic dimension. Patients with severe MS had small changes in the cubic dimension in comparison with the large LA size. The LA volume changes were similar among patients with AF and sinus rhythm. Thus, LA volume overload is an additional 2-D echo feature of severe MR.

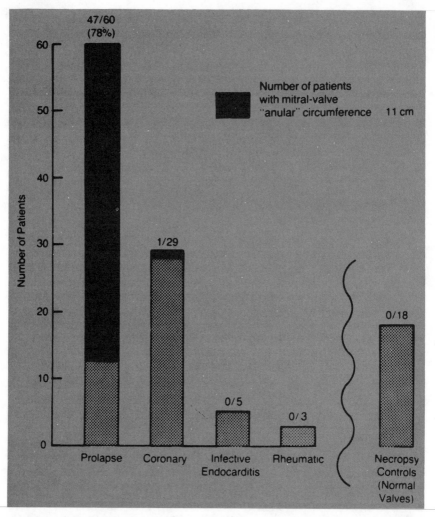

Fig. 5-3. Bar graph showing frequency of mitral valve "anular" circumference of greater than 11 cm in 4 conditions causing chronic, isolated, pure, mitral regurgitation in 97 patients with operatively excised valves. Normal mitral valves used as controls were excised from hearts of 18 necropsy patients who had no cardiac abnormalities. The frequency of men and women and age range was similar in the control and study patients. Reproduced with permission from Waller et al.[1]

Limitation of pulmonary wedge V waves in diagnosis

Fuchs and associates[3] from Baltimore, Maryland, studied the usefulness of large V waves in pulmonary capillary wedge tracings in establishing the diagnosis of MR in 1,021 consecutive patients in whom cardiac catheterization data were reviewed. Wedge tracings were obtained by Swan-Ganz catheters in 208 patients, usually because of suspected valve disease. Of the 208 patients, 102 had no trace of MR angiographically, 69 had mild to moderate and 37 had severe MR. V waves were graded as trivial (<5 mmHg), intermediate (5–10 mmHg), or large (≥10 mmHg above the mean wedge pressure). In the 50 patients with large V waves, 18 (36%) had no or trace MR; these included 5 with MS and 3 with mitral valve prosthesis, 4 with CAD and CHF, 2 with aortic valve disease and CHF, and 2 with a VSD. Of 37 patients with severe MR, 16 (43%) had large and 12 (32%) had trivial V waves. Thus, these data suggest that MR is the most common cause of large V waves; however, large V waves are neither sensitive nor specific for severe MR. Increased left atrial compliance can be associated with trivial V waves in the presence of severe MR. Mitral obstruction, CHF, and VSD may be associated with prominent V waves in the absence of important MR.

Pichard and associates[4] from New York City determined whether large V waves in the pulmonary capillary wedge tracing may be misleading in the diagnosis of MR. Of 237 consecutive patients with hemodynamic, angiographic, and echo data evaluated, 27 had large V waves (peak V wave 10 mmHg > than pulmonary wedge mean pressure). Ventriculograms were analyzed in blind fashion by 3 angiographers for evidence of MR; 17 patients had MR and 10 did not. The control group of 22 patients had normal V waves and no MR. Hemodynamic and echo variables were compared among the groups. The only significant difference between patients with and without MR with prominent V waves was in the slope of the ascent of the V wave (74.3 -vs- 141.9 mm/s, $p = 0.021$), also expressed as the MR index (6.01 -vs- 9.45, $p = 0.005$). A slope of 100 mm/second or slower had a sensitivity of 80% to confirm MR and a specificity of 70% to rule it out. The size of the V wave and the V/PW mean ratio were similar in patients in both groups and were not helpful in predicting the presence or absence of MR. In the patients without MR, those with large V waves had higher PW pressure (24 -vs- 16 mmHg, $p = 0.01$), a higher A wave (25 -vs- 16 mmHg, $p = 0.032$), a more elevated MR index (9.45 -vs- 3.99, $p = 0.001$), a larger left atrial size (25 -vs- 22 ml, $p = 0.05$), a greater V wave to pulmonary wedge mean pressure ratio (1.69 -vs- 1.10, $p = 0.001$), and a faster slope of ascent of the V wave (142 -vs- 53 mm/s, $p = 0.005$).

These data indicate that large V waves in the pulmonary wedge pressure tracing may be seen in the absence of MR. The size of the V wave is related to factors that determine left atrial compliance. Thus, caution is required in the diagnosis of MR by measurement of V wave amplitude in the pulmonary capillary wedge tracing.

Ultrasonic pulsed Doppler and 2-D echo for localizing regurgitant flow

Miyatake and associates[5] from Osaka, Japan, analyzed regurgitant flow in 40 patients with MR using combined ultrasonic pulsed Doppler technique and 2-D echo. Abnormal Doppler signals indicative of MR flow were detected in reference to the image of the long axis of the heart and the short axis at the level of the mitral orifice. The overall direction of the regurgitant flow into the left atrium was clearly seen in 28 patients and the localization of regurgitant flow in the mitral orifice in 38 patients. In patients with MVP involving the anterior or posterior leaflet, the regurgitant flow was directed posteriorly or anteriorly, respectively. When the prolapse occurred at the anterolateral commissure or posteromedial commissure, regurgitant flow was located near the anterolateral or posteromedial commissure, respectively, of the mitral orifice. In patients with rheumatic MR, the regurgitant flow was usually toward the central portion of the left atrium and was sited in the mid-part of the mitral orifice. The Doppler findings were consistent with left ventriculography. The ultrasonic pulsed Doppler technique combined with 2-D echo is useful for noninvasive analysis and preoperative assessment of MR.

Effects of arterial dilators

Greenberg and colleagues[6] from Portland, Oregon, studied 16 patients with severe MR to determine the acute effects of hydralazine on cardiac performance at rest and during exercise and to assess the long-term clinical response to therapy. Although arterial dilators favorably affect resting cardiac performance in MR by causing a redistribution and flow, patients often complain of symptoms that occur or worsen during exercise. The optimal dose of hydralazine ranged from 50–225 mg in this study and at rest reduced systemic vascular resistance (SVR) from 1,385–964 dyne/s/cm^5. Hemodynamics were monitored using the Swan-Ganz catheter introduced from a peripheral site and residing in the PA. As a result of oral hydralazine, PA wedge pressure decreased from 18–15 mmHg, cardiac index (CI) increased from 2.5–3.7 liters/min/m^2 and stroke volume index increased from 30–39 ml/m^2. The effects of hydralizine on exercise hemodynamics were further studied in 12 patients before treatment. The patients exercised at increasing work loads until they were limited by symptoms. After hydralazine therapy, exercise was repeated at a clinical work load. Although exercise alone resulted in a reduction in SVR from 1,385–1,111 dyne/s/cm^5, the addition of hydralazine caused a further reduction in resistance from 1,111 to 755 dyne/s/cm^5. Hydralazine reduced PA wedge pressure during exercise from 27–21 mmHg and increased CI from 3.7–4.9 liters/min/m^2. All 16 patients were discharged on hydralazine therapy and their clinical course was followed. Marked improvement was noted in symptoms according to New York Heart Association functional class 3–4 to class 1–2, which was sustained at ≥6 months and this occurred in 7 patients (44%). The mean follow-up in 8 patients was 13 ± 4 months. In 4 of the remaining 8 patients, hydralazine was discontinued because of internal side effects. Mitral surgery was performed in 3 of these patients as well as in 4 patients who demonstrated an initial hemodynamic response to therapy but did not have symptomatic improvement. Thus, these data demonstrate that hydralazine therapy results in substantial improvement in cardiac performance in patients with MR. The beneficial effects seen at rest are maintained during exercise. The acute improvement in hemodynamics resulted in sustained clinical improvement in half the patients. The other half needed valve surgery. Thus, arterial dilator therapy is of benefit for some patients with severe MR.

MITRAL VALVE PROLAPSE

Collagen dissolution as primary defect

The morphologic and histologic characteristics of redundant prolapsing mitral valves were studied by King and colleagues[7] from Columbus, Ohio. The mitral valves were obtained from 12 symptomatic patients with severe MR who required MVR. These findings were compared with those in 13 control valves. The mean surface area of the prolapsed mitral valve was > the control mitral valve; the mean longest diameter of the prolapsed valve, the mean shortest diameter, and the mean commissural diameter significantly exceeded those dimensions in the control valves. The density of the control valves was nearly uniform, whereas the mean density of the prolapsed valve was significantly reduced. Dissolution of elastin was only slightly more frequent in the prolapsed than in control valve. Myxomatous degeneration, noted in half of the controls was found in chordae and pars fibrosa only in prolapsed valves. Mucopolysaccharide infiltration was more severe in all sites except the anulus and prolapsed valves, and fragmentation of collagen was severe in either the pars fibrosa or the chorda of all prolapsed valves. Collagen dissolution in the pars fibrosa and chordae was present only in prolapsed valves which suggests the primacy of collage dissolution in mitral valves of patients with severe MR complicating the MVP syndrome. These investigators consider this process to be a disorder of collagen synthesis, content, or organization.

Association with low body weight and low blood pressure

Devereux and associates[8] from New York City determined whether body weight differed between individuals with inherited MVP and normal subjects. Their study consisted of examination of 177 relatives of 45 patients with MVP: 35 female and 19 male relatives had MVP and 51 female and 72 male relatives did not. There was no difference in mean height in relatives with and without MVP but those with MVP weighed significantly less. The BP also was significantly lower in relatives with MVP than in normal relatives (Fig. 5-4). It was suggested that the lower BP and the possible beneficial effects of lower weights on other cardiovascular risk factors might provide a selective advantage to carriers of the MVP gene, explaining its high prevalence in the general population. These findings may provide the first example of a

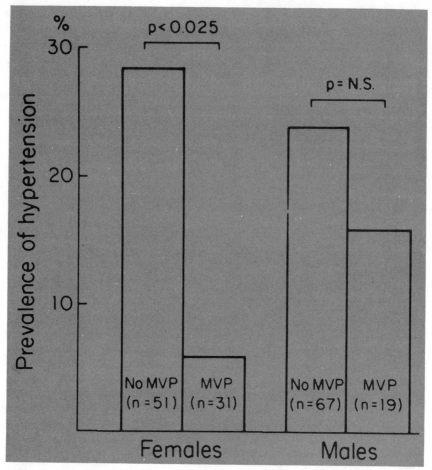

Fig. 5-4. Prevalence of hypertension (blood pressure over 140/90 mm Hg) among female and male relatives with MVP or without (No MVP). Reproduced with permission from Devereux et al.[8]

common inherited condition that is systematically associated with changes in body weight and BP. This study demonstrates highly significant differences in body weight in both sexes between subjects with and without MVP and confirms the frequent clinical observation that patients with MVP tend to be thin or asthenic.

Kagan[9] from Honolulu, Hawaii, took issue with Devereux and associates' proposed association between MVP and low BP and the finding of a lower prevalence of systemic hypertension in women with MVP compared with women without MVP. Because BP is strongly related to age, especially in females, and because the mean age of the women with MVP is lower than among women without MVP, Kagan took issue with the assertion of a difference in prevalence of systemic hypertension in females based on rates unadjusted for age. The statement, "differences in age between groups were not statistically significant," refers to what may be a quite significant biologic difference (37 -vs- 44) as age relates to BP in females. Insufficient data, according to Kagan, were presented by Devereux and associates for detailed analysis. Although sex-specific mean values for the systolic and diastolic BP were not given, some comparisons could be made. Comparison, for example, with published BP figures from the Framingham study suggest that the BP differences between MVP cases and non-MVP cases may be completely accounted for by the age difference. Thus, Kagan concluded on the question of whether MVP in females is associated with lower BP or with a lower prevalence of systemic hypertension the verdict must be "non-proven."

Increased left ventricular mass

Haikal and associates[10] from Columbia, Missouri, performed M-mode echo in 100 subjects with MVP and on 100 normal control subjects to determine if differences exist between the 2 groups in cardiac chamber size or LV performance or mass. Subjects with MVP had significantly greater LV mass than did control subjects. There were no significant differences in fractional LV shortening or LV end-diastolic volume. There was no significant difference in LV mass between asymptomatic subjects with MVP and those with chest pain, palpitations, syncope, or presyncope. Subjects with and without MR had no significant difference in LV mass. Thus, some patients with MVP have subtle LV hypertrophy that does not appear to be caused by other types of underlying organic heart disease.

Plasma catecholamine levels

The hypothesis that dysfunction of the autonomic nervous system may be responsible for some of the manifestations of MVP has recently been proposed. Such dysfunction, however, has long been suspected because of the occurrence of stress-related arrhythmias and of hyperkinetic ventricular contraction and because of the abnormal response of the autonomic nervous system to various maneuvers. Additionally, the frequent association of psychiatric symptoms and of sleep abnormalities has raised the possibility of an abnormality in central autonomic regulatory mechanisms. Pasternac and associates[11] from Montreal, Canada, measured total plasma catecholamine levels, plasma norepinephrine levels, heart rate, and systolic and diastolic BP in 15 symptomatic patients with MVP and in 19 patients in supine baseline conditions and in a standing position. In the 15 symptomatic patients, total plasma catecholamine levels and plasma norepinephrine levels were significantly elevated in both positions, and heart rate was lower than in normal subjects in the supine position but returned to normal in the upright position. Thus, symptomatic patients with MVP demonstrated increased resting sympathetic tone. In addition, the associated supine bradycardia suggested that increased vagal tone also might be present at rest. These observations support the hypothesis of a dual autonomic dysfunction in these patients and could account for some of the clinical manifestations of the MVP syndrome.

Abnormal first heart sound

In 52 patients with MVP, Tei and associates[12] from Los Angeles, California, studied the intensity of the first heart sound (S_1) in relation to the timing of the prolapse and to the presence of leaflet tip coaptation. Sixteen normal subjects served as controls. With 2-D echo, 3 distinct groups were identified. Sixteen patients had early systolic MVP coincident with initial mitral leaflet coaptation at the S wave on ECG; 21 had middle to late systolic MVP; 15 had flail mitral leaflet without normal leaflet coaptation at the free margins. The intensity of S_1 was expressed as the ratio of the S_1 amplitude to that of the aortic component of the second heart sound. This ratio was greater in the patients with early prolapse (6.2 ± 3.1, mean $\pm$ SD) than in the controls (1.4 ± 0.7, $p < 0.001$) (Fig. 5-5). The ratio was reduced in patients with flail valves (0.3 ± 0.5) and controls. Thus, the amplitude of S_1 may provide a clue to the type and timing of MVP.

Fig. 5-5. Schema of relations of 2-D echo appearance of mitral valve motion in early systole to amplitude of first heart sound (S_1). Panels A, B, and C show schema of 2-D echo of mitral valve at timing of S_1 or S wave on ECG (white arrow). Panel A shows early systolic appearance of mitral valve in normal subjects or patients with middle to late systolic prolapse. Mitral coaptation is normal, no prolapse is observed at this time, and the S_1 amplitude is normal. Panel B shows early-onset systolic prolapse with normal coaptation of leaflets at their free margins. The black arrow shows posterior mitral prolapse. Amplitude of S_1 is accentuated. Panel C shows flail mitral leaflet. Mitral valve leaflet has prolapsed into left atrium (LA) without normal coaptation at this time. The S_1 is markedly attenuated. Black arrow shows flail posterior mitral leaflet. LV denotes left ventricle and S_2 the second heart sound. Reproduced with permission from Tei et al.[12]

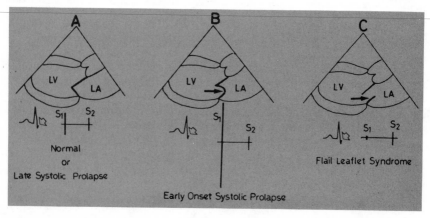

Exercise testing before and after beta blockade

Every positive exercise ECG test is not indicative of CAD, since MVP mimics CAD clinically and often in the ECG response to exercise. Abinader and Shahar[13] from Haifa, Israel, studied 12 patients with MVP in whom exercise testing was positive and then a second exercise test was done after beta blockade. All tracings returned to normal after adequate blockade, as was evident by a 17–22% reduction of resting and exercise heart rates. This study suggests that an exercise test after beta blockade should become part of the routine procedure in patients with MVP. The elimination of false positive ECG responses by beta blockade should help improve the specificity of the exercise test. Moreover, similar responses should lead to the suspicion of the presence of MVP. The 12 patients studied by these authors were among 38 with MVP who underwent exercise testing. The 12 were the only ones with initially positive exercise tests and their ages ranged from 24–55 years (mean, 42). All had both clinical and echo evidence of MVP. No patient had significant CAD by angiography.

Abnormal aortic valve echoes

Roger and Morley[14] from Glasgow, Scotland, described aortic valve echo features in 11 patients who had MVP. On 2-D echo, the aortic valve cusps were freely mobile but appeared thickened or folded. On M-mode echo, cuspal excursion was normal, systolic oscillation was well defined, and cuspal echoes were multiple and centrally positioned within the aortic root during ventricular diastole. Despite the abnormal aortic valve echo abnormalities, only 2 had AR. Thus, patients with MVP should have careful echo assessment of the aortic valve.

False negative supine M-mode echoes

Noble and associates[15] from Reno, Nevada, and Irvine, California, performed M-mode and 2-D echo during standing and after the inhalation of amyl nitrate in 17 patients (group 1) with auscultatory evidence of MVP but negative supine M-mode echo. To validate the standing M-mode echo technique 8 patients with classic auscultatory MVP with positive supine M-mode echo for MVP (group 2) and 15 control subjects (group 3) were studied. Standing M-mode echo elicited evidence of MVP in 14 of 17 (82%) of group 1—auscultatory evidence of MVP but negative supine M-mode echo; 2-D echo demonstrated MVP in 8 of 13 (62%) of the same patients. No clear advantage of 2-D echo long axis view over the apical 4-chamber view was found for diagnosis of MVP. Amyl nitrite was ineffective in eliciting echo evidence of MVP.

Risk of infective endocarditis

The absence of controlled evidence and the high prevalence of MVP have created substantial uncertainty about whether this condition is an important risk factor for bacterial endocarditis. Clemens and associates[16] from New Haven, Connecticut, evaluated this risk in a case control study of hospital inpatients who had undergone echo and who lacked any known risk factors for infective endocarditis, apart from MVP and isolated MR murmurs. Of 51 patients with infective endocarditis, 13 (25%) had MVP compared with only 10 (7%) of 153 matched controls without infective endocarditis. For the 51 matched case control sets, the odds ratio (8.2; 95% confidence interval, 2.4–28.4) indicated a substantially higher risk of infective endocarditis for persons with MVP than for those without it. This association remained statistically significant when parenteral drug abuse and routine antibiotic prophylaxis preceding dental work and other forms of instrumentation were taken into account. Furthermore, the risk may be higher than is indicated by this study, since 46% of the controls underwent echo for clinically suspected MVP, suggesting an overrepresentation of MVP in the control group. The results support the contention that MVP is a significant risk factor for infective endocarditis.

Combined with prolapse of another cardiac valve

Since patients with combined valvular prolapse appear to be more liable to become surgical candidates early in their lives than those with isolated MVP syndrome, Ogawa and colleagues[17] from Tokyo, Japan, examined the patterns of aortic and tricuspid valve motion in 50 patients with MVP by 2-D echo. Twelve patients had redundant aortic cusps bulging into the LV outflow tract during diastole, 8 of whom had AR and 7 had M-mode echo evidence of aortic valve cuspal prolapse. One patient underwent both MVR and AVR and the excised valves revealed marked myxomatous degeneration. Eight of 15 patients underwent contrast echo and had TR (systolic reflux of contrast material into the inferior vena cava persisting for >10 beats) and prolapse in the septal or anterior tricuspid leaflet or both. A similar tricuspid pattern was observed in 3 of 7 patients without TR. Tricuspid valve prolapse was identified in 20 patients (40% of the series). Nine patients had combined prolapse of mitral, aortic, and tricuspid valves. In 5 patients with mid-diastolic high pitched murmurs recorded along the left sternal border, tricuspid valve prolapse was demonstrated, and in 1 of them pulmonary regurgitation was confirmed by intracardiac phonocardiography.

With pseudoxanthoma elasticum

The association of MVP with various inherited disorders of connective tissue, such as Marfan's syndrome and Ehlers-Danlos syndrome, is well established. Although an association between pseudoxanthoma elasticum (PE) and MVP has been mentioned in previous published reports, the extent of the association has not been determined. Lebwohl and associates[18] from New York City therefore determined the prevalence of MVP in 14 patients with PE: 10 had an echo diagnostic of MVP. An association between the severity of skin lesions and the prevalence of MVP was absent. Because some cases of MVP are familial, the possibility that the findings in the present study merely represented a fortuitous association of familial MVP with inherited PE was considered. MVP was found in 4 members of a single family, but the presence of MVP in patients with PE who were from 7 different families made it unlikely that the association was fortuitous.

MITRAL STENOSIS

Cardiovascular responses to isometric exercise

Flessas and Ryan[19] from Worcester and Boston, Massachusetts, evaluated the hemodynamic response to isometric handgrip in 15 patients with MS, in 12 normal subjects, and in 13 with severe LV failure. Acceleration of heart rate and rise in LV systolic pressure were not significantly different among the 3 groups. The LV end-diastolic pressure did not change in normal subjects and patients with MS during handgrip, but it was raised markedly in patients with LV failure. Cardiac index increased in normal subjects but did not change in patients with MS and LV failure. Stroke index declined in patients with consumption and significant widening of the arteriovenous oxygen difference in patients with LV failure. In patients with MS, pulmonary capillary pressure increased by an average of 11 mmHg, with a parallel rise in mean PA pressure and no change in pulmonary vascular resistance. Thus, patients with MS have normal chronotropic and pressor responses to isometric exercise. Normal LV end-diastolic pressure response to isometric handgrip stress in patients with MS suggests good LV performance.

Morphometric investigations by 2-D echo

Schweizer and associates[20] from Aachen, West Germany, proposed a method for comparing the orifice size and the morphology of stenotic mitral valves removed intact at the time of replacement, with the preoperative 2-D echo cross-sections. The excised mitral valve was suspended on a specially constructed mounting. To avoid shrinkage, the orifice was stabilized with an air-filled balloon. A radiograph was taken directing the x-ray beam perpendicular to the valve orifice. In 40 of 51 patients, this method provided the means of relating the echo cross-sections to the valve morphology. Planimetry of the valve area compared favorably with the postoperatively determined orifice size. Agreement was found in 34 of 40 patients in orifice shape between preoperative echoes and x rays of the excised valve. The relation between intraoperative estimation of the size of the valve, using dilators with known diameters, and the postoperative results was less favorable. Areas of calcium were identified on echo as dense conglomerate echoes. In 30 patients (75%), the localization of calcific deposits and in 67% their extent was in agreement with the x rays of the valve taken after operation. In addition to determination of the area, 2-D echo allowed detailed studies of the stenotic valves, and was important for planning operative treatment.

With coronary narrowing

Chun and associates[21] from Washington, DC, and San Francisco, California, analyzed 82 patients with MS who underwent coronary angiography. Twenty-one (26%) had CAD. The mitral valve area, cardiac output, PA pressure, pulmonary vascular resistance, LV end-diastolic pressure, LV EF, and atypical chest pain did not correlate with findings of angina pectoris or of CAD; however, there was correlation with sex, age, and angina. Coronary artery disease occurred only after the age of 40 years and was more frequent in men with angina. Therefore CAD could not be ruled in patients with MS, especially those >40 years old without coronary arteriography.

Closed valvotomy

Closed mitral valvotomy is a well-established method for treatment of rheumatic mitral stenosis. It is a simple, safe, and effective means to provide long-term relief of symptoms and substantial improvement in survival. Commerford and associates[22] from the Republic of South Africa analyzed 680 patients aged ≥13 years who had closed mitral valvotomy between January 1965 and December 1977. There were 20 operation-related deaths (operative mortality, 3%). Four patients had early reoperation consisting of MVR for excessive MR produced at the time of the valvotomy. Actuarial survival for the whole group was 72% at 6 years without reoperation. A further 18% were alive but required another operation, either repeat valvotomy or MVR. Thus, the cumulative portion surviving 6 years was 90%, and 12 years, 78% (Fig. 5-6).

In 600 operations, operative findings were described: 475 had "suitable" valves and 125, "unsuitable" valves. Patients with surgically "unsuitable" valves died or required reoperation sooner than those with "suitable" valves. Similarly, clinical assessment of mitral valve mobility influenced subsequent survival. Those with ideal valves had projected survival to 12 years of 56%, as opposed to 30% for those with nonmobile valves. New York Heart Association functional class was significant in an ordered fashion. Those in class IV had a 58% 6-year survival and those in class III, a 78% 6-year survival. Patients having valvotomy during pregnancy (32 patients) had a significantly longer survival than those women operated upon when not pregnant. Age, sex, and cardiac rhythm at operation did not affect cumulative proportion surviving.

Repeat valvotomy was performed in 70 patients. The cumulative proportion surviving 12 years after repeat valvotomy appeared less than that after initial valvotomy, but the difference was not significant. The authors concluded that closed mitral valvotomy has a place where resources for treatment of MS are limited. This study spans a 12-year period beginning in 1965. Most North American centers reporting data for open mitral commissurotomy have an operative mortality approaching zero. The long-term survival patterns of these patients having open commissurotomy should be compared with this study from South Africa.

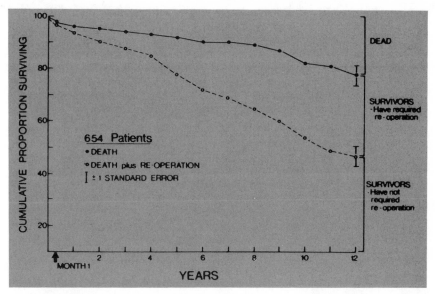

Fig. 5-6. Survival curve for whole group: upper curve indicates proportional cumulative survival, and lower curve indicates proportional cumulative survival without reoperation. Reproduced with permission from Commerford et al.[22]

MITRAL ANULAR CALCIUM

Conduction and rhythm disturbances

Mitral anular calcium is associated with high frequency of conduction defects. To delineate this association in patients with symptomatic bradyarrhythmias, 68 consecutive patients requiring pacemakers (group 1) and 56 matched controls (group 2) were studied by Nair and associates (23) from Omaha, Nebraska. The patients comprised 41 men and 27 women, whose ages ranged from 24–92 years (mean, 68). The control group consisted of 56 subjects without bradyarrhythmias, whose ages ranged from 30–86 years (mean, 70); there were 36 men and 20 women. Mitral anular calcium was detected in 59 patients (87%) with symptomatic bradyarrhythmias compared with 8 subjects (14%) in the control group. In group 1, 15 patients (22%) had complete AV block, 23 patients (34%) had AF with slow ventricular response, and 30 patients (44%) had intermittent sinus arrest. The frequency of mitral anular calcium was similar among these subgroups (93%, 83%, and 87%, respectively). This study confirms the strong association of mitral anular calcium with symptomatic bradyarrhythmias.

The clinical and echocardiographic findings in 123 patients with mitral anulus calcium were analyzed by Mellino and associates[24] from Cleveland, Ohio, and Pittsburgh, Pennsylvania. In all patients, M-mode echo demonstrated a dense band of echoes posterior to the mitral valve, moving parallel and anterior to the LV endocardium: 33% were classified as having minimal to mild mitral anulus calcification (<5 mm) and 67% had moderate to severe mitral anulus calcification (≥5 mm). There was a significant correlation between the degree of mitral anulus calcium and LA enlargement, CHF, aortic valve sclerosis, MR, AF, and AV fascicular conduction defects. The ECG evidence of conduction disturbances was significantly associated with mitral anular calcium ≥5 mm in width. Thus, the echo demonstration of moderate to severe mitral anular calcium is significantly associated with the clinical implications known to occur with this condition.

AORTIC VALVE STENOSIS

Value of measuring total 12-lead QRS amplitude in predicting transaortic systolic pressure gradient

Most ECG studies in patients with AS have involved living patients in whom the status of the LV myocardium, epicardial coronary arteries, and mitral valve was not precisely known. To determine the ECG findings attributable only to AS with or without AR, Siegel and Roberts[25] from Bethesda, Maryland, examined the 12-lead ECG recorded within 2 months of death in 50 patients aged 16–65 years (mean, 48) with peak systolic pressure gradients (PSPG) across the aortic valve from 52–180 mmHg (mean, 98) and anatomically normal mitral valves. Excluding 4 patients with complete left BBB, 44 (96%) of the other 46 patients had the usual voltage criteria for LV hypertrophy. Measurement of the total 12-lead QRS amplitude, which ranged from 144–417 mm (mean, 257), proved useful for it correlated directly with PSPG across the aortic valve and, when the 4 left BBB patients were excluded, with the peak LV systolic pressure. The total 12-lead QRS amplitude (mm) was similar in most patients to the LV systolic pressure (mmHg). Thus, subtraction of the indirect systemic arterial systolic pressure (mmHg) from the total 12-lead QRS amplitude (mm) provided a reasonable noninvasive prediction of the PSPG across the aortic valve in patients with moderate to severe AS (Fig. 5-7).

Diagnosis using estimation of peak LV systolic pressure by M-mode echo-determined end-diastolic relative wall thickness

In compensated hearts, LV systolic pressure (SP) can be estimated from the ratio of LV wall thickness to chamber radius (RWT). To determine the clinical value of such estimates, Reichek and Devereux[26] from Philadelphia,

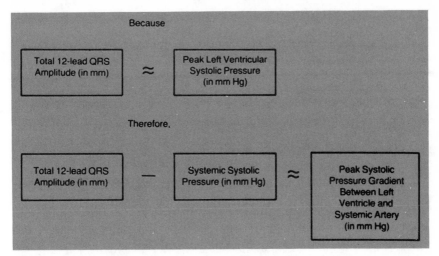

Fig. 5-7. Usefulness of measuring the total 12-lead QRS amplitude in predicting LV systemic arterial pressure gradient in AS unassociated with BBB. Reproduced with permission from Siegel and Roberts.[25]

Pennsylvania, examined echo RWT in an unscreened series of 81 individuals with aortic valve disease, hypertension, or normal hearts. Despite the presence, in many patients, of symptoms of congestive heart failure, reduced EF, or CAD, end-diastolic RWT correlated well with peak LV SP; 45 of 55 patients with LV SP ≥ 140 mmHg had end-diastolic RWT ≥ 0.45, whereas 26 of 26 with LV SP < 140 mmHg had lower values. End-diastolic RWT was ≥ 0.50 in 30 of 34 patients with LV SP ≥ 180 mmHg and in 6 of 21 with LV SP 140–180 mmHg. End-diastolic RWT correctly estimated LV SP range in 26 of 27 severe AS patients and, combined with echo aortic valve calcification, correctly recognized the presence or absence of severe AS in 99% of the series. The end-diastolic RWT for any given LV SP was higher in patients with antihypertensive treatment and lower in patients with severe aortic regurgitation. In contrast to series based on patients with normal LV function, end-systolic RWT correlated poorly with LV SP. This study shows that analysis of echo end-diastolic relative wall thickness is a useful guide to the severity of chronic LV pressure overloading if confounding factors such as antihypertensive therapy are absent. The combination of an elevated end-diastolic relative wall thickness with aortic valve calcium provides a specific and sensitive guide to the presence of severe AS in the adult.

Mechanism of angina with normal coronary arteries

The mechanism responsible for the development of angina pectoris in patients with severe AS and normal coronary arteries has not been identified. Using a specially designed Doppler probe, Marcus and associates[27] from Iowa

City, Iowa, measured the maximal velocity of coronary blood flow in the LAD coronary artery at the time of elective open heart surgery in 14 patients with AS and LV hypertrophy (13 had angina) and in 8 controls without LV hypertrophy. The ratio of peak velocity of coronary blood flow, after a 20-second occlusion, to resting velocity was decreased by >50% (p < 0.05) in the patients with AS. In 7 patients this ratio was decreased by >75%. Studies of the velocity of coronary blood flow in arteries perfusing the right ventricle showed only mild abnormalities. These data demonstrate a selective and marked decrease in coronary reserve in the hypertrophied left ventricle in patients with severe AS. The impairment in coronary reserve is probably an important contributor to the pathogenesis of angina pectoris in these patients.

Patterns of progression

Although AS is generally recognized as a progressive disease, the speed of the process varies and factors influencing the rate of progression have not been elucidated in the past. Wagner and Selzer[28] from San Francisco, California, examined factors that might affect progression in AS. These investigators reviewed serial hemodynamic studies in 50 adult patients: 7 patients had congenital, 22 rheumatic, and 21 degenerative calcific AS. The patients with calcific AS were older and had the onset of a murmur later in life. For all patients, average values at the first study was age, 54 years, peak gradient, 38 mmHg, and calculated aortic valve area, 1.3 cm^2. A mean of 3.5 years later, the gradient was 57 mmHg and aortic valve area was 0.8 cm^2. Peak LV pressure increased 9 mmHg and cardiac output decreased 0.5 liter/minute. Patients were further divided into rapid and slow progressors; the rates of change in aortic valve area were 0.3 and 0.02 cm^2/year, respectively. Degenerative calcific AS was observed in 76% of the rapid progressors and in 21% of the slow progressors. The groups also differed in that 48% of rapid progressors had a serial decrease in cardiac output of >1 liter/minute compared with 17% of slow progressors. All patients who progressed into the critical range of severity of AS (<0.5 cm^2) and developed LV failure had degenerative calcific AS. The investigators concluded that AS progresses more rapidly in patients with a degenerative etiology than in those with congenital or rheumatic disease.

Open aortic valvotomy: late results

Presbitero and associates[29] from London, England, analyzed 49 consecutive patients with AS aged 2–28 years at operations performed between 1961 and 1978. During this period, 3 patients later died, and 17 underwent reoperations (performed 2–14 years after the original open aortic valvotomy) for severe AS in 12 patients, AR in 3, and combined AS and AR in 2 (Fig. 5-8). Among the 12 patients requiring reoperation for severe AS, 5 aged >19 years had calcified aortic valves and normal aortic roots and each had AVR without complication. Seven had tunnel obstruction with a small aortic root, and

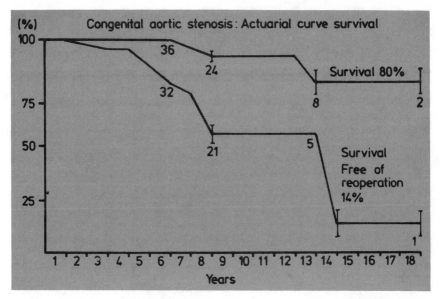

Fig. 5-8. Actuarial survival curves of 49 patients who had open aortic valvotomy: survival at 18 years of follow-up, upper curve reoperation; lower curve no reoperation. Bars show ± standard error at various points. Reproduced with permission from Presbitero et al.[29]

reoperation included total aortic root replacement in 4. Thus, the postoperative course after simple aortic valvotomy is determined by several factors, the most important being the anatomic form of the obstruction. Those presenting in the first decade of life with "lumpy" valves and small aortic roots tended to have a diffuse tunnel form of obstruction with residual stenosis after valvotomy. Older patients with pliable domed aortic valves slowly developed calcific deposits on the cusps, but since the aortic root was of good size operation was not a problem. Aortic valvotomy in children with congenital AS should be regarded as a palliative procedure, and most of these patients will subsequently require reoperation.

AORTIC REGURGITATION

Usefulness of pulsed Doppler echo

Ciobanu and associates[30] from Los Angeles, California, studied 27 patients attempting to detect and estimate the severity of chronic AR with pulsed Doppler echo. Twenty-five patients had associated AS, mitral valve disease, or both. A disturbed diastolic flow within the LV outflow tract was recorded in all but 1 patient; this finding suggests a sensitivity of the Doppler technique for detecting AR of 96%. The AR was clinically undetected in 3 patients (estimated clinical sensitivity of 89%). The Doppler technique allowed an estimation of the severity of AR by determining the distribution of diastolic flow within the LV outflow tract and body; a significant correlation between the Doppler method and angiographic estimation of AR was found (r = 0.88, p < 0.01). These data are encouraging regarding the ability of pulsed Doppler echo to detect and estimate the severity of chronic AR.

Effect of increasing heart rate

Firth and colleagues[31] from Dallas, Texas, determined whether increasing heart rate alters the severity of valvular AR in 12 patients with hemodynamically important AR. The LV volumes were measured with radionuclide ventriculographic techniques and forward cardiac index determined by thermodilution, both at rest and during atrial pacing at rates of 100 and 120 beats/minute. Atrial pacing resulted in a decremental reduction in LV end-diastolic and end-systolic volume indexes and radionuclide-determined stroke volume index, but no change in radionuclide-determined cardiac index or LV EF. Forward cardiac index increased with pacing at 120 beats/minute, despite a reduction in stroke volume index. There was a stepwise decrease in regurgitant volume/stroke from baseline to heart rates of 120 beats/minute, but no change in regurgitant volume/minute or regurgitant fraction. Mean femoral arterial, PA, and pulmonary capillary wedge pressures did not change with pacing.

These data suggest that atrial pacing in patients with AR results in a decrease in LV end-diastolic, end-systolic, stroke volume and in regurgitant volume/stroke, but no substantial change in forward cardiac output, regurgitant volume per/minute, regurgitant fraction, or LV EF. Although the reduction in LV volumes during pacing-induced tachycardia may be of some benefit, the data obtained suggest that the pressure in the pulmonary vascular bed is not altered by the tachycardia. Therefore pacing-induced tachycardia up to rates of 120 beats/minute offers little, if any, potential benefit in the patient with AR.

Myocardial contractility in asymptomatic patients

Schuler and associates[32] from Heidelberg, West Germany, studied 14 asymptomatic patients with isolated AR at rest and during maximal exercise stress. Nine normal volunteers served as a control group. The slope of the end-systolic pressure volume relation was determined noninvasively with equilibrium radionuclide ventriculography. Patients with AR did not differ from those in the control group with respect to LV EF at rest, 62 ± 8% -vs- 65 ± 6%, respectively. The slope of the end-systolic pressure volume relation was lower in the patients with AR (3.1 ± 1.1 compared with 4.1 ± 0.5, p < 0.05). Patients with AR could be classified into 2 subgroups with respect to the slope of the end-systolic pressure volume relation. Patients in subgroup A (n, 7) had a slope that fell within the normal range as defined by the control group and the LV exercise reserve was normal. Patients in subgroup B (n, 7) had a decreased slope indicating depressed myocardial contractility and all of these patients demonstrated LV dysfunction during exercise. These data suggest that the noninvasive determination of the end-systolic pressure volume relation identifies asymptomatic patients with AR with and without impaired myocardial contractility.

Radionuclide evaluation of left ventricular function

The rate of LV volume change during the first third of systole has been shown to be a more sensitive index of cardiac performance than EF in CAD. To test the hypothesis that a noninvasive index of ejection rate in early systole can also identify subtle abnormalities of LV performance in AR, Johnson and colleagues[33] from New York City evaluated the rate of change in LV counts during the first third of systole as measured by first-pass RNA in 34 AR patients and in 10 normal controls. By least squares analysis, a straight line was fit to the LV counts obtained at 0.025-second intervals during the first third of systole; the slope was divided by the average counts in the first third to give a rate constant proportional to LV volume change during early systole. The AR patients were divided into 2 groups based upon the response of EF to exercise. A normal response was defined as a rise ≥5%. Group 1 comprised 19 AR patients with a normal EF response to exercise, and group 2 comprised 15 AR patients with an abnormal EF response to exercise. The rate constant obtained at rest was 9.4 ± 2.8 for group 2, significantly lower than for group 1 (15.6 ± 3.9) or controls (14.9 ± 2.6). Using a rate constant of 12.0 as a cutoff, separation of the 2 AR groups was excellent with only 1 group 1 patient with rate constant <12.0 and 2 in group 2 with rate constant >12.0. When rate constant was plotted -vs- EF for all 44 individuals, there was a significant direct relationship, but with wide confidence limits. These data indicate that a noninvasive index of the rate of LV volume change during the first third of systole can identify abnormal LV reserve in AR patients with normal EF at rest.

Afterload mismatch and preload reserve

Ricci[34] in Vancouver, Canada, examined the interrelation of afterload, preload, and LV performance at 2 levels of systolic loading in 20 patients with AR to determine if the concept of afterload mismatch and preload reserve can be applied to this clinical entity. Two groups of patients were identified at different stages in the natural history of volume overload. Patients in group 1 had moderate LV enlargement with an end-diastolic volume (EDV) <150 ml/m^2 and patients in group 2 had severe LV enlargement with EDV >150 ml/m^2. Both groups had sufficient eccentric hypertrophy measured by LV mass, to keep afterload as measured by mean systolic LV wall stress only slightly above normal. The LV mean systolic wall stress was similar in each group. Patients in group 2 had a lower LV EF and velocity of circumferential fiber shortening than those in group 1 at a similar lower level of afterload. At a similar higher level of afterload, which increased EDV from 134–154 ml/m^2 in group 1 and from 191–218 ml/m^2 in group 2, patients in group 1 maintained their EF and forward stroke volume and had a significant increase in total LV stroke volume, whereas patients in group 2 had a decrease in EF and in forward stroke volume and no significant change in LV stroke volume. These data indicate that patients with moderate LV dilation during AR and sufficient hypertrophy to normalize afterload have a preload reserve that permits normal LV performance during a basal state as well as during acute increases in afterload. Patients with severe LV dilation, however, despite sufficient hypertrophy to normalize afterload, have afterload mismatch due to a depressed inotropic state, and have exhausted preload reserve such that acute increases in afterload worsen the afterload mismatch and cause further deterioration of LV performance. Thus, the concept of afterload mismatch and preload reserve appears to describe the natural history of hemodynamic alterations in chronic AR.

Secondary to systemic hypertension (without aortic dissection) requiring aortic valve replacement

Waller and associates[35] from Bethesda, Maryland, and Washington, DC, described clinical and morphologic observations in 4 patients who had severe AR from severe systemic hypertension unassociated with aortic dissection (Fig. 5-9). Each patient underwent AVR. Although AR of minimal or mild degree is well recognized to occur in patients with systemic hypertension, severe degrees of AR are rare in such patients, and AVR had not been previously reported. Why these 4 patients, however, had severe AR was not determined. Systemic hypertension must be added to the list of causes of severe pure AR. Additional patients with systemic hypertension associated with severe AR subsequently were reported by Waller and associates.[36,37]

Secondary to ankylosing spondylitis

Tucker and associates[38] from Stanford, California, studied 35 patients with ankylosing spondylitis (10 also had Reiter's syndrome) without clinically apparent cardiac involvement using phased array 2-D and sector-directed M-mode echo to determine the presence of aortic abnormalities. Aortic root dimensions were measured at the aortic anulus, at the tip of the cusps, and 0.5–1.5 cm above the cusps. The dimensions were compared with those in 20 normal men and among patient subgroups separated according to age, duration, and severity of ankylosing spondylitis, and presence of qualitative abnormalities. Two patients had aortic dimensions >4.2 cm at the valve (normal, ≤4.0 cm). Six patients had discrete areas of increased bright echoes below the left or noncoronary cusps suggestive of a subaortic "bump" and 2 of the 6 patients had increased aortic cuspal echoes suggesting aortic valve thickening or fibrosis or both. These changes occurred more commonly in older patients with more severe ankylosing spondylitis. These data suggest

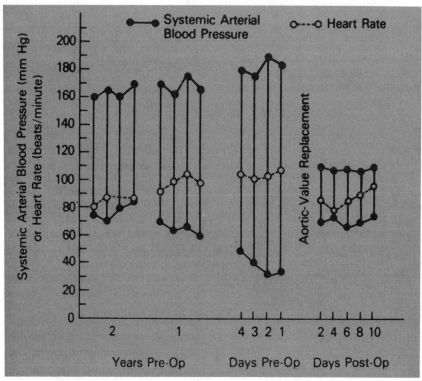

Fig. 5-9. Systolic and diastolic arterial pressures before (pre-op) and shortly after (post-op) aortic valve replacement. The pulse pressure decreased considerably after operation.

that aortic root changes suggestive of inflammation or fibrosis or both occur in asymptomatic patients with ankylosing spondylitis and may be detected by 2-D echo. Dilation usually does not occur without AR.

Treatment with nifedipine

Fioretti and associates[39] from Trieste, Italy, studied 12 patients with severe isolated AR to determine the efficacy of nifedipine (20 mg sublingually) in altering hemodynamic performance. The LV end-diastolic pressure decreased from 19 ± 8 (mean $\pm$ SD) to 9 ± 5 mmHg ($p < 0.0001$), mean aortic pressure from $98 \pm 12-80 \pm 9$ mmHg ($p < 0.0001$), systemic vascular resistance from $1,135 \pm 280-794 \pm 176$ dynes/s/cm^{-5} ($p < 0.0002$) and rate-pressure product from $11,732 \pm 1,727-10,022 \pm 1,103$ mmHg/beats/minute ($p < 0.01$). Forward cardiac index increased by 24%, but LV end-diastolic volume, EF, and total stroke work index did not change significantly. Regurgitant fraction, measured in 5 patients, changed in parallel with systemic vascular resistance. These data suggest that LV function was maintained while both preload and afterload were decreased by nifedipine. Thus, nifedipine exerts beneficial clinical effects in patients with important and isolated AR and may be useful in its chronic treatment.

Regression of left ventricular hypertrophy after aortic valve replacement

After AVR for chronic AR, LV mass may be reduced. A few patients achieved normal LV mass and others exhibit little or no regression of hypertrophy. The value of the ECG in assessing these structural changes has not been studied in detail. Carroll and associates[40] from Boston, Massachusetts, studied 21 patients before and after AVR for chronic AR. Muscle cross-sectional area derived from ECG dimension and from wall thickness data was used as an index of LV muscle mass. In 15 patients voltage was reduced after AVR; 7 had normal voltage, and 8 still had increased voltage. Patients with normal voltage had complete regression of hypertrophy by echo, whereas those who had persistently increased voltage had incomplete regression. Reduction in voltage generally occurred in the first 6 months after AVR.

There are practical advantages in using the ECG to evaluate the results of AVR. Lack of regression of LV hypertrophy manifested by persistently increased precordial voltage should draw attention to the possibility of paraprosthetic AR, systemic hypertension, patient prosthesis mismatch, or the presence of other cardiac lesions.

The parameters used in this study for precordial voltage ($SV_1 + RV_{5-6}$) plus echo cross-sectional area are easily obtainable preoperatively and postoperatively. The precordial voltage therefore seems a reliable and easy way to follow patients after AVR.

Depressed cardiac function after aortic valve replacement

To identify variables predictive of postoperative hemodynamic improvement, Donaldson and associates[41] from London, England, analyzed changes in LV mass, volume, morphology, and histochemistry in 67 patients undergoing AVR for chronic AR. Patients were divided into 2 groups: group A, 51 patients, with LV echo diameters returning to normal after operation; group B, 16 patients, with postoperative LV dilation. A preoperative biopsy was obtained in all patients; postoperative tissue samples were available in 13 patients (5 from group A, 8 from group B). Data were correlated with the postoperative clinical, hemodynamic state over a follow-up period of 3 years. Regression of LV hypertrophy was usually incomplete. Echo and angiographic data could not define the type and degree of dysfunction that was irreversible. Massive fiber hypertrophy (mean, 34.1 μm), moderately or severely increased interstitial fibrous tissue, reduced levels of the myofibrillar and mitochondrial enzymes adenosine triphosphates and succinate dehydrogenase in pre- and postoperative tissue samples correlated with persistent dilation, cardiac failure, and early death (group B). Irreversible morphologic and functional changes contributed to a depressed cardiac function after operation. Preoperative ventricular biopsies are thus of prognostic importance in patients with volume overloaded hearts.

REGURGITANT FRACTION IN PURE VALVULAR REGURGITATION

Janowitz and Fester[42] from Miami Beach, Florida, evaluated the ability of radionuclide ventriculography to quantitate LV regurgitant fraction utilizing first pass radionuclide ventriculography. They applied a measurement of the total number of counts ejected from the right and left ventricles (C_R and C_L) in the absence of any valve regurgitation and equal counting efficiency from each ventricle, $C_R/C_L = 1$. With valvular regurgitation in the left side of the heart, the regurgitant fraction was calculated as $(C_L - C_R)/C_L$, if no RV regurgitation was present. This approach was utilized in 5 normal volunteers, 7 patients studied with cardiac catheterization without regurgitation, and 22 patients with MR or AR or both. Excellent correlation was found with cardiac catheterization data in the group of patients with important left-sided valvular regurgitation ($r = 0.86$, n, 22). The authors concluded that this method was simple and accurate for measuring LV regurgitant fraction due to MR or AR or both. One note of caution needs to be added. Nicod and colleagues from Dallas, Texas, demonstrated that one may measure regurgitant fractions accurately in patients with normal ventricular function, but when ventricular function is depressed approaches such as those described by Janowitz and Fester do not accurately estimate the severity of valvular regurgitation (*J Nucl Med* 23:763, 1982).

Calculation of accurate stroke count ratios for the assessment of valvular regurgitation from equilibrium blood pool images has been difficult and has not permitted computation of regurgitant fractions (RF) because of contamination of RV stroke counts by right atrial activity. Henze and colleagues[43] from Los Angeles, California, described a new method to correct for this contamination by subtracting one-half of the right atrial counts from the RV counts, assuming that in the standard or modified left anterior oblique projection commonly used about one-half of the RA activity is superimposed to the right ventricle. This new method was tested in 20 patients without valvular disease or shunts. The LV/RV stroke count ratio approached unity (1.01 ± 0.14). The RV EF derived by this technique agreed well with those obtained by gated first-pass studies recorded in the right anterior oblique projection. In 9 normal subjects and 17 patients with moderately severe or severe AR (12 patients) or MR (7 patients), LV EF, RV EF, and RF were determined at rest and maximum exercise. In patients at rest, LV EF (56%) and RV EF (49%) did not differ significantly from LV EF (60%) and RV EF

(53%) in normal subjects. The calculated RF was negligible in normals (2%), but averaged 52% in patients with valvular disease. During exercise, LV EF fell significantly to 44% in patients but increased to 71% in normals. The RV EF increased in AR to 65% (similar to normals), but fell in MR to 37%. In both patient subsets RF decreased with exercise to 25% in AR and 39% in MR. These results indicate that this new approach permits assessment of RV EF and RF from gated equilibrium blood pool studies and is suitable to evaluate the hemodynamic response to physiologic and therapeutic interventions in patients with valvular regurgitation.

LEFT VENTRICULAR RELAXATION IN PURE VALVULAR REGURGITATION

Rousseau and associates[44] from Brussels, Belgium, studied LV relaxation in 57 patients; 27 with valvular regurgitation, 17 normal subjects, and 13 patients with CAD. The study assessed ventricular relaxation in patients with valvular regurgitation. Starting from a fixed level of wall stress (40 kdyne/cm^2), the incremental LV elastance (ratio P/V) and the changes in velocity of lengthening produced by a constant increase in LV volume (+20 ml/m^2) were determined. In patients with AR and MR, both the incremental elastance and the change in velocity lengthening were abnormal. The indexes also were impaired in patients with CAD. Significant correlations were found in the patients between incremental elastance and LV EF (r = 0.63), mean velocity of fiber shortening (r = 0.62), and LV end-systolic volume (r = 0.53), indicating a relation between impaired incremental elastance and alterations in inotropic state or afterload or both. This hypothesis was confirmed by the fact that patients with a peak systolic wall stress of <400 kdyne/cm^2 and a normal inotropic state also had normal incremental elastance. All but 1 patient with the same afterload but abnormal contractility had abnormal incremental elastance. These data suggest that abnormalities in early diastolic filling are common in patients with valvular regurgitation and are likely to be related to impaired LV relaxation.

INFECTIVE ENDOCARDITIS

Symposium

The February 1982 issue of the *Mayo Clinic Proceedings* contains a symposium with several papers on infective endocarditis. These papers include a general consideration of diagnosis and treatment,[45] pediatric endocarditis,[46] treatment of penicillin-sensitive streptococcal endocarditis,[47] enterococcal endocarditis,[48] and staphylococcal endocarditis.[49]

Echo diagnosis

Sensitivity, specificity, diagnostic accuracy, and prognostic implications of the M-mode echo pattern of vegetations were examined prospectively in consecutive patients referred with potential active infective endocarditis (IE) by Come and colleagues[50] from Boston, Massachusetts. A pattern of definite echo vegetations was present in 37% of 51 patients diagnosed clinically to have active IE. Specificity in 138 patients without IE was 96%. Diagnostic accuracy of a positive test was 76% and that of a negative test was 80%. Five of 6 false positive studies involved patients with prior IE or valvular thrombosis. If possible echo vegetations were included, sensitivity increased to 47% and specificity decreased to 89%. Echographic vegetations were significantly correlated with CHF and need for valve replacement and/or death. Seven of 8 patients with definite aortic valve vegetations died or required surgery, compared with 1 of 11 patients with mitral or tricuspid vegetations alone. Prognostic importance of echo documented vegetations depends upon their site within the heart. Thus, in conjunction with careful clinical assessment, echo evaluation of vegetations and valvular integrity appears to be an important modality for determining need for surgical intervention prior to the development of life-threatening complications.

Pringle and associates[51] from Belfast, Northern Ireland, compared clinical and echo findings to findings at operation in 18 patients with active infective endocarditis undergoing valve replacement for left-sided CHF. In 10 of 11 patients with clinically suspected severe AR and vegetations only on the aortic valve and in 2 of 3 patients with severe MR, echo provided confirmation of the clinical diagnosis. In the 3 patients with clinically suspected combined AR and MR, however, cardiac catheterization was necessary to confirm the severity of the valvular regurgitation. In an additional 3 patients, cardiac catheterization also was necessary to confirm the severity of the single valve lesion. Four patients had either a ring abscess or a VSD at operation and neither was detected by echo. Of the 18 patients, 14 (78%) survived valve replacement to leave the hospital. During follow-up to 44 months, reinfection, prosthetic dehiscence, or paravalvular leak did not occur. Thus, most patients with left-sided active infective endocarditis and continuing LV CHF resulting from severe valvular regurgitation did well postoperatively, and their preoperative status was assessed satisfactorily by echo.

Matsumoto and associates[52] from Osaka, Japan, described 2 patients with perforations in anterior mitral leaflet from active infective endocarditis and the perforations were clearly diagnosed preoperatively by both M-mode and 2-D echo. The echo observations were confirmed at operation.

Ginzton and associates[53] from Torrance, California, studied 16 patients with tricuspid valve endocarditis to define: 1) the clinical or echo subsets at risk for complications or need for tricuspid valve surgery, and 2) a long-term 2-D echo course of tricuspid vegetations. Among the 16 patients, there were 18 episodes of tricuspid endocarditis and 12 patients had a history of intravenous drug abuse. The most frequent organism responsible for tricuspid endocarditis was *Staphylococcus aureus* (11 patients). In patients who subsequently required tricuspid valve surgery, persistent endocarditis, cardiomegaly, and/or right-sided CHF were present. Ten patients had tricuspid valve vegetations by M-mode echo and all 16 had vegetations by 2-D echo. Vegetation size, right atrial enlargement, and abnormal septal motion were not of prognostic significance. These data suggest that: 1) 2-D echo increases the sensitivity for detection of tricuspid valve vegetations; 2) persistent infection and/or cardiomegaly and right-sided CHF identify subgroups of patients at increased risk who generally require surgery; 3) no M-mode or 2-D echo feature is of prognostic value; and 4) that tricuspid valve vegetations tend to resolve with time.

Pathology

Arnett and Roberts[54] from Bethesda, Maryland, reported a necropsy experience of 192 cases of fatal active infective endocarditis. The infection involved a right-sided cardiac valve in 40 patients (21%), only 1 or both left-sided valves in 114 patients (60%), 1 or more prosthetic cardiac valves in 30 patients (16%), and complicated congenital heart disease with a shunt in 6 patients (3%). *Staphylococcus* was the causative organism in 52% of the patients. Death was the result of cardiovascular damage in 72 patients, cerebral problems in 28, generalized sepsis in 25, and miscellaneous problems in 25.

Bacteremia and the heart

Stratton and associates[55] from Seattle, Washington, performed serial M-mode and 2-D echo at 1- to 2-week intervals in 57 patients with bacteremia to define the prevalence and course of cardiac abnormalities and the role of routine echo in patients with bacteremia. A control group of 23 patients with clinically suspected bacteremia but negative blood cultures was also studied. The mean number of echoes per patient was 2.4 in the bacteremic group and 2.2 in the control group. A total of 186 echoes were interpreted without any clinical knowledge of the presence of, and serial changes in, valvular vegetation, pericardial effusion, LV dysfunction, and other abnormalities.

Nine of 57 bacteremic patients had vegetations, whereas no vegetations occurred in the 23 nonbacteremic control patients (p < 0.05). In 4 of the 9 patients with vegetations, bacterial endocarditis was clinically unsuspected before echo, whereas the remaining 5 patients had clinically evident endocarditis. Of 9 bacteremic patients with a risk factor predisposing to endocarditis (intravenous drug abuse in 6, valvular heart disease in 3), 6 (67%) had a vegetation, whereas only 3 of 48 (6%) bacteremic patients without a risk factor had a vegetation (p < 0.001). Risk factors were present in 5 nonbacteremic control patients, none of whom had a vegetation. Pericardial effusions were noted in 19 (33%) of 57 bacteremic patients and in 4 (17%) of 23 nonbacteremic control patients (p = NS), but no patients had clinically evident tamponade of purulent pericarditis. Global LV dysfunction occurred in 11 (19%) of 57 bacteremic patients versus 3 (13%) of 23 nonbacteremic patients'(p = NS). On serial study, ventricular dysfunction improved in 6 of 11 bacteremic patients but in none of the nonbacteremic patients. Other lesions, including valvular prolapse and nonspecific valve thickening, were equally prevalent in both groups.

In unselected patients with bacteremia, serial echo rarely demonstrates findings that lead to a change in prognosis or therapy, and thus routine echo is not indicated. However, in bacteremic patients who have either a clear risk factor predisposing to endocarditis or a potential intravascular source of bacteremia, the authors recommend echo to detect otherwise unsuspected vegetations.

NECESSITY OF ROUTINE CARDIAC CATHETERIZATION BEFORE CARDIAC VALVE REPLACEMENT

This subject was extensively covered in *Cardiology 1982*. Subsequently, however, several additional papers appeared, most stressing the importance of cardiac catheterization in most patients before replacement of 1 or more cardiac valves.[56-62]

DIAGNOSIS OF RIGHT-SIDED VALVE DISEASE

Veyrat and associates[63] from Paris, France, studied 20 normal subjects and 18 patients with valvular heart disease whose lesions were independently assessed either by cardiac catheterization and/or operation. Each had pulsed Doppler echo combined with either M-mode or 2-D echo. Of the 82 patients, 41 had tricuspid lesions, including 31 with pure TR and 9 with tricuspid stenosis (TS). The tricuspid analogue flow velocity trace and the Doppler frequency spectrum (time interval histogram) were recorded (Fig. 5-10). Characteristic differences were found between the records from subjects with and without tricuspid lesions. In subjects with TR, there was a systolic negative wave on the analogue velocity display and broadening of the time interval histogram. In subjects with TS, there was an abnormal pattern, and significantly increased duration of the diastolic wave on the analogue velocity trace, again with broadening of the time interval histogram. Sensitivity and specificity ranged between 85% and 95%. The calculated ratio between the measured amplitudes of the systolic and diastolic waves correlated well with independently performed grading of the TR on a 3-point scale in 85% of cases. Grading of the severity of TS on a 3-point scale based on studies of the diastolic Doppler velocity anomalies was the same in 85% of cases as the grading based on established invasive techniques. The addition of 2-D echo to the pulsed Doppler technique increased the sensitivity for mild lesions.

Of the 59 patients with severe TR studied by Cha and associates[64] from Browns Mills, New Jersey, 88% had Carvallo's sign alone or in combination

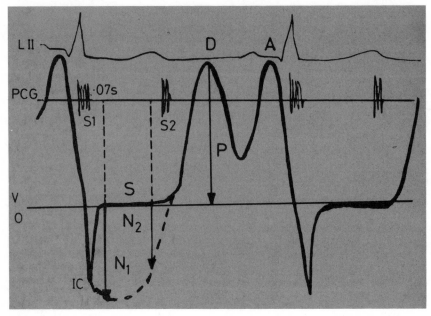

Fig. 5-10. Determination of N/P ratio. Reproduced with permission from Veyrat et al.[63]

with pulsatile liver or prominent jugular venous V waves, and 42% had the classic triad. Most patients had RA enlargement on chest x ray. The classic "ventricularization" pattern of RA pressure occurred in 30%, prominent V waves with rapid Y descent was present in 37%, and normal contour of RA waves with normal mean pressure occurred in 33%. The inspiratory maneuver was helpful to induce the ventricularization pattern or prominent V waves with rapid Y descent, especially in patients with normal RA pressure waves. Thus, right ventriculography is a sensitive and accurate method for detecting and quantitating TR in the absence of the diagnostic physical findings.

Despite the multiple advances in recent years in cardiac catheterization, confirmation of pulmonary regurgitation (PR) remains difficult, since the catheter must be placed across the pulmonic valve for PA injection. Miyatake and colleagues[65] from Osaka, Japan, studied 60 patients with PR by the pulsed Doppler technique combined with 2-D and M-mode echo. Patients with PR had abnormal Doppler signals just below the pulmonic valve in the RV outflow tract in diastole on the 2-D image. These signals were considered to indicate the regurgitant flow. There are 2 patterns of pulmonary regurgitant Doppler signals. In pulmonary hypertension, the maximal component of instantaneous flow velocity is sustained at about the same signal strength throughout diastole, but when the PA pressure is normal, the velocity slows down gradually from early diastole to end-diastole. In about half the patients, PR was detected by phonocardiography. In the remaining patients, the PR murmur could not be differentiated from an AR murmur or was masked by coexistent AR or PDA, whereas the Doppler technique indicated PR.

VALVULAR REGURGITATION OR STENOSIS IN SYSTEMIC CONDITIONS

Acute rheumatic fever in India

Although the incidence of acute rheumatic fever (ARF) in the USA has been greatly reduced in recent decades, this disease continues to be severe in India and other neighboring countries and temperate zones. Sanyal and associates[66] in New Delhi, India, examined the outcome of ARF in 85 children from North India who had received regular antistreptococcal prophylaxis after their initial attack. At the end of the 5-year follow-up, 33 patients had rheumatic heart disease (RHD); MR was the most common valvular disease and appeared in 91% of the patients, whereas MS developed in only 18%. Statistically, initial carditis CHF, cardiomegaly, or moderate to severe MR increased the risk of ARF. Most recurrences of ARF mimicked the first attack and produced further damage in 5 patients with carditis and in 1 patient with chorea. The cardiac status during the first attack of ARF and the continuity of prophylaxis were found to be major determinants of the outcome. Statistical comparisons disclosed that with continuous prophylaxis, the prevalence rate evolution and clinical spectrum of this sequelae of ARF in children from India did not differ significantly from those in the West.

Marfan's syndrome

Among 18 necropsy patients aged 15–52 years (mean, 34) with Marfan's syndrome studied by Roberts and Honig[67] from Bethesda, Maryland, 13 had fusiform aneurysms of the sinus and proximal tubular portions of the ascending aorta, severe AR, and severe aortic medial degeneration; 3 had dissection involving the entire aorta which was not dilated previously and the aortic media was normal histologically; and 2 patients had isolated mitral regurgitation with grossly and histologically normal aortas. Of the 13 with fusiform ascending aortic aneurysms, 2 ruptured spontaneously; of the remaining 11, 9 died after operations to correct severe AR. Of the 3 with aortic dissection, 2 had systemic hypertension before the dissection. Although the only cardiovascular manifestation of Marfan's syndrome was mitral regurgitation in 2 patients, 7 of the other 16 also had clinical evidence of mitral regurgitation and 11 of the total 18 had anatomic mitral abnormalities, including dilated (>11 cm) anuli (11 patients), prolapse (7 patients), ruptured chordae tendineae (5 patients), and mitral anular calcification (5 patients).

Analysis of 151 previously reported necropsy patients with Marfan's syndrome disclosed that 53 (35%) had fusiform ascending aortic aneurysms, 57 (38%) had aortic dissection, 33 (22%) had isolated or predominant mitral regurgitation, and 8 (5%) had miscellaneous conditions (mainly normal hearts and ascending aortas). The mean age at death in patients with either fusiform ascending aortic aneurysm or dissection was similar (28 years) and the mean age of patients with mitral regurgitation was much younger (12 years). Nearly three-fourths of the patients with mitral regurgitation were aged 15 years or younger, whereas the percentage of young patients with aneurysm or dissection was much less (15% and 7%, respectively). As with the patients studied by Roberts and Honig, the occurrence of dissection was infrequent in the previously reported patients with fusiform ascending aortic aneurysm. Dissection appeared to involve aortas that previously were of normal size or only mildly dilated, and the degree of "cystic medial necrosis" in them appeared to have been relatively mild. Thus, the aneurysmally dilated ascending aorta, the most common cause of AR in these patients, is generally not a candidate for dissection, but it is prone to complete rupture (Fig. 5-11). Finally, mitral anular dilation with or without leaflet prolapse appears to be the major cause of mitral regurgitation in patients with Marfan's syndrome.

Carcinoid syndrome

Callahan and associates[68] from Rochester, Minnesota, studied 19 patients with known carcinoid syndrome with M-mode and 2-D echo. Eight patients had no evidence of carcinoid heart disease by echo. Two had changes in the tricuspid valve echogram suggestive of early carcinoid heart disease, and the other 10 patients had the following echocardiographic findings: 1) the pattern of RV volume overload; 2) abnormal right-sided valves, including thickening and retraction and fixation in a semiopen position of the tricuspid valve and/or thickened, retracted pulmonic valve cusps; and 3) no obvious involvement of the left ventricle or the LV cardiac valves.

CARDIAC VALVE REPLACEMENT

In children

Gardner and associates[69] from Baltimore, Maryland, reviewed their experience with 64 patients, aged 1–19 years (mean, 14) who underwent replacement of aortic, mitral, or tricuspid valve between 1965 and 1980. Hospital mortality was 31% during the first 5-year period, 11% during the second, and from 1976–1980, it was 3% for 33 patients. Rheumatic valve

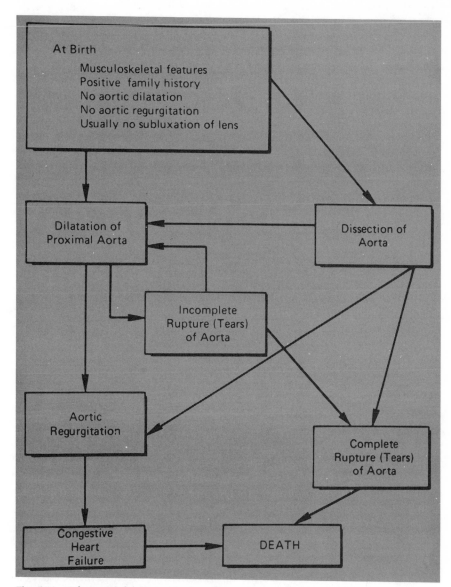

Fig. 5-11. Schema of development of cardiovascular complications in Marfan's syndrome. Reproduced with permission from Roberts and Honig.[67]

disease was present in 47% operated on from 1965–1975 and only 17% operated on from 1975–1980. Of 71 implanted prostheses, 51 were mechanical and 20 were porcine bioprostheses. Late follow-up (mean, 4.2 years) was available in 55 patients and in the group of 38 with mechanical prostheses, there were 2 thromboembolic episodes despite the fact that only 25 (68%) had been continuously anticoagulated. Thus, the overall incidence of thromboembolism was 0.8% per patient-year. Thromboembolism did not occur in the tissue valve group and 63% were free of valve failure at the sixth postoperative year, although 2 of 4 patients <12 years of age at operation, had accelerated degeneration. The authors demonstrated similar results for valve replacement in children as for older patients, except for accelerated tissue valve degeneration, which was most common in prepubertal patients. Their experience suggests that thrombus is less likely to develop on prosthetic valves in the young.

The desire for a valve replacement device free of the requirement for long-term anticoagulation has led many groups to employ bioprostheses. Experience with porcine bioprostheses in children indicates a high (many believe unacceptably so) incidence of premature degeneration and failure. Galioto and associates[70] from Philadelphia, Pennsylvania, reported the early failure of mitral Ionescu-Shiley bovine parietal pericardial prostheses in 2 children <1 year of age at operation. Failure requiring re-replacement occurred at 19 and 4 months postoperatively. Although pathologic examination showed mild changes in the cuspal tissue, there was extensive collagen deposition on the struts which interfered with cuspal mobility. This pathologic change is different from that observed with porcine bioprostheses, but casts doubt on the wisdom of employing this valve substitute in children.

Human and colleagues[71] from Capetown, South Africa, reviewed their results of 57 MVRs between 1972 and 1979 in 56 consecutive patients, aged 2–12 years (mean, 9.4) at operation. The etiology of the valve disease was rheumatic in 46, congenital in 8, and acute bacterial endocarditis in 2. Porcine bioprostheses were employed in 33 and mechanical prostheses in 24 patients. Overall hospital mortality was 1.7% and late mortality, 10.5%. Actuarial survival at 5 years was 92% for the bioprosthetic group and 77% for the mechanical group (p < 0.18). In the bioprosthetic group, serious thromboembolism occurred in 1 patient and severe calcific degeneration in 11 (33%) within 4 years after operation. In the mechanical group, multiple thromboemboli occurred in 1 patient and valve thrombosis in 1. Event-free curves showed only 10% of the bioprosthetic group complication free at 4 years compared with 84% of the mechanical group at 5 years (p < 0.0001). Thus, the porcine heterograft is an unsuitable device for MVR in children.

The lack of long-term durability of porcine heterograft bioprostheses in children has revived the use of mechanical valve substitutes in this group. Weinstein and associates[72] from San Francisco, California, reviewed their experience in 24 children ranging in age from 1–18 years (mean, 12.2) who underwent 27 operations for aortic, mitral, or combined valve replacement with 1 hospital death. Only 5 of the 23 survivors were placed on long-term anticoagulation with warfarin. The remaining 18 were given aspirin (plus dipyridamole in 5), 11 having a Björk-Shiley, 1 a Beall valve, and 6 a porcine bioprosthesis, which were used to replace the aortic valve in 10 and mitral valve in 8 patients. These 18 were followed between 1 and 59 months (mean, 20) and none experienced thrombotic, embolic, or bleeding complications.

There were 2 late deaths, 1 traumatic, and 1 related to congestive heart failure from a viral cardiomyopathy. The dosage of aspirin was 6 mg/kg/day up to 600 mg/day in older children and when dipyridamole was used, the dosage was 25 mg/day in children <12 years, 50 mg/day in those 12–18 years of age. The authors' experience and their review support the conclusion that aspirin may provide adequate protection against thromboembolism in children with prosthetic cardiac valves and avoids the hemorrhagic complications associated with warfarin.

Benmimoun and associates[73] from Geneva, Switzerland, reported hemodynamic variables and LV function in 44 children aged 3–17 years (mean, 12) after MVR with a Starr-Edwards (39 patients) or Hancock (5 patients) prosthesis. Postoperative study was 2–6 months (mean, 4) after operation. Residual gradients averaged 9 mmHg for the Hancock valve and 7 mmHg for the Starr-Edwards. Mean PA pressure and pulmonary wedge pressure decreased to normal or near normal levels in all but 5 patients, all of whom had paravalvular leak. The LV end-diastolic volume was measured in 27 patients and decreased from a mean value of 190 ml/M^2 preoperatively to 103 ml/M^2 after MVR; 11 of 27 had significant residual LV volume overload (LV end-diastolic volume >100 ml/M^2) and 4 of 11 with a large LV volume had either AR or residual MR. The LV EF averaged 57% before MVR and 56% after MVR; 9 of 27 had LV EF values <50% following MVR (3 with residual MR). These data indicate significant improvement in hemodynamics and LV volume overload after MVR in children, all findings to be expected. The disturbing feature is the residual LV volume overload and depressed LV EF in many patients despite MVR at a relatively young age. The problem of determining optimal timing for MVR before LV function deteriorates remains.

Miller and associates[74] from Stanford, California, reported on the durability of porcine xenograft valves in 87 hospital survivors, 40 receiving isolated valve replacement and 47 an extracardiac conduit. Long-term follow-up averaged 4.5 and 4.3 years, respectively. Among those who underwent valve replacement, 52% ± 13% were free of reoperation at 5 years, as were 80% ± 9% of those with extracardiac conduits. Twenty-two patients underwent reoperation because of valve or conduit failure, which was due to leaflet degeneration in 80% of the valve group compared with 13% of the conduit group. The most common cause of conduit failure was pseudointimal proliferation. A thorough discussion of the use of xenograft valves and conduits in children is presented and the authors reemphasize the need for superior biomaterials and valve substitute devices for use in the pediatric age group.

With bioprostheses (porcine aortic valve or bovine parietal pericardium)

Between June 1974 and September 1980, 46% of all valve replacements done by Geha and colleagues[75] from New Haven, Connecticut, were porcine xenografts. There were 325 adult and 31 pediatric survivors who were followed from 9–85 months (mean, 38). The authors again documented the limited durability of porcine bioprostheses in patients aged ≤20 years. Primary tissue failure occurred in 7 children between 21 and 48 months (23% of the pediatric series). In contrast, primary tissue failure occurred in only 2 of 325 adults. Thromboembolism occurred in 6 adults with bioprostheses in the mitral position, but did not occur in patients with bioprostheses isolated to the aortic or tricuspid valve positions. No thromboembolism occurred in patients with xenografts in the mitral position who were in sinus rhythm and received antiplatelet agents or in those in atrial fibrillation receiving warfarin. There is some controversy as to whether a large left atrium, AF, previous thromboembolism, or atrial thrombus at the time of surgery are incremental risk factors for thromboembolism subsequent to MVR. These authors believe this to be the case and administer warfarin sodium to all adult patients who have AF after MVR even when a xenograft is used. Their medium-term study suggests that tissue degeneration is only a rare event in adult patients followed up to 7 years. However, in a large group of patients having MVR, the threat of thromboembolism exists whether a xenograft or a prosthetic device is used. Thus, the need for anticoagulants mitigates to some extent one of the advantages of a tissue valve. Like so many other reports, the authors document early degeneration in tissue valves placed in children and suggest prostheses in such cases.

Craver and associates[76] from Atlanta, Georgia, reported on 1,093 patients who underwent cardiac valve replacement with porcine cardiac xenografts between May 1974 and July 1981. The hospital mortality for those patients with AVR was 3.7%, those with MVR, 7.8%, and those having both, 4.7%. Anticoagulation, although not routinely employed, was used in 7% of the AVR group, and 28% of the MVR group. Thromboembolism was infrequent: 8 episodes in 1,030 patients (0.78%) or 0.34% per patient-year. Fifty hospital survivors (4.8%) had valve dysfunction, 18 died, and 32 underwent reoperation. The incidence of the occurrence of valve dysfunction was more frequent in patients aged <35 years (Fig. 5-12). The authors concluded that the porcine valve functions well for 1–7 years with a low incidence of valve-related morbidity and mortality without routine anticoagulation in patients ≥35 years of age. An increased risk of valve dysfunction occurred >6 years after implantation. Most patients in this group were not anticoagulated and there was a low incidence of thromboembolism.

The data from 366 patients having MVR (250 single and 116 multiple) who received parietal pericardial xenografts between 1971 and 1982 were analyzed by Ionescu and colleagues[77] from Leeds, England. Cumulative duration of follow-up was 1,151 patient-years with a maximum duration of follow-up of 11 years. Actuarial survival at 11 years was 72 ± 14% (Fig. 5-13). Pericardial valve failure occurred in 7 patients (0.6 episodes per 100 patient-years). Actuarial freedom from valve failure at 11 years was 90 ± 9% for the entire series. Although 275 (75%) patients were in chronic AF, anticoagulants were not used in any patient beyond the first 6 postoperative weeks. The frequency of emboli was 0.6% per year. The actuarial freedom from embolism was 96 ± 1.5% at 6 and 11 years postoperatively (Fig. 5-14).

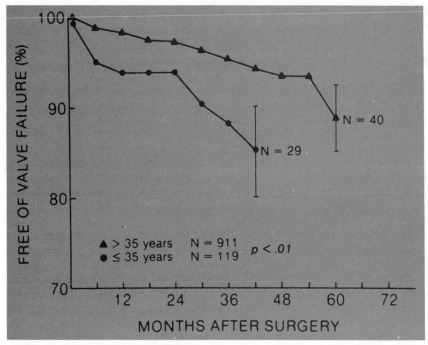

Fig. 5-12. Actuarial curves reflecting effect of patient age at implantation on freedom from xenograft failure. Reproduced with permission from Craver et al.[76]

Valve thrombosis was not encountered. When the authors addressed the issue of tissue valve durability, they compared the commercially prepared parietal pericardial xenograft with pericardial xenografts prepared in an earlier period at their own hospital and reported data from other institutions on other porcine valves. Their data suggest that the commercially prepared Ionescu-Shiley xenograft has better durability characteristics.

To determine the incidence and extent of calcification of implanted glutaraldehyde-treated porcine prosthetic heart valves, Cipriano and colleagues[78] from Stanford, California, examined 82 valves explanted from 73 patients for calcium by radiography and light microscopy. At the time of valve implantation, the patients ranged from 2–76 years and included 15 children and 58 adults. Valves explanted from children (average, 4.6 years) included 4 aortic, 5 mitral as well as 6 RV PA conduits and 1 LV abdominal aorta conduit. Valves explanted from adults (average time implanted, 3 years) included 32 aortic and 32 mitral as well as 1 triscuspid valve and 1 valve from a right ventricle-PA conduit. Calcification of explanted valves was graded from 0–4+ based on radiographs. All 16 valves in children were with grade 3+ or 4+ calcification in each of the aortic and mitral valves. In adult valves, calcification was present in 10 of 33 valves (30%) implanted for <3

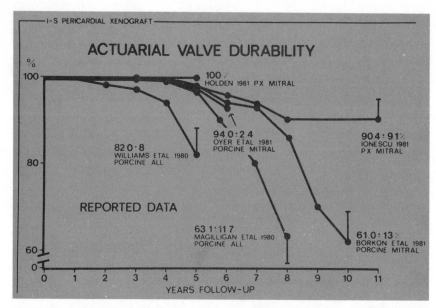

Fig. 5-13. Composite reported actuarial event-free curves for valve failure in patients with pericardial xenograft (PX) valves and in patients with porcine valves. Reproduced with permission from Ionescu et al.[77]

Fig. 5-14. Actuarial event-free curves for embolic complications in patients with mitral pericardial xenograft valve replacement. Separate curves are shown for patients with single and with multiple valve replacement. Numbers above horizontal axis denote number of patients at risk. Reproduced with permission from Ionescu et al.[77]

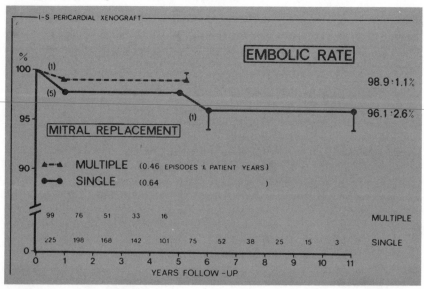

years, in 9 of 11 valves (82%) implanted for 3–5 years, and in 21 of 22 valves (96%) implanted for ≥5 years. Analysis of variance demonstrated calcification was strongly related to the duration that valves were implanted. Age at the time of valve implantation also had a strong effect on the amount of valvular calcification. Valves from children showed the most calcification and the amount did not change when valves were implanted in >30 years. Patient sex and valve position had no effect on the amount of calcification. Calcification in this study occurred at each right and left heart valve position most frequently at sites of commissural attachments.

Intrascuspal hematomas were found by Ishihara and associates[79] from Bethesda, Maryland, in 3 of 57 porcine valvular bioprostheses implanted as substitute cardiac valves in 50 patients and in 11 of 29 similar bioprostheses implanted in sheep. The 3 valves implanted in patients had been in the mitral position for 27, 65, and 107 months, respectively. Of the valves implanted in sheep, 6 had been in the mitral position and 5 in the tricuspid position from 20 minutes to 7 months. In each patient and in 4 of 11 sheep, the hematomas involved >1 cusp. These lesions were localized in the spongiosa, extended from the basal region toward the free edge of the cusp, and formed a plane of dissection which involved the spaces left in the spongiosa by the removal of proteoglycan material during preimplantation commercial processing. In one patient, the hematomas limited the mobility of the cusps and appeared to have been the cause of clinically significant prosthetic MS; in the other 2 patients and in the experimental animals, the hematomas were smaller and of uncertain hemodynamic significance. Intracuspal hematomas may become sites of eventual formation of calcific deposits. The pathogenesis of intracuspal hematomas is related to the entry of blood into the space between the sewing ring and the most basilar region of the bioprosthetic tissue. The blood penetrates into the space through the suture line between bioprosthetic tissue and sewing ring on the inflow surface of porcine valvular bioprostheses which have been mounted on AV type stents. Intracuspal hematomas were not found in bioprostheses mounted on aortic type stents, in which these sutures are more protected and more closely spaced, or in pericardial bioprostheses, which do not have a spongiosa.

With mechanical prostheses (Björk-Shiley or Starr-Edwards)

Schwarz and associates[80] from Heidelberg, West Germany, examined retrospectively 252 operated and 47 unoperated patients with isolated aortic valve disease. Aortic valve replacement was recommended to all patients based on clinical and hemodynamic findings. Preoperative hemodynamic and angiographic data were similar in operated and unoperated cohorts; 71% of patients received a Björk-Shiley prosthesis. Operative mortality was 7% for the entire surgical series. For patients with predominant AS, survival at 3 years was 87% in operated and 21% in unoperated patients. For patients with predominant AR, 5-year survival rate was 86% in operated and 87% in unoperated patients. The AVR improved long-term survival in patients with

AS who had normal or impaired LV function. In patients with AR and normal LV function, survival was not improved after AVR but those with LV dysfunction who were operated on tended to survive longer. Long-term survival of unoperated patients with AR was better than that in unoperated patients with AS. These investigators concluded that AVR improves long-term survival in patients with AS who have normal or abnormal LV function and that AVR does not change long-term survival in patients with AR, although those operated on with LV dysfunction tended to survive longer.

From London, England, Wain and associates[81] reported a follow-up of 1–14 years on 313 patients who underwent AVR with the Starr-Edwards caged-ball prostheses. Three different modifications of the Starr-Edwards device were used. Overall hospital mortality was 25%, and first year mortality, an additional 5%. Overall postoperative patient survival was 37%, with 19% free from any event at 14 years (Fig. 5-15). Thromboembolism was the most significant single event with the probability of 19% in 14 years (Table 5-1). Patients who had AVR before 1973 had a significantly greater probability of late death (31%) and of complications (47%) during the first 5 years. Those patients undergoing replacement after 1973 had a significantly greater probability of thromboembolic episodes (15%). There was no difference among the 3 series of Starr-Edwards prostheses with regard to probability of survival, nor for freedom from thromboembolism; however, patients with model 2300/2320 had a significantly higher incidence of hemolysis. Although the aortic allograft valve has been the first choice at their institution for isolated AVR, Wain and colleagues concluded that the Starr-Edwards device model 1260 was a rational and appropriate valve of second choice. This

Fig. 5-15. Actuarial curves of probabilities of patient survival and event-free survival after isolated aortic valve replacement with Starr-Edwards valves (1964–1980). Entering numbers of patients for each year are shown along abscissa. Reproduced with permission from Wain et al.[81]

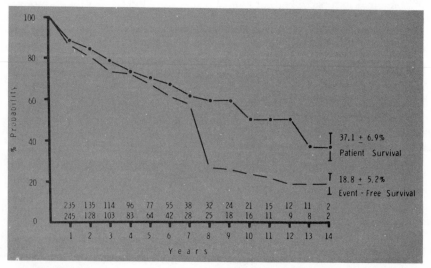

TABLE 5-1. *Causes of valve failure in patients with Starr-Edwards aortic valve replacements. Reproduced with permission from Wain et al.*[81]

CAUSE	# OF VALVES	# OF DEATHS
Thromboemboli	17	9
Paravalvular leak	16	3
Infection	12	8
Hemolysis	12	4
Cloth wear	2	0
Encapsulation	1	0
Obstruction	1	1
Total	61	25 (41%)

report is one of only a very few with >10 years follow-up after cardiac valve replacement. The hospital mortality suggests these were a high risk group of patients, but the 19% event-free survival at 4 years is a sobering reminder that this device, at least, seems only palliative. Recent studies concerning large numbers of patients having AVR have appreciably lower hospital mortality. This is undoubtedly due to a combination of factors, which include earlier operation, improved techniques of myocardial protection, and perhaps better devices. The present report may serve as a standard over the next 5–10 years for comparison of these newer prosthetic and tissue valves.

Fuster and associates[82] from Rochester, Minnesota, described late performance relative to thromboembolism for the Starr-Edwards prostheses in 302 patients followed 10–19 years after operation. Except for 7 patients with AVR and 3 patients with MVR, all patients received anticoagulants. Median follow-up was 15 years and 59% of patients in the aortic group and 56% in the mitral group were free of embolism (Fig. 5-16). After AVR, there were 4.6 embolic events per 100 patient-years, and 27% of patients with embolism had >1 embolus. After MVR, there were 4.2 embolic events per 100 patient-years, and 20% of patients with embolism had >1. The risk of embolism continued during the duration of follow-up. Modification of the silastic ball strut prosthesis apparently resulted in a decline in the yearly incidence of thromboembolism. Additionally, the adequacy of anticoagulation for patients with the mitral SE prosthesis, but not in patients with the aortic prosthesis, seemed to be related to subsequent freedom from thromboembolism. Thus, there is a continuing hazard of thromboembolism in patients having the Starr-Edwards prosthesis followed into their second decade. A lower incidence of thromboembolism in patients operated upon more recently may be related to earlier timing of operation, improved anticoagulation, including combinations with platelet-inhibitive drugs, and improved valve design.

Mintz and associates[83] from Philadelphia, Pennsylvania, evaluated the ability of auscultation, echophonocardiography and cinefluoroscopy to detect prosthetic valve malfunction in 81 patients with a Björk-Shiley prostheses in

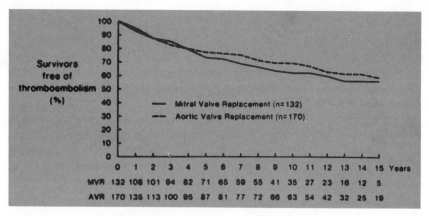

Fig. 5-16. Percentage of survivors free of thromboembolism plotted against time in years in patients with isolated Starr-Edwards mitral or aortic prostheses. The number of patients seen at each follow-up interval is given below horizontal axis. MVR = mitral valve replacement; AVR = aortic valve replacement. Reproduced with permission from Fuster et al.[82]

either the mitral or aortic positions or a Beall prosthesis in the mitral position. Thirty-two patients with abnormal prostheses in the mitral position proved by cardiac catheterization allowed the authors to determine a sensitivity of each of these variables in the detection of the prosthetic malfunction. The sensitivities were 94, 78, and 88% for auscultation, echophonocardiography, and cinefluoroscopy, respectively. In 25 patients with a normal prosthesis in the mitral position, the specificities were 96, 64, and 89%, respectively. Thus, auscultation detects almost all cases of malfunction of mechanical prosthetic valves. Echophonocardiography and cinefluoroscopy are sensitive, but false positive studies are common in the detection of prosthetic mitral valve dysfunction and both procedures are less useful in detecting malfunctioning prostheses in the aortic position.

The optimal method of myocardial protection during induced ischemic arrest has not been defined. Schaper and associates[84] from Giessen, West Germany, used electron microscopy to evaluate biopsies from hypertrophied muscle during 3 stages of operations to replace the aortic valve in 31 patients. Cold Kirsch solution was used as the cardioplegic agent. Kirsch solution contains 2.5% magnesium L-aspartate, 0.3% procaine, and 4.5% sorbitol. This was injected at a temperature of 4°C into the aortic root, and the average temperature of the subendocardium was 24°–28°C. The mean duration of cardiac arrest was 50 minutes. Biopsies were obtained: 1) before induction of cardiac arrest in the beating heart; 2) at the end of the ischemic interval; and 3) 20 minutes after the onset of reperfusion with the blood perfusate. Ultrastructural morphometry revealed cellular and especially mitochondrial swelling that occurred during the reperfusion phase, but not after the ischemia alone. The first biopsy showed numerous subcellular alterations typical of myocardial hypertrophy. The second biopsy showed disappearance of glycogen and the presence of intracellular edema. The third biopsy revealed recovery of the cell organelles; however, the quantitative morphometry indicated that there was persistence of mitochondrial swelling. There is a decrease in the volume density of contractile material, but the authors concluded that that reflected only the space-consuming process of mitochondrial swelling. This myocardial edema appeared only in the third biopsy after reperfusion. The authors suggested that these changes are indicative of incomplete myocardial protection by the method described. The Kirsch solution contains magnesium and procaine, but not potassium. Many other formulations of cardioplegic solutions are available but similar changes in cellular organelles and in cellular volume have been described after myocardial protection with the more frequently used potassium solutions. Whether these changes are a result of ischemia or reperfusion is unknown, and thus conclusions as to modification of the ischemia period or the event of reperfusion cannot be drawn.

Complications

Roberts[85] from Bethesda, Maryland, reviewed complications common to any valve site and most or all presently available mechanical or bioprosthetic valves and complications limited to a particular valve site irrespective of the type of prostheses utilized. The first group included prosthetic size disproportion, prosthetic thrombosis, paraanular prosthetic ring discontinuity (peribasilar leak), prosthetic degeneration or wear, suture overhang of prosthetic orifice, prosthetic endocarditis, entanglement of sutures beneath the occluder, incomplete removal of native valve or its calcific deposits preventing complete occluding of the prosthetic orifice by the occluder, dislodgment of portion of native cardiac valve during its excision, development of calcific deposits beneath site of attachment of a prosthetic valve ring, and hemolysis of blood elements. The complications limited to a particular valve site irrespective of type of prostheses utilized included disruption of connection between left atrium and left ventricle at mitral anulus with extravasation of blood into AV sulcus, excision of portion of LV free wall beneath papillary muscle during excision of papillary muscle with resulting rupture or aneurysmal formation, incision of LV free wall midway between mitral anulus and stump of LV papillary muscle during mitral valve excision, damage to LC coronary artery or coronary sinus during insertion of mitral prosthesis or during suture obliteration of entrance into LA appendage, contact of cage stent of mitral prosthesis with ventricular septum or LV free wall producing ventricular arrhythmia, diffuse or extensive LV fibrosis postmitral replacement, obstruction of coronary ostium by aortic prosthetic ring or stent, intimal thickening in aortic root post-AVR, and dissection of aorta post-AVR. Complications following combined mitral and AVR included contact of aortic valve poppet with stent or ring of mitral prosthesis causing AR and compression of anomalous LC coronary artery by mitral and aortic prosthetic fixation rings. This paper reviews in essence a personal experience by the author of 21 years of examining hearts of patients with ≥1 prosthetic valves.

Certain clinical and morphologic observations are described by Roberts and associates[86] from Bethesda, Maryland, in 10 patients who had MVR and lacerations of the LV free wall midway between the anulus of the mitral valve and the stumps of the LV papillary muscles. In 5 patients the lacerations led to LV free wall rupture, with immediate hemopericardium in 2 and delayed (2–4 days) rupture in the other 3. Of the other 5 patients, 3 developed aneurysm of the LV free wall, the mouth of which was located midway between mitral anulus and papillary muscle stumps, the sites of the lacerations observed in the other 7 patients (Fig. 5-17). The remaining 2 patients had midway lacerations that produced neither rupture nor aneurysmal formation. The midway LV lacerations are considered the result of LV incisions made at the time of mitral valve excision, generally in a setting

Fig. 5-17. Drawing showing a large submitral aneurysm, the mouth of which is located midway between mitral anulus and papillary muscle stumps. Wall of aneurysm is heavily calcified and was readily visible on chest radiograph during the last few years of life. Reproduced with permission from Roberts et al.[86]

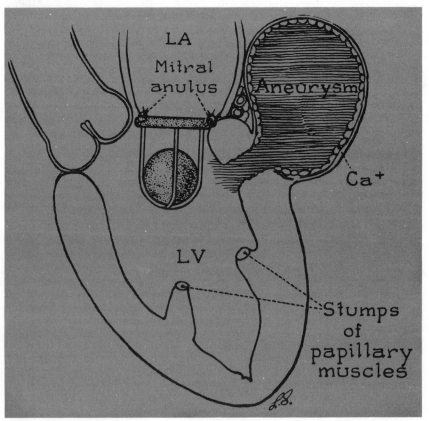

where the left-sided cardiac chambers were only mildly dilated or normal, and the tips of the blades of the scissors may have been inadequately visualized during mitral excision. This complication can be prevented by leaving the posterior mitral leaflet and its attached chordae intact or by applying exquisite care during the mitral excision procedure or both. The LV midway rupture may be the most common cause of death early after MVR and operatively induced LV laceration may lead to LV aneurysm late postoperatively.

References

1. WALLER BF, MORROW AG, MARON BJ, DEL NEGRO AA, KENT KM, McGRATH FJ, WALLACE RB, McINTOSH CL, ROBERTS WC: Etiology of clinically isolated, severe, chronic, pure mitral regurgitation: analysis of 97 patients over 30 years of age having mitral valve replacement. Am Heart J 104:276–288, Aug 1982.

2. GEHL LG, MINTZ GS, KOTLER MN, SEGAL BL: Left atrial volume overload in mitral regurgitation: a two dimensional echocardiographic study. Am J Cardiol 49:33–38, Jan 1982.

3. FUCHS RM, HEUSER RR, YIN FCP, BRINKER JA: Limitations of pulmonary wedge V waves in diagnosing mitral regurgitation. Am J Cardiol 49:849–854, March 1982.

4. PICHARD AD, KAY R, SMITH H, RENTROP P, HOLT J, GORLIN R: Large V waves in the pulmonary wedge pressure tracing in the absence of mitral regurgitation. Am J Cardiol 50:1044–1050, Nov 1982.

5. MIYATAKE K, NIMURA Y, SAKAKIBARA H, KINOSHITA N, OKAMOTO M, NAGATA S, KAWAZOE K, FUJITA T: Localization and direction of mitral regurgitant flow in mitral orifices studied with combined use of ultrasonic pulsed Doppler technique and two dimensional echocardiography. Br Heart J 48:449–458, Nov 1982.

6. GREENBERG BH, DeMOTS H, MURPHY E, RAHIMTOOLA SH: Arterial dilators in mitral regurgitation: effects on rest and exercise hemodynamics and long term clinical follow up. Circulation 65:181–187, Jan 1982.

7. KING BD, CLARK MA, BABA N, KILMAN JW, WOOLEY CF: "Myxomatous" mitral valves: collagen dissolution as the primary defect. Circulation 66:288–296, Aug 1982.

8. DEVEREUX RB, BROWN WT, LUTAS EM, KRAMER-FOX R, LARAGH JH: Association of mitral-valve prolapse with low body-weight and low blood pressure. Lancet 2:792–795, Oct 9, 1982.

9. KAGAN A: Mitral valve prolapse and blood pressure. Lancet 2:1408–1409, Dec 18, 1982.

10. HAIKAL M, ALPERT MA, WHITING RB, KELLY D: Increased left ventricular mass in idiopathic mitral valve prolapse. Chest 82:329–333, Sept 1982.

11. PASTERNAC A, TUBAU JF, PUDDU PE, KRÓL RB, DE CHAMPLAIN J: Increased plasma catecholamine levels in patients with symptomatic mitral valve prolapse. Am J Med 73:783–790, Dec 1982.

12. TEI C, SHAH PM, CHERIAN G, WONG M, ORMISTON JA: The correlates of an abnormal first heart sound in mitral-valve-prolapse syndromes. N Engl J Med 307:334–339, Aug 5, 1982.

13. ABINADER EG, SHAHAR J: Exercise testing in mitral valve prolapse before and after beta blockade. Br Heart J 48:130–133, Aug 1982.

14. RODGER JC, MORLEY P: Abnormal aortic valve echoes in mitral prolapse: echocardiographic features of floppy aortic valve. Br Heart J 47:337–343, Apr 1982.

15. NOBLE LM, DABESTANI A, CHILD JS, KRIVOKAPICH J: Mitral valve prolapse, cross-sectional and provocative M-mode echocardiography. Chest 82:158–163, Aug 1982.

16. Clemens JD, Horwitz RI, Jaffe CC, Feinstein AR, Stanton BF: A controlled evaluation of the risk of bacterial endocarditis in persons with mitral-valve prolapse. N Engl J Med 307:776–781, Sept 23, 1982.

17. Ogawa S, Hayashi J, Sasaki H, Tani M, Akaishi M, Mitamoura H, Sang M, Hoshino T, Handa S, Nakamura Y: Evaluation of combined valvular prolapse syndrome by 2 dimensional echocardiography. Circulation 65:174–180, Jan 1982.

18. Lebwohl MG, Distefano D, Prioleau PG, Uram M, Yannuzzi LA, Fleischmajer R: Pseudoxanthoma elasticum and mitral-valve prolapse. N Engl J Med 307:228–231, July 22, 1982

19. Flessas AP, Ryan TJ: Cardiovascular responses to isometric exercise in patients with mitral stenosis: comparison with normal subjects and patients with depressed ejection fraction. Arch Intern Med 142:1629–1633, Sept 1982.

20. Schweizer P, Bardos P, Krebs W, Erbel R, Minale C, Imm S, Messmer BJ, Effert S: Morphometric investigations in mitral stenosis using two dimensional echocardiography. Br Heart J 48:54–60, July 1982.

21. Chun PK, Gertz E, Davia JE, Cheitlin MD: Coronary atherosclerosis in mitral stenosis. Chest 81:36–41, Jan 1982.

22. Commerford PJ, Hastie T, Beck W: Closed mitral valvotomy: actuarial analysis of results in 654 patients over 12 years and analysis of preoperative predictors of long-term survival. Ann Thorac Surg 33:473–479, May 1982.

23. Nair CK, Sketch MH, Desai R, Mohiuddin SM, Runco V: High prevalence of symptomatic bradyarrhythmias due to atrioventricular node—fascicular and sinus node—atrial disease in patients with mitral anular calcification. Am Heart J 103:226–229, Feb 1982.

24. Mellino M, Salcedo EE, Lever HM, Vasudevan G, Kramer JR: Echographic-quantified severity of mitral anulus calcification: prognostic correlation to related hemodynamic, valvular, rhythm, and conduction abnormalities. Am Heart J 103:222–225, Feb 1982.

25. Siegel RJ, Roberts WC: Electrocardiographic observations in severe aortic valve stenosis: correlative necropsy study to clinical, hemodynamic, and ECG variables demonstrating relation of 12-lead QRS amplitude to peak systolic transaortic pressure gradient. Am Heart J 103:210–221, Feb 1982.

26. Reichek N, Devereux RB: Reliable estimation of peak left ventricular systolic pressure by M-mode echographic-determined end-diastolic relative wall thickness: identification of severe valvular aortic stenosis in adult patients. Am Heart J 103:202–209, Feb 1982.

27. Marcus ML, Doty DB, Hiratzka LF, Wright CB, Eastham CL: Decreased coronary reserve. A mechanism for angina pectoris in patients with aortic stenosis and normal coronary arteries. N Engl J Med 307:1362–1366, Nov 25, 1982.

28. Wagner S, Selzer A: Patterns of progression of aortic stenosis: a longitudinal hemodynamic study. Circulation 65:709–712, Apr 1982.

29. Presbitero P, Somerville J, Revel-Chion R, Ross D: Open aortic valvotomy for congenital aortic stenosis: late results. Br Heart J 47:26–34, Jan 1982.

30. Ciobanu M, Abbasi AS, Allen M, Hermer A, Spellberg R: Pulsed Doppler echocardiography in the diagnosis and estimation of severity of aortic insufficiency. Am J Cardiol 49:339–343, Feb 1982.

31. Firth BG, Dehmer GJ, Nicod P, Willerson JT, Hillis LD: Effect of increasing heart rate in patients with aortic regurgitation. Effect of incremental atrial pacing on scintigraphic hemodynamic and thermodilution measurements. Am J Cardiol 49:1860–1867, June 1983.

32. Schuler G, Olshausen K, Schwarz F, Mehmel H, Hofmann M, Hermann HJ, Lange D, Kübler W: Noninvasive assessment of myocardial contractility in asymptomatic patients with severe aortic regurgitation and normal left ventricular ejection fraction at rest. Am J Cardiol 50:45–52, July 1982.

33. Johnson LL, Marshall M, Johnson YE, Sciacca RR, Cannon PJ: Radionuclide angiographic

evaluation of left ventricular function by resting ejection rate during the first third of systole in patients with chronic aortic regurgitation. Am Heart J 104:92–100, July 1982.

34. Ricci DR: Afterload mismatch and preload reserve in chronic aortic regurgitation. Circulation 66:826–834, Oct 1982.

35. Waller BF, Zoltick JM, Rosen JH, Katz NM, Gomes MN, Fletcher RD, Wallace RB, Roberts WC: Severe aortic regurgitation from systemic hypertension (without aortic dissection) requiring aortic valve replacement. Analysis of four patients. Am J Cardiol 49:473–477, Feb 1982.

36. Waller BF, Kishel JC, Roberts WC: Severe aortic regurgitation from systemic hypertension. Chest 82:365–368, Sept 1982.

37. Waller BF, Roberts WC: Severe aortic regurgitation secondary to systemic hypertension (without aortic dissection). Cardiovasc Rev Reports 3:1504–1518, Oct 1982.

38. Tucker CR, Fowles R, Calin A, Popp RL: Aortitis in ankylosing spondylitis: early detection of aortic root abnormalities with two dimensional echocardiography. Am J Cardiol 49:681–686, March 1982.

39. Fioretti P, Benussi B, Scardi S, Klugmann S, Brower RW, Camerini F: Afterload reduction with nefedipine in aortic insufficiency. Am J Cardiol 49:1728–1732, May 1982.

40. Carroll JD, Gaasch WH, Naimi S, Levine HJ: Regression of myocardial hypertrophy: electrocardiographic-echocardiographic correlations after aortic valve replacement in patients with chornic aortic regurgitation. Circulation 65:980–987, May 1982.

41. Donaldson RM, Florio R, Rickards AF, Bennett JG, Yacoub MY, Ross DN, Olsen E: Irreversible morphological changes contributing to depressed cardiac function after surgery for chronic aortic regurgitation. Br Heart J 48:589–597, Dec 1982.

42. Janowitz WR, Fester A: Quantitation of left ventricular regurgitant fraction by first pass radionuclide angiocardiography. Am J Cardiol 49:85–92, Jan 1982.

43. Henze E, Schelbert HR, Wisenberg G, Ratib O, Schon H: Assessment of regurgitant fraction and right and left ventricular function at rest and during exercise: a new technique for determination of right ventricular stroke counts from gated equilibrium blood pool studies. Am Heart J 104:953–962, Nov 1982.

44. Rousseau MF, Pouleur H, Charlier AA, Brasseur LA: Assessment of left ventricular relaxation in patients with valvular regurgitation. Am J Cardiol 50:1028–1036, Nov 1982.

45. Wilson WR, Giuliani ER, Danielson GK, Geraci JE: General considerations in the diagnosis and treatment of infective endocarditis. Mayo Clin Proc 57:81–85, Feb 1982.

46. Johnson CM, Rhodes KH: Pediatric endocarditis. Mayo Clin Proc 57:86–94, Feb 1982.

47. Wilson WR, Giuliani ER, Geraci JE: Treatment of penicillin-sensitive streptococcal infective endocarditis. Mayo Clin Proc 57:95–100, Feb 1982.

48. Wilkowske CJ: Enterococcal endocarditis. Mayo Clin Proc 57:101–105, Feb 1982.

49. Thompson RL: Staphylococcal infective endocarditis. Mayo Clin Proc 57:106–114, Feb 1982.

50. Come PC, Isaacs RE, Riley MF: Diagnostic accuracy of M-mode echocardiography in active infective endocarditis and prognostic implications of ultrasound-detectable vegetations. Am Heart J 103:839–847, May 1982.

51. Pringle TH, Webb SW, Khan MM, O'Kane HOJ, Cleland J, Adgey AAJ: Clinical echocardiographic, and operative findings in active infective endocarditis. Br Heart J 48:529–537, Dec. 1982.

52. Matsumoto M, Strom J, Hirose H, Abe H: Preoperative echocardiographic diagnosis of anterior mitral valve leaflet fenestration associated with infective endocarditis. Br Heart J 48:538–540, Dec. 1982.

53. Ginzton LE, Siegel RJ, Criley JM: Natural history of tricuspid valve endocarditis: a two dimensional echocardiographic study. Am J Cardiol 49:1853–1859, June 1982.

54. Arnett EN, Roberts WC: Pathology of active infective endocarditis: a necropsy analysis of 192 patients. J Thorac Cardiovasc Surg 30:327–335, Dec 1982.

55. STRATTON RJ, WERNER JA, PEARLMAN AS, JANKO CL, KLIMAN S, JACKSON MC: Bacteremia and the heart: serial echocardiographic findings in patients with documented or suspected bacteremia. Am J Med 73:851–858, Dec 1982.

56. ROBERTS WC: No cardiac catheterization before cardiac valve replacement—a mistake. Am Heart J 103:930–933, May 1982.

57. ROBERTS WC: Reasons for cardiac catherization before cardiac-valve replacement. N Engl J Med 306:1291–1293, May 27, 1982.

58. Unsigned editorial: Echocardiography or catheterization? Lancet 1:998–1000, May 1, 1982.

59. O'ROURKE RA: Preoperative cardiac catheterization—its need in most patients with valvular heart disease. JAMA 248:745–750, Aug 13, 1982.

60. RAHIMTOOLA SH: The need for cardiac catheterization and angiography in valvular heart disease is *not* disproven. Ann Intern Med 97:433–439, Sept 1982.

61. ST. JOHN SUTTON M: Routine cardiac catheterization: a prerequisite for valve surgery? Int J Cardiol 1:320–323, 1982.

62. BOROW KM: When can cardiac surgery be performed without catheterization? J Cardiovasc Med 8:84–92, 1983.

63. VEYRAT C, KALMANSON D, FARJON M, MANIN JP, ABITBOL G: Non-invasive diagnosis and assessment of tricuspid regurgitation and stenosis using one and two-dimensional echopulsed Doppler. Br Heart J 47:596–605, June 1982.

64. CHA SD, DESAI RS, GOOCH AS, MARANHAO V, GOLDBERG H: Diagnosis of severe tricuspid regurgitation. Chest 82:726–731, Dec 1982.

65. MIYATAKE K, OKAMOTO M, KINOSHITA N, MATSUHISA M, NAGATA S, BEPPU S, PARK Y-D, SAKAKIBARA H, NIMURA Y: Pulmonary regurgitation studied with the ultra-sonic pulsed Doppler technique. Circulation 65:969–975, May 1982.

66. SANYAL SK, BERRY AM, DUGGAL S, HOOJA V, GHOSH S: Sequelae of the initial attack of acute rheumatic fever in children from North India. A prospective 5 year follow up study. Circulation 65:375–379, Feb 1982.

67. ROBERTS WC, HONIG HS: The spectrum of cardiovascular disease in the Marfan syndrome: A clinico-morphologic study of 18 necropsy patients and comparison to 151 previously reported necropsy patients. Am Heart J 104:115–135, July 1982.

68. CALLAHAN JA, WROBLEWSKI EM, REEDER GS, EDWARDS WD, SEWARD JB, TAJIK AJ: Echocardiographic features of carcinoid heart disease. Am J Cardiol 50:762–768, Oct. 1982.

69. GARDNER TJ, ROLAND JMA, NEILL CA, DONAHOO JS: Valve replacement in children: a fifteen-year perspective. J Thorac Cardiovasc Surg 83:178–185, Feb 1982.

70. GALIOTO FM JR, MIDGLEY FM, KAPUR S, PERRY LW, WATSON DC, SHAPIRO SR, RUCKMAN RN, SCOTT LP III: Early failures of Ionescu-Shiley bioprosthesis after mitral valve replacement in children. J Thorac Cardiovasc Surg 83:306–310, Feb 1982.

71. HUMAN DG, JOFFE HS, FRASER CB, BARNARD CN: Mitral valve replacement in children. J Thorac Cardiovasc Surg 83:873–877, June 1982.

72. WEINSTEIN GS, MAVROUDIS C, EBERT PA: Preliminary experience with aspirin for anticoagulation in children with prosthetic cardiac valves. Ann Thorac Surg 33:549–553, June 1982.

73. BENMIMOUN EG, FRIEDLI B, RUTISHAUSER W, FAIDUTTI B: Mitral valve replacement in children: comparative study of pre- and post-operative haemodynamics and left ventricular function. Br Heart J 48:117–124, Aug 1982.

74. MILLER DC, STINSON EB, OYER PE, BILLINGHAM ME, PITLICK PT, REITZ BA, JAMIESON SW, BAUMGARTNER WA, SHUMWAY NE: The durability of porcine xenograft valves and conduits in children. Circulation 66 (Suppl I):172–185, Aug 1982.

75. GEHA AS, HAMMOND GL, LAKS H, STANSEL HC JR, GLENN WWL: Factors affecting performance and thromboembolism after porcine xenograph cardiac valve replacement. J Thorac Cardiovasc Surg 83:377–384, March 1982.

76. CRAVER JM, JONES EL, MCKEOWN P, BONE DK, HATCHER CR JR, KANDRACH M: Porcine cardiac

xenograft valves: analysis of survival, valve failure, and explantation. Ann Thorac Surg 34:16–21, July 1982.

77. IONESCU MI, SMITH DR, HASAN SS, CHIDAMBARAM M, TANDON AP: Clinical durability of the pericardial xenograft valve: ten years' experience with mitral replacement. Ann Thorac Surg 34:265–277, Sept 1982.

78. CIPRIANO PR, BILLINGHAM ME, OYER PE, KUTSCHE LM, STINSON ED: Calcification of porcine prosthetic heart valves: a radiographic and light microscopic study. Circulation 66:1100–1104, Nov 1982.

79. ISHIHARA T, FERRANS VJ, BARNHART GR, JONES M, McINTOSH CL, ROBERTS WC: Intracuspal hematomas in implanted porcine valvular bioprostheses. Clinical and experimental studies. J Thorac Cardiovasc Surg 83:399–407, March 1982.

80. SCHWARZ F, BAUMANN P, MANTHEY J, HOFFMANN M, SCHULER G, MEHMEL HC, SCHMITZ W, KUBLER W: Effect of aortic valve replacement on survival. Circulation 66:1105–1109, Nov 1982.

81. WAIN WH, DRURY PJ, ROSS DN: Aortic valve replacement with Starr-Edwards valves over 14 years. Ann Thorac Surg 33:562–569, June 1982.

82. FUSTER V, PUMPHREY CW, McGOON MD, CHESEBRO JH, PLUTH JR, McGOON DC: Systemic thromboembolism in mitral and aortic Starr-Edwards prostheses: a 10–19 year follow-up. Circulation CV Surgery 1981 66:I-157–161, Aug 1982.

83. MINTZ GS, CARLSON EB, KOTLER MN: Comparison of noninvasive techniques in evaluation of the nontissue cardiac valve prosthesis. Am J Cardiol 49:39–44, Jan 1982.

84. SCHAPER J, SCHWARZ F, KITTSTEIN H, STAMMLER G, WINKLER B, SCHELD H, HEHRLEIN F: The effects of global ischemia and reperfusion on human myocardium: quantitative evaluation by electron microscopic morphometry. Ann Thorac Surg 33:116–122, Feb 1982.

85. ROBERTS WC: Complications of cardiac valve replacement: characteristic abnormalities of prostheses pertaining to any or specific site. Am Heart J 103:113–122, Jan 1982.

86. ROBERTS WC, ISNER JM, VIRMANI R: Left ventricular incision midway between the mitral anulus and the stumps of the papillary muscles during mitral valve excision with and without rupture or aneurysmal formation: analysis of 10 necropsy patients. Am Heart J 104:1278–1287, Dec 1982.

6

Myocardial Heart Disease

IDIOPATHIC DILATED CARDIOMYOPATHY

Cardiac work and substrate extraction

Thompson and associates[1] from London, England, measured LV pressure, cardiac output, coronary sinus blood flow, and myocardial substrate extraction in 10 patients with idiopathic dilated cardiomyopathy (IDC), and in 9 control patients who apparently had normal hearts. Coronary sinus blood flow and myocardial oxygen consumption were greater in the patients with IDC but were similar in the 2 groups when normalized for ventricular mass. Efficiency, estimated from the oxygen cost of external work, was grossly reduced in the IDC group. No differences in substrate extraction were demonstrated between the 2 groups. Myocardial lactate production was not observed in any patient with IDC. Free fatty acid and glycerol release were observed in several control subjects but in no patient with IDC. Measurements were repeated during pacing in 5 IDC patients and in each control. The latter showed a normal response to pacing, whereas in the IDC group, 4 sustained increases in end-diastolic LV pressure, 2 had large reductions in both cardiac output and coronary flow, and only 1 increased coronary flow during pacing. Despite the failure of coronary flow to increase, lactate extraction remained high. These results show that anaerobic carbohydrate metabolism is not an important energy source for inpatients with IDC and suggest that ischemia does not contribute to poor LV function. No gross abnormality of oxidative metabolism was identified, implying that low efficiency lay in the poor contractile performance of the IDC heart.

Reduced suppressor cell activity

The natural history and pathogenesis of idiopathic dilated cardiomyopathy (IDC) and myocarditis are unclear and a relation between the pathogenesis of these 2 diseases has not been resolved. Eckstein and colleagues[2] from Munich, West Germany, studied suppressor cell activity in 10 patients who had IDC, 13 who had myocarditis, and 98 healthy controls. Myocardial biopsy, coronary arteriography, and LV angiography were used to define and differentiate IDC and myocarditis. The suppressor component of the immune response was assessed by examining the in vitro responses of peripheral blood lymphoid cells under standard conditions. The lymphoid cells were incubated with concanavalin A to stimulate suppressor activity. Induced activity was measured by the ability of peripheral blood lymphocytes to inhibit ^{3}H-thymidine uptake of nonstimulated autologous cells when subsequently presented with allogenic or mitogenic stimuli. The IDC and the myocarditis groups were homogeneous and generally demonstrated low suppression values. Thus, these investigators speculated that the reduced suppressor cell activity may well be the common important predisposing condition for both myocarditis and IDC to either autoimmune diseases or viral infections.

Deficient natural killer cell activity

The importance of immune dysfunction in idiopathic dilated cardiomyopathy (IDC) has been postulated but remains to be demonstrated. Immunoregulatory dysfunction in IDC was suggested by the finding of defective in vitro suppressor activity in some patients. Natural killer (NK) cells are a subpopulation of circulating leukocytes whose part in defense against disease is being defined. The NK cell activity is present in normal individuals and associated with the large granular lymphocytes. Evidence is accumulating that these cells are important in immune surveillance, that they mediate natural resistance against tumors in vivo, certain virus and other microbial diseases, and allogeneic bone marrow transplants. Anderson and associates[3] from Salt Lake City, Utah, wondered whether abnormal NK cell responses might be associated with IDC. Augmented NK activity might mediate cytotoxicity to viral-infected or altered myocardial cells. Or a deficiency in NK activity might allow establishment and progression of myocardial lesions after initial injury by virus or other etiologic agents. Anderson and colleagues therefore compared NK activity in patients with IDC with that in normal blood donors and in patients with CHF from other causes. To evaluate NK activity in the patients with IDC, circulating peripheral blood mononuclear cells were obtained from 16 patients, from 54 normal blood donors, and from 14 patients with CHF due to other causes, primarily CAD. The NK activity was assessed as a lymphocyte/target cell ratio causing 50% killing (L/T_{50}). The L/T_{50} in normal blood donors was 17 ± 11. A normal L/T_{50} distribution also was noted in CHF controls (L/T_{50} = 20 ± 10) and 8 of 16 IDC patients (L/T_{50} = 18 ± 10). The NK activity was deficient (L/$T_{50} \geqslant 50$) in 8 of 16 patients with IDC but in only 2 of 54 normal persons ($p < 0.001$) and 0 of 14 CHF controls ($p < 0.01$). Of the several clinical and laboratory variables examined, only the frequency of the HLA-A3 tissue type was associated with NM deficiency. Thus, NK deficiency is an independent disease marker in about 50% of patients with IDC and should be evaluated for a possible role in its pathogenesis.

Cardiac neurons

Amorim and Olsen[4] from London, England, counted in a strip of right atrial wall adjacent to superior vena cava the number of ganglion cells in 7 hearts from patients with idiopathic dilated cardiomyopathy (IDC), in 7 hearts from normal subjects, and in 3 hearts of patients with fatal Chagas's heart disease. The number of neurons was significantly reduced in the patients with IDC compared with normal subjects, but not as reduced as in the patients with chronic Chagas's heart disease. Neither the mechanism nor the cause of the depopulation of neurons in the patients with IDC was determined.

HYPERTROPHIC CARDIOMYOPATHY

Overview

Goodwin[5] from London, England, reviewed developments in cardiomyopathies during the past 3 decades. He supported the hypothesis that HC results from abnormal catecholamine function in the developing heart. He challenged the concept of "obstruction" in HC on the basis that true obstruction to LV outflow is not present and that the pressure gradients often recorded are the result of elimination of the LV cavity as a result of powerful contraction of extensively hypertrophied muscle. He stressed the importance of impaired diastolic LV function with general and regional abnormalities of relaxation of a very complex nature. He reviewed the natural history of HC and its high incidence of sudden death in 250 patients studied in the past 20 years. His studies and others of antiarrhythmic therapy disclosed that, although neither beta adrenergic blocking agents nor calcium channel blocking agents control arrhythmias studied by ambulatory monitoring, amiodarone is highly effective. It remains to be seen how or whether amiodarone will reduce the frequency of sudden death among patients with HC. He also reviewed the mechanism of sudden death in the light of causes other than arrhythmias, such as impairment of LV filling and reduction in LV volume. He suggested a tentative scheme of therapy for HC patients based on control of symptoms with beta adrenergic blocking agents and management of arrhythmias with amiodarone.

In infants

Maron and associates[6] from Bethesda, Maryland, Rochester, Minnesota, Nashville, Tennessee, Salt Lake City, Utah, and Gainesville, Florida, described clinical and morphologic features of HC in 20 patients recognized as having this condition in the first year of life. Of the 20 infants, 14 were initially suspected of having heart disease solely because of a precordial murmur. Others had signs of marked CHF in the presence of nondilated ventricular cavities and normal or increased LV contractility and substantial cardiac enlargement on chest x ray. Other findings were considerably different from those usually present in older children and adults with HC (e.g., RV hypertrophy on ECG and cyanosis). Thus, in 14 infants, the initial clinical diagnosis was congenital cardiac malformation rather than HC. Of the 14 infants, 12 underwent left-sided cardiac catheterization and had substantial obstruction to LV outflow (peak systolic pressure gradient ⩾35 mmHg). Unlike older patients with HC, however, infants with HC commonly had marked obstruction to RV outflow (35–106 mmHg gradients) (9 patients); in 6 infants, the magnitude of obstruction to RV outflow was at least as great as that to LV outflow.

Of the 16 patients who had echo or necropsy examination, the ventricular septum was thicker than the LV free wall in all. Ventricular septal thickening was substantial in patients studied both before and after 6 months of age (mean, 16 mm) indicating that in patients with HC, marked LV hypertrophy may be present early in life and is probably present from the time of birth. The clinical course in these patients was variable but the onset of marked CHF in the first year of life appeared to be an unfavorable prognostic sign (Fig. 6-1). Of the 11 infants with CHF, 9 died within the first year of life. In infants with HC, unlike older children and adults with this condition, sudden death was less common (2 patients) than death due to progressive CHF (5 patients).

Natural history

McKenna and associates[7] from London, England, assessed the natural history of ECG LV hypertrophy in relation to clinical factors, treatment with propranolol, and prognosis in 100 patients with HC who were followed 5–20 years. Seventy-one patients received propranolol 120–800 mg/day (average, 240). At diagnosis, the voltage measurement from $SV_1 + RV_5$ was 37 mm, the R wave in aVL was 12 mm, and the mean frontal plane voltage was 15 mm. After 5 years, these values were increased to 43, 14 and 17 mm, respectively. Neither a LV outflow tract gradient nor propranolol treatment influenced these voltage changes. Twenty patients had an increase of >10 mm in $SV_1 + RV_5$ which was associated with exertional chest pain and death.

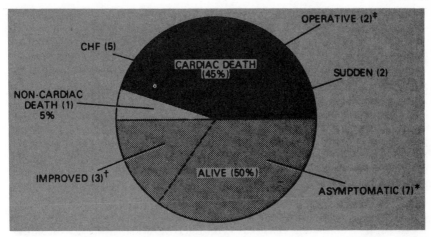

Fig. 6-1. Clinical course of 20 infants with HC. *Includes 1 patient who underwent combined septal myotomy-myectomy and resection of RV outflow tract muscle. †Includes 1 patient who underwent septal myotomy-myectomy. ‡Includes 2 patients who underwent resection of RV outflow tract muscle. Reproduced with permission from Maron et al.[6]

Four patients had a decrease of >10 mm in SV_1 + RV_5. Two of them received high dose propranolol, 1,720 mg a day for 12 years, and another received 800 mg/day for 12 years. No other patient received more than 480 mg of propranolol daily. Thus, in HC there is ECG evidence of progressive hypertrophy that is associated with a poor prognosis and, as shown in this study, is not influenced by treatment with propranolol in moderate dosage. Thus, regression of hypertrophy is rare and may be related to long-term treatment with high dose propranolol.

With ventricular septal hypertrophy localized to the apical region

Maron and associates[8] from Bethesda, Maryland, described clinical and morphologic features in a unique subgroup of 7 patients with HC. Five either died suddenly or are alive but severely symptomatic. In each patient, ventricular septal hypertrophy was demonstrated by 2-D echo or at necropsy to be virtually confined to its apical one-half. Conventional M-mode echo was unreliable in identifying this site of hypertrophy because it was often inaccessible to the path of the M-mode beam. Apical distribution of septal hypertrophy does not constitute a separate disease entity, but rather appears to be part of the morphologic spectrum of HC as judged from 2 findings; 1) genetic transmission of HC in relatives of each study patient, and 2) marked disorganization of cardiac muscle cells in the LV wall of the 2 patients studied at necropsy. Apical distribution of septal hypertrophy in these patients was associated with relatively mild T-wave inversion on ECG and characteristic angiographic LV appearance with mid-ventricular constriction and a small, often poorly contractile apical segment. These ECG and angiographic features differ from those previously described in Japanese patients with "apical HC" in whom "giant" T-wave inversion and a "spade-like" LV appearance were characteristic.

Diastolic function

Beta adrenergic blocking drugs in HC provide symptomatic relief, but their effect on long-term prognosis is uncertain. Alvares and Goodwin[9] from London, England, studied 30 patients noninvasively by simultaneously recordings of echo, apexcardiogram, phonocardiogram, and ECG to assess diastolic abnormalities on and off oral beta adrenergic blocking drugs. While on treatment, the patients had a mean dosage of propranolol of 200 mg/day. The treatment was stopped for 1 week and then noninvasive assessment was repeated. The following diastolic time intervals were studied: isovolumic relaxation period (A_2-mitral valve opening), rapid relaxation period (A_2-O point of the apexcardiogram), and the period from mitral valve opening to the O point of the apexcardiogram (Mo-O) when most of the filling of the LV occurs (Fig. 6-2). The prolongation of the rapid relaxation period reflects a reduced rate of fall of the LV pressure when the pressure differential does not change between A_2 and the O point of the apexcardiogram, and in this study this period was prolonged in 19, shortened in 8, and remained the same in 3 patients after beta blockade. The Mo-O point was prolonged in 22, shortened in 7, and unchanged in 1 patient after beta adrenergic blocking drugs. All these results were independent of heart rate. Thus, the response of diastolic time intervals to beta blocking drugs in HC was variable but there was a significant number of patients in whom the time available for filling of the LF was prolonged, suggesting better filling possibly because of improved distensibility of the LV after beta adrenergic blocking drugs.

Sudden death

Maron and associates[10] from Bethesda, Maryland, analyzed the clinical profile of 78 patients with HC who died suddenly or had cardiac arrest and survived. At the time of the cardiac event, 71% were <30 years old, 54% had no functional limitations, and 61% were performing sedentary or minimal physical activity. Of the 78 patients, 19 (24%) were taking propranolol in apparently adequate doses. No clinical or morphologic variable was reliable in identifying patients at risk for sudden death. Of 62 patients who died suddenly, 48 (77%) had a markedly increased ventricular septal thickness of ≥20 mm. Septal thickness, however, was similar in patients who died suddenly (25 mm) and in age- and sex-matched control patients with HC who survived (24 mm). An abnormal ECG was present as often in patients who died suddenly as in control patients who survived. Thus, in these patients with HC and cardiac arrest no characteristic cardiac symptom or hemodynamic variable was identified and propranolol did not appear to provide absolute protection against sudden death.

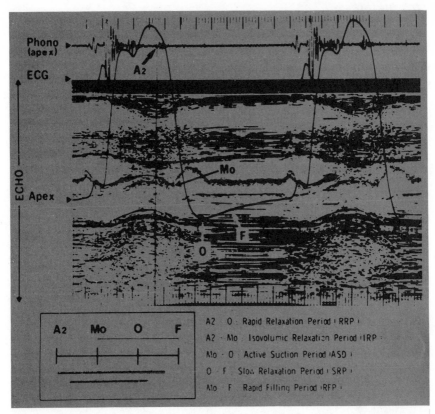

Fig. 6-2. Simultaneous recording of phonocardiogram (phono), electrocardiogram (ECG), apexcardiogram (apex), and echocardiogram (echo) in a patient with HC. Diagram shows diastolic time intervals measured. A_2, aortic component of second heart sound; Mo, mitral valve opening. O and F points of the apexcardiogram. Reproduced with permission from Alvares et al.[9]

Familial in Iceland

Bjarnason and associates[11] from Reykjavik, Iceland, used an abnormally thick ventricular septum (≥1.3 cm) as an echo marker to find the inheritance pattern of HC among relatives of 8 patients who had HC at necropsy. Fifty-eight family members were examined and 18 (41%) of the 44 first degree relatives had HC. The overall inheritance pattern was consistent with an autosomal dominant genetic disorder. The diagnosis of HC was difficult in that only 13% of the 18 patients had serious symptoms and only 30% had precordial murmurs. The ECG was abnormal in 87% of those who had an abnormally thick ventricular septum. Symmetric septal hypertrophy occurred in 30% of their patients with HC and only 17% had clinical evidence of LV outflow obstruction.

HLA linkage

Human leukocyte antigen (HLA) tissue-typing studies on patients with genetically transmitted HC have demonstrated an HLA linkage in white and black patient groups and an HLA-DR locus association in a Japanese population group. To confirm whether a specific HLA antigen or antigens might serve as a marker for HC, Gardin and associates[12] from Chicago, Illinois, and Bethesda, Maryland, performed tissue-typing studies on 50 unrelated, normotensive North American whites with HC. Patients were subdivided into 3 hemodynamic subgroups: obstructive (35 patients), provocative gradients (10 patients), and nonobstructive (5 patients). Although there was an increased frequency of the B12 and AW32 HLA antigens in the total group, after correction of p values for the number of antigens studied, the associations were not statistically significant. Analysis of the HLA antigen frequencies in the 3 hemodynamic subgroups yielded no statistically significant HLA-A, B, or C locus associations, and no unusual deviation in linkage disequilibrium between A and B locus antigens was observed. These authors concluded that, although on the sixth chromosome there may be a susceptibility gene for HC, which segregates with a specific haplotype in a given family, no specific HLA-A, B, or C locus antigen was found useful as a marker. HLA-Dr locus antigen typing might prove useful in this population.

Catenoidal shape of the ventricular septum

Morphologic observations have indicated that the ventricular septum in patients with HC has a catenoid shape (1 that is concave to the left in the transverse plane and convex to the left in the sagittal plane). Silverman and associates[13] from Baltimore, Maryland, studied 6 patients to determine if such a septal configuration is present in living adults. Utilizing phased array 2-D echo, LV wall segment curvature, thickness, and motion were compared with values in 6 patients with LV hypertrophy secondary to systemic hypertension and to 6 normal subjects. Patients with HC had a septum that had a catenoidal configuration and showed significantly less septal curvature in a curvature thickness index during the cardiac cycle that occurred in control groups ($p < 0.05$). The LV free wall had significantly greater change of curvature thickness index over the cardiac cycle in patients with HC ($p < 0.05$). The LV free wall appeared to account for systolic anterior motion of the anterior mitral leaflet. The catenoid shape of the septum in HC may account for the asymmetric hypertrophy and septal immobility.

Postextrasystolic changes in systolic time intervals

To determine if postextrasystolic changes in systolic time intervals can be used to estimate the severity of resting or provocative LV outflow pressure gradient in HC, Stefadouros and associates[14] from Augusta, Georgia, studied cardiac catheterization records of 42 patients with HC looking for VPC preceded by control sinus beats and followed by postpremature sinus beats. There were 75 such instances in 25 patients. In comparison to the control beat, the preejection period (PEP) in the postpremature beat was shorter by $\Delta PEP = -20 \pm 11$ ms in 73 of 75 instances, and remained unchanged in 2. The ejection time (ET) in the postpremature beat was invariably longer by $\Delta ET = 37 \pm 20$ ms (range, 10–85 ms) and the PEP/ET ratio lower than control by $\Delta(PEP/ET) = -0.10 \pm 0.05$ (range, -0.10 to -0.25). Total electromechanical systole (EMS) in the postpremature beat was shorter (11 of 75), the same (10 of 75), or longer (53 of 75) than in the control beat, the overall change being $\Delta EMS = 18 \pm 22$ ms. Both ΔPEP and $\Delta(PEP/ET)$ correlated poorly with the systolic peak (LV-aortic pressure gradient in either the control beat (Gc) or the postpremature beat (Gx), and also with the change in gradient (ΔG) from the control to the postpremature beat. In contrast, significant linear correlations were found between ΔEMS and either Gc, Gx, or ΔG, and also between ΔET and either Gc, Gx, or ΔG. Since internal and external measurements of ET are known to be almost identical, the regression equation ($\Delta G = 1.65 \ \Delta ET - 9$) relating ΔET and ΔG should be useful for the noninvasive assessment of the magnitude of provocative LV outflow pressure gradient in patients with HC with spontaneous or externally induced VPC.

ECG in echo-unaffected relatives

Loperfido and asssociates[15] from Rome, Italy, analyzed the ECG and vectorcardiographic features of first degree relatives of patients with documented familiar HC. Nine affected members and 29 relatives were examined in 4 families. The subjects were considered to be affected when the ventricular septal to LV free wall thickness ratio >1.3 by M-mode echo. Four relatives have asymmetric septal hypertrophy (ASH). Among 25 relatives without ASH, 2 >20 years and 10 <20 years of age had increased voltage of QRS anterior forces on the orthogonal ECG. The vectorcardiographic data of the relatives <20 years of age without evidence of ASH (18 subjects) were compared with those of 38 normal control subjects of comparable age range. The young relatives without ASH had significantly greater Q amplitude and Q/R ratio than the normal controls. In contrast, the echo data were not significantly different. The authors suggest that the ECG finding of abnormal anterior forces in ≥1 first degree relatives of subjects with documented HC may constitute a valuable aid in ascertaining the genetic transmission of the disease and in recognizing affected members without echo evidence in HC.

Cardiac arrhythmias

Bjarnason and associates[16] from Reykjavik, Iceland, assessed the prevalence of cardiac arrhythmias in 22 relatives of patients who had come to necropsy with HC. Fifty close relatives of 8 deceased patients were examined: the ventricular septal thickness in 22 relatives by echo was ≥1.3 cm and in 28 it was less than that. A comparison of the prevalence and types of cardiac arrhythmias, as shown by 24-hour ambulatory ECG monitoring, was made between the 2 groups and also a third apparently healthy group of 40 persons. The patients with HC had a significant increase in supraventricular extrasystoles per 24 hours, supraventricular arrhythmias, high grade ventricular arrhythmia, and the number of patients with >10 VPC every 24 hours when compared with the other groups. There was no significant difference between normal relatives and controls. The prevalence and types of arrhythmia in these patients were similar to those found by other investigators using different diagnostic criteria. These results support the contention that patients with HC and all close relatives of necropsy-proved cases of HC should be examined by echo and subsequently by ambulatory ECG monitoring if the ventricular septum is ≥1.3 cm in thickness.

Nifedipine effect on diastolic properties

Lorell and associates[17] from Boston, Massachusetts, studied the effect of nifedipine on LV isovolumic relaxation and diastolic filling properties and systemic and LV hemodynamics in 15 patients with HC. After administration of 10 mg nifedipine sublingually, the prolonged LV isovolumic time was assessed by echo and decreased from 112–23 ms and the LV pressure decay as measured by time constant improved from 63–49 ms. The LV filling dynamics are also improved as assessed by a return toward normal in the depressed peak rate of LV diastolic filling (dimension change 72–101 mm/s) and peak rate of posterior wall thinning (47–68 mm/s). These changes were accompanied by hemodynamic evidence of improved diastolic function shown as a decrease in LV end-diastolic pressure and a downward shift in the LV diastolic pressure dimension relation suggesting improved LV distensibility. After nifedipine, there was a slight increase in heart rate and a decrease in systemic arterial BP with no depression of the LV percent fractional shortening or cardiac index. Abnormal LV relaxation and diastolic filling rates in HC are dynamic and favorably modified by nifedipine and this effect is not related to a depression of LV systolic function.

Nifedipine and propranolol

Landmark and associates[18] from Olso, Norway, studied the hemodynamic effects of nifedipine alone compared with the combined administration of both nifedipine and propranolol in 12 patients with HC. The combined administration of nifedipine and propranolol appeared to be superior to that of nifedipine alone. The spontaneous heart rate was reduced in most cases after nifedipine plus propranolol, and at atrial pacing the following results were obtained: LV peak systolic pressure decreased from 200 ± 39–157 ± 30 mmHg; a positive correlation was found between the predrug LV end-diastolic pressure and the magnitude of reduction in LV end-diastolic pressure; systolic BP was reduced from 125 ± 31–111 ± 27 mmHg, and total peripheral resistance was reduced from 1,403 ± 307–1,160 ± 209 dynes^{-1}/cm^{-5}. The combined administration reduced the resting LV outflow gradient from 76 ± 19–45 ± 26 mmHg, while cardiac index was left unchanged. The effects on mean pulmonary arteriolar resistance and mean pulmonary arteriolar and mean pulmonary capillary venous pressure were in most cases slight and insignificant. The results indicate an improved hemodynamic condition in patients with HC after the combined administration of nifedipine and propranolol.

Effect of disopyramide in HC

The LV outflow pressure gradient in patients with HC may be affected by changes in myocardial contractility, systemic vascular resistance, and ventricular volume. Propranolol has little effect on the pressure gradient at rest, but it may diminish the increment that occurs with exercise. Verapamil has a greater effect than propranolol in reducing the gradient at rest, but it has less effect on patients with large such gradients. Recent studies have shown that the antiarrhythmic drug disopyramide has potent negative inotropic properties and therefore should reduce the pressure gradient in HC. Pollick[19] from Toronto, Canada, described the effect of disopyramide in 5 patients with HC. The drug was administered intravenously to 4 patients during cardiac catheterization, and in each the basal pressure gradient was abolished (Fig. 6-3). Oral disopyramide was subsequently given in 3 further studies during noninvasive evaluation. This treatment resulted in reductions of the systolic anterior motion of the anterior mitral leaflet, of the precordial murmur, and of the LV ejection time, indicating a decrease in the resting pressure gradient. Subsequent maintenance therapy with oral disopyramide in 3 patients resulted in improved exercise tolerance and increased functional capacity.

Aortic regurgitation after operative treatment

Wiener and associates[20] from Rochester, New York, described a 51-year-old man who developed AR that was first noted 12 years after partial septotomy and septectomy for HC. At the time of septotomy-septectomy the aortic valve was normal and the patient never had infective endocarditis. This case report is important because it suggests that AR may be a fairly frequent problem late after relief of the LV outflow pressure gradient operatively in HC. The simple manipulation, that is, touching the aortic valve cusps by the operator's finger, causes deendothelization of the surfaces of the aortic valve cusps, and these surfaces heal apparently initially by platelet deposits and later fibrous tissue proliferation. The 3 aortic valve cusps in the patient were excised and the aortic valve replaced with a prosthesis. The excised aortic valve cusps were thickened by fibrous tissue and were smaller than normal. Because many patients with HC who undergo septotomy-septectomy are relatively young, AR potentially can be a problem years later.

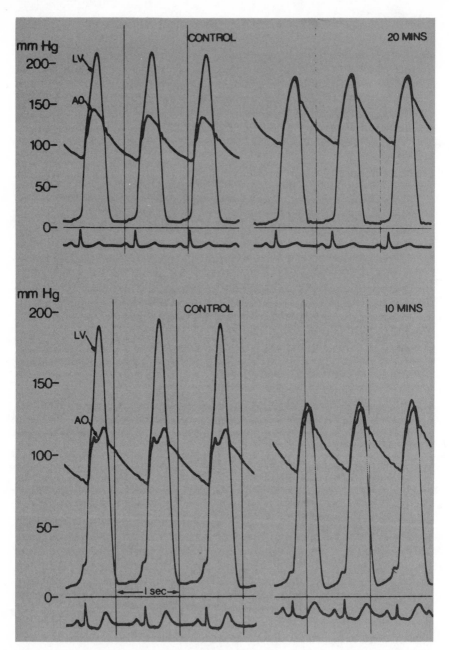

Fig. 6-3. Simultaneous LV and aortic pressures before (control) and 20 min after disopyramide (100 mg i.v.) in patient 1 (upper panel) and before and 10 min after disopyramide in patient 2 (lower panel). Pressure gradient fell from 73 mmHg to 0 in patient 1 and from 70 mmHg to 3 mmHg in patient 2. Reproduced with permission from Pollick.[19]

CARDIAC AMYLOIDOSIS

Voltage/mass relation

Carroll and associates[21] from Boston, Massachusetts, evaluated 14 patients with biopsy-proved systemic amyloidosis utilizing noninvasive cardiac testing to assess the presence and severity of cardiac amyloidosis. There was a definite tendency for ECG voltage to be low and for echo muscle cross-sectional area to be increased (11 ± 3 cm^2/m^2; normal range, 6–10). When both the ECG and echo were combined, a distinctive pattern emerged for these patients in contrast to patients with pericardial disease (n, 8) or aortic valve disease (n, 24). There was an inverse correlation between voltage and muscle cross-sectional area ($r = -0.79$) in patients with amyloidosis; moreover, marked derangement of the voltage/cross-sectional area relation was associated with clinical symptoms and mortality. Patients with amyloidosis and cardiac symptoms had abnormal LV chamber radius to wall thickness ratios consistent with infiltration of the myocardium by amyloidosis.

Positive myocardial technetium-99m pyrophosphate scintigraphy

Wizenberg and colleagues[22] from Detroit, Michigan, studied 10 consecutive patients with tissue-proved amyloidosis, 7 of whom presented with CHF, and were found to exhibit intense diffuse uptake of technetium-99m pyrophosphate on cardiac radionuclide imaging. The patients exhibited echo and systolic time interval abnormalities suggestive of combined restrictive and dilated cardiomyopathic changes. On M-mode echo, there was symmetrically increased thickness of the ventricular septum and LV posterior wall in diastole, decreased fractional shortening of the LV minor axis diameter in systole, and decreased percent thickening of the septum and LV free wall in systole. Three patients had enlarged LV end-diastolic diameter. All 10 patients had abnormally increased preejection period related to LV ejection time. When combined with noninvasive tests of LV performance, positive myocardial pyrophosphate scanning provides a new and useful adjunt in the diagnosis of cardiac amyloidosis.

Left ventricular dysfunction determined by computerized M-mode echo

St. John Sutton and colleagues[23] from Rochester, Minnesota, and Philadelphia, Pennsylvania, assessed LV function in cardiac amyloid using computer-assisted analysis of M-mode echo from 20 patients with biopsy proved amyloid and compared them with similar data from 20 normal subjects. Patients with cardiac amyloid had a consistent characteristic set of quantitative echo findings: 1) LV cavity size was normal or small, 2) peak rate of diastolic cavity filling was decreased, 3) isovolumic relaxation was prolonged, 4) fractional shortening and peak circumferential rate were decreased, and 5) peak rates of both systolic thickening and diastolic thinning of the septum and posterior LV wall were decreased. The LV function in patients with cardiac amyloid was compared with that in patients with AS and normal coronary arteries, who were used as models of similar wall thickness and cavity size. There was significantly greater impairment of regional and global LV function in amyloid, that is, more than could be accounted for by increased wall thickness alone, indicating that the further abnormalities of LV function were caused by an intramyocardial restriction secondary to amyloid deposition per se. The LV function also was compared in amyloid and in patients with nonobstructive HC, since these 2 groups of patients may be confused both clinically and by ECG. The technique used differentiated between these 2 disorders in terms of cavity and regional LV dynamics when patients were considered as a group, but with less certainty when patients were considered individually, due to overlap between the 2 groups. The severity and consistency of the echo abnormalities in cardiac amyloid are of value in establishing the diagnosis, which can be confirmed directly by tissue biopsy.

ENDOMYOCARDIAL FIBROSIS WITH AND WITHOUT EOSINOPHILIA

Idiopathic hypereosinophilic syndrome

Fauci and associates[24] from Bethesda, Maryland, reviewed their extensive experience with patients with the idiopathic hypereosinophilic syndrome (IHS). This syndrome represents a hetergeneous group of disorders with the common features of prolonged eosinophilia of an undetectable cause and organ system dysfunction. Fifty patients with the IHS were studied over 11 years at the National Institutes of Health. Multiple organ systems were involved; bone marrow hypereosinophilia was common to all patients, but the most severe clinicopathologic involvement was of the heart and nervous system. Necropsy gross examination of the hearts of patients with IHS and nonidiopathic hypereosinophic syndrome suggested that the common mechanism of cardiac disease is the eosinophilia. Endomyocardial biopsy findings showed that the endothelial cells in the endocardium and of the microvasculature were the primary targets of the tissue damage. This damage appears to initiate the mural thrombosis which appears to be the precursor of endocardial fibrosis and restrictive endomyocardopathy. In vitro culture of circulating eosinophil colony-forming units showed some normal studies, some studies showing increased progenitor cells committed to eosinophil development, and others showing an excess production of eosinophil colony-stimulating factor. Chemotherapy to lower the eosinophil counts has resulted in marked improvement in prognosis in patients with IHS, as have aggressive surgical approaches to cardiovascular complications.

Patients with the idiopathic hypereosinophilic syndrome (IHS) present a variety of serious clinical problems. One is progressive and often acute deterioration of cardiac function associated with severe thickening of the mural ventricular endocardium of 1 or both ventricles. Clinically detectable heart disease eventually occurs in most patients with IHS, and cardiac involvement is the most common cause of morbidity and mortality. Mural endocardial thickening and superimposed thrombus, the characteristic anatomic features of IHS, often lead to a restrictive cardiomyopathy, which may be accompanied by AV valve regurgitation. Valve replacement in patients with IHS, however, has been infrequent. Harley and associates[25] from Bethesda, Maryland, described 3 patients with IHS, each of whom had severe AV valve regurgitation causing intractable CHF and each underwent MUR or tricuspid valve replacement or both. After valve replacement, all 3 patients had striking improvement in exercise tolerance and control of the CHF. Thus, AV valve replacement may be beneficial in selected patients with CHF associated with the endocardial process of IHS.

Davies and associates[26] from London, England, studied M-mode and 2-D echoes in 9 patients with eosinophilic endomyocardial disease who had undergone cardiac angiography. In 7 patients, amplitude processed 2-D echoes showed regions where the relative intensity of endomyocardial echoes was greater than normal and their distribution corresponded to known areas of fibrosis. Standard 2-D echo was normal in all but 3 patients. In 8 patients, M-mode echo showed only nonspecific abnormalities, but appeared to be useful in assessing the functional consequences of myocardial or mitral valve disease. After digitalization, a reduction in the duration and an increase in the peak rate of dimension increase during filling occurred in 4 patients, in 2 others the peak rate of dimension increase was reduced and filling was prolonged. Thus, amplitude processed 2-D echo may be useful in diagnosing the extent and severity of eosinophilic endomyocardial disease. These noninvasive techniques may provide a means for early diagnosis of endomyocardial fibrosis and could be useful in assessing its progression or response to treatment.

Endomyocardial fibrosis of Africa

Endomyocardial fibrosis is one of the most common forms of heart disease in certain portions of Africa. George and associates[27] from Lagos, Nigeria, described M-mode echo findings in 21 patients with endomyocardial fibrosis. The M-mode features associated with RV endomyocardial fibrosis included exaggerated motion and thickening of the anterior RV wall, increased RV end-diastolic dimension, and paradoxical motion of the ventricular septum. An echo-free space behind the LV wall indicative of pericardial effusion was present in 3 patients. The tricuspid valve was recorded easily in all 21 patients. Six patients with LV endomyocardial fibrosis had diminished LV end-diastolic dimension. Three had echo features of pulmonary hypertension. Fine fluttering of the anterior mitral leaflet and tricuspid leaflet were noted in 2 patients.

TOXIC CARDIOMYOPATHY

Doxorubicin (Adriamycin) was administered by continuous infusion by Legha and associates[28] from Houston, Texas, to reduce plasma levels and thus lessen cardiac toxicity. Cardiotoxicity was monitored by noninvasive methods, and endomyocardial biopsy specimens were studied by electron microscopy. Cardiotoxicity was compared in 21 patients receiving doxorubicin intravenously over 48 or 96 hours and in 30 control patients treated by standard intravenous injection. Both groups were studied prospectively and were well matched by risk factors for doxorubicin cardiotoxicity. The median cumulative dose for those receiving continuous infusion was 600 mg/m^2 body surface area (range, 360–1,500) compared with 465 mg/m^2 (range, 290–680) in the control group (p = 0.002). Of the 30 patients in the control group, 14 had severe morphologic changes in the biopsy specimens, precluding further doxorubicin administration, compared with 2 of 21 patients receiving the drug by continuous infusion (p < 0.02). The mean morphologic score for the infusion group, 0.9, was lower than the mean for the control group, 1.6 (p = 0.004). Antitumor activity was not compromised. Thus, decreasing peak plasma levels of doxorubicin by continuous infusion reduces cardiotoxicity.

NEUROGENIC CARDIOMYOPATHY

Friedreich's ataxia

Features of HC, including increased septal to free wall ratio and dynamic LV outflow tract obstruction, have been described as characteristic cardiac findings in Friedreich's ataxia. To characterize the cardiac abnormality in Friedreich's ataxia, 25 such patients were studied by echo by Gottdiener and associates[29] from Washington, DC. Concentric (symmetric) thickening of the ventricular septum and the LV posterior wall was present in 13 (52%) of the 25 patients; only 1 patient had an increased septal to free wall ratio. In these patients, the magnitude of LV hypertrophy was related to the severity of the neurologic abnormality. Systolic anterior motion of the anterior mitral leaflet was not present in any patient, suggesting the absence of resting LV outflow tract obstruction. The LV end-diastolic dimension was normal in 17 patients and decreased in 7; the remaining patient manifested increased LV end-diastolic dimension, decreased LV fractional shortening, and CHF. The LA dimension was increased in 6 (43%) of the 14 patients with LV wall thickening. By echo, LV wall thickness was normal in 15 asymptomatic first degree relatives of patients with Friedreich's ataxia (who had LV hypertrophy), suggesting that the cardiac abnormality in this disease is not transmitted independently of the neurologic disorder. Hence, in patients with Friedreich's ataxia and cardiac involvement, LV wall thickening is most commonly concentric (symmetric) but not independently genetically transmitted, and evidence of dynamic LV outflow tract obstruction is absent. Cardiac involvement in Friedreich's ataxia dose not appear to be a manifestation of HC.

Myotonia atrophica

Myotonia atrophica, a neuromuscular disease marked by autosomal dominant transmission and delayed relaxation of skeletal muscle, has been associated with CHF, conduction abnormality, and MVP. To determine the relaxation rate of cardiac muscle, LV size and function, and the presence of MVP, 30 patients with myotonia atrophica were studied by Gottdiener and associates[30] from Washington, DC, and Bethesda, Maryland, using digitized M-mode echo. Intracardiac conduction intervals were determined by noninvasive His bundle recording from surface electrodes using a high resolution, R-wave triggered, signal averaging computer. Neurologically unaffected first degree relatives of the patients with myotonia atrophica also were studied to determine if cardiac abnormalities were present in the absence of neurologic manifestations of the disease. Peak normalized diastolic endocardial velocity in patients with myotonia atrophica did not differ from unaffected first degree relatives or normal subjects. Systolic LV function and LV dimensions on echo were normal in both groups. However, MVP was present in 7 (29%) of 24 patients who could be evaluated but not in unaffected first degree relatives. Despite normal LV systolic and diastolic function, infranodal intracardiac conduction was prolonged in patients with myotonia atrophica but not in neurologically unaffected relatives. Delay in proximal intracardiac conduction also was found in patients with myotonia atrophica but not in neurologically unaffected relatives. Hence, cardiac findings in myotonia atrophica include proximal and distal conduction delay by external His bundle recording even in the absence of abnormality of the standard 12-lead ECG. There also may be an increased frequency of MVP; however, early diastolic relaxation of the LV is unimpaired, and cardiac manifestations of myotonia are not transmitted independently of neurologic abnormality.

Duchenne's muscular dystrophy

Hunsaker and associates[31] from Columbus, Ohio, evaluated the progression of cardiac involvement in Duchenne's muscular dystrophy using systolic time intervals, determined if the degree of cardiac involvement bore a relation to the severity of skeletal muscle disease, and described M-mode and 2-D echo findings. In 1970, systolic time intervals were studied in 16 patients. During the 10-year interim, 2 patients were lost to follow-up study and 5 died. The 9 remaining patients were restudied in 1980 by M-mode and 2-D echo as well as systolic time intervals. The peak ejection period/LV ejection time of these 9 patients increased from 0.37 ± 0.05 (mean, ±SD) in 1970 to 0.47 ± 0.07 (p < 0.005) in 1980. Three patients remained ambulatory, and their peak ejection period/LV ejection time (0.41 ± 0.04) was significantly better than that of the nonambulatory patients (0.50 ± 0.07, p < 0.05). The M-mode echo percentage diameter change was also worse in the nonambulatory group (21 ± 4% -vs- 34 ± 7%, p < 0.02). The 5 patients who were noambulatory in 1970 died in the intervening 10 years. This study demonstrated that the heart disease of Duchenne's muscular dystrophy is progressive and that the severity of skeletal muscle disease is probably associated with the degree of cardiac dysfunction.

MYOCARDITIS

Heikkila and Karjalainen[32] from Helsinki, Finland, studied 185 consecutive soldiers aged 18–38 years (mean, 20) with ECG changes arousing a suspicion of myocarditis in connection with an acute infectious disease. Of the 185 patients, 160 were classified into 7 ECG groups; definite or probable myocarditis was observed in 104 patients. The ECG patterns considered characteristic for acute myocarditis were: ST-segment elevations followed by T-wave inversions; gradually changing T-wave inversions not corrected by beta blockade therapy, and VPC > 10/minute triggered by acute infection (Fig. 6-4). Of the 81 patients without myocarditis, 39 had functional T-wave abnormalities that were completely normalized by beta blockade or stable T-wave inversions. The most frequent symptoms in the patients with acute myocarditis were fatigue and chest pains; loud S_3 gallop, paradoxical cardiac pulsation, pericardial friction rub, or cardiac enlargement. Echo disclosed segmental wall motion abnormalities related to the T-wave inversions. Serum creatine kinase MB fraction increased in 70% of the acute myocarditis

Fig. 6-4. Schematic representation of serial ST-T patterns of myopericarditis, myocarditis, and non-myocarditis states. Reproduced with permission from Heikkila and Karjalainen.[32]

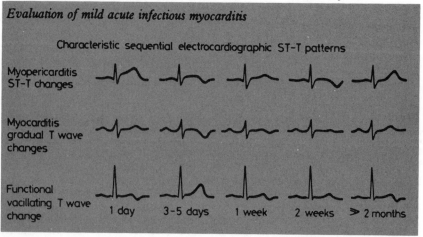

Evaluation of mild acute infectious myocarditis

Characteristic sequential electrocardiographic ST-T patterns

Myopericarditis ST-T changes

Myocarditis gradual T wave changes

Functional vacillating T wave change

1 day   3–5 days   1 week   2 weeks   ≥ 2 months

patients during the ST-segment elevation stage. In the nonmyocarditis groups, the clinical and pertinent laboratory findings remained normal. Thus, in patients with mild acute infectious myocarditis, early signs of myocardial dysfunction usually are present.

Peripartum cardiomyopathy may be considered the new presentation of primary myocardial disease during pregnancy or during the 5 months after pregnancy. Melvin and associates[33] from London, England, reported 3 consecutive patients with peripartum cardiomyopathy. Each had signs and symptoms of CHF in the absence of any known previous medical illness. All underwent detailed investigations, including complete virologic studies for possible Coxsackie B virus infection. Acute inflammatory myocarditis was diagnosed by histologic examination of cardiac tissue obtained by endomyocardial biopsy during cardiac catheterization. Immunosuppressive treatment with prednisone and azathioprine resulted in dramatic clinical improvement associated with the disappearance of the inflammatory infiltrate in all 3 patients. Thus, this report documents the presence of myocarditis as the condition responsible for the cardiomyopathy associated with pregnancy in their 3 patients. The explanation for the myocarditis in their patients was unclear.

ASSOCIATION WITH A SYSTEMIC DISEASE

Carnitine deficiency

Waber and associates[34] from Baltimore, Maryland, studied a 3.5-year-old boy with dilated cardiomyopathy (cardiothoracic ratio, 0.72) and a brother who died at 23 months with a large heart. Skeletal muscle and plasma carnitine were 2% and 10% of normal, respectively. Treatment with oral L-carnitine resulted in dramatic clinical improvement with cardiothoracic ratio decreased to 0.57 in 2 months and digoxin and diuretic therapy discontinued. These authors present the second case of familial cardiomyopathy associated with carnitine deficiency. Tripp et al (*N Engl J Med* 305:385, 1981) also reported a family of Germanic origin (similar to this patient) in whom cardiomyopathy occurred early, was much more severe than skeletal muscle weakness, and responded equally dramatically to oral carnitine. There may yet be significant numbers of subsets of patients in the morass of "idiopathic" dilated cardiomyopathy whose etiology will be discovered and specific therapy instituted.

Hyperthyroidism

Forfar and associates[35] from Edinburgh, Scotland, assessed the effects of exercise and beta adrenoceptor blockade on LV EF measured by radionuclide ventriculography in 9 patients with uncomplicated hyperthyroidism. Patients were studied in both the hyperthyroid and euthyroid states. The hyperthyroid state was characterized by a high LV EF at rest but, paradoxically, by a significant fall (p < 0.01) in LV EF during exercise. At the same work load and at the same heart rate, patients had a restoration of the normal rise in LV EF during exercise when they were euthyroid. The LV EF was greater during exercise (p < 0.02) when the patients were euthyroid than when they were hyperthyroid. Pretreatment with propranolol caused similar reductions in resting LV EF in the hyperthyroid and euthyroid states; the drug attenuated the rise in LV EF during exercise when the patients were euthyroid, but did not influence the exercise-induced reduction in LV EF in hyperthyroidism. The abnormal LV function observed during exercise in hyperthyroidism suggests a reversible functional cardiomyopathy, independent of beta adrenoceptor activation, that is presumably a direct effect of an excess in circulating thyroid hormones.

Polymyositis-dermatomyositis

Haupt and Hutchins[36] from Baltimore, Maryland, studied clinical records of 16 patients with polymyositis-dermatomyositis syndromes to determine the nature and extent of the cardiac involvement. The patients had an average age of 56 years; 2 were children aged 2 and 10 years. The duration of the disease ranged from 1–72 months (average, 21). Nine patients had dermatomyositis, 5 had dermatomyositis with malignancy, and 2 had an overlap syndrome. Seven patients had clinical evidence of CHF, 4 of whom had microscopic evidence of myocarditis. Two patients had BBB; in 1 there was direct involvement of the conduction system by myositis and contraction band necrosis. Four patients had evidence of active myocarditis and all had CHF. Focal myocardial fibrosis was present in 4. Vascular alterations were present in the coronary arteries in 5: 3 had active vasculitis, 1 had intimal proliferation, and 1 had medial sclerosis with calcification. All patients with active myocarditis had skeletal muscle involvement. Nine patients had myositis without myocarditis. These data suggest that cardiac involvement is common in patients with polymyositis. Congestive heart failure or conduction abnormalities may be indicative of myocarditis.

Diabetes mellitus in children

Friedman and associates[37] from Chicago, Illinois, performed M-mode echo in 33 children with type 1 diabetes mellitus (DM) and in 51 normal children. Abnormalities of myocardial performance were present in many children with DM. The mean end-systolic LV volume was greater in diabetics than in controls. Mean EF, minor axis shortening, and velocity of circumferential fiber shortening were decreased in diabetics. No evidence of increased myocardial mass was observed in the diabetics. No correlation occurred between myocardial dysfunction, clinical assessment of control, or glycohemoglobin in the diabetic children.

Osteogenic sarcoma

Seibert and associates[38] from Bethesda, Maryland, studied at necropsy 20 patients with fatal osteogenic sarcoma, 4 of whom had metastases to the heart. One had recurrent VT, 1 had anatomic evidence of AR due to massive periaortic neoplastic infiltration that prevented coaptation of the aortic cusps during ventricular diastole, 1 had massive invasion of the perisuperior vena caval tissues and typical clinical features of the superior vena caval syndrome, and 1 had neoplastic obstruction of the inferior vena cava as it entered the thorax. Among patients with either primary or secondary neoplasms to the heart, osteogenic sarcoma is unique because the metastases contain bone and therefore may be radiographically visible; they are usually large and often intracavitary.

MECHANISM OF CHEST PAIN

To clarify the pathogenesis of chest pain in patients with cardiomyopathies, Pasternac and associates[39] from Boston, Massachusetts, compared coronary blood flow (CBF) and other indicators of ischemia at rest and during pacing-induced tachycardia in 9 patients with cardiomyopathy (4 HC, 5 dilated) and in 5 control subjects. The CBF was reduced at rest and during pacing in cardiomyopathy patients compared with controls. In patients with HC, pacing induced chest pain in all, increased ST depression in 3, and increased coronary venous lactate concentration. With pacing, 2 of 5 patients with dilated cardiomyopathy had chest discomfort and 3 had increased ST depression but coronary venous lactate concentration did not change significantly. In both groups of cardiomyopathies, the ratio of the systolic and diastolic pressure-time indexes tended to increase more than in controls with pacing. Thus, myocardial perfusion is decreased in patients with certain cardiomyopathies both at rest and during pacing. Changes detected during pacing point to subendocardial ischemia as the likely mechanism for angina in HC and possibly in dilated cardiomyopathy.

ENDOMYOCARDIAL BIOPSY

Nippoldt and associates[40] from Rochester, Minnesota, described findings in the first 100 consecutive patients to undergo RV endomyocardial biopsy at the Mayo Clinic. The patients were divided retrospectively into 5 groups, depending on the prebiopsy clinical diagnosis, and the biopsies were reviewed histologically in a single-blind format. Group 1 consisted of 34 patients with a diagnosis of unexplained CHF and a dilated heart; of these, 4 (12%) had active myocarditis by biopsy. Of the 6 patients in group 2 with a clinical diagnosis of myocarditis, only 1 (17%) had biopsy evidence of inflammation, but 2 (33%) had changes that, in the clinical setting, were suggestive of cardiomyopathy. Group 3 consisted of 27 patients with arrhythmia, syncope, or cardiac arrest but without CHF; of these, 4 (15%) had active myocarditis by biopsy, and 8 (30%) had changes that, with the clinical history, were consistent with cardiomyopathy. Group 4 included 19 patients with unexplained CHF and a nondilated heart; 4 (21%) had cardiac amyloid on biopsy. Group 5 was a diverse group of 14 patients with possible cardiac involvement with a known systemic disease; myocardial disease was documented by biopsy in 7 (50%). On the basis of these findings, the authors recommended endomyocardial biopsy 1) in patients with dilated cardiomyopathy in whom myocarditis was suspected, 2) in patients with the clinical diagnosis of active myocarditis in whom tissue documentation was indicated before treatment with anti-inflammatory or immunosuppressive drugs, 3) in patients with clinically unexplained life-threatening arrhythmias in whom myocarditis or cardiomyopathy could be present, and 4) in patients with apparent hypertrophic or restrictive cardiomyopathy in whom cardiac amyloid might be present.

The clinical diagnosis of active lymphocytic myocarditis is often difficult because of its nonspecific clinical presentation. In an attempt to define specific criteria for diagnosis of this type of myocarditis, Edwards and associates[41] from Rochester, Minnesota, counted the number of interstitial lymphocytes in 20 high power (×400) microscopic fields in each of 170 endomyocardial biopsy specimens. The normal mean number of myocardial lymphocytes was determined to be fewer than 5.0/high power field, and mean values greater than this were considered to represent active lymphocytic myocarditis. With the use of these histologic criteria, the endomyocardial biopsy may be helpful in the detection of active myocarditis and in the evaluation of treatment.

Overview

In an editorial Fowles and Mason[42] from Stanford, California, reviewed their indications for myocardial biopsy. Their clinical indications for endomyocardial biopsy included suspected cardiac allograft rejection; suspected myocarditis; monitoring of therapy for myocarditis; detection and monitoring of doxorubicin cardiotoxicity; diagnosis of secondary cardiomyopathies, such as cardiac amyloidosis, sarcoidosis, hemochromatosis, glycogen storage disease; detection of endocardial fibrosis; and differentiation between restrictive myocardial and constrictive pericardial disease.

References

1. THOMPSON DS, NAQVI N, JUUL SM, SWANTON RH, WILMSHURST P, COLTART DJ, JENKINS BS, WEBB-PEPLOE MM: Cardiac work and myocardial substrate extraction in congestive cardiomyopathy. Br Heart J 47:130–136, Feb 1982.

2. ECKSTEIN R, MEMPEL W, BOLTE H-D: Reduced suppressor cell activity in congestive cardiomyopathy and in myocarditis. Circulation 65:1224–1229, June 1982.

3. ANDERSON JL, CARLQUIST JF, HAMMOND EH: Deficient natural killer cell activity in patients with idiopathic dilated cardiomyopathy. Lancet 2:1124–1127, Nov 20, 1982.

4. AMORIM DS, OLSEN EGJ: Assessment of heart neurons in dilated (congestive) cardiomyopathy. Br Heart J 47:11–18, Jan 1982.

5. GOODWIN JF: The frontiers of cardiomyopathy. Br Heart J 48:1–18, July 1982.

6. MARON BJ, TAJIK AJ, RUTTENBERG HD, GRAHAM TP, ATWOOD GF, VICTORICA BE, LIE JT, ROBERTS WC: Hypertrophic cardiomyopathy in infants: clinical and natural history. Circulation 65:7–17, Jan 1982.

7. MCKENNA WJ, BORGGREFE M, ENGLAND D, DEANFIELD J, OAKLEY CM, GOODWIN JF: The natural history of LV hypertrophy in HC: an electrocardiographic study. Circulation 66:1233–1240, Dec 1982.

8. MARON BJ, BONOW RO, SESHAGIRI TNR, ROBERTS WC, EPSTEIN SE: Hypertrophic cardiomyopathy with ventricular septal hypertrophy localized to the apical region of the left ventricle (apical hypertrophic cardiomyopathy). Am J Cardiol 49:1839–1847, June 1982.

9. ALVARES RF, GOODWIN JF: Non-invasive assessment of diastolic function in hypertrophic cardiomyopathy on and off beta adrenergic blocking drugs. Br Heart J 48:204–212, Sept 1982.

10. MARON BJ, ROBERTS WC, EPSTEIN SE: Sudden death in HC: A profile of 78 patients. Circulation 65:1388–1394, June 1982.

11. BJARNASON I, JONSSON S, HARDARSON T: Mode of inheritance of hypertrophic cardiomyopathy in Iceland: echocardiographic study. Br Heart J 47:122–129, Feb 1982.

12. GARDIN JM, GOTTDIENER JS, RADVANY R, MARON BJ, LESCH M: HLA linkage vs association in hypertrophic cardiomyopathy. Chest 81:466–472, Apr 1982.

13. SILVERMAN KJ, HUTCHINS GM, WEISS JL, MOORE GW: Catenoidal shape of the interventricular septum in idiopathic hypertrophic subaortic stenosis: two dimensional echocardiographic confirmation. Am J Cardiol 49:27–32, Jan 1982.

14. STEFADOUROS MA, CANEDO MI, ABDULLA AM, KARAYANNIS E, BAUTE A, FRANK MJ: Postextrasystolic changes in systolic time intervals in the assessment of hypertrophic cardiomyopathy. Br Heart J 47:261–269, March 1982.

15. LOPERFIDO R, FIORILLI R, DIGAETANO A, DI GENNARO M, SANTARELLI P, BELLOCCI B, COPPOLA E, ZECCHI P: Familial hypertrophic cardiomyopathy: vector cardiographic findings in echocardiographically unaffected relatives. Br Heart J 47:588–595, June 1982.

16. BJARNASON I, HARDARSON T, JONSSON S: Cardiac arrhythmias in hypertrophic cardiomyopathy. Br Heart J 48:198–203, Sept 1982.

17. LORELL BH, PAULUS WJ, GROSSMAN W, WYNNE J, COHN PF: Modification of abnormal LV diastolic properties by nifedipine in patients with HC. Circulation 65:499–507, March 1982.

18. LANDMARK K, SIRE S, THAULOW E, AMLIE JP, NITTER-HAUGE S: Hemodynamic effects of nifedipine and propranolol in hypertrophic obstructive cardiomyopathy. Br Heart J 48:19–26, July 1982.

19. POLLICK C: Muscular subaortic stenois. Hemodynamic and clinical improvement after disopyramide. N Engl J Med 307:997–999, Oct 14, 1982.

20. WIENER MW, VONDOENHOFF LJ, COHEN J: Aortic regurgitation first appearing 12 years after successful septal myectomy for hypertrophic obstructive cardiomyopathy. Am J Med 72:157–160, Jan 1982.

21. CARROLL JD, GAASCH WH, MCADAM KPWJ: Amyloid cardiomyopathy: characterization by a distinctive voltage/mass relation. Am J Cardiol 49:9–13, Jan 1982.

22. WIZENBERG TA, MUZ J, SOHN YH, SAMLOWSKI W, WEISSLER AM: Value of positive myocardial technetium-99m-pyrophosphate scintigraphy in the noninvasive diagnosis of cardiac amyloidosis. Am Heart J 103:468–473, Apr 1982.

23. ST. JOHN SUTTON MG, REICHEK N, KASTOR JA, GUILIANI ER: Computerized M-mode echo analysis on LV dysfunction in cardiac amyloid. Circulation 66:790–799, Oct 1982.

24. FAUCI AS, HARLEY JB, ROBERTS WC, FERRANS VJ, GRALNICK HR, BJORNSON BH: The idiopathic hypereosinophilic syndrome. Clinical, pathophysiologic, and therapeutic considerations. Ann Intern Med 97:78–92, July 1982.

25. HARLEY JB, McINTOSH CL, KIRKLIN JJW, MARON BJ, GOTTDIENER J, ROBERTS WC, FAUCI AS: Atrioventricular valve replacement in the idiopathic hypereosinophilic syndrome. Am J Med 73:77–81, July 1982.

26. DAVIES J, GIBSON DG, FOALE R, HEER K, SPRY CJF, OAKLEY CM, GOODWIN JF: Echocardiographic features of eosinophilic endomyocardial disease. Br Heart J 48:434–440, Nov 1982.

27. GEORGE BO, GABA FE, TALABI AI: M-mode echocardiographic features of endomyocardial fibrosis. Br Heart J 48:222–228, Sept 1982.

28. LEGHA SS, BENJAMIN RS, MACKAY B, EWER M, WALLACE S, VALDIVIESO M, RASMUSSEN SL, BLUMENSCHEIN GR, FREIREICH EJ: Reduction of doxorubicin cardiotoxicity by prolonged continuous intravenous infusion. Ann Intern Med 96:133–139, Feb 1982.

29. GOTTDIENER JS, HAWLEY RJ, MARON BJ, BERTORINI TF, ENGLE WK: Characteristics of the cardiac hypertrophy in Friedreich's ataxia. Am Heart J 103:525–531, Apr 1982.

30. GOTTDIENER JS, HAWLEY RJ, GAY JA, DiBIANCO R, FLETCHER RD, ENGEL WK: Left ventricular relaxation, mitral valve prolapse, and intracardiac conduction in myotonia atrophica: assessment by digitized echocardiography and noninvasive His bundle recording. Am Heart J 104:77–84, July 1982.

31. HUNSAKER RH, FULKERSON PK, BARRY FJ, LEWIS RP, LEIER CV, UNVERFERTH DV: Cardiac function in Duchenne's muscular dystrophy: results of a 10-year follow-up study and noninvasive tests. Am J Med 73:235–238, Aug 1982.

32. HEIKKILA J, KARJALAINEN J: Evaluation of mild acute infectious myocarditis. Br Heart J 47:381–391, Apr 1982.

33. MELVIN KR, RICHARDSON PJ, OLSEN EGJ, DALY K, JACKSON G: Peripartum cardiomyopathy due to myocarditis. N Engl J Med 307:731–734, Sept 16, 1982.

34. WABER LJ, VALLE D, NEILL C, DiMAURO S, SHUG A: Carnitine deficiency presenting as familial cardiomyopathy: a treatable defect in carnitine transport. J Pediatr 101:700–705, Nov 1982.

35. FORFAR JC, MUIR AL, SAWERS SA, TOFT AD: Abnormal left ventricular function in hyperthyroidism. Evidence for a possible reversible cardiomyopathy. N Engl J Med 307:1165–1170, Nov 4, 1982.

36. HAUPT HM, HUTCHINS GM: The heart and cardiac conduction system in polymyositis-dermatomyositis: a clinicopathologic study of 16 autopsied patients. Am J Cardiol 50:998–1006, Nov 1982.

37. FRIEDMAN NE, LEVITSKY LL, EDIDIN DV, VITULLO DA, LACINA SJ, CHIEMMONGKOLTIP P: Echocardiographic evidence for impaired myocardial performance in children with type 1 diabetes mellitus. Am J Med 73:846–850, Dec 1982.

38. SEIBERT KA, RETTENMIER CW, WALLER BF, BATTLE WE, LEVINE AS, ROBERTS WC: Osteogenic sarcoma metastatic to the heart. Am J Med 73:136–141, July 1982.

39. PASTERNAC A, NOBLE J, STREULENS Y, ELIE R, HENSCHKE C, BOURASSA MG: Pathophysiology of chest pain in patients with cardiomyopathies and normal coronary arteries. Circulation 65:778–788, Apr 1982.

40. NIPPOLDT TB, EDWARDS WD, HOLMES DR Jr, REEDER GS, HARTZLER GO, SMITH HC: Right ventricular endomyocardial biopsy. Clinicopathologic correlates in 100 consecutive patients. Mayo Clin Proc 57:407–418, July 1982.

41. EDWARDS WD, HOLMES DR Jr, REEDER GS: Diagnosis of active lymphocytic myocarditis by endomyocardial biopsy. Quantitative criteria for light microscopy. Mayo Clin Proc 57:419–425, July 1982.

42. FOWLES RE, MASON JW: Myocardial biopsy. Mayo Clin Proc 57:459–461, July 1982.

Congenital Heart Disease

ATRIAL SEPTAL DEFECT, SECUNDUM TYPE

Meyer and associates[1] from Cincinnati, Ohio, studied 51 children before and after repair of secundum ASD with M-mode echo. Age at operation was 2–17 years (mean, 7) and postoperative studies were obtained within 3 months in 42, from 3–12 months in 17, at 24 months in 11, and 3–5 years postrepair in 13. An initial decrease in RV size in the first 3 months after repair occurred in all patients, but persistent RV dilation remained in 80% followed ≤ 5 years after operation. The RV septal motion returned to normal in 55% by 3 months and in 89% with subsequent follow-up. The LV size and function were normal early and late after operation.

These data document significant residual RV enlargement after ASD closure in many children. The residual enlargement is small in degree, however, and may be of no functional significance. In addition, echo is only grossly quantitative in terms of RV size. There is no argument with early closure of ASD with significant left-to-right shunt (generally Qp/Qs > 1.8), but, in contrast with these authors, many would favor waiting until 5–6 years of age. Many children have enough of a decrease in ASD (and shunt) size from infancy to 5 years to obviate the need for surgery.

Sinus node dysfunction in patients after repair of the secundum ASD has been attributed to surgical damage. Clark and Kugler[2] in Omaha, Nebraska, studied 15 consecutive patients with ASD before operative intervention. Noninvasive testing included 24-hour ECG monitoring and a standard 13-lead ECG. Invasive electrophysiologic techniques included corrected sinus node recovery time (CSRT), sinoatrial conduction time, His bundle recording to measure A-H and H-V intervals, atrial pacing rate at which AV node Wenckebach occurred and AV node refractory period. The ECG revealed an ectopic atrial rhythm in 2 patients. Electrophysiologic studies demonstrated an abnormal CSRT in 10 patients, 5 patients revealed evidence of AV nodal dysfunction with prolonged A-H interval or abnormal atrial pacing rate at which AV Wenckebach occurred. Thus, these investigators demonstrated that sinus node dysfunction or AV node dysfunction in patients with ASD can be present before surgical intervention.

Electrophysiologic studies were performed in 17 unselected patients (mean age, 20 years) with ASD, secundum type, by Sobrino and associates[3] from Madrid, Spain. Signs of AV nodal dysfunction were absent in 53%, 7 (41%) had prolonged effective refractory period of the AV node and 5 (29%) had AV nodal tachycardia and reentry. Three of the 4 cases showed antegrade conduction (A_e-H interval) faster than retrograde conduction (H-A_e interval) during the tachycardia. In 1 patient with reentry, a similar phenomenon was observed. In the remaining patient the conduction time was reversed (A_e-H longer than H-A_e). In 2 patients infra-His and intra-His block (first and second degree) with persistence of the tachycardia was observed. Thus, abnormalities in both sinus and AV nodal function are a frequent finding in patients with ASD, and in the sinus node, any kind of significant abnormality can be found.

ATRIOVENTRICULAR CANAL

Surgical results for corrective repair of patients with complete AV canal defects have progressively improved in recent years. Chin and associates[4] from Boston, Massachusetts, reported an experience with 43 patients < 24 months of age who were surgically repaired between 1975 and 1980. Hospital mortality was 62% (8 of 13) for patients operated from 1975 to 1977 and 17% (2 of 30) for patients operated from 1978 to 1980. Late mortality was 7% and 6%, respectively. Seventeen unselected patients underwent cardiac catheterization 10–19 months postoperatively and 5 (29%) had moderate or severe MR. One had a significant residual shunt. Anatomic features that adversely affected the outcome were 1) deficient valve tissue, 2) ventricular hypoplasia and AV valve malalignment, 3) presence of an accessory valve orifice, 4) presence of solitary LV papillary muscle group, and 5) multiple VSD. Thus, although surgical results continue to improve, mitral dysfunction remains the major cause of operative mortality and late disability.

The natural history of patients with complete AV (canal) defects predicts the early development of severe pulmonary vascular disease and early death. This and dissatisfaction with PA banding led Bender and associates[5] from Nashville, Tennessee, to advise corrective repair during the first year of life for those with heart or growth failure, or pulmonary hypertension. They reported 24 consecutive infants with 2 (8%) hospital deaths and 1 late death, all in patients with associated defects. Survivors followed 7–60 months have been free of reoperation for valvular dysfunction and have shown an increased rate of growth. Postoperative catheter studies showed pulmonary vascular resistance <3 units · m^2 in each and MR, which was mild in 2, moderate in 1. One patient developed complete heart block 1 year after repair. The authors continue to recommend repair by leaflet division and attachment to a single patch used to close the atrial and ventricular septal defects during the first year of life.

Most serious observers recognize a wide spectrum of pathologic anatomy in hearts categorized as AV septal (canal) defects. Studer and associates[6] from Birmingham, Alabama, presented a meticulous study of 310 patients undergoing repair between 1967 and 1982. They characterized these hearts as having a deficiency of the atrial septum just above the AV valves and of the inlet portion of the ventricular septum (whether or not interatrial or interventricular communications coexisted). The AV valves were abnormal, being composed of left and right lateral, superior, and inferior (6) leaflets, and a common orifice was present in 139 patients and a 2 orifice AV valve in 171 patients. The variability of the interatrial and interventricular communications, AV valve leaflets and orifice, accessory orifice, major and minor associated defects, age, preoperative functional class, and degree of MR were analyzed to determine incremental risk factors for hospital death and late survival. Earlier date and younger age at operation, increased preoperative level of disability and degree of MR, and the presence of VSD or accessory valve orifice were risk factors for hospital death. The incremental risk factors of young age disappeared after 1976. Their experience shows the probability of hospital death in 1981 for patients with AV septal defects and VSD with mild to moderate MR was 5% and was independent of age at operation. It was 13% if MR was severe. Postoperatively, 99% of 239 late survivors were New York Heart Association functional class 1 or 2. Incremental risk factors for premature late death (n, 19) were increased preoperative level of disability and degree of MR, and the presence of an accessory orifice or Down's syndrome. Left AV valve repair failure (32 of 310) markedly reduced late survival and was related to the severity of preoperative MR, functional status, the type of surgical repair and was more common in those without VSD. The authors believe the architecture of the AV valve is best preserved by repair using a 2-patch technique, taking cognizance of the variable morphology and the varied etiology of preexisting MR. Corrective repair is advised during the first year of life.

VENTRICULAR SEPTAL DEFECT

Effects of increasing hemoglobin concentration in left-to-right shunting

The influence of severe chronic anemia on cardiovascular dynamics has long been recognized. The decreased blood viscosity and vascular tone that accompany the reduced oxygen-carrying capacity lead to increased venous return and preload with increased cardiac output. When oxygen demand exceeds oxygen supply, CHF develops. In the absence of cardiac disease, mild anemia is generally well tolerated through such compensatory mechanisms as the increased cardiac output and a decreased affinity of hemoglobin for oxygen. The combination of anemia with an intracardiac defect, however, may enhance or precipitate cardiopulmonary compromise-effects not antici-pated with a normal heart. Lister and associates[7] from New Haven, Connecticut, studied the acute effects of increasing hemoglobin concentra-tion and blood hematocrit on the pulmonary and systemic circulations of 9 infants with large left-to-right shunts. After isovolumic exchange transfu-sion, which was designed to raise hemoglobin but keep blood volume constant, a consistent rise in systemic and pulmonary vascular resistances occurred. This rise was comparable to those previously found in isolated circulations showing a linear relation between hematocrit and log of the vascular resistance. These changes in resistance were accompanied by decreases in systemic and pulmonary blood flow and a marked decline in left-to-right shunting. Despite the decrease in systemic blood flow, there was no decline in systemic oxygen transport, and there may have been a marginal decrease in LV stroke work. These observations help explain why the newborn with a large VSD and a high hemoglobin concentration does not have clinical signs of a large left-to-right shunt, and they also suggest that the postnatal decline in hematocrit has a substantial role in the normal fall in pulmonary vascular resistance after birth.

Effects of hydralazine

Beekman and associates[8] from Ann Arbor, Michigan, studied the acute effects of 0.2 mg/kg hydralazine intravenously on pulmonary flow (Qp), systemic flow (Qs), pulmonary arteriolar resistance (Rpa), and systemic resistance (Rsa) in 7 infants with VSD and large left-to-right shunt (Qp/Qs, 3.4 ± 0.4; RV/LV pressure ratio, 0.83 ± 0.08; mean, ± SEM). Qs uniformly increased from 4.5 ± 0.2–6.7 ± 0.5 liters/min/M^2 and Rsa fell from 13.9 ± 0.7–9.5 ± 0.7 units/M^2. Qp and Rpa were unchanged but both Qp/Qs ratio and left-right shunt fell by 32% and 24%, respectively. These findings indicate that hydralazine may be useful in management of infants with large left-to-right shunts.

Infants with a large VSD and refractory CHF now can be repaired with a low mortality (< 5%) and a dramatic, early "cure" of all the signs and symptoms of a large shunt. Thus, afterload therapy is not of major importance in this setting. Nevertheless, special circumstances may dictate prolonged medical therapy and hydralazine may prove useful. It does, however, have pulmonary vasodilating properties and documentation of the effect on Qp, Rpa, Qs, and Rsa should be obtained before chronic therapy is begun. Some infants with complete AV canal do not respond favorably to hydralazine.

Multiple defects

Fellows and associates[9] from Boston, Massachusetts, reported angiographic data from 364 infants with VSD. Multiple VSD was found in 56 (15%): 18 of 111 (16%) with isolated VSD with or without PDA, 14 of 39 (36%) with VSD plus coarctation of the aorta, 8 of 117 (7% in TF), 8 of 43 (19%) in TGA plus VSD, and 8 of 54 (15%) in common AV canal. Axially angled views in either the long axis oblique or hepatoclavicular projections were satisfactory in most patients, but a reciprocal right anterior oblique view was useful for demonstrating defects in the extreme anterior part of the septum in 2 patients. In 13 of 15 patients with preoperative angiograms, multiple VSD was correctly diagnosed. These authors present excellent documentation of the use of angled angiograms using the methods of Bargeron et al (*Circulation* 56: 1075, 1977) to detect multiple VSD. The cardiologist now should be able to give the surgeon precise preoperative information on the size and location of all VSD.

Conduction defects and arrhythmias late after closure

Blake and associates[10] from London, England, reported follow-up data on 187 patients with VSD closure by surgical ventriculotomy between 1958 and 1975. The age at operation ranged from 2–44 years (mean, 13), and the mean follow-up period, from 1–21 years (mean, 11). Additional defects included: RV outflow obstruction 38 (20%), AR 19 (10%), PDA 8 (4%), and ASD 30 (16%). Preoperative systolic PA pressure was >40 mmHg in 103 (55%), but only 74 (40%) had PA/aortic pressure ratios ⩾0.5. Postoperatively, 119 (64%) had right BBB and 42 (22%) had left axis deviation with or without right BBB. Complete heart block developed in 8 (4%) patients with 4 deaths; 3 of 8 developed this complication 13–15 years postrepair. Ventricular arrhythmia (grade 1–4) occurred in 39 (21%) with 11 deaths. Sudden unexpected death occurred in 8 patients aged 4–44 years; 4 patients had heart block and 4 had documented ventricular arrhythmia.

These disturbing data point up the need for late assessment of conduction and rhythm in patients who have had VSD closure. Patients at higher risk for these complications include those with transient postoperative heart block and any documented episodes of ventricular arrhythmia. Other possible risk factors include operation without adequate myocardial protection (applies mostly to patients operated upon before 5–6 years age), ventriculotomy, older age at operation, significant residual hemodynamic abnormalities, and development of right BBB plus left anterior hemiblock. The last risk factor has been discussed in detail in postoperative TF patients and most investigators have felt it was unrelated to late sudden deaths.

UNIVENTRICULAR HEART

Angiography

Axial angiograms of 54 patients aged 1 day to 18 years were evaluated by Soto and associates[11] from Birmingham, Alabama, to determine the views most useful for demonstrating anatomic details. The 4-chamber and the long axis oblique views were found most helpful in imaging the main chamber, the outlet chamber when present, outlet chamber obstruction, AV and ventriculoarterial connections.

This article should be studied by all angiographers who do this work. It is extremely frustrating to patient, parents, and physicians to perform a catheterization and not obtain all the necessary data to make appropriate surgical decisions in the patients with a univentricular heart. Precatheterization 2-D echo can be of great help in determining AV connections, atrial anatomy, venous anomalies, and valvular malformation. The angiographic data then can be focused on ventricular and great artery anatomy and connections and most patients subjected to only 1 preoperative catheterization.

Septation

Patients with a single ventricle and 2 AV valves may be treated with a variety of palliative surgical procedures or more definitively by a modified Fontan (ventricular exclusion) operation or ventricular septation. McKay and associates[12] from Birmingham, Alabama, reported their surgical experience with 16 patients who underwent septation of a single left ventricle with 2 AV valves and a left subaortic outlet chamber between 1967 and 1981. Each of 5 patients who had associated severe subaortic obstruction from a small VSD died from low cardiac output (mortality, 44%). In contrast, only 2 of 11 patients without this died in hospital and both of them had a small ventricle. Heart block occurred in 10 patients. Multivariate analysis identified small ventricular size and subaortic stenosis as incremental risk factors for both hospital mortality and postoperative low cardiac output. There were no late deaths among 9 survivors followed between 2 months and 4 years (median, 1.5 years) and each patient was New York Heart Association class I. The authors believe that suitable patients for ventricular septation must have a moderately enlarged ventricle without the severe hypertrophy that accompanies important subaortic obstruction. They recommend preparing those patients with associated PS and a small ventricle by constructing an initial systemic PA shunt. Thus, planned initial palliation, appropriate patient selection, timing of repair, and improving surgical methods should further reduce hospital mortality. The good late functional results support continuation of this surgical option in patients with suitable anatomy.

Controversy persists regarding the choice of ventricular septation -vs- a modified Fontan operation as the best definitive procedure for this group. One must recall, however, that <50% of these patients are candidates for the Fontan type operation using usual criteria. For those in whom it is a possible option, further experience and longer follow-up studies are necessary to resolve this dilemma. The Birmingham group has had no hospital mortality for the septation operation among 17 similar patients with a moderately enlarged ventricle without subaortic stenosis through August 1982.

AORTOPULMONARY DEFECTS

Echo assessment

Smallhorn and associates[13] from London, England, used suprasternal 2-D echo to assess PDA in 94 patients aged 28 weeks gestation to 8 years. A control group of 37 patients without PDA were compared. Reliable assessment of patency was possible in 87 (93%) cases; 7 (7%) with a PDA <2 mm in size were falsely negative. There were no false positive diagnoses. These data demonstrate the reliability of echo diagnosis of significant sized PDA by suprasternal echo in children. The technique is not easy and considerable attention must be given to avoiding a false positive diagnosis when demonstrating echo dropout where the left lower lobe PA crosses the aorta. Nevertheless, with time and experience, PDA diagnosis probably will be as accurate and reliable as VSD diagnosis and only defects <2–3 mm will be missed.

Serwer and associates[14] from Durham, North Carolina, compared Doppler retrograde/forward flow ratios (R/F) to radionuclide estimates of pulmonary/systemic (Qp/Qs) flow ratios in 13 patients aged 2 weeks to 9 years, including 2 preterm infants with PDA. The R/F ratio correlated well with Qp/Qs ratio (r^2 0.82, p < 0.01). After PDA ligation, the R/F ratio fell markedly. This interesting demonstration of a fairly tight relation between Qp/Qs and Doppler R/F ratio provides another noninvasive measurement for evaluating infants with PDA. It could prove extremely useful in the preterm infant to detect early PDA shunting and change in ductal shunt and to estimate degree of shunt.

Fisher and associates[15] from Chicago, Illinois, observed diastolic fluttering of the pulmonic valve cusps on M-mode echo in 15 (38%) of 39 infants and children with confirmed isolated PDA. The authors postulated that this flutter was caused by high velocity jet of blood from the PDA directed at the pulmonic valve resulting in fluttering of the valvular cusps throughout the cardiac cycle, most remarkable during ventricular diastole. In patients with left-sided cardiac volume overload, this finding increased the specificity of M-mode echo in the diagnosis of PDA.

Rice and associates[16] from Rochester, Minnesota, demonstrated the usefulness of 2-D echo in 2 patients in diagnosing aortopulmonary window. The direct communication between the PA and ascending aorta were demonstrated in both patients by high parasternal short axis scanning with superior tilting of the transducer to visualize the proximal aorta and pulmonary trunk (Fig. 7-1).

In premature infants

Mikhail and associates[17] from Denver, Colorado, reviewed their experience with 734 premature infants with PDA of whom 428 were medically and 306 surgically treated between 1976 and 1981. Medical treatment consisted of fluid restriction, diuretics, respiratory support, and rarely digoxin; surgical ligation was done in the 42% who remained unresponsive to this regimen. The surgically treated group had lower weight, a higher incidence of respiratory distress syndrome, and a larger echo left atrial/aorta ratio, yet required a shorter duration of intubation. There was no mortality directly related to operation; however, hospital death from complications of prematurity occurred in 9% of the surgical group -vs- 11% of the medical group, and considering only those patients <1.5 kg was 11% and 23%, respectively (p < 0.005). Necrotizing enterocolitis occurred in 0.3% of those surgically

Fig. 7-1. Diagram of typical tomographic echo features of aortopulmonary window. *Left*, Short-axis view at level of aortic and pulmonary valves shows normal relationship of pulmonary artery wrapping around ascending aorta. *Right*, High-parasternal, short-axis view above semilunar valves shows direct communication between aorta and main pulmonary artery just proximal to bifurcation of right and left pulmonary arteries (i.e., aortopulmonary window). Reproduced with permission from Rice et al.[16]

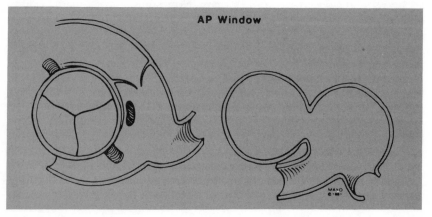

AP Window

treated -vs- 11% of those medically treated (p < 0.001) and was fatal in 57%. The authors concluded that surgical treatment was advisable for refractory PDA in premature infants, since it is associated with a reduced incidence of enterocolitis, shorter duration of intubation, and a higher hospital survival.

Indomethacin therapy

A hemodynamically important shunt through a PDA is a major problem among premature infants. Mahony and associates[18] from San Francisco, California, performed a double-blind, controlled study of prophylactic indomethacin therapy in 47 premature infants (<1,700 g) who had subclinical PDA. They received either indomethacin or placebo at a mean age of 2.9 days. Among the 25 infants weighing >1,000 g, a hemodynamically important ductus shunt developed in only 4 of the 14 given placebo. The incidence of important shunts, the number of surgical ligations, and the duration of oxygen therapy were not appreciably different between the study groups. In contrast, among the 22 infants who weighed ≥1,000 g, a major ductus shunt developed in 10 of the 12 given placebo. In the smaller infants, indomethacin therapy was associated with a significantly lower incidence of major shunts, fewer surgical ligations, a decreased duration of oxygen therapy, and fewer days necessary to regain birth weight. Thus, prophylactic indomethacin therapy in infants weighing <1,000 g prevents the later development of large ductus shunts and decreases morbidity.

PULMONIC STENOSIS

Percutaneous balloon valvuloplasty

Although percutaneous transluminal balloon angioplasty (PTBA) has been accepted as a nonsurgical technique for dilation of stenotic arteries in the peripheral, renal, and coronary circulations, application of the balloon dilation principle to intracardiac valves had not been described until Kan and associates[19] from Baltimore, Maryland, dilated the stenotic pulmonic valve of an asymptomatic 8-year-old child with isolated congenital pulmonic valve stenosis. Before angioplasty the peak RV systolic pressure was 60 and after angioplasty, it was 28 mmHg. The procedure was performed by utilizing a #7 French balloon wedge catheter that was advanced into the pulmonary trunk from the right femoral vein. A 200 cm exchange tight "J" guide wire was passed through the catheter into the PA of the left lower lobe of the lung. The dilation catheter, specifically developed for balloon valvuloplasty, consisted of a #9 French catheter with a polyethylene balloon, 14 by 40 mm. It was advanced over the exchange guide wire and positioned across the stenotic pulmonic valve. The guide wire was left in place in the left PA to stabilize the tip of the dilation catheter. The balloon was briefly inflated by hand with dilute contrast material to a pressure of 45 psi while RV and systemic arterial pressures were recorded. During the time that the balloon was inflated, there was a rise in RV pressure and a fall in systemic arterial pressure. The inflation-deflation cycle lasted 20–30 seconds, with <10 seconds of complete occlusion of the RV outflow. At the end of the occlusion period, mild sinus bradycardia with an ectopic atrial pacemaker and an occasional PVC were present. There was a return to sinus rhythm immediately upon deflation of the balloon. After deflation, there was a transient rise in the RV pressure, then a gradual decrease over 15 minutes to a stable value of 28 mmHg; the systemic arterial pressure was unchanged. Cardiac catheterization also was performed 4 months after the balloon dilation procedure and the RV peak systolic pressure was 38 and the PA peak systolic pressure was 18. The PA peak systolic pressure before angioplasty was 12 so the preoperative gradient was 48 mmHg.

The authors subsequently performed balloon valvuloplasty in 4 other patients 3 months, 18 months, 3 years, and 14 years of age, with immediate reductions in the ratio of RV to systemic-arterial pressures. These later 4 patients have, however, not yet had follow-up cardiac catheterizations to assess the long-term effectiveness of the procedure.

Pepine and associates[20] from Gainesville, Florida, described similarly successful treatment in an adult (59-year-old woman) with pulmonic valve stenosis.

Operative valvotomy

Griffith and associates[21] from Pittsburgh, Pennsylvania, reviewed their experience with pulmonic valvotomy without infundibular resection in 78 children >2 months of age. Patients judged to have associated fixed obstruction either by pulmonary anular or fibrous infundibular stenosis were excluded. The angiographic systolic diameter of the infundibulum (I) was related to the valve anulus (V) and the I/V ratio was <0.2 in 11 (group A), 0.2–0.5 in 12 (group B), and >0.5 in 55 (group C) patients. Peak RV pressure measured intraoperatively after valvotomy fell from a mean of about 135–104 mmHg in group A, 100–90 mmHg in group B, and 95–40 mmHg in group C. One patient in A required secondary infundibular resection to permit weaning from bypass. Ten patients restudied from 2–10 years postoperatively had an average peak RV pressure of 30 mmHg with resolution of infundibular stenosis. The authors concluded that in the absence of fixed infundibular obstruction or peak RV pressure >200 mmHg, concomitant resection of infundibular hypertrophy is not advisable. The authors again have demonstrated that high early postrepair peak RV pressure will regress late postoperatively after valvotomy alone. One (ADP) wonders, however, if the high postrepair RV pressure found in groups A and B would not contribute to increased morbidity in a larger series. Since no information is given to condemn concomitant infundibular resection in these subsets and since it can be safely accomplished without RV incision, many tend to recommend it.

Closed transventricular valvotomy in 24 infants with severe valvar PS was evaluated by Daskalopoulos and associates[22] from Buffalo, New York. Their ages ranged from 1 day to 11 months (median, 53 days); 21 (88%) were <6 months and 10 (42%) were <1 month old. There were 4 hospital deaths (16%) and the 20 survivors were followed for 3–133 months (median, 54). There were no late deaths and each survivor was free of cyanosis and CHF at follow-up. Five of the 20 had persistent RV hypertrophy. Postoperatively, the peak RV/LV pressure ratio decreased from a mean of 1.31 to a mean of 0.42 in the 12 restudied patients 7–85 months (mean, 50) later, and only 1 had a ratio >0.70. RV end-diastolic volume was measured preoperatively in 17 patients and was normal or enlarged in 12 (no hospital deaths) and smaller than normal in 5 (2 hospital deaths, $p = 0.075$). Mean age at operation, however, was 100 days and mean arterial saturation was 92% in the normal or enlarged RV group and 17 days ($p < 0.05$) and 68% ($p < 0.1$) in the small RV group. The authors believe that closed valvotomy is preferable to operations requiring the use of cardiopulmonary bypass and demonstrate good late results after the transventricular approach. Their data suggest that small RV size is a preoperative incremental risk factor for hospital death. They believe additional studies comparing systemic-to-pulmonary artery shunting (with or without valvotomy) and valvotomy alone, in those with small RV size, are needed.

PULMONIC VALVE ATRESIA WITH INTACT VENTRICULAR SEPTUM

Echo detection

Huhta and associates[23] from Rochester, Minnesota, compared 2-D echo and angiographic data on detection of true right main PA and measurement of the right main PA size in 65 patients (aged 16 months to 54 years) with pulmonary atresia without VSD. Suprasternal short axis and long axis views were used for measurements. True right PA with confluent PAs was identified correctly in 52 of 53 patients by echo; there were 3 false positives (aorticopulmonary collateral artery misdiagnosed as true right PA). Thus, among 12 patients with nonconfluent PAs, echo correctly predicted the absence of a central right PA in 9 of 12. Echo measurements of PA size correlated well with angiography ($r = 0.95$) and operative ($r = 0.84$) measurements. This study demonstrates how this technique can be used to detect true PAs and more importantly provides a noninvasive method to follow PA size after palliative surgery and aid in timing angiographic study and subsequent reparative operation.

Left ventricular function

Although much attention has been given to study of the right ventricle in patients with pulmonary atresia and intact ventricular septum, Sideris and associates[24] from Albany, New York, and Toronto, Canada, assessed LV systolic function and compliance in 15 patients 1 day to 7 weeks of age. Systemic arterial oxygen saturation (SAO_2) ranged from 25%–84% (mean, 52). Balloon atrial septostomy, and a systemic to PA shunt and/or a closed pulmonary valvotomy, was performed in each patient. The LV end-diastolic volume and pressure were used to calculate the compliance index (dv/dp) for each patient and provided separation of them into 2 distinct groups. Group I consisted of 7 patients with impaired LV compliance and none survived infancy, 6 having died in hospital and 1 at 9 months of age. Each of the 8 patients in group II had normal LV compliance and 2 died in hospital (p = 0.03) and none later. There was no difference in RV size, tricuspid valve size and function, presence of a PDA, preoperative SAO_2, or atrial pressure gradients between the 2 groups. Each patient had a satisfactory rise in postoperative SAO_2 and was free of transatrial gradients, yet low cardiac output was the most common cause of early death. Thus, preoperative evaluation of LV compliance might be of significant prognostic value for early survival in these patients.

Necropsy features

Bull and associates[25] from London, England, studied 32 autopsy specimens and 46 angiograms from neonates with pulmonary atresia and intact ventricular septum and concluded that massive hypertrophy of the RV wall resulted in RV hypoplasia. The hypertrophy was sufficient to obliterate the trabecular and/or infundibular portion of the RV chamber in one-third of the hearts. From these data, the authors suggested a classification based on a tripartite RV chamber with an inlet (sinus) part, a trabecular part, and a conus (infundibular) part. The absence of the trabecular and conus parts correlated well with measured tricuspid valve diameter and RV hypertrophy.

The tripartite RV cavity was developed by Goor and Lillehei (*Congenital Malformation of the Heart.* New York, Grune & Stratton, 1975, p 11). Its application to this very difficult to manage lesion may prove useful. Current management still should be directed to RV decompression by opening up the valve and/or outflow tract as soon as feasible after first providing adequate pulmonary blood flow with a shunt. This is not always possible with extremely diminutive ventricles. Major questions remain with regard to selection of patients and optimal timing of such a procedure, potential growth of the ventricle in different subsets, potential for tricuspid valve and anulus growth, and the severity and significance of RV and LV ischemia and fibrosis present before operation. The authors' classification system should aid in providing a more unified method for reporting results based on similar patient subsets.

Surgical management

The most effective surgical management of neonates with pulmonary atresia and intact ventricular septum (PAIVS) has been controversial. DeLeval and associates[26] from London, England, retrospectively reviewed their experience with 60 patients treated between 1970 and 1980 with a variety of surgical procedures. Preoperative angiograms were analyzed and of 24 patients who had inlet, trabecular, and infundibular portions (tripartite) of the RV, 12 died; of 11 without a trabecular portion, 3 died; and of 11 with only an inlet portion, 3 died; the overall hospital mortality was 39%. Early mortality after a variety of surgical procedures fell from 17 of 31 (55%) before 1977 to 1 of 15 (7%) afterward (p < 0.01). During the more recent period, prostaglandin infusion was employed preoperatively in each patient, and 5 underwent transpulmonary valvotomy with or without formalin infiltration of the ductus with 1 death, 3 had only a systemic pulmonary artery shunt with no deaths, and 7 had a shunt plus pulmonary valvotomy without mortality. The data justify the conclusion that however favorable the RV anatomy appears, reliable augmentation of pulmonary blood flow requires a systemic-to-pulmonary connection.

Later definitive repair was performed in 9 patients with 2 early and 2 late deaths. Of 7 patients without a trabecular cavity, a Fontan-type operation was used in 4 with 1 early and 1 late death, and in 3 a valvotomy with or without a patch or ASD closure was used with 1 early and no late deaths. In 2 others with tripartite ventricles a valvotomy with ASD closure was employed with 1 late death. Late actuarial survival at 5 years was 36% compared with 55% for a group of 21 patients with critical pulmonary stenosis. Serial postoperative angiographic estimates of tricuspid valve (TV) diameter were available in 12 patients. Of 6 in whom RV to PA continuity had been achieved, 3 demonstrated a normal rate of TV growth compared with 6 others without demonstrated RV to PA continuity who had little or no increase in TV diameter.

The authors recommend a transpulmonary valvotomy plus shunt for all patients with PAIVS and a RV infundibulum who have a hypoplastic TV. For those with tripartite ventricles and adequate TV size, primary complete repair should be considered. When the infundibular portion is absent, a right-sided shunt alone is advised so as to avoid ductal distortion and a preoperative balloon atrial septostomy is done if the ASD is restrictive.

Surgical options for definitive repair include: 1) complete repair when there is a normal (or near normal) TV diameter and RV is tripartite or without an infundibular portion, and 2) a Fontan-type operation when TV diameter is small (predicted gradient > 3 mmHg). A theoretic relation between TV diastolic gradient, diameter, and cardiac output was presented.

TETRALOGY OF FALLOT

Case for preoperative coronary angiography

If a major coronary artery is severed during an operation for complex congenital heart disease, disastrous consequences may occur. McManus and associates[27] from Bethesda, Maryland, discussed in an editorial how this fatal complication might be prevented. One approach would be to perform coronary angiography preoperatively in all patients with complex congenital heart disease in whom ventriculotomy was planned, and at least 5 reasons appeared to justify this approach: 1) An operatively important coronary anomaly is sufficiently frequent in patients with many complex congenital cardiac anomalies (Fig. 7-2); 2) an anomalous coronary artery coursing across the RV outflow tract may not be identifiable at operation (Fig. 7-3); 3) damage to a coronary artery at operation may have serious or fatal consequences; 4) knowledge of the presence of a significant coronary

Fig. 7-2. Most common coronary arterial origins and distributions in patients with TF. The anomalous arteries which could be damaged by right ventriculotomy are stippled. Reprinted with permission from McManus et al.[27]

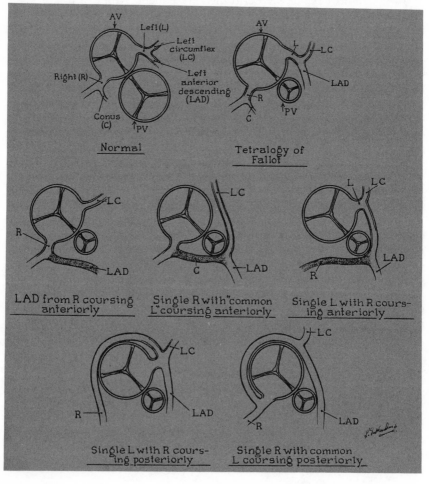

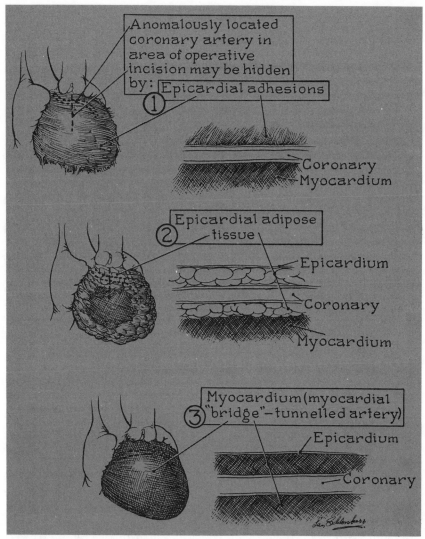

Fig. 7-3. Ways in which an anomalous artery may be hidden from view at operation. Reprinted with permission from McManus et al.[27]

anomaly may alter the timing and type of operative procedure performed; and 5) coronary angiography is a safe procedure in these patients.

Because major anomalous coronary arteries are frequent and their damage at operation may produce disastrous consequences; because they cannot be predictably identified at operation without preoperative angiography; because knowledge of their presence may alter the timing of, and the type of, operative procedures performed; and because coronary angiography is a safe procedure in patients with cyanotic congenital heart disease, it appears that preoperative coronary angiography is warranted in all patients with complex congenital heart disease.

Late operative results

Katz and associates[28] from Birmingham, Alabama, reviewed the long-term results of 414 patients who underwent repair of TF between 1967 and 1977. There were 9 late deaths, 6 cardiac related, and the 8-year actuarial survival of 96% was similar to but significantly less than that of 98% for the age, sex, and race-matched general population. Each of 8 patients (2%) who underwent reoperation required this within the first 5 years of repair. Arrhythmic symptoms were present in 10 patients (5%) and CHF in 8 (3%). Incremental risk factors for late events, including death, were older age at operation, high $P_{RV/LV}$ measured immediately after repair and the presence of a Potts shunt. Late $P_{RV/LV}$ measured in 33 restudied patients without important residual shunts was 0.55 ± 0.2, which was lower than the 0.61 ± 0.2 measured in the operating room ($p = 0.03$). The authors believe a $P_{RV/LV}$ <0.7 late postoperatively is well tolerated as long as the pulmonary valve is competent and therefore accept a value of <0.85 immediately after repair. When necessary, simple transanular patching rather than valve insertion is appropriate, since, at least within 10–20 years postoperatively, no unfavorable effect on survival and symptoms has been demonstrated.

Ventricular arrhythmias after repair

Sudden death is now a recognized complication in patients who have undergone operative repair of TF. Although earlier studies suggested that late cardiac arrest was related to progression of bifascicular block to complete heart block, recent reports strongly suggest that patients with manifest ventricular arrhythmias are at higher risk for sudden death. Of 72 patients who had undergone surgical correction of TF >5 years previously and evaluated by Webb Kavey and associates[29] from Syracuse, New York, 30 (42%) manifested serious ventricular arrhythmias on treadmill exercise and/or 24-hour ambulatory ECG monitoring. Four patients with documented ventricular arrhythmias had subsequent cardiac arrest; an additional patient was admitted in VT. Patients with ventricular arrhythmias (group II) were significantly older than patients without arrhythmias (group I), both at surgery and at evaluation. The incidence of residual elevation of RV systolic or diastolic pressure on postoperative catheterization did not differ between the 2 groups. VPC on standard ECG were significantly more frequent in patients with documented ventricular arrhythmias. Thus, chronic serious ventricular arrhythmias are common in patients after TF repair, and treadmill exercise testing and ambulatory ECG monitoring should be an integral part of the long-term postoperative assessment in these patients. After repair of TF, the prognosis for patients with documented ventricular arrhythmias is clearly impaired; all such patients should be treated with antiarrhythmic medications.

Sudden death late after surgery for congenital heart disease is usually attributed to ventricular arrhythmias, which may be difficult to suppress. Webb Kavey and associates[30] from Syracuse, New York, evaluated 19 consecutive patients with VPC documented by 24-hour ambulatory ECG monitoring treated with phenytoin orally. Sixteen patients had undergone previous repair of TF; 3 had undergone aortic valve surgery. Nine children had been unresponsive to previous antiarrhythmic therapy. Before treatment, 4 patients had VT, 3 had couplets, 6 had frequent multiform VPC, 4 had infrequent multiform VPC, and 2 had frequent uniform VPC. During treatment with phenytoin, the arrhythmia was decreased in all 19 patients and was completely suppressed in 15; the 4 remaining patients had only uniform VPC on repeat ambulatory ECG. The mean serum level was 16.8 μg/ ml (range, 12–25) with a mean dose of 3.4 mg/kg (range, 2–4). In 1 patient, a skin rash led to discontinuation of phenytoin; no other side effects occurred. Thus, phenytoin was used successfully to suppress ventricular arrhythmias in 19 consecutive patients with VPC late after surgery for congenital heart disease. Phenytoin thereby appears to be the drug of choice for this patient group.

With aortic regurgitation

Capelli and associates[31] from London, England, reported AR occurring in 18 patients aged 12–42 years with TF or pulmonary atresia with VSD. Multiple causes contributed to AR including: long-standing volume overload 14, infective endocarditis 6, and surgical sutures in the right coronary cusp 2. Aortic valve surgery was required in 13, 6 at the time of repair of TF and 7 as a second operation. There were 5 deaths: 2 post-AVR, 1 with severe AR and CHF post-TF repair without AVR, and 2 with inoperable TF.

This problem fortunately is rare in the young patient. Early operation in childhood should prevent severe AR. In older patients coming to operation, ascending aortography as suggested by the authors appears warranted so that the surgeon can be aware of the problem and assess the need for AVR at the time of TF repair.

Reoperation

The early and late results of surgical repair of TF have progressively improved over the years. Some patients, however, do have persistent important hemodynamic abnormalities that necessitate secondary repair. Uretzky and associates[32] from Rochester, Minnesota, reviewed 41 patients who underwent reoperation between 1962 and 1979. A residual VSD was closed in 28, residual pulmonic stenosis was relieved in 11, tricuspid valve repair or replacement was done in 6, and in 5 patients a RV aneurysm was repaired. An extracardiac RV-PA conduit was placed in 5, an orthotopic pulmonary valve in 3, closure of ASD in 3, repair of a residual surgical shunt in 3, and in 1 each MVR or AVR. The surgical mortality decreased from 25% before 1970 to 0% from 1971–1979 (p = 0.02). There was 1 late death.

The authors recommend reoperation when an RV-PA gradient ⩾50 mmHg or an isolated VSD with a QP/QS >1.5 is present. When service TR coexists with pulmonic regurgitation and RV dilation, tricuspid and pulmonic valve replacement is indicated. The RV outflow tract aneurysms were more related to the incompleteness of repair than to the type of outflow patch material used.

TRANSPOSITION OF THE GREAT ARTERIES

Left ventricular wall thickness

The attractiveness of arterial switching for patients with TGA prompted Huhta and associates[23] from Rochester, Minnesota, to study LV wall thickness in 92 autopsy specimens. This measurement corresponds to systolic LV thickness in living subjects as measured by echo. The LV wall thickness was normal at birth in 30 patients with TGA and intact ventricular septum, but between 2 and 4 months first began to become significantly and progressively thinner than normal. Wall thickness at various ages in 39 hearts with TGA plus VSD fell within the 95% confidence limits of normal, although the slope of the regression line was different from normal (p < 0.01) by covariance analysis. The wall thickness of 23 hearts with TGA plus VSD plus pulmonary stenosis increased normally up to age 16 years. The data suggest that patients with TGA and intact septum >2 months of age may have inadequate LV thickness to support systemic afterload. If LV thickness correlates with potential ventricular function, its measurement by echo, combined with clinical data, may aid in selecting suitable patients for arterial switching.

Tricuspid valve abnormalities

Since tricuspid valve (TV) abnormalities can alter the surgical options available to manage patients with TGA and VSD, Huhta and associates[34] from Rochester, Minnesota, reviewed 121 autopsy specimens to define their frequency and type. Forty structural abnormalities of the TV were found in 38 specimens (33%) and 17 (14%) were judged surgically important. Tricuspid valve straddling with chordal insertion into the left ventricle was present in 2 and TV replacement would be required to effect VSD closure, or a modified Fontan-type operation could be considered. Tricuspid valve dysplasia was present in 2, a double orifice valve in 1, and accessory TV tissue prolapsed through the VSD to cause subpulmonary stenosis in 3. Abnormal insertion of single or multiple TV chordae was the most common abnormality, present in 33 specimens (27%), 12 judged to prevent utilization of the VSD for a Rastelli-type repair. An overriding pulmonary trunk (Taussig-Bing anomaly) was present in 25 specimens and 9 (36%) had surgically significant chordal abnormalities. Thus, abnormalities of the TV in patients with TGA and VSD may affect the surgical options. These may be detected in some patients by preoperative angiographic and echo studies and should prompt the surgeon to consider transatrial intracardiac inspection before committing the patient to a specific type of repair.

Echo-assisted balloon atrial septostomy

Allan and associates[35] from London, England, reported the use of 2-D echo to guide balloon atrial septostomy (BAS) in 5 patients with TGA. After echo diagnoses of TGA, catheterization was carried out to record hemodynamic data. Then BAS was performed without fluoroscopy. A subcostal echo window allowed simultaneous visualization of right atrium, left atrium, ASD, mitral and tricuspid values. The balloon can be observed creating the ASD and the difference between a torn or stretched foramen ovale is apparent immediately.

Perry and associates[36] from Washington, DC, reported their experience with echo-assisted BAS in 10 patients, including a 5-month-old whose echo suggested a thin atrial septum. Diagnoses included TGA, tricuspid atresia, pulmonic atresia or stenosis, and total anomalous pulmonary venous return. All septostomies were successful in abolishing atrial gradients and improving systemic oxygen saturation. There were no complications.

Both groups presented excellent data on the use of 2-D echo to perform BAS with more accurate localization of the catheter than is possible with fluoroscopy. As more centers gain experience and confidence with this technique, BAS under echo guidance probably will become the procedure of choice. It should prove faster, safer, and more predictive of what has been accomplished with closed atrial defect enlargement.

Anatomic operative correction

Jatene and associates[37] from Sao Paulo, Brazil, reviewed their experience with 33 patients who underwent arterial switch operations for TGA since 1975 when they first reported success with this technique. Systemic LV pressure was present in 32, VSD in 29 with associated PDA in 6, isolated PDA in 3, and 1 patient had neither PDA or VSD. Overall hospital mortality was 52%, but in the most recent 12 patients, only 2 died (17%). Retrospectively, 10 patients who died were considered unsuitable for repair because of a hypoplastic LV in 1 and severe pulmonary vascular disease in 9. There were 2 late reoperations among the 16 survivors: for recurrent VSD in 1 and for pulmonary stenosis (PS) 5 years later in the other. The remaining patients have had a very satisfactory late result and do not have AR.

The authors continue to advise the venous switch for patients with intact ventricular septum and low LV pressure and anatomic correction for those with systemic LV pressure and large pulmonary flow. When subvalvar PS coexists with TGA and VSD, they advise arterial switching when the obstruction can be surgically removed and a Rastelli repair when it cannot. They recommend division of the pulmonary trunk at its bifurcation, and of the aorta, more distally, which currently permits primary great artery reconstruction without prosthetic material. The anastomosis of the new aorta is made before selection of the sites of coronary artery reimplantation which are dependent also upon the position of the new pulmonary trunk, relative to the aorta.

Radionuclide angiography after repair

Hurwitz and associates[38] from Boston, Massachusetts, and Indianapolis, Indiana, studied 29 patients by RNA after repair of TGA. Age at operation ranged from 2 days to 165 months (median, 19 months) and time from surgery to RNA ranged from <3 weeks to >3 years. Operations were: Mustard in 23, Senning in 3, and Rastelli in 3. Comparisons were made with catheterization data, and RNA correctly detected right-to-left shunting in 3 of 3, caval obstruction in 9 of 10, and provided similar information on Qp/Qs in 9 of 9 patients with left-to-right shunting.

These authors demonstrate the use of RNA to provide noninvasive clinically relevant information on postoperative TGA patients. A 2-D echo with Doppler or contrast also can be used to detect caval obstruction, and RNA can be used to quantify RV and LV function. Thus, most information needed to evaluate postoperative TGA patients (exclusive of pulmonary pressure) can be obtained noninvasively.

Right ventricular function during exercise after repair

Benson and associates[39] from Toronto, Canada, studied RV EF by gated RNA at rest and with supine bicycle exercise in 19 asymptomatic patients from 3.7–14.8 years (mean, ± SEM; 6.4 ± 2.7 years) after Mustard's operation for TGA. The mean age at surgery was 2.0 ± 1.0 years; 16 patients were in sinus rhythm. The mean RV EF at rest was 44 ± 12% and was 46 ± 11% at peak exercise. Eleven patients (58%) showed an abnormal EF response: either no change or a fall in EF by ≥5%. Heart rate increased 84% but systolic BP increased only 16% at peak exercise. No correlation was found between exercise response and age at surgery or interval since surgery.

These data indicate that clinically well children after an intraatrial repair of TGA may have abnormal systemic ventricular function with exercise. Previous studies on resting RV EF (Graham et al *Circulation* 52:678, 1975; Hagler et al, *Am J Cardiol* 44:276, 1979) and the RV response to an afterload stress (Borrow et al, *Circulation* 64:878, 1981) have also shown abnormalities in most TGA patients postrepair. The alternative operation (arterial switch) still has a prohibitive mortality for TGA repair in most centers. Further follow-up data on patients who have had repairs by the Senning or Mustard techniques in infancy with optimal myocardial preservation techniques and avoidance of severe, prolonged preoperative hypoxemia are urgently needed to determine if late RV function can be significantly improved with these measures.

Impeded coronary flow after anatomic correction

Goor and associates[40] from Tel-Hashomer and Tel-Aviv, Israel, focused attention on improving operative methods to translocate the left and right coronary arteries during anatomic correction of TGA. They reported 6 patients who underwent anatomic repair ≤9 months of age and 1 at 3½ years, with 4 hospital survivors. In 5 of the 7 patients, obstruction of the left or right coronary artery was detected, each having wide QRS complexes and 3 having visible cyanotic areas of the left ventricle. In 2, a kinked left or right coronary artery was corrected with return of the QRS complex to normal. In 2 survivors, coronary obstruction was demonstrated at postoperative angiography, which also showed ventricular contraction abnormalities. The authors believe that coronary obstruction plays a major role in the high mortality of the arterial switch operation. They indicate that the new aortic anastomosis should be completely constructed and the aortic cross-clamp released to permit selection of the definitive site of coronary transfer upon the normally distended aorta.

Sinus node function after Mustard operation

Cardiac rhythm disturbances are common following the Mustard operation for TGA. The most frequent arrhythmias are due to the sick sinus syndrome, characterized by tachyarrhythmias and/or bradyarrhythmias. Because sinoatrial node dysfunction may be progressive, and since such patients are susceptible to symptoms or sudden death as a result of their arrhythmia, a sensitive method is needed to identify those children with sinus node disease. To screen for sinoatrial node dysfunction following the Mustard procedure for TGA, Hesslein and associates[41] from Houston, Texas, studied the chronotropic response to graded maximal treadmill exercise in 29 patients at mean 6.7 years after operation. Although 93% of patients had normal resting heart rate, 83% had significant depression of maximum heart rate and/or recovery heart rate after termination of exercise. These findings were similarly present among a subset of 13 with normal exercise tolerance. Resting and exercise-induced heart rate in 10 patients receiving chronic digoxin therapy was no different than in 19 patients without medication. Sixteen patients with abnormal chronotropic responses to exercise had intracardiac electrophysiologic evaluation that confirmed sinoatrial node dysfunction in 9. Abnormal heart rate responses did not correlate with clinical symptoms, cardiac arrhythmias, or postoperative hemodynamics. Thus, maximal exercise testing appears to be a sensitive noninvasive method to identify sinoatrial node dysfunction in postoperative children.

CORRECTED TRANSPOSITION:—
OPERATIVE TREATMENT

Westerman and colleagues[42] from Boston, Massachusetts, reviewed their experience with 23 patients with corrected transposition (C-TGA) who underwent repair of coexisting intracardiac anomalies from 1974 through 1981. A VSD was closed in 20, pulmonary stenosis managed by valvotomy and/or resection in 10, by an extracardiac conduit in 9, and anatomic tricuspid valve regurgitation was treated in 5. Hospital mortality was 9% and among 18 patients with S, L, L segmental anatomy, 6 (46%) of 13 with normal sinus rhythm preoperatively developed surgical heart block. Three patients (14%) died late postoperatively, 2 from severe pulmonary vascular disease and 1 from arrhythmia. Postoperative cardiac catheterization studies were performed in 14 patients 3 days to 4 years postoperatively (mean, 12 months), which demonstrated a trivial VSD in 3, important residual pulmonic stenosis in 5 after resection or valvotomy, and severe anatomic TR in 3 after VSD closure. Eight secondary operations were required to relieve subpulmonary obstruction in 5 and replace an incompetent anatomic tricuspid valve in 2 and a degenerated tricuspid valve bioprosthesis in 1, without hospital mortality.

In patients with S, L, L hearts, an extracardiac conduit is usually (12 of 14 patients) required to relieve subpulmonary stenosis. In this subset improved knowledge of the conduction tissue should further reduce the frequency of surgically created heart block.

LEFT VENTRICULAR OUTFLOW
OBSTRUCTION

Natural history of discrete subaortic stenosis

Shem-Tov and associates[43] from Tel Hashomer, Israel, report follow-up data over 1–17 years (mean, 6) in 21 patients with mild discrete subaortic stenosis (gradient <50 mmHg). Age at diagnosis was 1–19 years. During this follow-up interval, 17 (81%) developed ≥1 of the following complications: infective endocarditis in 3 (14%), AR in 5 (27%), hyperactive asymmetric LV contraction in 3 (14%), or increase in mean gradient from 35–77 mmHg in 7 (33%, 7 of 8 in whom repeat catheterization was performed).

The complications encountered by these authors corroborate previous data by Neufeld et al (*Am J Cardiol* 38:53, 1976) regarding progression of this disease in children. It is still not clear as to optimal management of the patient with a relatively mild gradient (e.g., 30–50 mmHg). Some patients operated upon early will require repeat operation later. It does seem reasonable to liberalize somewhat any "gradient criteria" for operation and to observe these patients closely for progression of the gradient.

Left ventricular outflow enlargement by the Konno procedure

Patients with congenital AS associated with a small aortic anulus may be managed by a variety of surgical procedures. Misbach and associates[44] from San Francisco, California, reported experience with 18 patients who underwent AVR with patch enlargement of the ventricular septum, aortic valve anulus, and ascending aorta as described by Konno. They ranged in age from 4–58 years and each had a LV-aortic gradient >50 mmHg. Valvar AS with a hypoplastic anulus was present in 10, subaortic stenosis in 6, and 2 patients had previously placed small aortic valve prostheses. One or multiple previous cardiac operations had been done in 14 patients.

The authors recommend suturing the Dacron patch to the LV side of the septum and bolstering it with Teflon felt strips on the RV side of the septum. This patch is used to enlarge the aortic anulus by 35–50%. A second patch of parietal pericardium is used not only to widen the RV incision, but also to roof the entire exposed portion of the Dacron patch upon the ascending aorta, an effort to minimize postoperative bleeding (Fig. 7-4).

This method permitted enlargement of the diameter of the anulus by ≥4 mm and the use of a prosthesis ≥21 mm in each patient. No significant residual gradients were present. There was 1 hospital death (6%) from intraabdominal bleeding in a 7-year-old child who had a previously placed LV-abdominal aortic conduit with a degenerated porcine valve. There was 1 late death from bacterial endocarditis and 1 had complete heart block. The remaining patients are well and without evidence of residual VSD.

This experience again demonstrates this technique as an effective method of enlarging the LV outflow tract and small aortic anulus and also presents useful technical modifications to reduce intraoperative bleeding and the chance of residual defects.

With ventricular septal defect

Discrete narrowing of the LV outflow tract in association with VSD was found in 13 patients by Shore and associates[45] from London, England. Associated defects included coarctation of aorta (2 patients), TF (1 patient), and complete AV canal defect (1 patient). Four patients had the diagnosis made only after VSD closure. A 2-D echo performed in 8 patients clearly demonstrated a fibromuscular shelf and its relation to the VSD in each patient. These authors as well as Fisher and associates[46] demonstrated the use of 2-D echo to make the diagnosis of subaortic stenosis before VSD repair. Frequently, pressure data and angiography may not yield the correct diagnosis. The fibromuscular shelf probably should be excised even in the absence of a preoperative gradient.

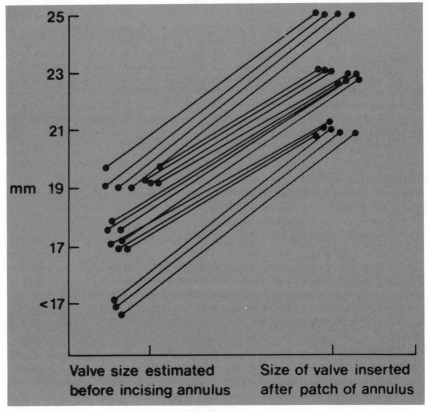

Fig. 7-4. *Left,* Prosthetic valve size which was estimated could be placed by incising anulus in noncoronary cusp in 18 patients. *Right,* Size of valve actually inserted after placing a patch in right coronary cusp and septum using Konno procedure. Reproduced with permission from Misbach et al.[44]

ECHOCARDIOGRAPHY

Assessment of left ventricular volume and ejection fraction

Mercier and associates[47] from Los Angeles, California, reported comparisons of 2-D echo and biplane angiographic estimations of LV volumes and EF in 25 children with CHD. Eight different algorithms were tested using multiple short and long axis views. Methods using both long and short axis ("biplane") data were superior to "uniplane" methods, and all methods underestimated both end-diastolic and end-systolic volumes. An ellipsoid biplane method requiring only the direct measurement of the LV diameter on the short axis view at the level of the tips of the papillary muscles and the LV diameter longest length on the apical 4-C view. With this method, the correlation with the angiographic LV end-diastolic volume was r = 0.97, end-systolic volume r = 0.93, and EF r = 0.91.

These studies provide data on the ease with which one can calculate LV volumes and EF in children: measure 2 diameters 1 length and a calculator provides the data in seconds. Silverman et al (*Circulation* 62: 548, 1980) showed similar correlations with slightly different views. The methods are easy; the real problem is in obtaining precise measurements from well-delineated endocardial surfaces at reproducible points. The reader who wants to quantify echo volumes and EF should study the original articles in detail.

Assessment of main coronary arteries in coronary artery fistula

Yoshikawa and colleagues[48] in Kobe, Japan, used real-time cross-section echo to study the main coronary arteries in 20 normal subjects, 12 patients with patent DA, and 14 patients with coronary artery fistula in whom the diagnosis was established by angiography. In 12 patients, the coronary artery that formed the fistula was dilated, the right coronary artery was involved in 8 and the left coronary artery in 4 patients. The dilated coronary artery appeared as 2 dominant parallel echoes of wide lumen, originating from the aorta and the region of the involved artery. The echo diameter of the coronary artery correlated well with the angiographically estimated diameter of the artery. In the normal subjects and the patients with patent DA, these investigators found no echo findings of coronary artery dilation. Thus, this study demonstrates that cross-sectional echo can be useful in identifying the dilated coronary artery and coronary artery fistula and distinguishing this entity from patent DA.

Of truncus arteriosus

Rice and associates[49] from Rochester, Minnesota, demonstrated the feasibility of 2-D echo to diagnose truncus arteriosus in 9 patients who had the diagnosis of truncus confirmed by cardiac catheterization and usually also by operation. They emphasized that 2-D echo is very useful in diagnosing truncus arteriosis and involves demonstration of the origin of the PA from the truncal root by the use of high parasternal short axis views and scanning superiorly above the truncal valve (Fig. 7-5).

Of systemic venous anomalies

Huhta and associates[50] from London, England, performed 2-D echo on 800 consecutive children with congenital heart disease without prior knowledge of diagnosis. The sensitivity for correct echo diagnosis was: right

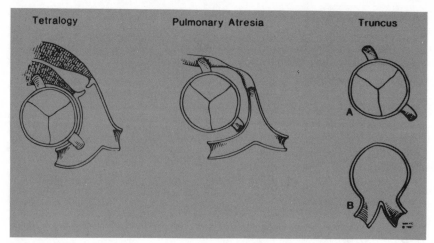

Fig. 7-5. Differential echo features of TF, pulmonary atresia, and truncus arteriosus. *Tetralogy of Fallot*, (1) infundibular stenosis and (2) direct visualization of an often thickened and stenotic pulmonary value. *Pulmonary atresia*, (1) infundibular and valvular atresia and (2) hypoplastic or absent pulmonary arteries. *Truncus arteriosus*, (1) absent RV outflow tract and pulmonary valve and no visible pulmonary arteries at truncal valve level (A) and (2) direct continuity of truncal root and pulmonary arteries by high-parasternal scan (B). Reproduced with permission from Rice et al.[49]

superior vena cava (SVC) 792 of 792, left SVC 46 of 48 (96%), bilateral SVC 38 of 40 (95%), bridging innominate vein with bilateral SVC 13 of 18 (72%), SVC connection to coronary sinus or either atrium 100%, absence of suprarenal inferior vena cava (IVC) 31 of 33 (94%), and total anomalous hepatic venous connection 23 of 23. Specificity was 100% except for 1 child with exomphalos. Precatheterization data on systemic venous anomalies can aid considerably in planning the study, particularly in children with complex heart disease. One may even arrive at a fairly specific diagnosis in many instances, such as abnormal hepatic venous connection indicating polysplenia. In addition, information on abnormal drainage of the coronary sinus and the presence or absence of a good-sized bridging innominate vein is useful to the surgeon in planning repair. This article should be studied by everyone performing cardiac catheterization in children.

In dextrocardia

Huhta and associates[51] from Rochester, Minnesota, prospectively evaluated 40 patients with a clinical diagnosis of dextrocardia using 2-D echo. An adequate examination was possible in 33 (80%). Findings were confirmed by cardiac catheterization and angiography in 31 patients and at operation in 26. Atrial situs was defined accurately in all 33, pulmonary venous connections in 27, and AV and ventriculoarterial connections, in all 33 patients. Twenty patients had 2 separate well-developed ventricles and 13 had univentricular hearts; all 33 were identified correctly.

These authors show that the segmental approach can be utilized effectively to diagnose complex congenital heart disease. The 2-D echo and angiography were found comparable and complimentary with respect to determination of ventricular morphology and ventriculoarterial connections. Angiography was superior to echo in defining ventriculoarterial connections in the presence of pulmonic valve atresia or near atresia and echo was superior to angiography in defining AV anatomy and associated anomalies, such as AV valve straddling. Current pediatric cardiology practice should include a careful 2-D echo before angiocardiography for the study to be carried out most efficiently and to minimize the number of angiograms necessary to determine the complete anatomy.

Of conotruncal malformations

Sanders and associates[52] from Boston, Massachusetts, presented data using subxiphoid 2-D echo in 113 infants with conotruncal malformations. Of the 113, 109 infants could be examined successfully using this technique and 104 of the 109 had a correct diagnosis substantiated at angiocardiography. All patients with TGA had a correct diagnosis, and 10 of 11 patients with double outlet right ventricle were correctly diagnosed. Tetralogy of Fallot was correctly diagnosed in 34 of 36 patients, pulmonic atresia with VSD in 8 of 9 patients, and truncus arteriosus in 5 of 6 patients.

This approach allows one to display ventricles and great arteries simultaneously and facilitates diagnosis of conotruncal malformations. Potential sources of error include misidentification of the great artery. In most patients combined precordial and subcostal imaging is necessary to provide an accurate diagnosis.

EBSTEIN'S ANOMALY

Management of recurrent tachycardia

Smith and associates[53] in Durham, North Carolina, evaluated 22 patients with Ebstein's anomaly because of recurrent tachycardia. A total of 30 accessory pathways were present in 21 of 22 patients. Twenty-six accessory pathways were of the AV type, whereas 4 were Mahaim fibers. Multiple accessory pathways were present in 8 patients. Of the 26 accessory AV pathways, 25 were right-sided either in the posterior septum or the posterolateral free wall. At surgery, preexcitation was invariably localized to the atrialized ventricle. Accessory AV pathways were successfully sectioned with no deaths in 13 of 15 patients.

These data suggest that certain ECG findings found in patients with recurrent tachycardia should suggest the possibility of associated Ebstein's anomaly. Specifically, surface ECG alterations suggesting preexcitation of the right posterior septum or right posterolateral free wall, as well as the combination of a long V-A interval and right BBB during reciprocating tachycardia, suggest this possibility.

Surgical treatment

Westaby and colleagues[54] from Birmingham, Alabama, reported a surgical experience with 24 patients with Ebstein's malformation, operated between 1967 and 1981. Tricuspid valve replacement was done in 16 patients with 4 hospital deaths (17%) and 3 of these 4 were among 6 patients who were preoperatively New York Heart Association functional class IV. Plication of the atrialized portion of the right ventricle was performed in 2 patients who also underwent tricuspid valve replacement. The ASD was closed in each patient and was the only procedure done in 8 patients with no or mild TR. There were 3 late deaths, 1 from noncardiac causes and 2 from persistent TR in patients without valve replacement. There were no late deaths or valve-related complications in those who underwent valve replacement. Arrhythmias were present in 20 patients preoperatively, were surgically treated in 4 patients, and late postoperatively 10 of the 16 survivors with preoperative arrhythmias were improved. The authors believe that intraoperative assessment of the degree of TR is not always accurate and that tricuspid valve replacement should be employed unless certainty exists that the valve is competent. Tricuspid valve replacement provides good early and late results if it is done before advanced symptomatic deterioration occurs.

Danielson[55] from Rochester, Minnesota, described his experience with 42 consecutive patients with Ebstein's anomaly who underwent surgical repair. They ranged in age from 11 months to 62 years. A plastic repair was accomplished in 34 (81%), RV plication and valve replacement in 6 (14%), and a modified Fontan-type procedure in 2. Three patients had interruption of accessory conduction pathways. There were 3 hospital deaths (7%), 2 of which were the result of sudden VF in patients with massive cardiomegaly. There were 2 late deaths in patients with large hearts and major preoperative ventricular arrhythmias. Late follow-up data were obtained in the first 22 survivors between 2.5 and 10 years postoperatively. Most before operation were New York Heart Association class III or IV and all but 3 improved to class I or II at follow-up. The author believes the surgical choice of plication with anuloplasty -vs- tricuspid valve replacement can be decided by preoperative echo. Plastic repair is preferred with closure of the ASD for patients in class III or IV. Thorough preoperative electrophysiologic studies are advised when a history of arrhythmias is suspected.

AORTICO-LEFT VENTRICULAR TUNNEL

Although aortico-LV tunnel is a rare congenital malformation, it is 1 in which prompt diagnosis and early surgical treatment results in a complete cure and prevents the development of AR and progressive LV dilation. Thus,

Levy and associates[56] from Tel-Aviv, Israel, described a patient and reviewed 38 patients previously reported. Aortico-LV tunnel is a tubular connection from the right aortic sinus, superior to the right coronary ostia, which passes anterior to the aortic valve anulus, through the outflow portion of the ventricular septum to enter the left ventricle. The lesion is present at birth and must be seriously considered in an infant or small child with clinical signs of severe AR. True valvular AR usually appears much later in life and PDA ruptured sinus of Valsalva, coronary artery fistula, VSD with AR, and TF with absent pulmonic valve must be distinguished by catheterization studies. Aortico-LV tunnel in older subjects may result in aortic anular and cuspal distortion with true AR, a complication presumably prevented by early operation. These patients often have huge hearts and may die suddenly or of CHF during medical treatment. Of 26 patients operated upon, 21 survived. The operation is best done by patch or suture closure of the aortic orifice of the tunnel (as opposed to closure of the LV side of the tunnel) and is advised by the authors upon diagnosis, even at young age.

AORTIC ARCH ANOMALIES

Repair of coarctation in infants

Although the method of subclavian flap repair of coarctation of the aorta (C of A) was reported in 1966 by Waldhausen, only more recently have many surgical groups developed experience with this method. Bergdahl and associates[57] from Birmingham, Alabama, reviewed their experience with 55 infants < 1 year of age. From 1967–1977, 21 were operated by resection and end-to-end anastomosis and 4 by patch graft angioplasty. From 1977–1981 the subclavian flap method was exclusively employed in 30 consecutive infants. Hospital mortality for 16 patients with isolated C of A was 6%, for 20 with associated VSD, 20% (p = 0.25), and for 19 with other major associated cardiac anomalies, 58%. Although the latter were uniformly distributed, the mortality for those repaired by resection and end-to-end anastomosis was 62% (13 of 21) and by the subclavian flap method was 7% (2 of 30), p < 0.0001. The authors believe that only an aortoplasty with viable tissue, as the subclavian flap, can uniformly relieve the aortic obstruction of very young infants with C of A and provide the lowest probability of future recurrence.

Echo in interruption

Two-D echo findings in 8 infants with interrupted aortic arch were presented by Riggs and colleagues[58] from Chicago, Illinois. The echo diagnosis of aortic interruption was correctly made in 7 of 8 patients before angiocardiography. Echo images from the suprasternal notch or from a high parasternal approach demonstrated interruption and continuation of the

PDA into the descending aorta. The characteristic conal VSD was readily visualized from an apical 2-chamber view or from a subcostal sagittal view. These authors demonstrate the practical usefulness of 2-D echo for precatheterization diagnosis of interrupted aortic arch. Smallhorn and associates[59] reported similar findings in 7 patients. These data can be very useful in planning diagnostic studies and in early institution of prostaglandin therapy. Angiography is probably still necessary in most patients to be certain of the anatomic details before surgery.

MISCELLANEOUS TOPICS IN PEDIATRIC CARDIOLOGY

Pregnancy outcome in congenital heart disease

Whittemore and associates[60] from New Haven, Connecticut, prospectively followed 233 women with congenital heart disease (118 postoperative, 115 not operated) through 482 pregnancies. There was no maternal mortality, infective endocarditis, brain abscess, or stroke. Pregnancies resulting in live born infants did not differ between operated and nonoperated patients and averaged 77%. The number and size of live-born infants, however, was greater in mothers operated upon for cyanotic heart disease than those unoperated. In addition, the number of infants born alive to mothers in good to excellent cardiovascular condition was greater than those in fair to poor condition. The latter also had a higher prevalence of interrupted pregnancies and cardiovascular complications during pregnancy. When corrected for familial or known heritable defects, the prevalence of congenital heart disease in offspring was 14% and was highest in mothers with obstruction to ventricular outflow (23%).

These data suggest that the prevalence of congenital cardiac anomalies in children of mothers with congenital heart disease without a known history of affected first degree relatives is considerably higher than previous estimates of 3%–5%. Similar information on fathers with congenital heart disease would be of great interest. If these data are corroborated by other studies, genetic counseling figures in this setting will have to be revised upward.

Radionuclide assessment of pulmonary vascular reactivity in left-to-right shunt with pulmonary hypertension

Fujii and associates[61] from Boston, Massachusetts, used RNA to study pulmonary vascular reactivity in 8 patients (9 studies) with a large, relatively unrestrictive intracardiac defect and PA hypertension. The RNA was performed first with the patient breathing room air and then after 10 minutes of breathing a mixture containing $\geq 90\%$ oxygen. The pulmonary-to-systemic flow ratios obtained by gamma variate analysis of the radionuclide time-activity curves were compared with those calculated from the Fick principle at cardiac catheterization. A good correlation existed between the 2 methods both in room air studies (r = 0.88) and in those obtained with ≥90% oxygen (r = 0.94). All 6 studies (in 5 patients) with a reactive pulmonary vasculature, as judged by pulmonary vascular resistance at cardiac catheterization, of <6 units/m^2 with oxygen, had a radionuclide-determined pulmonary-to-systemic flow ratio of ≥3.0 with oxygen. Three patients with a nonreactive pulmonary vasculature had a radionuclide-determined pulmonary-to-systemic flow ratio of ≤2.3 with oxygen, a value that was unchanged from the room air value. These data suggest that radionuclide ventriculography may be useful for assessing pulmonary vascular reactivity in patients with large, relatively unrestrictive intracardiac defects.

Myocardial injury in infants with congenital heart disease

Creatine kinase (CK)-MB activity was measured by Boucek and associates[62] from Nashville, Tennessee, in 282 children with congenital heart disease of various types. Elevated CK-MB activity was found in symptomatic patients with large left-to-right ventricular shunts and in symptomatic infants with coarctation of the aorta (C of A) or AS. In contrast, patients with only moderate left-to-right ventricular shunts (Qp/Qs ≤ 2.0), patients with ASD, and asymptomatic children with C of A or AS did not differ from controls in CK-MB activity. Preoperative patients with TGA and TF also had elevated CK-MB activity with TGA patients having a higher activity and a lower systemic oxygen saturation than TF patients.

These studies suggest that myocardial injury can occur preoperatively in patients with severe hemodynamic impairment and/or cyanosis. Such injury could be an important determinant for postoperative cardiac function. Further data correlating measurements reflecting cardiac injury, degree and duration of preoperative hemodynamic abnormality, and degree and duration of cyanosis with postoperative function should be extremely valuable in evaluating current therapy.

Pulmonary hypoplasia in Down's syndrome

Cooney and Thurlbeck[63] from Vancouver, Canada, studied the lungs of 7 patients of various ages who had Down's syndrome (mongolism) to determine whether they had abnormalities in pulmonary development. Six of the 7 had hypoplastic lungs. Pulmonary hypoplasia was of equal severity, irrespective of the presence (5 patients) or absence (2 patients) or the type of congenital heart disease. Three other patients with congenital heart disease but without Down's syndrome had lungs that were equally diminished in volume. However, these lungs lacked the structural abnormalities seen in Down's syndrome, which consisted of a diminished number of alveoli in relation to acini and enlarged alveoli and alveolar ducts. The patients with Down's syndrome also had a smaller total number of alveoli and a smaller alveolar surface area. It appears that the smaller alveolar surface area is accompanied by loss of capillary surface area, which is responsible for the aggravation of pulmonary hypertension in patients with Down's syndrome.

MISCELLANEOUS TOPICS IN PEDIATRIC CARDIAC SURGERY

Blade atrial septostomy

A collaborative study from 5 institutions on the use of blade atrial septostomy was reported by Park and associates[64] from Pittsburgh, Pennsylvania. Fifty-three procedures were performed: TGA in 31, mitral atresia in 10, tricuspid atresia in 5, and miscellaneous anomalies in 6. Patients' ages ranged from 1 day to 12 years (mean, 13 months). Improvement was documented in 79% by improvement in systemic oxygen saturation (TGA), reduction of atrial pressure gradient, or measured enlargement of the ASD. Major complications occurred in 5 patients: myocardial perforation in 2 with 1 death, and central nervous system insult in 3. Four additional patients had excessive blood loss requiring transfusion.

The authors present encouraging results with this technique for patients who need an enlarged ASD after the neonatal period when balloon septostomy usually will not suffice. Fortunately, the patients who need such a procedure are rare; TGA patients with small ASD can be repaired and tricuspid atresia patients rarely require ASD enlargement. Nevertheless, selected patients (particuarly those with mitral atresia) may be candidates for blade septostomy. They usually have small left atrial chambers that makes the procedure more difficult. Obviously, experienced pediatric cardiologists should consult directly with these investigators before attempting blade septostomy in such patients.

Classic shunting operations

Arciniegas and associates[65] from Detroit, Michigan, reported an experience with 297 systemic-PA shunts constructed over a 9-year period. The overall hospital mortality for 200 Blalock-Taussig shunts was 5.5%, for 84 Waterston shunts, 13%, and for 13 Potts shunts, 7.6%. Group I consisted of 176 patients with TF with either pulmonary stenosis or atresia and group II, of 121 patients with a variety of complex congenital defects. Hospital mortality for group I was 2.5% (3 of 120) and for group II it was 10% (8 of 80) after a Blalock-Taussig shunt (p < 0.02), and 5.5% (3 of 54) and 27% (8 of 30), respectively, after a Waterston shunt (p < 0.01). Hospital mortality was unrelated to age at operation in either group, regardless of the type of shunt. Shunt revision was required in 1.5% of the Blalock-Taussig group and 16.6% of the Waterston group and nonfatal early complications were similar, although 1 patient in the former group did have severe limb ischemia with hand contracture.

All shunts constructed during the first month of life remained patent during the first postoperative year and subsequently 23% required a second shunt procedure. Although the need for secondary shunting was greater for patients initially treated during the first month than for older patients (p < 0.005), the average period of adequate palliation was similar for all age groups. The authors favor the use of the classic Blalock-Taussig shunt because of its low risk and good functional result even in very young infants, its lower incidence of serious late postoperative complications, and its ease of future surgical closure.

Glenn shunt

In contrast to a systemic-PA shunt, a superior caval right PA (Glenn) anastomosis provides a larger effective pulmonary blood flow without increasing ventricular volume and work. Its use in recent years has diminished because of broader application of corrective type operations. Di Carlo and associates[66] from Toronto, Canada, reviewed their experience with 83 patients, aged 17 days to 15 years (mean, 4.8 years), who underwent a Glenn shunt between 1961 and 1980. Tricuspid atresia was present in 36, TGA-VSD-PS in 23, single ventricle in 13, and a variety of complex defects in 11. Follow-up was made in 100% and ranged from 6 months to 17 years (mean, 9.4 years), with postoperative catheterization studies available in 36 patients. Overall hospital mortality was 10%, but was 2% in the last 42 patients (p = 0.02), and 15 (20%) died late postoperatively, 9 associated with total repair. Hospital mortality was greater in patients < 18 months of age. At 9.4 years (mean follow-up time), actuarial survival, excluding hospital mortality, was 84% and 58% continued to be satisfactorily palliated by the Glenn shunt without the need for further operative intervention. Children >5 years at operation had prolonged palliation and at 11 years, 71% were without additional surgery, compared with 33% of those <5 years. Shunt patency without gradient was demonstrated in 35 of 36 patients restudied and mean superior vena cava pressure was 11 mmHg. Pulmonary arteriovenous fistulas were not detected. The authors believe the Glenn shunt should be considered for palliation of patients with complex heart disease not amenable to total repair, and it is most useful for patients >5 years of age.

Atriopulmonary anastomosis

Multiple surgical methods have been described to bypass the right ventricle since the original report by Fontan and Baudet in 1971. Kreutzer and associates[67] from Buenos Aires, Argentina, have contributed importantly in this area, and they reviewed their surgical experience since 1971 with 29 patients, 21 with tricuspid atresia and 8 with other types of single ventricle. Three of the 4 surgical techniques used over a 10-year period consisted of an anterior anastomosis of the right atrial appendage to the 1) pulmonary trunk with interposition of an aortic homograft or Dacron tube in 4 patients, 2) to the pulmonary trunk with its attached valve in 5, or 3) to the RV infundibulum in 9. Method 4 was a direct posterior anastomosis between the upper part of the right atrium and the main and right PA used in 11 patients. There were 5 (17%) hospital deaths and 1 late death (the first patient in this series) related to degeneration of an irradiated aortic homograft 8 months after operation. Twenty-one of the survivors are New York Heart Association functional class I. The authors enthusiastically support this operation for suitable patients with tricuspid atresia and other types of single ventricle. In their experience, method 4 can be employed regardless of the great artery anatomy and is currently preferred.

Ben Shachar and associates[68] from Minneapolis, Minnesota, studied 8 of 11 late survivors of the Fontan procedure performed for tricuspid atresia. Age at operation was 5–26 years (mean, 15 years). All patients had a valved conduit to provide direct continuity between the right atrium and PA. Cardiac index at rest was 2.3 ± 0.6 and during supine bicycle exercise, 4.9 ± 1.1. Heart rate, pulmonary vascular resistance, and LV filling pressure were normal at rest and with exercise. Right atrial pressure at rest was 15 ± 4 mmHg and with exercise, 25 ± 4 mmHg. Conduit gradients at rest were 2.3 ± 2 and with exercise, 8 ± 5 mmHg. These data clearly show an abnormal exercise response with high systemic venous pressure in tricuspid atresia patients who were without symptoms at rest and were studied 4–25 months post-Fontan. Hopefully, better long-term results will be obtained with earlier operation, avoidance of conduits, and use of the patient's own right ventricle and pulmonic valve when possible. Continuation of detailed, long-term follow-up studies at rest and with exercise is essential to the evolution of the optimal management for patients with tricuspid atresia.

Williams and associates[69] from Rochester, Minnesota, studied the hemodynamic response to dopamine and nitroprusside infusions in 9 patients early after connecting the right atrium to the rudimentary right ventricle (outlet chamber) or directly to the PA. Four patients had tricuspid atresia, 4 had a univentricular heart, and 1 had a double outlet right ventricle with dextrocardia. Cardiac index (CI) increased from 1.98 ± 0.86 liters/min/m^2 to 2.75 ± 1.05 in those receiving dopamine alone at 7.5 μg/kg/min, to 2.57 ± 0.78 for those on nitroprusside alone up to 5 μg/kg/min, and to 2.74 ± 0.84 for those on both drugs (p < 0.001 for each). The RA pressure (P_{RA}) fell from 21 ± 4–15 ± 3 mmHg (p < 0.001) with nitroprusside alone, but was unchanged with dopamine. Pulmonary arteriolar resistance index decreased significantly with either or both agents. These data indicate that nitroprusside alone is prefereable to increase CI after this operation, since it also reduces P_{RA}, which will decrease the severity of postoperative fluid retention.

Seven patients were evaluated by Janos and colleagues[70] from Cincinnati, Ohio, using RNA following Fontan-like procedures for complex cyanotic congenital defects (tricuspid atresia in 5 patients). Both first pass and ECG gated equilibrium angiography were performed in each. Residual right-to-left shunts, RA outflow and PA obstruction, and LV dysfunction were demonstrated by these techniques. In addition, RA EF by gated equilibrium scan was measured in each patient. Relatively low RA EF was seen in conjunction with residual obstruction to pulmonary flow. A RNA is useful in the postoperative evaluation of patients after Fontan procedures.

Fibrous "peels" in right-sided valved conduits

Obstruction within extracardiac valved conduits can occur at the anastomosis sites, at the level of the valve or within the conduit itself from fibrous tissue growth. In an effort to study further the histology of fibrous "peels" and to speculate upon the possible mechanisms of their development, Agarwal and associates[71] from Rochester, Minnesota, reviewed 14 autopsy specimens containing porcine valved RV-PA conduits that had been placed for a variety of cardiac defects 1 day to 5 years earlier. "Neointima" began developing as early as the first postoperative day as a thin layer of platelet-fibrin thrombus, and between 2–3 weeks became organized by fibroblastic migration and proliferation from both proximal and distal anastomotic sites. Incomplete development frequently led to fenestrations. "Peels" >1 month old did not change, having a densely fibrous luminal surface and thrombus with necrotic debris adjacent to the Dacron cloth. This observation supports the concept that progressive thickening of the "peel" primarily occurs at the "peel"-Dacron interface, rather than at the "peel"-lumen interface. Improved conduit materials clearly are needed to permit secure anchoring of the "peel" to the tube, which might limit further "peel" thickening, without increasing conduit bleeding in the heparinized patient.

"Correction" of truncus arteriosus using a nonvalved conduit

Classically an extracardiac conduit containing a homograft or more commonly a porcine bioprosthesis has been employed during corrective repair of patients with truncus arteriosus. Degeneration of these valved conduits and their general unavailability in sizes <12 mm, prompted Peetz and associates[72] from Ann Arbor, Michigan, to repair 2 patients aged 4 days using a nonvalved 8 and 10 mm polytetrafluoroethylene tube. Both patients convalesced normally. This small experience raises serious question of the desirability of using a porcine valve in these conduits, recognizing their progressive future failure. Small subjects will outgrow their initial conduit, be they valved or unvalved, and will require future re-replacement at which time the use of a valve can be reconsidered. The authors have demonstrated that a competent pulmonic valve is not completely necessary for survival after repair of this defect in a neonate.

One wonders if in a larger experience, hospital mortality would be greater when a nonvalved tube is used during repair of truncus. Efforts to develop more durable tissue valves should be intensified, since from experience with patients having repair of TF with transanular patching, some series demonstrate higher hospital mortality in small subjects and a greater incidence of later reduced exercise tolerance and symptoms of CHF [ADP].

Repair of toral anomalous pulmonary venous connection

Byrum and associates[73] from Ann Arbor, Michigan, reviewed their experience with 11 consecutive infants <6 months of age at the time of repair of total anomalous pulmonary venous connection (TAPVC). There was 1 hospital death (9%) and 2 late deaths (18%) from bradyarrhythmia in 1 and recurrent pulmonary venous obstruction in the other over a 3.5 year period. Seven of 8 long-term survivors and 3 additional patients underwent postoperative catheterization studies that showed PA pressure and resistance at normal or nearly normal values. The LV diastolic volume was normal before operation in 5 patients and at follow-up study in 9. Sinus node function was normal in each of the 7 late survivors studied and AV conduction was normal in 3 of 4. The authors' experience confirms the safety of repair of patients with TAPVC early in infancy and demonstrates normal hemodynamics, LV size, and in most patients normal cardiac electrophysiology later.

References

1. MEYER RA, KARFHAGEN JC, COVITZ W, KAPLAN S: Long-term followup study after closure of secundum atrial septal defect in children: an echocardiographic study. Am J Cardiol 50:143–148, July 1982.

2. CLARK EB, and KUGLER JD: Preoperative secundum atrial septal defect with coexisting sinus node and atrioventricular node dysfunction. Circulation 65:976–979, May 1982.

3. SOBRINO JA, DE LONBERA F, DEL RIO A, PLAZA I, MATE I, SOTILLO J, HERNANDEZ-LANCHAS CH, SOBRINO N: Atrioventricular nodal dysfunction in patients with atrial septal defect. Chest 81:477–482, Apr 1982.

4. CHIN AJ, KEANE JF, NORWOOD WI, CASTANEDA AR: Repair of complete common atrioventricular canal in infancy. J Thorac Cardiovasc Surg 84:437–445, Sept 1983.

5. BENDER HW, HAMMON JW, HUBBARD SG, MUIRHEAD J, GRAHAM TP: Repair of atrioventricular canal malformation in the first year of life. J Thorac Cardiovasc Surg 84:515–522, Oct 1982.

6. STUDER M, BLACKSTONE EH, KIRKLIN JW, PACIFICO AD, SOTO B, CHUNG GKT, KIRKLIN JK, BARGERON LM JR: Determinants of early and late results of repair of atrioventricular septal (canal) defects. J Thorac Cardiovasc Surg 84:523–542, Oct 1982.

7. LISTER G, HELLENBRAND WE, KLEINMAN CS, TALNER NS: Physiologic effects of increasing hemoglobin concentration in left-to-right shunting in infants with ventricular septal defects. N Engl J Med 306:502–506, March 4, 1982.

8. BEEKMAN RH, ROCCHINI AP, ROSENTHAL A: Hemodynamic effects of hydralazine in infants with a large ventricular septal defect. Circulation 65:523–528, March 1982.

9. FELLOWS KE, WESTERMAN GR, KEANE JF: Angiocardiography of multiple ventricular septal defects in infancy. Circulation 66:1094–1099, Nov 1982.

10. BLAKE RS, CHUNG EE, WESLEY H, HALLIDIE-SMITH KA: Conduction defects, ventricular arrhythmias, and late death after surgical closure of ventricular septal defect. Br Heart J 47:305–315, Apr 1982.

11. SOTO B, PACIFICO AD, DISCIASCIO G: Univentricular Heart: an angiographic study. Am J Cardiol 49:787–794, March 1982.

12. McKAY R, PACIFICO AD, BLACKSTONE EH, KIRKLIN JW, BARGERON LM JR: Septation of the univentricular heart with left anterior subaortic outlet chamber. J Thorac Cardiovasc Surg 84:77–87, July 1982.

13. SMALLHORN JF, HUHTA JC, ANDERSON RH, McCARTNEY FJ: Suprasternal cross-sectional echocardiography in assessment of patent ductus arteriosus. Br Heart J 48:321–330, Oct 1982.

14. SERWER GA, ARMSTRONG BE, ANDERSON PAW: Continuous wave Doppler ultrasonographic quantitation of patent ductus arteriosus flow. J Pediatr 100:297–299, Feb 1982.

15. FISHER EA, SEPEHRI B, BARRON S, HASTREITER AR: Echocardiographic diastolic flutter of the pulmonic valve in patent ductus arteriosus. Chest 81:74–77, Jan 1982.

16. RICE MJ, SEWARD JB, HAGLER DJ, MAIR DD, TAJIK AJ: Visualization of aortopulmonary window by two-dimensional echocardiography. Mayo Clin Proc 57:482–487, Aug 1982.

17. MIKHAIL M, LEE W, TOEWS W, SYNHORST DP, HAWES CR, HERNANDEZ J, LOCKHART C, WHITFIELD J, PAPPAS G: Surgical and medical experience with 734 premature infants with patent ductus arteriosus. J Thorac Cardiovasc Surg 83:349–357, March 1982.

18. MAHONY L, CARNERO V, BRETT C, HEYMANN MA, CLYMAN RI: Prophylactic indomethacin therapy for patent ductus arteriosus in very-low-birth-weight infants. N Engl Med 306:506–508, March 4, 1982.

19. KAN JS, WHITE RI, MITCHELL SE, GARDNER TJ: Percutaneous balloon valvuloplasty: a new method for treating congenital pulmonary valve stenosis. N Engl J Med 307:540–542, Aug 26, 1982.

20. PEPINE CJ, GESSNER IH, FELDMAN RL: Percutaneous balloon valvuloplasty for pulmonic valve stenosis in the adult. Am J Cardiol 50:1442–1445, Dec 1982.

21. GRIFFITH BP, HARDESTY RL, SIEWERS RD, LERBERG DB, FERSON PF, BAHNSON HT: Pulmonary valvulotomy alone for pulmonary stenosis: results in children with and without muscular infundibular hypertrophy. J Thorac Cardiovasc Surg 83:577–583, Apr 1982.

22. DASKALOPOULOS DA, PIERONI DR, GINGELL RL, ROLAND JA, SUBRAMANIAN S: Closed transventricular pulmonary valvotomy in infants. J Thorac Cardiovasc Surg 84:187–191, Aug 1982.

23. HUHTA JC, PIEHLER JM, TAJIK AJ, HAGLER DJ, MAIR DD, JULARVD PR, SEWARD JB: Two dimensional echocardiographic detection and measurement of the right pulmonary artery in pulmonary atresia—ventricular septal defect: angiographic and surgical correlation. Am J Cardiol 49:1235–1240, Apr 1982.

24. SIDERIS EB, OLLEY PM, SPOONER E, FARINA M, FOSTER E, TRUSLER G, SHAHER R: Left ventricular function and compliance in pulmonary atresia with intact ventricular septum. J Thorac Cardiovasc Surg 84:192–199, Aug 1982.

25. BULL C, DE LEVAL MR, MERCANTI C, MACARTNEY FJ, ANDERSON RH: Pulmonary atresia and intact ventricular septum: a revised classification. Circulation 66:266–272, Aug 1982.

26. DELEVAL M, BULL C, STARK J, ANDERSON RH, TAYLOR JFN, MACARTNEY FJ: Pulmonary atresia and intact ventricular septum: surgical management based on a revised classification. Circulation 66:272–280, Aug 1982.

27. MCMANUS BM, WALLER BF, JONES M, EPSTEIN SE, ROBERTS WC: The case for preoperative coronary angiography in patients with tetralogy of Fallot and other complex congenital heart diseases. Am Heart J 103:451–456, March 1982.

28. KATZ NM, BLACKSTONE RH, KIRKLIN JW, PACIFICO AD, BARGERON LM, JR: Late survival and symptoms after repair of tetralogy of Fallot. Circulation 65:403–410, Feb 1982.

29. WEBB KAVEY R-E, BLACKMAN MS, SONDHEIMER HM: Incidence and severity of chronic ventricular dysrhythmias after repair of tetralogy of Fallot. Am Heart J 103:342–350, March 1982.

30. WEBB KAVEY R-E, BLACKMAN MS, SONDHEIMER HM: Phenytoin therapy for ventricular arrhythmias occurring late after surgery for congenital heart disease. Am Heart J 104:794–798, Oct 1982.

31. CAPELLI H, ROSS D, SOMERVILLE J: Aortic regurgitation in tetralogy of Fallot and pulmonary atresia. Am J Cardiol 49:1979–1983, June 1982.

32. URETZKY G, PUGA FJ, DANIELSON GK, HAGLER DJ, MCGOON DC: Reoperation after correction of tetralogy of Fallot. Circulation 66 (Suppl I):202–208, Aug 1982.

33. HUHTA JC, EDWARDS WD, FELDT RH, PUGA FJ: Left ventricular wall thickness in complete transposition of the great arteries. J Thorac Cardiovasc Surg 84:97–101, July 1982.

34. HUHTA JC, EDWARDS WD, DANIELSON GK, FELDT RH: Abnormalities of the triscuspid valve in complete transposition of the great arteries with ventricular septal defect. J Thorac Cardiovasc Surg 83:569–576, Apr 1982.

35. ALLAN LD, LEANAGE R, WAINWRIGHT R, JOSEPH MC, TYNAN M: Balloon atrial septostomy under two dimensional echocardiographic control. Br Heart J 47:41–43, Feb 1982.

36. PERRY LW, RUCKMAN RN, GALIOTO FM, SHAPIRO SR, POTTER BM, SCOTT LP: Echocardiographically assisted balloon atrial septostomy. Pediatrics 70:403–408, Sept 1982.

37. JATENE AD, FONTES VF, SOUZA LCB, PAULISTA PP, NETO CA, SOUSA JEMR: Anatomic correction of transposition of the great arteries. J Thorac Cardiovasc Surg 83:20–26, Jan 1982.

38. HURWITZ RA, PAPANICOLASU N, TREVES S, KEANE JF, CASTENADA A: Radionuclide angiography in evaluation of patients after repair of transposition of the great arteries. Am J Cardiol 49:761–765, March 1982.

39. BENSON LN, BONET J, McLAUGHLIN P, OLLEY PM, FEIGLIN D, DRUCK M, TRUSLER G, ROWE RD, MORCH J: Assessment of right ventricular function during supine bicycle exercise after Mustard's repair. Circulation 65:1052–1059, June 1982.

40. GOOR DA, SHEM-TOV A, NEUFELD HN: Impeded coronary flow in anatomic correction of transposition of the great arteries: prevention, detection, and management. J Thorac Cardiovasc Surg 83:747–754, May 1982.

41. HESSLEIN PS, GUTGESELL HP, GILLETTE PC, McNAMARA DG: Exercise assessment of sinoatrial node function following the Mustard operation. Am Heart J 103:351–357, March 1982.

42. WESTERMAN GR, LANG P, CASTANEDA AR, NORWOOD WI: Corrected transposition and repair of associated intracardiac defects. Circulation 66 (Suppl I):197–202, Aug 1982.

43. SHEM-TOV A, SCHNEEWEISS A, MOTRO M, NEUFELD HN: Clinical presentation and natural history of mild discrete subaortic stenosis: followup of 1–17 years. Circulation 66:509–512, Sept 1982.

44. MISBACH GA, TURLEY K, ULLYOT DJ, EBERT PA: Left ventricular outflow enlargement by the Konno procedure. J Thorac Cardiovasc Surg 84:696–703, Nov 1982.

45. SHORE DF, SMALLHORN J, STARK J, LINCOLN C, DeLEVAL MR: Left ventricular outflow tract obstruction coexisting with ventricular septal defect. Br Heart J 48:421–427, Nov 1982.

46. FISHER DJ, SNIDER AR, SILVERMAN NH, STANGER P: Ventricular septal defect with discrete subaortic stenosis. Pediatr Cardiol 2:265–269, June 1982.

47. MERCIER JC, DiSESSA TG, JARMAKANI JM, NAKANISHI T, HIRAISHI S, ISABEL-JONES J, FRIEDMAN WF: Two-dimensional echocardiographic assessment of left ventricular volumes and ejection fraction in children. Circulation 65:962–969, May 1982.

48. YOSHIKAWA J, KATAO H, YANAGIHARA K, TAKAGI Y, OKUMACHI F, YOSHIDA K, TOMITA Y, FUKAYA T, BABA K: Noninvasive visualization of the dilated main coronary arteries in coronary artery fistulas by cross-sectional echo. Circulation 65:600–603, March 1982.

49. RICE MJ, SEWARD JB, HAGLER DJ, MAIR DD, TAJIK AJ: Definitive diagnosis of truncus arteriosus by two-dimensional echocardiography. Mayo Clin Proc 57:476–481, Aug 1982.

50. HUHTA JC, SMALLHORN JF, MACARTNEY FJ, ANDERSON RH, DeLAVAL M: Cross-sectional echocardiographic diagnosis of systemic venous return. Br Heart J 48:388–403, Oct 1982.

51. HUHTA JC, HAGLER DJ, SEWARD JB, TAJIK AJ, JULSRUD PR, RITTER DG: Two-dimensional echocardiographic assessment of dextrocardia: a segmental approach. Am J Cardiol 50:1351–1360, Dec 1982.

52. SANDERS SP, BIERMAN FZ, WILLIAMS RG: Conotruncal malformations: diagnosis in infancy using subxiphoid 2-dimensional echocardiography. Am J Cardiol 50:1361–1367, Dec 1982.

53. SMITH WM, GALLAGHER JJ, KERR CR, SEALY WC, KASELL JH, BENSON DW, REITER MJ, STERBA R, GRANT AO: The electrophysiologic basis and management of symptomatic recurrent tachycardia in patients with Ebstein's anomaly of the tricuspid valve. Am J Cardiol 49:1223–1234, Apr 1982.

54. WESTABY S, KARP RB, KIRKLIN JW, WALDO AL, BLACKSTONE EH: Surgical treatment in Ebstein's malformation. Ann Thorac Surg 34:388–395, Oct 1982.

55. DANIELSON GK: Ebstein's anomaly: editorial comments and personal observations. Ann Thorac Surg 34:396–400, Oct 1982.

56. LEVY MJ, SCHACHNER A, BLIEDEN LC: Aortico-left ventricular tunnel: collective review. J Thorac Cardiovasc Surg 84:102–109, July 1982.

57. BERGDAHL LAL, BLACKSTONE EH, KIRKLIN JW, PACIFICO AD, BARGERON LM JR: Determinants of early success in repair of aortic coarctation in infants. J Thorac Cardiovasc Surg 83:736–742, May 1982.

58. RIGGS TW, BERRY TE, AZIZ KV, PAUL MH: Two-dimensional echocardiographic features of the aortic arch. Am J Cardiol 50:1385–1390, Dec 1982.

59. SMALLHORN JF, ANDERSON RH, MACARTNEY FJ: Cross-sectional echocardiographic recognition of interruption of aortic arch between left carotid and subclavian arteries. Br Heart J 48:229–235, 1982.

60. WHITTEMORE R, HOBBINS JC, ENGLE MA: Pregnancy and its outcome in women with and without surgical treatment of congenital heart disease. Am J Cardiol 50:641–651, Sept 1982.

61. FUJII AM, RABINOVITCH M, KEANE JF, FYLER DC, TREVES S: Radionuclide angiocardiographic assessment of pulmonary vascular reactivity in patients with left to right shunt and pulmonary hypertension. Am J Cardiol 49:356–361, Feb 1982.

62. BOUCEK RJ, KASSELBERG AG, BOERTH RC, PARRISH MD, GRAHAM TP: Myocardial injury in infants with congenital heart disease: evaluation by creatine kinase MB isoenzyme analysis. Am J Cardiol 50:129–135, July 1982.

63. COONEY TP, THURLBECK WM: Pulmonary hypoplasia in Down's syndrome. N Engl J Med 307:1170–1173, Nov 4, 1982.

64. PARK SC, NECHES WH, MULLINS CE, GIROD DA, OLLEY PM, FALKOWSKI G, GARIBJAN VA, MATTHEWS RA, FRICKER FJ, BEERMAN LB, LENOX CC, ZUBERBUHLER JR: Blade atrial septostomy: collaborative study. Circulation 66:258–266, Aug 1982.

65. ARCINIEGAS E, FAROOKI ZQ, HAKIMI M, PERRY BL, GREEN EW: Classic shunting operations for congenital cyanotic heart defects. J Thorac Cardiovasc Surg 84:88–96, July 1982.

66. DI CARLO D, WILLIAMS WG, FREEDOM RM, TRUSLER GA, ROWE RD: The role of cava-pulmonary (Glenn) anastomosis in the palliative treatment of congenital heart disease. J Thorac Cardiovasc Surg 83:437–442, March 1982.

67. KREUTZER GO, VARGAS FJ, SCHLICHTER AJ, LAURA JP, SUAREZ JC, CORONEL AR, KREUTZER EA: Atriopulmonary anastomosis. J Thorac Cardiovasc Surg 83:427–436, March 1982.

68. BEN SHACHAR G, FUHRMAN BP, WANG Y, LUCAS RV, LOCK JE: Rest and exercise hemodynamics after the Fontan Procedure. Circulation 65:1043–1048, June 1982.

69. WILLIAMS DB, KIERNAN PD, SCHAFF HV, MARSH HM, DANIELSON GK: The hemodynamic response to dopamine and nitroprusside following right atrium-pulmonary artery bypass (Fontan procedure). Ann Thorac Surg 34:51–57, July 1982.

70. JANOS GG, GELFAND MJ, SCHWARTZ DC, KAPLAN S: Postoperative evaluation of the Fontan procedure by radionuclide angiography. Am Heart J 104:785–793, Oct 1982.

71. AGARWAL KC, EDWARDS WD, FELDT RH, DANIELSON GK, PUGA FJ, McGOON DC: Pathogenesis of nonobstructive fibrous peels in right-sided porcine-valved extracardiac conduits. J Thorac Cardiovas Surg 83:584–589, Apr 1982.

72. PEETZ DJ, SPICER RL, CROWLEY DC, SLOAN H, BEHRENDT DM: Correction of truncus arteriosus in the neonate using a nonvalved conduit. J Thorac Cardiovasc Surg 83:743–746, May 1982.

73. BYRUM CJ, DICK M, BEHRENDT DM, ROSENTHAL A: Repair of total anomalous pulmonary venous connection in patients younger than 6 months old. Late postoperative hemodynamic and electrophysiologic status. Circulation 66 (Suppl I):208–214, Aug 1982.

8

Chronic Congestive Heart Failure: Treatment And Related Topics

---

DIGITALIS GLYCOSIDE

The view that digitalis clinically benefits patients with CHF and sinus rhythm lacks support from a well-controlled study. Using a randomized, double-blind, crossover protocol, Lee and associates[1] from Boston, Massachusetts, compared the effects of oral digoxin and placebo on the clinical courses of 25 outpatients without AF. According to a clinicoradiographic scoring system, the severity of CHF was reduced by digoxin in 14 patients; in 9 of whom improvement was confirmed by repeated trials (5 patients) or right-sided cardiac catheterization (4 patients). The other 11 patients had no detectable improvement from digoxin. Patients who responded to digoxin had more chronic and more severe CHF, greater LV dilation and EF depression, and a third heart sound (Fig. 8-1). Multivariate analysis showed

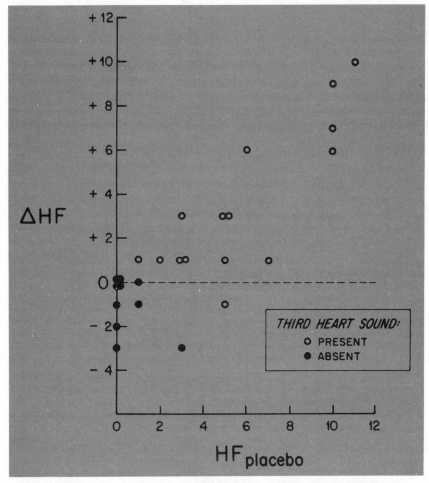

Fig. 8-1. Change in heart failure score (ΔHF [i.e., $HF_{placebo} - HF_{digoxin}$]) plotted against heart-failure score during placebo administration. The linear relation between ΔHF and $HF_{placebo}$ is described by the following equation: $\Delta HF = 0.81\ HF_{placebo} - 1.3$; ($r = 0.85$; $p < 0.001$). Patients whose ΔHF was positive were considered to have responded clinically to digoxin and had associated third heart sound. Reproduced with permission from Lee et al.[1]

that the third heart sound was the strongest correlate of the response to digoxin ($p < 0.0001$). These data suggest that long-term digoxin therapy is clinically beneficial in patients with CHF unaccompanied by AF whose CHF persists despite diuretic treatment and who have a third heart sound.

To assess the efficacy of digitalis in patients with chronic clinically compensated CHF and normal sinus rhythm, Fleg and associates[2] from Baltimore, Maryland, performed a double-blind crossover study with digoxin and placebo in 30 consecutive outpatients. Serum digoxin levels, clinical symptoms and signs, and objective indexes of cardiac function were monitored. No patient's clinical condition deteriorated during 3 months of placebo administration. Discontinuation of digoxin resulted in a small increase in echo-determined resting LV end-diastolic dimension (1.8 ± 0.6 mm, $p < 0.001$) and a similar decrease in velocity of circumferential fiber shortening ($-0.08 ± 0.04$ circ/s, $p < 0.05$) from the corresponding values of 56 ± 2 mm and 0.90 ± 0.08 circ/second during digitalis therapy. Resting LV EJ and preejection period were prolonged by digoxin withdrawal. Maximal exercise capacity was unchanged. No clinical exacerbation of CHF attributable to digitalis withdrawal occurred over a follow-up period averaging 19 months. Thus, long-term digoxin therapy has only a minor effect on cardiac performance that is without apparent clinical importance in ambulatory patients treated with cardiac glycosides.

VASODILATORS (ISOSORBIDE DINITRATE, NITROGLYCERIN, HYDRALAZINE, NITROPRUSSIDE, MINOXIDIL)

The influence of oral isosorbide dinitrate on exercise performance in 11 patients with CHF was evaluated by Hecht and associates[3] from Los Angeles, California. Patients underwent rest and supine bicycle exercise equilibrium radionuclide ventriculography and hemodynamic measurements before and after oral isosorbide dinitrate, 40 mg 4 times a day for 24 hours. Ninety minutes after the last dose, isosorbide dinitrate increased the duration of exercise by 28%, total work performed by 32%, and fewer patients terminated exercise because of dyspnea ($p < 0.05$). The LV EF increased after isosorbide dinitrate by 14% ($p < 0.02$) and there were decreases in mean PA pressure (-23%, $p < 0.02$), mean systemic arterial pressure (-8%, $p < 0.05$), systemic vascular resistance (-18%, $p < 0.05$), and pulmonary vascular resistance (-46%, $p < 0.001$). Isosorbide dinitrate decreased pulmonary capillary wedge pressure (-19%, $p < 0.001$), mean PA pressure (-23%, $p < 0.001$), mean systemic arterial pressure (-7%, $p < 0.001$), heart rate (-5%, $p < 0.01$), systemic vascular resistance (-20%, $p < 0.01$), and pulmonary vascular resistance (-37%, $p < 0.01$), and increased cardiac index by 15%, stroke volume index by 19%, while not changing EF during exercise. Thus, oral isosorbide dinitrate reduces both preload and afterload, resulting in beneficial acute effects on LV performance during exercise in patients with important CHF.

Haq and associates[4] from Toronto, Canada, studied 12 patients with chronic severe CHF refractory to conventional therapy to document the response to vasodilator therapy. The choice of vasodilator therapy was made according to the patient's hemodynamic subset during the control period with oral isosorbide dinitrate or topical nitroglycerin given to 1 group of patients and hydralazine intravenously and oral or topical nitrates given to another group. Cardiac output and intraarterial and pulmonary capillary wedge pressures were recorded continuously to assess the hemodynamic responses to the vasodilators used. Control and post-treatment M-mode echo and radionuclide ventriculograms were obtained to assess the change in LV size and EF occurring with hemodynamic improvement. Vasodilator therapy caused a 33% decrease in pulmonary capillary wedge pressure ($p < 0.001$) and a 35% increase in cardiac index ($p < 0.001$), but no significant change in LV end-diastolic or end-systolic chamber size by echo or in EF measured with radionuclide ventriculography. In this study, M-mode echo and radionuclide ventriculography were not helpful in monitoring the actual hemodynamic response to vasodilator therapy acutely in patients with a LV EF of <30%.

It is known that hydralazine reduces impedance to LV ejection and therefore produces substantial short-term improvement in cardiac performance in patients with severe CHF. Although sustained hemodynamic effects of hydralazine in patients with severe CHF have been reported, it remains unclear whether tolerance to hydralazine may occur in patients who do not benefit clinically. Packer and associates[5] from New York City performed hemodynamic studies in 11 patients with severe chronic CHF whose symptoms had returned to their pretreatment status after 37 ± 15 weeks (mean, $\pm$SEM) of therapy with hydralazine. The cardiac index increased from 1.8–3.5 liters/min/M^2 body surface area, and systemic vascular resistance decreased from 1,748–754 dynes $\cdot$ sec $\cdot$ cm^{-5} (both $p < 0.01$) during initial hydralazine administration but returned to pretreatment values on repeat evaluation; withdrawal of the drug produced no hemodynamic deterioration. Responsiveness to hydralazine could not be restored by doubling the oral dose or by intravenous administration; tolerance was associated with fluid retention in 5 patients but was not reversed by intensive diuresis. In contrast, the responses to nitroprusside evaluated before and after the development of hydralazine tolerance were unaltered; other oral vasodilators were still effective. Thus, drug-specific tolerance may account for the lack of clinical improvement in some patients with severe CHF who receive long-term treatment with hydralazine.

Magorien and colleagues[6] in Columbus, Ohio, evaluated the acute effects of oral hydralazine on coronary vascular resistance (CVR), coronary blood flow (CBF) and myocardial oxygen consumption (MVO$_2$) in 10 patients with chronic nonischemic CHF. Oral hydralazine was administered 1 mg/kg body weight and CBF estimated using the coronary sinus thermodilution technique. Central hemodynamic responses demonstrated a modest decrease in mean arterial pressure, pulmonary capillary wedge pressure, and systemic vascular resistance while the cardiac index increased from 2.3–3.1 and the LV stroke work index from 24–28. Heart rate and diastolic filling time did not change. CBF increased approximately 50%, from 144–218 ml/minute and CVR decreased from 0.55–0.36 mmHg/ml/minute. Oral hydralazine increased MVO$_2$ by 33%, from 15–20 ml/minute. Despite this modest augmentation in MVO$_2$, the arterial-coronary sinus oxygen difference decreased from 104–94 and the myocardial extraction ratio decreased from 71%–64%. The ratio of CVR and systemic vascular resistance decreased with hydralazine therapy while CBF increased from 3.5%–4.3% of total cardiac output. Thus, in some patients with dilated cardiomyopathy, hydralazine exerts a favorable effect on coronary circulation and improves the critical myocardial oxygen supply/demand ratio.

Arterial oxygen (O_2) transport derived from cardiac output (CO) and arterial O_2 content may be decreased in CHF. Rubin and associates[7] from Los Angeles, California, examined the determinants of arterial O_2 transport in 15 patients with chronic severe CHF at rest and during bicycle ergometry. During control therapy at rest, arterial O_2 tension was normal and increased slightly during exercise. During hydralazine therapy at rest, arterial O_2 tension was slightly higher and also increased during exercise. Hydralazine did not increase arterial O_2 tension but exercise did. Arterial O_2 saturation and content were normal and did not change under any condition or treatment. During the control therapy, at rest, arterial O_2 transport was low and remained abnormally low during exercise. During hydralazine therapy, arterial O_2 transport was higher at rest and during exercise. Hydralazine increased arterial O_2 transport because it increased stroke volume at rest and during exercise but it did not change arterial oxygenation. Arterial oxygenation is normal in chronic CHF at rest and during exercise. Hydralazine thus increases CO and arterial O_2 transport without changing arterial oxygenation.

Firth and associates[8] from Dallas, Texas, studied 12 patients with severe, chronic CHF and a marked LV dilation to determine whether changes in noninvasively determined LV EF, volume, or dimension reliably reflected alterations in intracardiac pressure and flow. Sodium nitroprusside was used to decrease LV volumes and improve hemodynamic parameters, multigated radionuclide ventriculography ("MUGA") to measure LV volumes and EF and invasive hemodynamic monitoring to identify alterations in hemodynamics. Nitroprusside caused a decrease in mean systemic arterial, mean PA, and mean pulmonary capillary wedge pressure and an increase in forward cardiac index. Simultaneously, LV end-diastolic and end-systolic volume indexes decreased, but the scintigraphically determined cardiac index did not change significantly. The LV EF averaged 0.19 ± 0.05 before nitroprusside and increased by <0.05 units in response to nitroprusside in 11 of 12 patients. The only significant correlation between scintigraphically and invasively determined variables was between the percent change in end-diastolic volume index and percent change in pulmonary capillary wedge pressure ($r = 0.68$, $p = 0.01$). Nitroprusside produced changes in scintigraphically determined LV EF, end-systolic volume index, and cardiac index, but these alterations did not have a predictable relation to changes in intracardiac pressure, forward cardiac index, or vascular resistance. In addition, nitroprusside, produced a considerably greater percent change in the invasively measured variables than in the scintigraphically determined ones.

Therefore, in patients with marked cardiac dilation and severe CHF small changes in LV volumes, filling pressures, and cardiac output may not be detected by currently existing scintigraphic methods. Failure to demonstrate a beneficial effect of a particular regimen using noninvasive measurements does not guarantee that a small hemodynamic improvement actually occurred.

The hemodynamic response to minoxidil, an orally active, potent vasodilator, was evaluated by McKay and colleagues[9] from San Francisco, California, in 11 patients with severe chronic CHF. The hemodynamic response was determined following single doses of 10, 15, 20, 25, and 30 mg of minoxidil. The hemodynamic response was characterized by marked increases in cardiac index (+63%) and stroke volume index (+52%) and by decrease in systemic vascular resistance (−38%). There was also a slight decrease in pulmonary capillary wedge pressure from an average of 24–21 mmHg. Although the average mean initial arterial pressure remained unchanged, 1 patient developed significant hypotension. Chronic minoxidil therapy (8 patients) was associated with fluid retention and weight gain. In 4 patients in whom fluid retention could be minimized with larger doses of diuretics, a sustained clinical and hemodynamic improvement was observed. These findings suggest that minoxidil has the potential to improve cardiac function and may be useful in chronic vasodilator therapy of CHF, provided fluid retention can be controlled.

Nathan and associates[10] from Los Angeles, California, evaluated the effects of acute and chronic oral administration of minoxidil on hemodynamics, oxygen consumption, exercise performance, and clinical status in 10 patients with severe, chronic heart failure refractory to digitalis and diuretic therapy. Cardiac index was 2.0 ± 0.4 liters/min/M^2 at rest and 2.9 ± 0.8 at symptom-limited maximal exercise on conventional therapy, compared with 2.6 ± 0.3 liters/min/M^2 at rest and 3.6 ± 0.8 at maximal exercise after short-term minoxidil administration ($p < 0.02$, control -vs- minoxidil at both rest and exercise). Stroke volume was increased after minoxidil treatment without significant effect on heart rate. Systemic vascular resistance was decreased by minoxidil from $2,050 \pm 722$–$1,325 \pm 374$ dynes/s/cm^{-5} at rest and from $1,500 \pm 830$–$1,206 \pm 589$ dynes/s/cm^{-5} at maximal exercise ($p = 0.01$, control -vs- minoxidil). Minoxidil did not significantly alter LV filling, right atrial, or mean PA pressure, but pulmonary vascular resistance decreased both at rest and during exercise ($p < 0.05$). Maximal exercise oxygen consumption increased from 8.9 ± 3.2 ml/kg/minute on conventional therapy to 10.5 ± 2.4 on minoxidil therapy ($p < 0.03$), median maximal exercise work load increased from 25–50 W and median exercise duration increased from 6–9 minutes. During chronic minoxidil administration in all 5 patients who completed a schedule of 6-week follow-up demonstrated symptomatic improvement. However, worsening edema developed in all patients, requiring increased diuretic dosage and close supervision. In addition, in 10 patients with CAD, symptoms worsened in 2.

These data suggest that minoxidil is a useful vasodilating agent in some patients with severe chronic heart failure, but it has important side effects and it may cause a worsening of symptoms in patients with CAD.

ANGIOTENSIN-CONVERTING ENZYME INHIBITORS (CAPTOPRIL) AND COMPARISON TO OTHER AGENTS

Twelve patients with severe chronic CHF underwent simultaneous evaluation of the pharmacokinetic, pharmacodynamic, and neurohumoral actions of a single 25 mg oral dose of the angiotensin-converting enzyme inhibitor, captopril, as carried out by Cody and associates[11] from New York City. Following drug administration, which raised plasma renin activity (PRA) and thereby indicated significant angiotensin-converting enzyme inhibition, both free (unchanged) and total captopril (including active metabolites) were detectable in the blood within 40 minutes and peak blood levels of the agent were recorded 1 hour after captopril. Total captopril concentration was higher and persisted longer than free captopril, which became virtually nondetectable 8 hours after ingestion. Concomitantly, LV function was markedly augmented by the oral angiotensin-converting enzyme inhibition in all patients, with the magnitude of this improvement being closely related to the baseline PRA. Thus, the overall hemodynamic response to captopril, which rapidly appears in the bloodstream following drug intake in patients with advanced CHF, is a function of the extent of baseline renin-angiotensin-aldosterone activity.

The efficacy of chronic ambulatory captopril therapy was evaluated by Creager and associates[12] from Boston, Massachusetts, over an 18-month period in 36 patients with refractory CHF utilizing cardiac catheterization, treadmill exercise, nuclear scintigraphy, echo, and symptomatology. Clinical improvement to New York Heart Association functional class I or class II was observed in 63% of patients (20 of 32) after 2 months of treatment; this amelioration of CHF symptoms was sustained in 63% of patients (10 of 16) at 18 months. Exercise tolerance increased in 64% of patients (16 of 25) at early follow-up and in 79% (11 of 14) at late follow-up. Univariate analysis revealed that the precaptopril and postcaptopril stroke work index and the postcaptopril cardiac index related to favorable long-term clinical response. Fourteen CHF patients (39%) died during the 18-month follow-up. Univariate analysis revealed that the pretreatment stroke work index, RA pressure, plasma norepinephrine concentration, and echo-shortening fraction were significant predictors of mortality. Multivariate analysis indicated that the stroke work index was the principal determinant of survival: the 18-month cumulative survival rate for CHF patients with a stroke work index < 32 $gm \cdot m/M^2$ was 44% compared with 88% when the stroke work index was $>$ $32 \ gm \cdot m/M^2$. Thus, captopril results in sustained symptomatic and functional improvement in patients with advanced CHF, but the mortality remains high and is primarily related to the severity of cardiac dysfunction.

In a placebo controlled study, Cowley and associates[13] from Nottingham, England, gave captopril to 10 patients with severe CHF whose symptoms were not controlled with digoxin and diuretics. The exercise tolerance in them was significantly improved. Serial measurements of forearm vascular resistance, an indirect index of arteriolar tone, and of venous tone were made. Improvement in exercise performance was correlated significantly with reduction in forearm vascular resistance caused by captopril.

Fouad and associates[14] from Cleveland, Ohio, evaluated the long-term effects of captopril by sequential hemodynamic study over a 6-month period in 19 patients with resistant CHF. Initial improvement during the first week of therapy was noted only in 11 of the 19 patients and was marked by significant increases in cardiac output, stroke volume, reduction in heart rate, and reduction in total peripheral resistance. In the remaining 8 patients, 7 improved subsequently with maintained therapy so that by the end of 3 months of treatment only 1 patient failed to respond significantly. The hemodynamic index that reflected response best was a shortening in mean pulmonary transit time. Associated with the hemodynamic alterations, there was an increase in plasma renin activity and a significant reduction in plasma aldosterone, but these changes did not differ significantly between patients who responded markedly and those who responded moderately to captopril. These data suggest that the response of patients with CHF to captopril can occur gradually. Improvement was related to peripheral hemodynamic changes that led to a reduction in both total peripheral vascular resistance and cardiopulmonary volume. Measurements of plasma aldosterone-renin activity provide an efficient means of testing compliance to the drug regimen.

Awan and colleagues[15] from Davis, California, studied the 6-month extended vasodilator efficacy of captopril by sequential cardiac catheterization, nuclear scintigraphy, echo, treadmill exercise, and symptomatology in 9 patients with severe chronic LV failure. Captopril lowered LV filling pressure from 23–14 mmHg acutely and to 14 mmHg with continuous 6-month therapy; concomitantly captopril raised cardiac index from 2.03–2.46 liters/min/M^2 initially and to 2.33 at 6 months (Fig. 8-2). Simultaneously, captopril raised LV EF from 0.21–0.25 acutely and to 0.30 at 6 months, and lowered LV end-diastolic dimension from 65–61 mm acutely and to 60 mm at 6 months. These beneficial actions of captopril on LV pump function raised treadmill exercise duration from 339–426 seconds initially, and to 499 seconds at 6 months, while considerably reducing CHF symptomatology. Thus, captopril provides markedly beneficial sustained hemodynamic and clinical improvement in advanced LV failure without fluid accumulation or late vasodilator drug tolerance.

Cody and associates[16] from New York City evaluated in 24 patients the interaction of cardiac function and sympathetic tone in severe CHF by assessing the cardiac index/plasma norepinephrine. Potential changes were assessed during first-dose and long-term captopril therapy, including sympathetic responsiveness to the gravitational stress of head-up tilt. Baseline cardiac index and norepinephrine levels demonstrated a significant inverse correlation (r = −0.640, p < 0.001). Norepinephrine decreased from 803 ± 116–635 ± 76 pg/ml following first-dose captopril therapy (p < 0.02), with

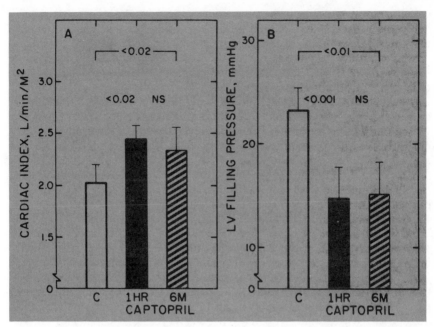

Fig. 8-2. Hemodynamic effects of oral captopril on cardiac index *(panel A)* and *LV* filling pressure *(panel B)* 1 h after initial drug ingestion and after 6 months *(6 M)* of continuous 3 times daily oral therapy. *C* = control. Reproduced with permission from Awan et al.[15]

overall hemodynamic improvement. Significant first-dose correlations were not observed. During long-term therapy, norepinephrine decreased from 694 ± 118–457 ± 106 pg/ml, associated with improvement of symptoms and exercise tolerance. The extent of cardiac index increase was matched by norepinephrine reduction, so that their correlation was maintained (r = −0.540, p < 0.02). First-dose and long-term therapy were associated with improved responsiveness of sympathetic tone to the reduction of cardiac index induced by the gravitational stress of tilt. In summary, sympathetic tone was increased in severe CHF, correlating inversely with cardiac function. Although there was improvement of cardiac function with first-dose captopril therapy, significant correlations of supine improvement with reduction of sympathetic tone were noted primarily with long-term therapy. Responsiveness of sympathetic tone to the stress of tilt, however, was evident during first-dose and long-term therapy.

In 15 patients with chronic CHF produced by CAD, Chatterjee and associates[17] from San Francisco, California, measured cardiac output and right-sided cardiac pressures before and after the oral angiotensin-converting enzyme inhibitor, captopril, which was administered in increasing doses. In 12 of 15 patients, coronary blood flow and in 11 patients myocardial oxygen extraction and consumption and lactate extraction also were determined before and after captopril therapy. Cardiac index and stroke volume index increased by an average of 25% and 27%, respectively. Pulmonary capillary wedge pressure also decreased in all patients (mean, 27%), suggesting improved LV function. The rate-pressure product, coronary blood flow, and myocardial oxygen consumption decreased significantly. In 1 of 11 patients there was myocardial lactate production, despite decreased myocardial oxygen demand and consumption. These findings suggest that in patients with chronic CHF, improved LV function with captopril is generally associated with decreased metabolic cost and that deterioration of metabolic function occurs infrequently.

Kugler and associates[18] from New York City studied the acute hemodynamic metabolic effects of captopril therapy in 12 patients with severe CHF during maximal exercise performed on an upright bicycle ergometer. During the control period, exhaustion occurred after 4.2 minutes of exercise, cardiac index (CI) increased from 1.5–3.4 liters/min/M^2 at exhaustion. Systemic arteriovenous oxygen difference (A-VO$_2$) increased (from 9–13 ml/100 ml) and oxygen uptake (VO$_2$) increased (from 3–11 ml/kg/min). The PA oxygen (O$_2$) content decreased (from 7–4 ml/100 ml) and femoral vein oxygen (FVO$_2$) content decreased (from 5–3 ml/100 ml). During captopril therapy, CI significantly increased both at rest (1.9 -vs- 1.5) and during maximal exercise (3.7 -vs- 3.4 liters/min/M^2). The A-VO$_2$ decreased significantly at rest (from 9–8 ml/100 ml) and during maximum exercise (from 13–12 ml/100 ml). The PAO$_2$ at exhaustion was significantly higher during captopril therapy than during the control period, whereas the FVO$_2$ was unchanged. Captopril therapy did not significantly increase maximal VO$_2$ or exercise duration. Thus, the acute administration of captopril to patients with severe CHF does not increase exercise capacity despite improved cardiac performance. Furthermore, captopril therapy does not acutely result in metabolic benefits to skeletal muscles during exercise.

The resting hemodynamic effects of captopril in CHF are relatively well known but little information is available on the hemodynamic response to exercise or changes in noninvasive measurements of the size and function of both ventricles. Massie and associates[19] from San Francisco, California, administered 25 mg of oral captopril to 14 stable New York Heart Association class III patients. Rest and exercise hemodynamic measurements and blood pool scintigrams were performed simultaneously before and 90 minutes after captopril. The radionuclide studies were analyzed for LV and RV end-diastolic volumes (EDV), end-systolic volumes (ESV), EF, and pulmonary blood volume (PBV). The primary beneficial responses at rest were decreased in LV EDV and RV EDV from 388–350 ml and from 52–43 volume units, respectively, and their corresponding filling pressures from 24–17 mmHg and 10–6 mmHg. Although stroke volume did not increase significantly, both LV EF and RV EF increased slightly from 19%–22% and from 25%–29%, respectively. During exercise, similar changes were noted in both hemodynamic and radionuclide indexes. Thus, with moderate symptomatic limitation from chronic CHF, captopril predominately reduces ventricular volume and filling pressure with a less significant effect on cardiac output. These effects persist during exercise, when systemic vascular resistance is already very low. Furthermore, radionuclide techniques are valuable in assessing the drug effect, particularly when ventricular volumes also are measured.

In 42 patients with moderate to severe CHF, the acute hemodynamic and neurohumoral response to captopril and teprotide were measured by Levine and Cohn[20] from Minneapolis, Minnesota. Plasma renin activity (PRA) was elevated and correlated with control plasma norepinephrine but not with any control hemodynamics. Acutely, converting enzyme inhibitors significantly decreased RA, PA capillary wedge, and mean arterial pressures, total systemic vascular resistance, pulmonary vascular resistance, and heart rate, and increased cardiac index. Control PRA correlated with the degree of hemodynamic change for PA pressure, pulmonary capillary wedge pressure, mean arterial pressure, systemic vascular resistance, and pulmonary vascular resistance. Long-term captopril therapy in 12 patients resulted in symptomatic improvement and a marked increase in exercise tolerance (7.4–10.4 minutes). These data suggest that converting enzyme inhibitors effect beneficial acute hemodynamic improvements in depressed LV function, leading to substantial reduction in disabling symptomatology and augmentation of exercise capacity in patients with stable severe CHF. Thus, captopril appears to provide well-tolerated, effective long-term ambulatory vasodilator therapy for advanced cardiac dysfunction.

The effects of long-term therapy with captopril were studied by Kugler and colleagues[21], from New York City in 11 patients with severe CHF. At initiation of therapy, cardiac index increased from 1.88–2.12 liters/min/M^2, whereas pulmonary capillary wedge pressure decreased from 28–18 mmHg. This improvement in resting cardiac performance was maintained during maximal exercise; however, maximal oxygen uptake was not acutely increased by captopril. During chronic therapy, 6 of the 11 patients showed symptomatic improvement; however, only 3 of these 6 patients demonstrated an increase in maximal oxygen uptake, which was measured at an average of 13 weeks following initiation of therapy. Five patients did not improve clinically during chronic therapy. In these patients, hemodynamic measurements that had improved initially after captopril returned to baseline values during chronic therapy. The addition of prazosin to chronic captopril therapy elicited a beneficial hemodynamic response in all 5 patients. Thus, the results of long-term therapy with captopril are variable in patients with severe CHF, and symptomatic improvement does not always correlate with objective measurement of exercise capacity. Combined alpha adrenergic blockade and angiotensin-converting enzyme inhibition appears safe in patients who fail to exhibit a sustained improvement on captopril alone.

Kluger and associates[22] from New York City studied 20 patients to determine the contribution of sympathetic tone and the renin-angiotensin system to the pathogenesis of CHF. In 20 paired studies of the same 10 patients, the baseline hemodynamic and hemodynamic and humoral correlates of CHF and the response to alpha adrenergic blockade with prazosin and captopril were assessed. Baseline renin activity ranged from normal to very elevated and baseline plasma catecholamine levels always were elevated. Baseline plasma norepinephrine values reflected the severity of CHF, correlating inversely with baseline cardiac index before administration of the drugs. Improvement in hemodynamic function occurred after acute therapy with either prazosin or captopril, but baseline renin and norepinephrine did not predict the response to prazosin. Baseline renin values did predict the response to captopril: pulmonary wedge pressure ($r = 0.776$, $p < 0.01$), stroke index ($r = 0.752$, $p < 0.02$), systemic vascular resistance ($r = 0.673$, $p < 0.05$). These data suggest that elevated levels of plasma norepinephrine correlates inversely with baseline cardiac function, but norepinephrine levels do not always change despite improved control of CHF following prazosin therapy. The renin-angiotensin system exhibited a wide spectrum of activity, and hemodynamic improvement following captopril was related to this activity. Absence of correlation between plasma norepinephrine and plasma renin activity suggested that their contributions to vasoconstriction were not interdependent. Increased sympathetic tone was consistently found in patients with severe CHF, whereas renin-angiotensin activity differed widely. From these data, it appears that the hemodynamic response to captopril can be used to identify a subset of patients with severe CHF and angiotensin-renin abnormalities.

Halperin and associates[23] from New York City evaluated the coronary hemodynamic effects of vasodilator therapy with captopril and teprotide in 11 patients with CAD and severe CHF. During 2 hours of therapy, systemic vascular resistance was reduced from 2,408 ± 240 to 1,715 ± 170 dynes/s/cm^{-5} ($p < 0.001$) and cardiac output improved by 19%, resulting in lower arterial pressure (101 ± 8–86 ± 5 mmHg, $p < 0.001$) and LV filling pressure (30 ± 2–21 ± 2 mmHg, $p < 0.001$). Coronary sinus thermodilution blood flow paralleled perfusion pressure did not vary overall in response to these agents. Coronary vascular resistance also was unchanged. There was no change in the coronary arteriovenous oxygen content difference or calculated oxygen consumption. Heart rate and systolic BP product decreased significantly in response to these interventions ($p < 0.02$). These data suggest that hemodynamic improvement from captopril and teprotide are dependent on a reduction in the angiotensin-mediated ventricular afterload and preload. These agents produce no effect on coronary vasomotor tone in patients with advanced CHF from CAD.

The hemodynamic effects of captopril alone and in combination with the beta adrenergic receptor agonist terbutaline were evaluated by Awan and colleagues[24] from Davis, California, in 10 patients with severe chronic CHF. The heart rate remained unchanged, whereas captopril lowered mean systemic BP from 86–64 mmHg, and decreased LV filling pressure markedly from 27–19 mmHg. The addition of terbutaline produced no further change in these variables. Simultaneously, captopril augmented cardiac index from 2.1–2.9 liters/min/M^2 and stroke index from 27–37 ml/beat/M^2. Concomitant captopril plus terbutaline further raised cardiac index to 3.2 liters/min/M^2

and stroke index to 40 ml/beat/M^2. Further, the captopril-effected decline in total systemic vascular resistance from 1,577–841 dynes · s · cm^{-5} was not reduced additionally by captopril plus terbutaline combination. These results indicate that both captopril and terbutaline markedly augment cardiac function in CHF. Moreover, the salutary effects of the systemic vasodilator appear additive to the beneficial actions of the beta adrenergic receptor agonist, thereby providing substantial augmentation of the function of the failing heart.

Rouleau and colleagues[25] from San Francisco, California, evaluated changes in coronary hemodynamics, myocardial metabolism, and LV function in 14 patients with CHF after the administration of captopril, prazosin, and hydralazine. Eleven patients received captopril in incremental doses until the arterial pressure decreased by 10 mmHg, 11 patients received prazosin, and 10 patients received hydralazine. The control hemodynamics and metabolic variables before each drug were similar. All 3 vasodilators increased cardiac index (captopril 19%, prazosin 29%, and hydralazine 36%) and decreased the pulmonary capillary wedge pressure (captopril 24–17 mmHg, prazosin 20–13 mmHg, and hydralazine 19–16 mmHg) thus indicating improved LV function with all 3 agents. The average rate-pressure product decreased after captopril and prazosin by 27% and 14%, respectively, but only captopril decreased the myocardial oxygen consumption significantly (19%). There was myocardial lactate production, indicating ischemia in 1 patient with captopril, 2 patients with prazosin, and 2 patients with hydralazine. Thus, in patients with chronic CHF only captopril consistently improved LV function at a decreased metabolic cost. Despite improved hemodynamics and LV function, metabolic function can deteriorate during vasodilator therapy in some patients with chronic CHF from CAD.

Four studies were conducted by Packer and associates[26] from New York City in 36 patients with severe chronic CHF to compare the central hemodynamic effects of captopril to other vasodilator agents. Although captopril produced less marked increases in cardiac output than did hydralazine (n, 14), nitroprusside (n, 15), or prazosin (n, 7), it produced decreases in LV filling pressures similar to nitroprusside and prazosin but more than hydralazine. Captopril and isosorbide dinitrate (n, 11) produced similar decreases in systemic vascular resistance and LV filling pressure. However, cardiac output increased less with captopril than with nitrates, because heart rate slowed during captopril therapy. In addition, mean RA pressure decreased less with captopril than with nitrates, because captopril had minimal effects on limb venous capacitance and pulmonary arteriolar resistance. Alterations in LV pressure-volume relations likely contributed to the marked decreases in LV filling pressures with captopril. Thus, the central hemodynamic effects of captopril differ significantly from other vasodilator drugs used in the treatment of CHF. These effects cannot be characterized simply in terms of balanced peripheral arterial and venous vasodilation; captopril exerts highly complex effects on peripheral vessels as well as having actions independent of its peripheral vasodilator effects.

SALBUTAMOL

Since the efficacy of oral long-acting sympathomimetic drugs is not well established, Mifune and colleagues[27] from Tokyo, Japan, investigated the hemodynamic effects of orally administered salbutamol in 8 CHF patients. Cardiac index, heart rate, BP, and LV filling pressure were monitored for 6 hours after a single oral administration of 4–8 mg salbutamol and placebo. In patients who had received salbutamol, a 40% increase in cardiac index was noted 1 hour postadministration; a 44% increase occurred at 2 hours; and a significant increase persisted for 6 hours. Changes in heart rate showed a similar time course; however, the increase was less pronounced (+27%). The changes in BP were slight and no patient developed complications. After placebo administration, no consistent changes in the hemodynamic parameters were noted. This study suggests that, due to its sustained positive action on cardiac output, the oral administration of salbutamol may be efficacious in ambulatory patients with low cardiac output due to CHF.

AMRINONE

In 6 patients with severe CHF refractory to conventional therapy, including vasodilators, Maskin and associates[28] from New York City treated with oral amrinone for 20–72 weeks (mean, 41). At initiation of therapy, the cardiac index increased from 1.7 ± 0.3–2.6 ± 0.5 liters/min/M^2 ($p < 0.01$) and pulmonary capillary wedge pressure decreased from 26 ± 3–19 ± 5 mmHg ($p < 0.05$). Symptoms were alleviated and exercise capacity increased from 6 ± 4–11 ± 4 minutes ($p < 0.05$). During long-term therapy, exercise capacity remained constant in 3 patients, whereas it decreased in 3. All patients had an increase in heart size. Withdrawal of amrinone therapy precipitated severe CHF at rest and hemodynamic deterioration in all 6 patients. The cardiac index decreased from 1.9 ± 0.5–1.3 ± 0.3 liters/min/M^2 ($p < 0.05$) and pulmonary capillary wedge pressure rose from 21 ± 3–29 ± 6 mmHg ($p < 0.05$). These changes were reversed by reinstitution of therapy. Thus, amrinone-dependent hemodynamic benefits were demonstrated during long-term therapy without tachyphylaxis. Additionally, progression of the underlying cardiac disease was observed in every patient.

PROSTACYCLIN

Yui and colleagues[29] from Kyoto, Japan, evaluated the acute hemodynamic effects of intravenous prostacyclin in 9 patients with severe CHF refractory to digitalis and diuretics. After prostacyclin infusion, pulmonary capillary wedge pressure decreased from 21 ± 8–15 ± 7 mmHg, mean arterial pressure from 99 ± 13–76 ± 7 mmHg, systemic vascular resistance from 2,574 ± 384–1,368 ± 283 dynes/s/cm^{-5}, pulmonary vascular resistance from 1,008 ± 451–443 ± 135 dynes/s/cm^{-5}, and pulmonary arteriolar resistance from 330 ± 111–189 ± 73 dynes/s/cm^{-5} (p < 0.001). Heart rate increased from 78 ± 21–82 ± 24 beats/minute, cardiac index from 2.0 ± 0.37–3.2 ± 0.59 liters/min/M^2, and stroke index from 28 ± 9–42 ± 0.6 cc/M^2) (p < 0.001). Thus, prostacyclin infusion does improve the hemodynamics in patients with CHF refractory to traditional therapy.

TERBUTALINE

The hemodynamic effects of terbutaline infusion at rates of 0.15, 0.3, and 0.45 μg/kg/minute were studied and compared in 8 patients with severe CHF by Wang and colleagues[30] from Hartford, Connecticut. Terbutaline infusion at 0.15 μg/kg/minute infusion produced insignificant effects at 30 minutes. At 0.3 μg/kg/minute infusion, highly significant beneficial hemodynamic effects were observed: at 60 minutes cardiac index increased from 1.79–3.60 liters/min/M^2 and stroke volume index increased from 20.1–36.7 ml/beat/M^2; mean PA wedge pressure fell from 28–19 mmHg; systemic vascular resistance fell from 2,624–1,455 dynes · s · cm^{-5}/M^2; and pulmonary vascular resistance, from 248–150 dynes · s · cm^{-5}/M^2. Mean arterial pressure and oxygen uptake did not change significantly; however, mean heart rate increased from 93–103 beats/minute and plasma potassium fell from 3.86–3.12 mEq/liter. The 0.45 μg/kg/minute infusion at 30 minutes produced no greater hemodynamic changes than that from 0.3 μg/kg/minute. This study suggests that intravenous terbutaline produces beneficial effects and may be useful in the acute management of severe CHF.

RELATED TOPICS

Catecholamine activity

Francis and associates[31] from Minneapolis, Minnesota, studied 14 patients with CHF to evaluate the activity of the sympathetic nervous system during dynamic upright exercise. Plasma norepinephrine and epinephrine levels were measured in the basal upright posture before and during maximal exercise. Results were compared with those in 6 healthy control subjects before and during maximal exercise. Plasma norepinephrine increased during exercise from a mean (±SE of the mean) of 650–1,721 pg/ml in the group with CHF. This increase was significantly less than that of the control group (318 ± 36–3,230 ± 418 pg/ml). However, for equivalent levels of body oxygen consumption, the group with CHF had higher levels of plasma norepinephrine than the control group. Plasma norepinephrine was similar in the 2 groups in the basal upright position, but it increased more during exercise in the normal subjects than in the group with CHF. These data demonstrate alterations in the sympathetic nervous system during exercise in patients with CHF. Norepinephrine increases in patients with CHF to a greater extent than in normal subjects with lower levels of exercise, but the extremely high levels of norepinephrine and epinephrine generated by normal subjects during maximal exercise do not occur in patients with CHF.

Levine and associates[32] from Minneapolis, Minnesota, studied 55 hospitalized patients with CHF to make resting hemodynamic measurements and obtain plasma for catecholamine and renin determinations. Plasma norepinephrine values (mean ±SE of the mean, 594 ± 51 pg/ml; range, 153–1,868) and plasma renin activity (mean, 12.9 ± 2.4 ng/ml/hr; range, 0.6–85.2) were significantly higher than in normal subjects (p < 0.01). Twenty-six of these patients had plasma norepinephrine and renin determinations on 3 successive days and these values did not change significantly. In contrast, plasma epinephrine (mean, 138 ± 26 pg/ml; range, 24–1,099) increased significantly at the time of an invasive hemodynamic study, probably because of stress-induced mechanisms. Baseline plasma norepinephrine values, when compared with resting hemodynamic values, demonstrated significant correlations with: right atrial pressure (r = 0.44), PA pressure (r = 0.45), pulmonary capillary wedge pressure (r = 0.42), pulmonary vascular resistance (r = 0.55), pulmonary arteriolar resistance (r = 0.41), cardiac index (r = 0.42), systemic vascular resistance (r = 0.30), and heart rate (r = 0.52). Plasma renin activity was only weakly correlated with plasma norepinephrine (r = 0.38) and did not correlate significantly with any hemodynamic measurement. These data are from subsets of patients with CHF in whom the severity of CHF correlated with neurohumoral activity. Sympathetic responses appear to be either a marker of or a contributor to the hemodynamic derangements in such patients. Since hemodynamic abnormalities did not correlate with plasma renin activity, it appears that the renin-angiotensin and catecholamine systems are activated independently in patients with CHF.

Seventeen patients with chronic CHF were studied by Francis and colleagues[33] from Minneapolis, Minnesota, to assess the relation of resting LV function, as measured by noninvasive and invasive methods, to maximal exercise capacity, as measured by peak total body oxygen consumption (VO_2). Supine basal plasma norepinephrine also was measured to evaluate its relation to the severity of CHF and to determine whether it may be a better predictor of exercise capacity in CHF patients than the more commonly employed noninvasive and invasive tests of LV function. Of the 17 patients, 14 underwent upright bicycle exercise to their symptomatic maximum. There was no significant correlation between peak VO_2 and the noninvasive measurements of LV performance obtained at rest, including cardiothoracic ratio, LV internal dimension by M-mode echo, percent shortening of the minor axis by M-mode echo, and radionuclide EF. Hemodynamic measurements were performed in 16 patients. The hemodynamic measurements at rest also failed to correlate with exercise capacity. The supine basal plasma norepinephrine, which was elevated in 17 patients, had an inverse relation with stroke work index and stroke index, and a positive correlation with RA pressure. Although both noninvasive and invasive measurements at rest failed to correlate significantly with peak $\dot{V}O_2$ during exercise, the plasma norepinephrine had a significant inverse correlation with peak exercise $\dot{V}O_2$. The basal supine plasma norepinephrine therefore is elevated in patients with CHF, is a marker for the severity of CHF as measured by hemodynamics performed at rest, and is a better predictor of exercise capacity than standard noninvasive and invasive tests performed at rest.

Perhaps the most likely location for a primary abnormality in cardiac failure is in the specialized cellular components that modulate calcium flux, some of which reside in the sarcolemma. One component of this system is the beta adrenergic receptor; through combination with a hormone agonist, this receptor may stimulate the enzyme adenylate cyclase to form cyclic AMP, which in turn may promote transmembrane calcium flux. Although a fully functioning beta adrenergic system is not necessary for normal cardiac function in nondiseased hearts performing under basal conditions, beta adrenergic stimulation does contribute to the mechanical response to stress and is important in supporting cardiac function in CHF. Thus, an abnormality of the beta adrenergic receptor pathway might explain the presence of effort-induced symptoms and stress-related performance abnormalities in patients with myocardial dysfunction and might explain the clinical deterioration that occurs once heart muscle disease has developed. To identify the role of the myocardial beta adrenergic pathway in CHF, Bristow and associates[34] from Stanford, California, examined beta adrenergic receptor density, adenylate cyclase and creatine kinase (CK) activities, muscle contraction in vitro, and myocardial contractile protein levels in the left ventricles of failing and normally functioning hearts from cardiac transplant recipients or prospective donors. Eleven failing left ventricles had a 50%–56% reduction in beta receptor density, a 45% reduction in maximal isoproterenol-mediated adenylate cyclase stimulation, and a 54%–73% reduction in maximal isoproterenol-stimulated muscle contraction, compared with 6 normally functioning ventricles ($p < 0.05$ for each comparison). In contrast, cytoplasmic CK activity, adenylate cyclase activities stimulated by fluoride ion and by histamine, histamine-stimulated muscle contraction, and levels of contractile protein were not different in the 2 groups ($p > 0.05$). Thus, in failing human hearts a decrease in beta receptor density leads to subsensitivity of the beta adrenergic pathway and decreased beta agonist-stimulated muscle contraction. Regulation of beta adrenergic receptors may be an important variable in cardiac failure.

Antidiuretic hormone

In advanced CHF, severe edema develops associated with hyponatremia. In 20 patients with severe CHF, Riegger and associates[35] from Würzburg,

West Germany, studied plasma antidiuretic hormone (ADH) concentrations related to hemodynamics and plasma osmolality. Prazosin was used to test the acute response to changes in atrial receptors and hemofiltration to test the response to changes in volume receptors. One group of patients had inappropriately high ADH values (14.5 ± 8.8 pg/ml) in relation to their plasma osmolality, which was well below normal values (276 ± 23 mosmol/ kg water) with no apparent osmoregulatory control. The other group showed a normal relation of ADH and plasma osmolality (3.9 ± 1.0 pg/ml; 289 ± 8 mosmol/kg water). Only in the normally regulating group did lowering of LA pressure by prazosin result in a rise in ADH related to the decrease in pressure. Inappropriately high ADH secretion could be reversed by hemofiltration. This suggests that the syndrome of "dilutional hypo-osmolality" in severe CHF may be caused by an inappropriately high ADH secretion in which the osmoreceptor system is dominated by nonosmolar stimuli; however, it cannot be ruled out that associated hemodynamic effects in the kidney or other intrarenal or hormonal factors contribute to this mechanism.

Hyponatremia

The renin-angiotensin system may play an important homeostatic role in both experimental and clinical CHF. Increased circulating angiotensin II could contribute to systemic vasoconstriction which supports BP but also might adversely affect LV performance. Plasma renin activity (PRA) varies widely in patients with CHF but the mechanism of its stimulation in some patients and not in others is unclear. Hemodynamics, renal failure, or volume factors all might be expected to stimulate the renin-angiotensin system. Because a beneficial hemodynamic response in patients with CHF to agents that block the activity of the renin-angiotensin system has been observed, an understanding of the factors that stimulate it in CHF and the recognition of clinical correlates of high PRA appear to have important therapeutic implications. Accordingly, Levine and associates[36] from Minneapolis, Minnesota, explored the possible influence of hemodynamic and renal functional factors on PRA in 36 patients with moderate to severe CHF. A thermodilution Swan-Ganz flow-directed balloon-tipped catheter was inserted and placed into the PA where it was inflated to occlude a PA branch. The brachial artery also was cannulated. In 6 other patients a catheter was placed for the central venous pressure recording.

Resting hemodynamic, renal functional, and electrolyte data were obtained from all 42 patients. The low cardiac index and high right atrial and pulmonary capillary wedge pressures reflected the severity of the CHF. Renal function was moderately diminished, as was evident from the slightly increased blood urea nitrogen and creatinine. Serum sodium correlated inversely with PRA. The degree of CHF measured by RA pressure, pulmonary capillary wedge pressure, cardiac index, and systemic vascular resistance did not correlate with PRA. Similarly, renal function as measured by blood urea nitrogen, creatinine, and urinary sodium excretion did not correlate with PRA. In a prospectively screened group, 7 patients with CHF who were found to be hyponatremic had PRA > 15 ng/ml/hour. Serial determinations in 1 patient showed PRA to vary inversely with the serum sodium. Thus, serum sodium can be used to identify those patients with CHF who have a high PRA. The value of identifying these high renin CHF patients was seen in their response in 4 cases to specific therapy with a converting enzyme inhibitor.

Hypocalcemia

Calcium ions have a key role in the excitation and the contraction of cardiac muscle cells. Calcium also influences the renal excretion of sodium. The importance of sodium retention in the pathogenesis of CHF has been well described. It is therefore suprising that clinical evidence of CHF is observed so infrequently in calcium-deficiency states. A few patients with hypocalcemia who acquired cardiomegaly and CHF that appeared to be refractory to therapy until the serum calcium concentration was raised have been described. The relation between the level of serum calcium and recovery, however, has not been defined. Furthermore, the effect of hypocalcemia on cardiac function in patients with known underlying heart disease has not been well described. Connor and associates[37] from Baltimore, Maryland, studied a 76-year-old woman with hyperparathyroidism who became refractory to conventional therapy for CHF after hypocalcemia occurred. The CHF resolved only when the hypocalcemia was corrected. This sequence of events, which was observed on 3 separate occasions, indicates that CHF may be refractory in the presence of hypocalcemia. The observations in their patient indicate that in patients with unexplained or refractory CHF, the possibility of unrecognized hypocalcemia as a contributing factor should be considered.

Cardiac reserve and functional status

Muscular work requires the integration of cardiopulmonary mechanisms for gas exchange and oxygen delivery. The response of these mechanisms may be impaired in patients with chronic cardiac failure and the pattern of oxygen utilization and gas exchange during exercise can provide an objective assessment of the severity of CHF. Weber and colleagues[38] from Philadelphia, Pennsylvania, examined the rates of air flow, oxygen uptake, CO_2 elimination, and minute ventilation during progressive treadmill exercise in 62 patients with stable CHF. Exercise cardiac output, systemic oxygen extraction, and lactate production were measured directly in 40 patients with CHF of varying severity. As the severity of the CHF increased from class A to class D, there was a progressive decrease in exercise capacity from 1,157–373 seconds and maximum oxygen utilization from 23–8 ml/min/kg. These decreases corresponded with the reduced maximum oxygen output and stroke volume during exercise. The appearance of anaerobic metabolism and the corresponding anaerobic threshold, determined noninvasively, were reproducible and correlated with the rise in mixed venous lactate concentration. No apparent untoward effects were experienced during or after the

420 • CARDIOLOGY 1983

progressive exercise tests. These investigators concluded that the measurement of respiratory gas exchange and air flow during exercise is an objective reproducible and safe noninvasive method for characterizing cardiac reserve and functional status in patients with chronic CHF.

References

1. LEE DCS, JOHNSON RA, BINGHAM JB, LEAHY M, DINSMORE RE, GOROLL AH, NEWELL JB, STRAUSS HW, HABER E: Heart failure in outpatients. A randomized trial of digoxin versus placebo. N Engl J Med 306:699–705, March 25, 1982.

2. FLEG JL, GOTTLIEB SH, LAKATTA EG: Is digoxin really important in treatment of compensated heart failure? A placebo-controlled crossover study in patients with sinus rhytym. Am J Med 73:244–250, Aug 1982.

3. HECHT HS, KARAHALIOS SE, SCHNUGG SJ, ORMISTON JA, HOPKINS JM, ROSE JG, SINGH BN: Improvement in supine bicycle exercise performance in refractory congestive heart failure after isosorbide dinitrate: radionuclide and hemodynamic evaluation of acute effects. Am J Cardiol 49:133–140, Jan 1982.

4. HAQ A, RAKOWSKI H, BAIGRIE R, McLAUGHLIN P, BURNS R, TIHAL H, HILTON D, FEIGLIN D: Vasodilator therapy in refractory congestive heart failure: a comparative analysis of hemodynamic and noninvasive studies. Am J Cardiol 49:439–444, Feb 1982.

5. PACKER M, MELLER J, MEDINA N, YUSHAK M, GORLIN R: Hemodynamic characterization of tolerance to long-term hydralazine therapy in severe chronic heart failure. N Engl J Med 306:57–62, Jan 14, 1982.

6. MAGORIEN RD, BROWN GP, UNVERFERTH DV, NELSON S, BOUDOULAS H, BAMBACH D, LEIER CV: Effects of hydralazine on coronary blood flow and myocardial energetics in CHF. Circulation 65:528–533, March 1982.

7. RUBIN SA, BROWN HV, SWAN HJC: Arterial oxygenation and arterial oxygen transport in chronic myocardial failure at rest, during exercise and after hydralazine treatment. Circulation 66:143–148, July 1982.

8. FIRTH BG, DEHMER GJ, MARKHAM RV, WILLERSON JT, HILLIS LD: Assessment of vasodilator therapy in patients with severe congestive heart failure: limitations of measurements of left ventricular ejection fraction and volumes. Am J Cardiol 50:954–959, Nov 1982.

9. McKAY CR, CHATTERJEE K, PORTS TA, HOLLY AN, PARMLEY WW: Minoxidil therapy in chronic congestive heart failure: acute plus long-term hemodynamic and clinical study. Am Heart J 104:575–580, Sept 1982.

10. NATHAN M, RUBIN SA, SIEMIENCZUK D, SWAN HJC: Effects of acute and chronic minoxidil administration on rest and exercise hemodynamics and clinical status in patients with severe, chronic heart failure. Am J Cardiol 50:960–966, Nov 1982.

11. CODY RJ, COVIT A, SCHAER G, WILLIAMS G: Captopril pharmacokinetics and the acute hemodynamic and hormonal response in patients with severe chronic congestive heart failure. Am Heart J 104:1180–1183, Nov 1982.

12. CREAGER MA, FAXON DP, HELPERIN JL, MELIDOSSIAN CD, McCABE CH, SCHICK EC, RYAN TJ: Determinants of clinical response and survival in patients with congestive heart failure treated with captopril. Am Heart J 104:1147–1154, Nov 1982.

13. COWLEY AJ, ROWLEY JM, STAINER KL, HAMPTON JR: Captopril therapy for heart failure. A placebo controlled study. Lancet 2:730–732, Oct 2, 1982.

14. FOUAD FM, TARAZI RC, BRAVO EL, HART NJ, CASTLE LW, SALCEDO EE: Long-term control of

congestive heart failure with captopril. Am J Cardiol 49:1489–1496, Apr 1982.

15. AWAN NA, AMSTERDAM EA, HERMANOVICH J, BOMMER WJ, NEEDHAM KE, MASON DT: Long-term hemodynamic and clinical efficacy of captopril therapy in ambulatory management of severe chronic congestive heart failure. Am Heart J 103:474–479, Apr 1982.

16. CODY RJ, FRANKLIN KW, KLUGER J, LARAGH JH: Sympathetic responsiveness and plasma norepinephrine during therapy of chronic congestive heart failure with captopril. Am J Med 72:791–797, May 1982.

17. CHATTERJEE K, ROULEAU JL, PARMLEY WW: Hemodynamic and myocardial metabolic effects of captopril in chronic heart failure. Br Heart J 47:233–238, March 1982.

18. KUGLER J, MASKIN C, FRISHMAN WH, SONNENBLICK EH, LEJEMTEL TH: Regional and systemic metabolic effects of angiotensin-converting enzyme inhibition during exercise in patients with severe heart failure. Circulation 66:1256–1261, Dec 1982.

19. MASSIE B, KRAMER BL, TOPIC N, HENDERSON SG: Hemodynamic and radionuclide effects of acute captopril therapy for heart failure: changes in left and right ventricular volumes and function at rest and during exercise. Circulation 65:1374–1381, June 1982.

20. LEVINE TB, COHN JN: Determinants of acute and long-term response to converting enzyme inhibitors in congestive heart failure. Am Heart J 104:1159–1164, Nov 1982.

21. KUGLER J, MASKIN CS, FRISHMAN W, SONNENBLICK EH, LEJEMTEL TH: Variable clinical response to long-term angiotensin inhibition in severe heart failure: demonstration of additive benefits of alpha-receptor blockade. Am Heart J 104:1154–1159, Nov 1982.

22. KLUGER J, CODY RJ, LARAGH JH: The contributions of sympathetic tone and the renin-angiotensin system to severe chronic congestive heart failure: response to specific inhibitors (prazosin and captopril). Am J Cardiol 49:1667–1674, May 1982.

23. HALPERIN JL, FAXON DP, CREAGER MA, BASS TA, MELIDOSSIAN CD, GAVRAS H, RYAN TJ: Coronary hemodynamic effects of angiotensin inhibition by captopril and teprotide in patients with congestive heart failure. Am J Cardiol 50:967–972, Nov 1982.

24. AWAN NA, NEEDHAM KE, LUI H, RUTLEDGE J, AMSTERDAM EA, MASON DT: Complementary combined captopril and terbutaline therapy in severe chronic congestive heart failure. Am Heart J 104:1224–1228, Nov 1982.

25. ROULEAU JL, CHATTERJEE K, BENGE W, PARMLEY WW, HIRAMATSU B: Alterations in LV function and coronary hemodynamics with captopril, hydralazine, and prazosin in chronic ischemic heart failure: a comparative study. Circulation 65:671–678, Apr 1982.

26. PACKER M, MEDINA N, YUSHAK M: Contrasting hemodynamic responses in severe heart failure: comparison of captopril and other vasodilator drugs. Am Heart J 104:1215–1223, Nov 1982.

27. MIFUNE J, KURAMOTO K, UEDA K, MATSUSHITA S, KUWAJIMA I, SAKAI M, IWASAKI T, MOROKI N, MURAKAMI M: Hemodynamic effects of salbutamol, an oral long-acting beta-stimulant, in patients with congestive heart failure. Am Heart J 104:1011–1015, Nov 1982.

28. MASKIN CS, FORMAN R, KLEIN NA, SONNENBLICK EH, LEJEMTEL TH: Long-term amrinone therapy in patients with severe congestive heart failure: drug-dependent thermodynamic benefits despite progression of the disease. Am J Med 72:113–118, Jan 1982.

29. YUI Y, NAKAJIMA H, KAWAI C, MURAKAMI T: Prostacyclin therapy in patients with congestive heart failure. Am J Cardiol 50:320–324, Aug 1982.

30. WANG RYC, TSE TF, YU DYC, LEE PK, CHOW MSS: Beneficial hemodynamic effects of intravenous terbutaline in patients with severe heart failure. Am Heart J 104:1016–1021, Nov 1982.

31. FRANCIS GS, GOLDSMITH SR, ZIESCHE SM, COHN JN: Response of plasma norepinephrine and epinephrine to dynamic exercise in patients with congestive heart failure. Am J Cardiol 49:1152–1156, Apr 1982.

32. LEVINE TB, FRANCIS GS, GOLDSMITH SR, SIMON AB, COHN JN: Activity of the sympathetic nervous system and renin-angiotensin system assessed by plasma hormone levels and their

relation to hemodynamic abnormalities in congestive heart failure. Am J Cardiol 49:1659–1666, May 1982.

33. Francis GS, Goldsmith SR, Cohn JN: Relationship of exercise capacity to resting left ventricular performance and basal plasma norepinephrine levels in patients with congestive heart failure. Am Heart J 104:725–731, Oct 1982.

34. Bristow MR, Ginsburg R, Minobe W, Cubicciotti RS, Sageman WS, Lurie K, Billingham ME, Harrison DC, Stinson EB: Decreased catecholamine sensitivity and beta-adrenergic-receptor density in failing human hearts. N Engl J Med 307:205–211, July 22, 1982.

35. Riegger GAJ, Liebau G, Kochsiek K: Antidiuretic hormone in congestive heart failure. Am J Med 72:49–52, Jan 1982.

36. Levine TB, Franciosa JA, Vrobel T, Cohn JN: Hyponatremia as a marker for high renin heart failure. Br Heart J 47:161–166, Feb 1982.

37. Connor TB, Rosen BL, Blaustein MP, Applefeld MM, Doyle LA: Hypocalcemia precipitating congestive heart failure. N Engl J Med 307:869–872, Sept 30, 1982.

38. Weber KT, Kinasewitz GT, Janicki JS, Fishman AP: Oxygen utilization and ventilation during exercise in patients with chronic cardiac failure. Circulation 65:1213–1223, June 1982.

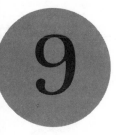

Miscellaneous Topics

PERICARDIAL HEART DISEASE

Subepicardial fat producing extra echo spaces

Of 844 patients having echoes, Wada and associates[1] from Yokohama and Kanagawa, Japan, found 700 with clinically inexplicable extra echo spaces. Of these 700 patients, 50 had computerized tomography of their hearts which showed the extra echo spaces to be caused either by anterior or posterior subepicardial fat. Its frequency increased with age (Table 9-1). Thus, subepicardial fat should be recognized as the cause of such extra echo spaces.

ECG criteria for diagnosis

The differentiation of the ECG changes of acute pericarditis from the normal variant with early repolarization has long been a problem for clinicians and electrocardiographers. Ginzton and Laks[2] from Torrance, California, examined the quantitative ECG differentiation of acute pericarditis from normal variant ST/T changes. The ECGs of 19 patients with acute pericarditis were compared with those of 20 subjects with typical normal variant changes. Patients were excluded if their ECGs demonstrated condi-

TABLE 9-1. *Extra echo spaces by age. Reproduced with permission from Wada et al.*[1]

| | | EXTRA ECHO SPACES | | |
| | | | POSTERIOR | |
DECADE	# OF PATIENTS	ANTERIOR	SYSTOLIC	SYSTOLIC/ DIASTOLIC
0–9	9	0	0	0
10–19	32	15 (46.8%)	0	0
20–29	57	33 (57.8%)	7 (12.2%)	0
30–39	98	79 (80.6%)	25 (25.5%)	13 (13.2%)
40–49	158	146 (92.4%)	69 (43.6%)	40 (25.3%)
50–59	139	135 (97.1%)	60 (43.1%)	49 (35.2%)
60–69	101	97 (96.0%)	42 (41.5%)	37 (36.6%)
70–79	82	78 (95.1%)	23 (28.0%)	42 (51.2%)
80–89	24	24 (100%)	3 (12.5%)	19 (79.1%)
Total	700	607 (86.7%)	229 (32.7%)	200 (28.5%)

tions that markedly altered repolarization. The positive and negative predictive values of previously recorded criteria were not high. In the present study, a T-wave amplitude in lead V_6 < 0.3 mV was diagnostic of acute pericarditis with high statistical significance, but there was overlap of patients between the groups. The ratio of the amplitude of the onset of the ST segment to the amplitude of the T wave in that lead (ST/T ratio in V_6) proved to be the most reliable discriminator. An ST/T ratio >0.25 was diagnostic in all patients with acute pericarditis. The ST/T ratio >0.25 mV in V_4 and V_5 as well as I were also significant discriminators. If V_6 is unavailable, an ST/T ratio >0.25 in V_4 V_5 or I is highly suggestive of acute pericarditis. An ST/T ratio >0.25 mV in V_6 discriminated the ECGs of all patients with acute pericarditis from normal variants in this study.

Diastolic collapse of the right ventricle with tamponade

Armstrong and associates[3] from Indianapolis, Indiana, evaluated a newly described echo sign for the detection of cardiac tamponade retrospectively in 91 patients. M-mode echo was reviewed in 86 patients, 36 of whom had concurrent 2-D echo examinations; in 5 patients, only 2-D echo was performed. Cardiac tamponade was present clinically in 17 patients, 14 of whom had abnormal posterior motion of the RV free wall in early diastole. Two of the 17 patients with tamponade had equivocally abnormal motion and 1 had normal wall motion. The patient with normal wall motion was later proved to have predominately constrictive pericardial disease. In all cases, the abnormal wall motion reverted to normal after a definitive drainage procedure. The 2-D echo confirmed that the abnormal RV wall motion represented a true collapse of the RV cavity in early diastole. Of the 69 patients without clinical cardiac tamponade, only 7 had abnormal RV wall motion. Detection of abnormal diastolic RV wall motion may be a sensitive indicator of a hemodynamically significant pericardial effusion. Conversely, the presence of normal motion of the RV free wall appears to be a reliable indicator that the pericardial effusion is exerting little effect on overall cardiac function.

Left ventricular volume and function during and after tamponade

To determine the causes of cardiac failure during cardiac tamponade in man, Grose and associates[4] from New York City studied LV volume and function in 8 patients during pericardiocentesis using gated equilibrium radionuclide ventriculography. In the 7 patients with clinical and hemodynamic evidence of cardiac tamponade, end-diastolic (EDV) and end-systolic volumes (ESV) increased progressively as the initial 500 ml of fluid were removed. The most marked increase occurred during the removal of the first 200 ml of pericardial fluid. After removal of 500 ml of pericardial fluid, the EDV increased from 52–111 ml and ESV from 17–34 ml. Additional aspiration of fluid resulted in no further changes in LV volume. The EF averaged 70% before removal of fluid and was unchanged by pericardiocentesis. In the patient who did not have hemodynamic evidence of tamponade, there were only minor changes in LV volumes and EF. These data suggest that LV pump function is well preserved in cardiac tamponade and that the diminution in stroke volume and consequent cardiovascular collapse in tamponade are due to marked LV underfilling.

Volume expansion plus nitroprusside -vs- pericardial Centesis in tamponade

Acute cardiac tamponade is a medical emergency that requires urgent therapy. Removal of the pericardial fluid obviously is affective but delays may occur while the catheterization laboratory or operating room is being prepared. Alternative methods would be useful as interim therapy, if they were also effective. The time-honored emergency therapy for acute cardiac tamponade is intravascular volume expansion. Vasodilator drugs also have been recommended, especially in combination with volume expansion. These recommendations, however, are based on studies in nonhuman animals. There is a surprising paucity of relevant data on humans. Thus, Kerber and associates[5] from Iowa City, Iowa, assessed the hemodynamic effects of 2 recommended interventions, volume expansion and nitroprusside infusion, in 11 patients with acute cardiac tamponade. They found that these interventions effected virtually no hemodynamic or symptomatic improvement, in contrast to the major benefits of pericardial fluid withdrawal. Thus, the definitive emergency therapy for tamponade remains pericardiocentesis or surgical drainage and the use of these procedures should not be delayed in the expectation that other interventions will confer major hemodynamic benefit.

Treatment by subxiphoid pericardiotomy

Alcan and associates[6] from New York City treated by subxiphoid pericardiotomy performed under local anesthesia 18 patients with cardiac tamponade. This group included 9 patients with uremic pericarditis, 5 with metastatic cancer, 2 with trauma, 1 with tuberculosis, and 1 of unknown cause. Immediate relief of the acute tamponade was achieved in all 18 patients with only minor and self-limiting postoperative complications, including supraventricular arrhythmias (5 patients) and fever (5 patients). None died in either the operative period or from reaccumulation of the pericardial fluid. The drainage period averaged 10 days (range, 3–28). The authors consider subxiphoid pericardiotomy to be a safe and effective method for the management of pericardial effusion of diverse causes. Because the surgeon was able to obtain a biopsy of the parietal pericardium and because the procedure was safe, the authors considered this procedure superior to both needle pericardiocentesis and pericardiectomy in the acutely ill patient.

Immune reactions in tuberculous and constrictive pericarditis

Maisch and associates[7] from Würzburg, West Germany, studied 12 patients with exudative tuberculous pericarditis, 10 with constrictive pericarditis due to previous tuberculosis, 10 with viral pericarditis, 20 with pulmonary tuberculosis, and 98 healthy donors to analyze humoral immune reactions to these processes. Pericarditis occurred in 12.5% of patients with tuberculosis; the incidence of tuberculosis in the 149 patients with pericarditis was 8%. Pericardial effusions of >500 ml with impending cardiac tamponade required repeated pericardiocentesis in 4 patients.

Antimyolemmal antibodies, a muscle-specific type of antisarcolemmal antibody, were found in all patients with exudative tuberculous pericarditis and viral perimyocarditis, in only 1 of 12 patients with constrictive pericarditis, and in no patient with pulmonary tuberculosis. Antifibrillary antibodies, primarily the antimyosin type, were not found in patients with viral heart disease, but were demonstrated in 75% of patients with tuberculous pericarditis. Sera with complement-fixing antimyolemmal antibodies of the immunoglobulin type in titer >1:40 induced cytolysis of vital adult heterologous cardiocytes isolated and enriched by silica sol gradient centrifugation. These data suggest that antimyolemmal antibodies are diagnostic indicators of perimyocardial involvement in tuberculous pericarditis and that such antibodies may play a role in its pathogenesis.

Constriction as a complication of cardiac surgery

Kutcher and associates[8] from Atlanta, Georgia, evaluated 5,207 adult patients undergoing cardiac surgery. Constrictive pericarditis developed in 11 patients (0.2% frequency). Seven had undergone CABG and 4 had valve replacements; the parietal pericardium was left open in all cases. The average interval between surgery and presentation with pericardial constriction was 82 days (range, 14–186). M-mode echo revealed epicardial and pericardial thickening in 7 patients and variable degrees of posterior pericardial effusion in 5 patients. Cardiac catheterization demonstrated diastolic pressures with a characteristic early diastolic dip and late plateau pattern. Two patients responded to medical therapy for chronic pericarditis, 1 had a limited parietal pericardiectomy, and the remaining 8 patients required radical pericardiectomy. These data suggest that chronic constrictive pericarditis occurs in a very small number of patients who have undergone previous cardiac surgery despite their having an open pericardium. This possibility needs to be considered in patients presenting with chest pain or alterations in ventricular function after open heart surgery.

Echo in congenital absence of parietal pericardium

The M-mode and 2-D echo features of congenital absence of the pericardium were described in 2 cases by Nicolosi and associates[9] from Trieste, Italy. M-mode echo showed RV dilation and abnormal systolic motion of the ventricular septum. Echo contrast studies with peripheral injection of saline solution revealed normal persistence of microbubbles in the right side of the heart. Two-D short axis parasternal views showed some RV dilation with anterior displacement of the LV cavity in systole, which appeared to be wider than the posterior motion of the ventricular septum toward the posterior wall. The resulting positive motion of the ventricular septum toward the transducer could account for the abnormal pattern on M-mode echo.

Metastatic neoplasms

Adenle and Edwards[10] from St. Paul, Minnesota, analyzed 60 cases of pericardial metastatic disease, including 26 with significant effects on the cardiovascular system. Pericardial metastases were suspected clinically in 18 of the patients. The most common features reported were exertional dyspnea and pleural effusion. Although they were nonspecific, ECG ST-T changes and low voltage QRS complexes were helpful in suspecting pericardial metastases. Thoracic roentgenograms were not helpful unless there was a large pericardial effusion.

PULMONARY HYPERTENSION

Smooth muscle content of pulmonary arterial media

The number of smooth muscle cells per unit of surface area of the media of muscular pulmonary arteries was assessed by Wagenvoort and Wagenvoort[11] from Amsterdam, The Netherlands, and expressed as an index of medial smooth muscle density. The relative medial thickness of these arteries also was established. Subjects were 10 children and 10 adults in each of the following conditions: normal, congenital heart defect with a left-to-right shunt (CHD), primary pulmonary hypertension (PPH), and MS. A total of 80 persons were studied. The density of medial smooth muscle was generally the same in normal control subjects and in patients with CHD or PPH and was independent of the medial thickness. The index also was the same in children with MS, but significantly reduced in adult patients with MS, apparently by a prominent contribution of collagen and edematous ground substance to the media. This may partially explain the discrepancy, often observed in adult patients with MS, of a very thick media associated with mild elevation of pressure. The differences in medial structure also may account for some hemodynamic differences between adults and children with MS.

In the sickle hemoglobinopathies

Although pulmonary hypertension has been suspected in patients with sickle hemoglobinopathies, documentation of elevation in PA pressures is rare. Indeed, Collins and Orringer[12] from Chapel Hill, North Carolina, searched medical reports and found only 1 patient with sickle cell anemia reported in whom the PA pressure was elevated (47/19 mmHg). In 2 additional reported patients with sickle hemoglobinopathies, both clinical and autopsy findings disclosed pulmonary vascular disease and cor pulmonale but hemodynamic studies were not performed. From their own institution, Collins and Orringer found 3 patients with pulmonary hypertension documented by cardiac catheterization and sickle hemoglobinopathy. The PA systolic pressures ranged from 55–82 mmHg. The authors pointed out that pulmonary hypertension in patients with sickle cell anemia has an extremely poor prognosis and therefore application of experimental modalities, such as continuous oxygen therapy, partial exchange transfusion, or even limited phlebotomy, may be justified.

Treatment with hydralazine

Packer and associates[13] from New York City treated 13 consecutive patients with either primary or secondary pulmonary hypertension who had normal LV function with hydralazine to reduce pulmonary vascular resistance and clinical symptoms. Despite marked decreases in systemic vascular resistance (40%; $p < 0.001$), hydralazine produced only moderate decreases in pulmonary arteriolar resistance (21%), without improving stroke volume or PA pressure. Instead, mean systemic arterial pressure fell markedly (17 mmHg, $p < 0.01$) in association with a reflex increase in heart rate (11 beats/min, $p < 0.01$). Four patients became symptomatically hypotensive within 24 hours of the initiation of treatment 2 required pressors for circulatory support, and 1 died. Progressive renal insufficiency developed in 1 patient, and a symptomatic decrease in systemic arterial oxygen saturation occurred in another; both changes were reversed upon discontinuation of the drug. Thus, hydralazine fails to produce consistent hemodynamic and clinical benefits in patients with primary and secondary pulmonary hypertension, and it frequently causes serious adverse reactions.

In an accompanying editorial by Kadowitz and Hyman[14] from New Orleans, Louisiana, the study of Packer and associates is contrasted to a previous study by Rubin and Peter (*N Engl J Med* 302:69–73, 1980) and to 1 by Lupi-Herrera and associates.[15] Hydralazine, alone or in combination with diuretics and beta blocking agents, is, of course, widely used in the treatment of systemic hypertension and has recently been shown to have vasodilating activity in the pulmonary vascular bed. Since hydralazine increases cardiac output and dilates resistance vessels, it is not surprising that this agent was found to decrease pulmonary vascular resistance in the studies of Rubin and Peter. It is likely that calcium entry blockers will be more useful in treatment of patients with pulmonary hypertension.

Pulmonary arterial hypertension of unknown etiology remains a challenging clinical problem and in recent years vasodilator therapy has been tested in these individuals. Lupi-Herrera and associates[15] from Mexico City, Mexico, administered hydralazine to 12 patients with primary pulmonary hypertension (PPH). All patients were studied at rest and 9 during exercise. On the basis of hydralazine response at rest, the patients were divided into 2 groups. In 6 patients, group A, pulmonary arteriolar resistance (R_p) decreased. Cardiac index increased and systemic resistance (R_s) decreased. The R_p/R_s ratio did not change significantly after hydralazine. In the remaining 6 patients, group B, R_s decreased significantly but the other variables did not change. These observations suggested that the pulmonary vasodilatory effect of hydralazine caused a marked reduction of RV afterload in group A. In group B, a marked systemic vasodilatory effect occurred and RV afterload was not reduced. On the basis of the previous hemodynamic response, only group A patients were treated with hydralazine. Hemodynamic measurements were repeated 48 hours after the drug, both at rest and during exercise as well as 8 months later. The beneficial hemodynamic effects of hydralazine persisted; thus, these data suggest that hydralazine can reduce R_p in selected patients with PPH.

Kronzon and associates[16] from New York City treated 2 patients with primary pulmonary hypertension (PPH) with hydralazine and the PA pressure increased further and the symptoms worsened. The mechanism of this adverse effect was a decrease of systemic vascular resistance attended by an increase in cardiac output without a fall in the pulmonary vascular resistance. These authors recommended hemodynamic monitoring in patients undergoing vasodilator therapy for PPH.

Hydralazine reduced pulmonary vascular resistance (PVR) in patients with primary and secondary pulmonary hypertension, but the effects on RV function of a change in resistance without a reduction in PA pressure remain unknown. Rubin and colleagues[17] from Durham, North Carolina, evaluated hemodynamic effects of hydralazine 50 mg administered orally every 6 hours for 48 hours in 14 patients with RV failure and pulmonary hypertension resulting from various etiologies. Hydralazine reduced mean RV end-diastolic pressure (EDP) from 17–11 mmHg and increased cardiac output and stroke volume by >40%. In 9 patients who had no change in mean PA pressure with hydralazine, total PVR decreased from 16–11 and cardiac index increased from 2–3 liters/min/M^2. There was a close correlation between the reduction in total PVR and RV EDP. These data suggest that hydralazine can increase cardiac output and reduce RV EDP even when PA pressure remains unchanged.

Treatment with captopril

Rich and associates[18] from Chicago, Illinois, gave captopril, an angiotensin-converting enzyme inhibitor to 4 patients with primary pulmonary hypertension (PPH) to see if it would lower PA pressure or pulmonary vascular resistance. The patients were studied at rest and during supine bicycle exercise, before and after 48 hours of captopril treatment (≤450 mg/day). During treatment, each patient was monitored: systemic and pulmonary pressures were measured hourly and cardiac output, every 2–4 hours. They found no significnt effect of captopril, either at rest or with exercise, on the cardiac output, PA pressure, or pulmonary vascular resistance, measured at the end of 48 hours of treatment. During the 48-hour period, all patients showed pronounced swings in their PA and systemic artery pressures and cardiac outputs that had no relation to the administration of captopril or the time of day. Thus, captopril appears to be ineffective in causing a sustained reduction in PA pressure or pulmonary vascular resistance in patients with PPH. It appears, however, that these patients have spontaneous variability in their pulmonary resistance from hour to hour.

Ikram and associates[19] from Christchurch, New Zealand, treated 5 patients with primary pulmonary hypertension (PPH) with captopril for 4 days. To ensure accuracy of hemodynamic and hormone data, the patients were studied under conditions of constant body posture, regulated dietary sodium and potassium intake, and unchanged diuretic therapy. Captopril reduced mean PA pressure in parallel with plasma angiotensin II levels. The RV EF recordings increased considerably in 3 patients. Systemic arterial pressure fell but there was no change in RA pressure, cardiac output, or heart rate. The decline in plasma and urine aldosterone levels presumably contributed to the positive cumulative potassium balance and to the rise in the plasma potassium. These results suggest that converting enzyme inhibitors warrant a larger trial with prolonged follow-up in the treatment of PPH.

Treatment with prostacyclin

To evaluate the effects of prostacyclin on pulmonary vascular tone in primary pulmonary hypertension (PPH), Rubin and associates[20] from Durham, North Carolina, and Denver, Colorado, performed right-sided cardiac catheterization on 7 patients with PPH and made hemodynamic measurements before and after infusing incremental doses of prostacyclin. In maximal doses of 2–13 ng/kg/minute prostacyclin reduced mean PA pressure from 62–55 mmHg and total pulmonary resistance from 17–10 units. Cardiac output increased from 4.2–6.6 liters/minute. Heart rate increased from 83–94 beats/minute and mean systemic arterial pressure decreased from 90–77 mmHg. Three patients who received a continuous infusion of prostacyclin for 24–48 hours had sustained reductions in total pulmonary resistance during the infusion period. Thus, these data demonstrate that prostacyclin can increase cardiac output and reduce PA pressure and total pulmonary resistance in patients with PPH.

CHRONIC OBSTRUCTIVE PULMONARY DISEASE

Nocturnal hypoxemia and associated ECG changes

The advent of ear oximetry, which allows noninvasive measurement of arterial oxygen saturation (SaO_2), has generated fresh interest in the role of hypoxemia in the pathogenesis of pulmonary hypertension and cardiac arrhythmias. Tirlapur[21] from Cardiff, Wales, studied ECG effects of hypoxemia during the night in patients with chronic obstructive airways disease (COAD). He recorded both SaO_2 and the ECG during the night. In 7 "blue bloater" patients, the mean basal SaO_2 was <80%, and it fell by >10% during 29 episodes of transient hypoxemia. Only 5 such episodes occurred in 3 of 5 "pink-puffer" patients. All "blue bloaters" with low basal mean SaO_2 had multiple atrial premature contraction and VPC and a high heart rate at rest; 6 patients had a prolonged QTc, 3 had ST-T depression, and 1 had right BBB. Oxygen therapy increased basal mean SaO_2, reduced ectopic activity, abolished ST-T changes and BBB, significantly reduced the resting heart rate and the amplitude of the R and S waves, and shortened the QTc in 4 nonsmokers. These results suggest that sustained hypoxemia contributes to myocardial dysfunction and CHF in "blue bloater" patients.

Correlation with right ventricular ejection fraction

Brent and associates[22] from New Haven, Connecticut, evaluated 20 patients with chronic obstructive pulmonary disease to determine the physiologic correlates of RV EF. Radionuclide and hemodynamic measurements were obtained simultaneously. In 7 patients, studies were repeated after the intravenous administration of sodium nitroprusside. Seventeen of the 20 patients had a RV EF <45%. There was a strong inverse linear correlation between RV EF and afterload as assessed by peak or mean PA pressure (r = −0.81) and pulmonary vascular resistance index (r = −0.73). The RV EF also correlated, although less strongly, with preload as assessed by RV end-diastolic volume index (r = −0.56) and mean right atrial pressure (r

= −0.51). The RV EF did not correlate with cardiac index, the ratio of peak PA pressure to RV end-systolic volume index, arterial oxygen tension, or LV EF. After nitroprusside, mean arterial pressure, peak PA systolic pressure, and pulmonary vascular resistance index decreased significantly. The slope and volume intercept of each pressure-volume line were determined; the administration of dobutamine resulted in a leftward shift from the end-systolic pressure-volume line. There were poor correlations between the slope and RV EF as well as between the slope and the control ratio between PA systolic pressure and end-systolic volume index. These data suggest that RV EF is highly dependent on afterload, but less dependent on preload. The RV EF is a relatively poor indicator of the slope of the systolic pressure-volume relation, thus raising questions concerning its usefulness as an independent index of RV contractility.

Treatment with terbutaline

Brent and associates[23] from New Haven, Connecticut, evaluated the influence of the selective beta$_2$ adrenoreceptor agonist, terbutaline, in a well-defined group of 8 patients with chronic obstructive pulmonary disease, abnormal RV performance, and elevated pulmonary vascular resistance. Radionuclide and hemodynamic data were obtained simultaneously using first-pass radionuclide ventriculography and thermodilution PA catheterization. Terbutaline increased RV EF from 35 ± 10–46 ± 5%. The changes in RV EF were greatest in patients with the highest level of pulmonary vascular resistance and the lowest control EF. The LV EF also increased significantly from 62 ± 10–71 ± 10. These data demonstrate that terbutaline results in substantial increases of RV performance. This effect is mediated at least partially through alterations in pulmonary vascular resistance.

To assess RV and LV responses to the subcutaneous administration of terbutaline sulfate, a beta$_2$ selective agonist, Hooper and colleagues[24] from San Diego, California, evaluated 14 patients with chronic obstructive pulmonary disease (COPD) with equilibrium RNA. Before injection, 8 patients (57%) had an abnormal RV EF, 4 (29%) had a low LV EF, and 3 (21%) had low EF of both ventricles. After terbutaline injection, RV EF increased in 13 of 14 patients (93%) by 17% and LV EF increased in all patients by 15%. Both LV and RV end-diastolic volumes decreased, whereas stroke volume was unchanged. Cardiac output rose by 0.8 liters/minute, primarily due to the increase in heart rate (10 beats/min), since stroke volume did not significantly change. It is concluded that in patients with COPD subcutaneous terbutaline has significant beta$_1$ cardiac effects; it increases the heart rate and decreases cardiac size.

Treatment with theophylline

Although oral theophylline is a widely used bronchodilator in chronic obstructive pulmonary disease (COPD), its effects upon cardiac performance have not been fully established. Accordingly, the effect of slow release oral theophylline upon RV EF and LV EF was evaluated by Matthay and colleagues[25] from New Haven, Connecticut, using first-pass quantitative RNA in 15 patients with COPD. After 72 hours of therapy, oral theophylline significantly increased RV EF (42–48%). In 7 of 10 patients with depressed baseline RV performance, including 2 with cor pulmonale, RV EF normalized (≥45%). After long-term therapy, an average of 16 weeks, RV EF also increased (43–48%). The LV EF improved significantly from 64%–68% at 72 hours and from 61%–65% after long-term therapy. These data indicate that oral theophylline produces a sustained modest enhancement of resting biventricular performance in COPD.

PULMONARY EMBOLISM

Bell[26] from Baltimore, Maryland, summarized signs and symptoms in 327 patients with pulmonary embolism. He pointed out that pulmonary emboli are the most frequent cause of death of all recognized pulmonary diseases and may be the third most common cause of death in the USA. This statement is much different from my (WCR) experience. He goes on to state that pulmonary emboli afflict more than 500,000 persons in the USA each year. I (WCR) simply cannot believe that pulmonary emboli are a more common cause of pulmonary death than chronic obstructive lung disease. He reasons that the disease presents such a perplexing problem because of the difficulty in diagnosis. There is simply no component of the history, physical examination, or noninvasive laboratory findings that are specific. He emphasizes that the symptoms and signs, although uniformly nonspecific, may be of some help (Table 9-2). If a patient, for example, is initially suspected of having pulmonary emboli but does not have chest pain, dyspnea, or tachypnea, the diagnosis is unlikely. He emphasizes that the only definitive technique to establish the diagnosis of pulmonary emboli before death is angiography. Although pulmonary angiography is unparalleled in accuracy, a better technique is needed because of the number of professional personnel, time, and expensive equipment required, as well as the inherent risk to the patient. Until this is found, the physician must rely on the findings of history, physical examination, arterial blood gases, and ventilation-perfusion lung scanning to reach a diagnosis. If after these tests, diagnosis is still in doubt, angiography should be performed promptly. He also urged that angiography should be performed when 1) any surgical technique is contemplated; 2) an increased risk from using thrombolytic or anticoagulant therapy exists (the presence of occult bleeding before institution of therapy); or 3) there is a past history of recurrent episodes of possible pulmonary emboli without documentation of diagnosis.

The most significant advance in the management of thromboembolic disease has been in therapy. The advent of thrombolytic therapy (streptokinase or urokinase) has for the first time made it possible not only to induce the dissolution of thrombi, but also to return cardiopulmonary and peripher-

TABLE 9-2. *Signs and symptoms of 327 patients with pulmonary embolism.*

	TOTAL SERIES N = 327	MASSIVE EMBOLI N = 197 vs	SUBMASSIVE EMBOLI N = 130
Symptoms			
Chest pain	83	79	89*
Pleuritic	74	67	82†
Nonpleuritic	14	16	13
Dyspnea	84	85	82
Apprehension	59	65†	50
Cough	53	53	52
Hemoptysis	30	23	40†
Sweats	27	29	23
Syncope	13	20‡	4
Signs			
Respirations > 16/min	92	95	87
Rales	58	57	60
↑ S_2P	53	58*	45
Pulse > 100/min	44	48	38
Temperature > 37.8°C	43	43	42
Phlebitis	32	36	26
Gallop	34	39†	25
Diaphoresis	36	42†	27
Edema	24	23	25
Murmur	28	28	27
Cyanosis	19	25‡	9
Associated Conditions			
Current venous disease	45	47	42
Immobilization	58	60	55
CHF and chronic lung disease	38	36	40
Malignant neoplasm	6	8	5

All figures are precents, ↑ S_2P = increased intensity of the pulmonic component of the second heart sound. * Statistically significant (p < 0.05). † Statistically significant (p < 0.01). ‡ Statistically significant (p < 0.001). Based on chi-square test with continuity correction.

al vascular hemodynamics rapidly back to normal. Benefit from the use of thrombolytic agents has already been established for patients with: 1) massive pulmonary emboli (>2 lobar arteries involved); 2) pulmonary emboli accompanied by shock, and 3) submassive pulmonary emboli superimposed on underlying cardiopulmonary dysfunction resulting in physiologic decompensation.

He cautions that there is no universally accepted regimen for prophylactic treatment of patients likely to experience pulmonary emboli. Regimens employing low dose heparin, low dose heparin plus dihydroergotamine, oral anticoagulants, antiplatelet agents, elastic stockings, and electromechanical and pneumatic exercise devices are currently in vogue, but none is proved.

Early mobilization is the most important form of prophylaxis that has been identified.

To evaluate factors associated with the correct ante mortem diagnosis of pulmonary embolism, Goldhaber and associates[27] from Boston, Massachusetts, reviewed 1,455 autopsy reports at the Peter Bent Brigham Hospital from 1973–1977. Of 54 patients identified with anatomically major pulmonary embolism at necropsy, 16 (30%) had correct ante mortem diagnosis. Accuracy was far greater in postoperative patients (64%) (p = 0.02) and in patients with autopsy-proved venous thrombosis (55%) (p = 0.005). Lung scanning (82%) (p = 0.0002) and pulmonary angiography (80%) (p = 0.05) during the 10 days before death also were associated with an increased tendency to correct clinical diagnosis of pulmonary embolism. In contrast, among 21 patients with autopsy-proved major pulmonary embolism who also had pneumonia, no pulmonary embolism was diagnosed before death (p = 0.0001). Furthermore, among patients ≥70 years of age, only 10% with pulmonary embolism at necroscopy had a correct diagnosis before death (p = 0.02). In patients with pneumonia or in elderly patients, an increased awareness of the possibility of pulmonary embolism and more frequent use of lung scanning and pulmonary angiography may increase the accurate clinical diagnosis of pulmonary embolism.

Iwasaki and associates[28] from Nishinomiya, Japan, studied echo findings in 5 patients with pulmonary embolism and found that the tricuspid echo showed abnormalities in valve motion (a monophasic triangular wave during diastole) and an increased RV dimension. An "a" dip of the pulmonic valve echo also occurred in all 5 patients. Later, tricuspid echo regained the normal M-shaped configuration. The authors speculated that the monophasic triangular pattern of the tricuspid valve during RV diastole was probably related to the shorter duration of tricuspid valve opening compared with that of the mitral valve.

BRONCHIAL ASTHMA

To explain the mechanism of paradoxical pulse in severe bronchial asthma, Jardin and colleagues[29] from Boulougne, France, performed hemodynamic studies and measured esophageal pressure in 9 patients who had status asthmaticus and clinical paradoxical pulse. Two-D echo allowed simultaneous assessment of cyclic changes in RV and LV size throughout the respiratory cycle. Esophageal pressure varied from a markedly negative level during inspiration (−24 cm water) to a positive level during expiration (7.6 cm water). Competition between right and left heart chambers for pericardial space during inspiration was suggested by the reduced LV cross-sectional area at end-systole and end-diastole, the leftward septal shift, and the increased RV internal diameter at end-systole and end-diastole. Competition from filling, however, could not entirely account for the paradoxical pulse, for systemic and pulmonary pulse pressures were almost in phase: both were

minimal at inspiration and maximal at expiration. The increase in impedance to RV ejection is another factor reducing LV preload at inspiration. This
reduction in preload was shown to be the predominant mechanism for the
decrease in LV stroke output at inspiration.

ECHO TOPICS

Unreliability of M-mode left ventricular dimensions for calculating stroke volume and cardiac output without heart disease

Single-dimension LV echo measurements are currently being used in
investigational studies as the basis for evaluting cardiac output parameters in
normal subjects, even though validity of the method for normal subjects has
not been established. Rasmussen and associates[30] from Indianapolis, Indiana, prospectively compared stroke volume derived from M-mode LV
internal dimensions to Fick stroke volume in 20 patients with no objective
evidence of cardiac disease. Based on simultaneous studies, stroke volume by
Fick ranged from 39–121 ml and cardiac output, from 3.9–10.4 liters/
minute. Comparing the LV internal dimension cubed method with Fick, the
correlation coefficient was $r = 0.47$ for stroke volume and $r = 0.36$ for
cardiac output. The LV internal dimension absolute error in cardiac output
ranged from $-2.11-+3.21$ liters/minute. Use of other published formulas for
calculating stroke volume from internal dimension did not improve accuracy. These data indicate that stroke volume and cardiac output cannot be
accurately measured or reliably estimated from M-mode LV internal dimensions.

Measurement of left ventricular ejection fraction

Two-D echo is increasingly being used to determine LV EF. There remain,
however, important questions concerning the 2D-echo determination of EF:
1) which 2-D echo formulae correlate best with contrast ventriculography; 2)
how often can a particular formula be applied to a large group of patients;
and 3) what effect does 2-D echo quality or the presence of segmental wall
motion abnormalities have on the accuracy of echo determined EF? To
answer these questions, Stamm and colleagues[31] from Charlottesville, Virginia, prospectively determined the 2-D echo EF utilizing 10 different formulae
in 65 consecutive patients undergoing contrast ventriculogram within the
following 24 hours. They also sought to examine the ability of trained
observers to estimate EF from 2-D echo. The 2-D echo EF formulae that
utilized biplane areas were generally more accurate than single plane area or
diameter only formulae, but were obtainable in fewer patients. The biplane
Simpson's rule yielded a correlation with ventriculogram of $r = 0.89$, but was

available in only 34 patients. Although the single plane formulae were slightly less accurate, they were measured in more patients; ellipsoid single plane apical 4-chamber r = 0.80, n, 56, and short ellipse r = 0.86, n, 47. The measured EF in patients with akinetic segments yielded a greater standard error of the mean, although correlations remained adequate when compared with the normal patient population. The EF from patients with poor quality compared with good quality echo studies had a slightly greater standard error, but correlations were little affected. Thus, biplane formulae for calculating EF yield better correlations, but are available from fewer patients than single plane formulae. An estimate of EF was sufficiently accurate for most clinical situations and was available in 98% of patients. The presence of abnormal wall motion or a poor quality 2-D echo study increased the standard error slightly, but had little effect on the correlation with contrast ventriculogram.

Limitations of determination of left ventricular volume by echo

Schnittger and associates[32] from Palo Alto, California, measured LV volumes in 18 patients utilizing 2-D echo recordings and fluoroscopic measurements in patients with abnormal wall motion and previously implanted myocardial markers. There was a good correlation between the echo values for volume and those derived from myocardial markers (r = 0.87) and there was no statistically significant differences in values obtained with the 2 methods at end-diastole or end-systole. The EF obtained with 2-D echo (mean ± SD, 46 ± 7%) and with fluoroscopic recordings of the markers (41 ± 9%) did not differ significantly.

These results were compared with those in another 18 patients (9 with abnormal wall motion) having 2-D echo within 24 hours of a 30° right anterior oblique contrast left ventriculogram. In these studies, 2-D echo ventricular volumes correlated well with angiographic volumes (r = 0.85), although angiocardiographic end-diastolic volume was consistently underestimated by echo. The EF by echo also was less than that obtained with angiography (47 ± 8 -vs- 60 ± 7%, respectively; p < 0.001). This study suggests less underestimation of volume with echo, even in very abnormal ventricles, than has been reported previously. The authors speculate that perhaps some improvement in echo methodology is responsible.

Estimation of right ventricular volume

Watanabe and associates[33] from Kyoto, Japan, studied 23 consecutive patients to determine the ability of 2-D echo to estimate RV volumes. Biplane 2-D echoes that were perpendicular to each other were obtained from the apical approach. The echo RV volume was calculated using Simpson's rule. The echo dimensions of the RV long, short, and maximal short axes also were measured in each view. Volumes and dimensions were compared with both the angiographic RV body volumes calculated by applying Simpson's rule with the echo values in each group. Correlation between the echo and the angiographic RV body volumes (r = 0.94 at end-diastole, r = 0.84 at end-systole) was good and better than between echo RV dimensions and angiographic RV body volumes. Echo measurements of RV body volume were helpful in distinguishing patients with and without RV volume overload. These data suggest that a correlation between echo dimensions of the RV long axis and angiographic RV volumes is poor, whereas that between echo dimensions of the RV short or maximal short axis and angiographic RV volumes is good. The data suggest the estimation of RV volume and morphology by 2-D echo may be useful.

Abnormalities of ventricular septal motion postoperatively

To evaluate whether the postoperative abnormalities in septal motion observed by M-mode echo are due to changes in either ventricular shape or of total cardiac motion within the thorax, Kerber and Litchfield[34] from Iowa City, Iowa, obtained preoperative and early and late postoperative M-mode echo and 2-D echo on 25 patients undergoing cardiac surgery. No patient had CAD. All patients had normal preoperative septal motion; 11 patients retained normal (group N) septal motion on postoperative M-mode echo; 14 patients developed abnormal (group A) septal motion. Comparison of these 2 groups revealed that group A patients had a greater degree of posterior epicardial motion toward the chest wall during systole. This indicates a greater anterior motion of the entire heart within the thorax, which produces the observed septal motion abnormality by carrying the septum forward passively as the whole heart moves anteriorly. This excessive forward cardiac motion may be due to fixation of the heart anteriorly by postoperative sternal-cardiac adhesions. No changes in LV shape, size, or function were found to be associated with abnormal septal motion, nor was septal contraction impaired. Changes in intrathoracic cardiac motion are the probable cause of septal motion abnormalities after cardiac surgery.

TOPICS IN NUCLEAR CARDIOLOGY

Measuring left ventricular volume

Since the introduction of the angiographic method for quantitating LV volume by Dodge and Sandler, this technique employing either biplane or single plane projections has been a standard for LV dimensional analysis. Links and associates[35] from Baltimore, Maryland, described a new method for obtaining absolute LV volume from gated blood pool studies in 35 patients who also underwent single plane contrast ventriculography. Gated 40° left anterior oblique (LAO) and static anterior views were required. LV volume and end-diastole was calculated from the ratio of the attenuation corrected end-diastolic count rate from the gated study to the count rate per millimeter from a blood sample. The attenuation correction was made by dividing the end-diastolic count rate by e^{-ud}, where u is the linear attenuation coefficient of water and d is the distance from the skin marker to the center of the LV and the anterior view divided by sign 40° to yield the depth of LV and left anterior oblique view. In phantom studies, the correlation between RN and true volume was 0.99 (RN, 1.03 true volume–3 ml) with a standard error of estimate of 8 ml. In the patient studies, the RN end-diastolic volume was used to calibrate the LV time activity curve which yielded LV volume throughout the cardiac cycle. The correlation between RN and angiographic end-diastolic and end-systolic volume was 0.95 and a standard error of estimate of 33 ml. Thus, these investigators described a centigraphic method for direct determination of absolute LV volume without assumptions about the shape of the ventricle or the necessity of using regression equation to convert volume units to true volume.

First-pass left ventriculograms were obtained by Tobis and colleagues[36] from Orange, California, using digital subtraction angiography in 24 patients after intravenous injection of 30–40 ml of iodinated contrast material. An image processing computer was used to enhance the iodine signal in the image relative to the background soft tissue by digitizing each new frame of the fluoroscopic exposure and subtracting from it a stored mask image. Digital left ventriculograms were obtained in the 30° right anterior oblique position using high fluoroscopic exposure levels (8 mA and 70–90 kVp) and compared with 30° right anterior oblique cineangiograms obtained at cardiac catheterization. Standard cineangiograms were performed in 33 patients at cardiac catheterization but 6 (18%) were excluded because of runs of VT initiated by the standard intraventricular injection of 40 ml of contrast media. Digital subtraction angiography was attempted in the 33 patients and left ventriculograms of clinically useful quality were obtained in 30 (91%). There were close correlations between end-diastolic volumes, end-systolic volumes, and EF. Multiple VPC occurred in a total of 10 (30%) of 33 patients during standard intraventricular cineangiography but did not occur in any patient during the intravenous first-pass technique. Wall motion abnormalities were visualized as well by digital angiography as by the standard method. Digital angiography appears to be an important new addition to diagnostic cardiology because it provides a less invasive outpatient method for obtaining contrast left ventriculograms that have much greater spatial resolution than radionuclide cineangiograms.

Measuring right ventricular volume

Dehmer and associates[37] from Dallas, Texas, developed methodology allowing accurate measurement of RV volumes using nongeometric radionuclide techniques. Sixty patients without clinical or hemodynamic evidence of right-sided regurgitation were studied with simultaneous measurements of RV stroke volume obtained using gated radionuclide ventriculography and thermodilution techniques. Three techniques for the acquisition of the radionuclide studies were evaluated and radionuclide ventriculograms were obtained with a 25° rotating slant hole collimator positioned in a 10–15° left anterior oblique projection with a collimator slanted toward the cardiac apex along the axis of the ventricular septum. Excellent agreement between thermodilution stroke volume and radionuclide ventriculographic stroke volume estimates were found using this scintigraphic approach. Thus, RV volumes may be measured accurately with gated radionuclide ventriculography and without geometric assumptions utilizing this approach.

Korr and associates[38] from Providence, Rhode Island, evaluated the ability of equilibrium gated radionuclide ventriculography to measure RV function in 60 patients. Radionuclide measurements of RV EF were correlated with RV hemodynamics. There was a significant negative linear correlation between RV EF and mean PA pressure (r = −0.82) and between RV EF and RV end-diastolic pressure (r = −0.67). Patients with an elevated RV end-diastolic pressure and mean PA pressure had a more severely depressed EF than did those with an elevated mean PA pressure alone. The mean RV EF in 20 normal subjects was 53 ± 6%, a value that agrees well with previous data from both radionuclide and contrast angiographic studies. The data obtained in this evaluation suggest that an abnormal RV EF in the absence of primary RV volume overload suggests abnormal pressures in the right side of the heart, whereas a normal value excludes severe PA hypertension and an elevated RV end-diastolic pressure.

Detecting wall motion abnormalities

The value of phase analysis of multiple gated acquisition blood pool images for identifying wall motion abnormalities due to stress-induced ischemia was examined by Ratib and colleagues[39] from Los Angeles, California. Myocardial segments with an abnormal phase (delayed onset of wall motion) were localized on a phase distribution image of the left ventricle and the synchrony of LV systolic wall motion was assessed from histograms of the LV phase distribution, i.e., the standard deviation (SD) from the mean of this peak, termed SDP. Its upper limits of normal at rest and exercise were established in 7 normal subjects as the mean ±2 SD and were 12° at rest and 10° at maximum exercise. Of the 56 patients, 37 had CAD, 11 had valvular heart disease and normal coronary arteries, and 8 had either cardiomyopathy or typical angina and normal coronary arteries and normal cardiac valves. In the CAD patients, SDP was abnormal in 95% during exercise, whereas only 86% had had an abnormal EF response and/or exercise-induced wall motion abnormalities by visual interpretation. By contrast, in the 11 valvular heart disease patients, SDP was abnormal in only 2, despite exercise-induced wall motion abnormalities in 5 and an abnormal EF response in all 11. Thus, although an abnormal EF response to exercise is a sensitive indicator of cardiac disease, it is, however, like exercise-induced wall motion abnormalities, not specific for CAD. By contrast, phase analysis not only permitted separation of wall motion abnormalities induced by ischemia from those associated with valvular disease, but was also an objective, highly sensitive, and specific indicator of regional myocardial ischemia.

PHARMACOLOGIC TOPICS

Effect of beta blockade and stimulation on stage fright

Stage fright is an ubiquitous problem that most people find bothersome and unpleasant. To a performing musician, however, stage fright may not be the trivial problem that it is to the physician. Because tachycardia, sweaty palms, cardiac irregularities, tremors, systemic hypertension, tight breathing, nausea, and the urge to urinate are true physical impediments to musical performance, stage fright may disable a recital artist. Pharmacologic control of these effects has been achieved by the use of alcohol and/or tranquilizers, often at the expense of the brilliance and sensitivity of the performance itself. Since, from a physiologic standpoint, stage fright is the fight or flight reaction mediated by the sympathetic adrenal axis, Brantigan and associates[40] from Denver, Colorado, and Omaha, Nebraska, investigated the effects of beta blockade on musical performance with propranolol in a double-blind fashion, and the effects of beta stimulation using terbutaline. Stage fright symptoms were evaluated in 2 trials, which included 29 subjects, by questionnaire and by State Trait Anxiety Inventory. The quality of musical performance was evaluated by experienced music critics. Beta blockade eliminated the physical impediments to performance caused by stage fright and even eliminated the dry mouth so frequently encountered. The quality of musical performance, furthermore, as judged by experienced music critics was significantly improved. This effect was achieved without tranquilizers. Beta stimulating drugs, on the other hand, increased stage fright problems and were detrimental to musical performance. Thus, another use for beta blockers.

Treatment of life-threatening digitalis intoxication with digoxin-specific Fab antibody fragments

In 1976, Smith and associates[41] from Boston, Massachusetts, utilized specific digoxin antibodies in the treatment of advanced digoxin toxicity and reported the initial clinical use of purified digoxin-specific Fab fragments. On the basis of that favorable experience, Smith and associates initiated a multicenter clinical trial using purified digoxin-specific Fab fragments from sheep for the treatment of advanced digitalis toxicity resistant to conventional therapeutic measures. He and his associates from 20 centers in the USA described their experience in the first 26 patients treated under this protocol. All 26 patients had advanced cardiac arrhythmias and, in some cases, hyperkalemia that was resistant to conventional therapy. All patients had an initial favorable response to doses of Fab fragments calculated to be equivalent, on a molar basis, to the amount of cardiac glycoside in the patient's body. In 4 patients treated after prolonged hypotension and low cardiac output, death ensued from cerebral or myocardial hypoperfusion. In

1 patient, the available Fab fragment supply was inadequate to reverse a massive suicidal ingestion of digoxin, and the patient died from ventricular arrhythmias. In the remaining 21 patients, cardiac rhythm disturbances and hyperkalemia were rapidly reversed, and full recovery ensued. There were no adverse reactions to the treatment. Thus, the use of purified digoxin-specific Fab fragments is a safe and effective means to reverse advanced, life-threatening digitalis intoxication.

Effect of verapamil on serum digoxin

Since many patients receiving verapamil also are being treated with digitalis, Klein and colleagues[42] from Tel Aviv, Israel, and Whippany, New Jersey, studied the effect of verapamil on the pharmacokinetics of digoxin in 49 patients with chronic AF. A daily dose of 240 mg verapamil was given to patients receiving a stable dose of digoxin. Serum digoxin levels rose from 0.76–1.31 ng/ml during verapamil treatment. This effect was dose dependent, as shown in 7 patients who received 160 mg and later 240 mg of verapamil. There was a stepwise rise in serum digoxin concentration from a control value of 0.60–0.84 ng/ml and 1.24 ng/ml. The effect of verapamil developed gradually within the first few days in 7 subjects in whom serum digoxin concentration reached within 7 days 90% of the increase observed 14 days after onset of verapamil. Renal digoxin clearance decreaed significantly in 6 patients in whom serum digoxin concentration increased. Creatinine clearance did not change in any of these 7 patients. Among the 49 patients, verapamil resulted in the development of signs and symptoms that suggested digitalis toxicity in 7. Thus, verapamil significantly increases serum digoxin concentration. The process appears to be dose dependent and gradual and is at least partially explained by reduced renal clearance without reduction in glomerular filtration. The dose of digoxin may need readjusting in patients who are concomitantly receiving verapamil.

Pharmacokinetics of verapamil

Reiter and associates[43] from Durham, North Carolina, evaluated the kinetic characteristics of verapamil in 9 patients after a single intravenous dose. The intravenous regimen was designed to maintain a plasma verapamil concentration of 150 ng/ml by providing a loading bolus of 10 mg over 2 minutes, followed by a rapid loading infusion (0.375 mg/min) for 30 minutes, and a maintenance infusion of 0.125 mg/minute. This regimen was tested in 7 patients for 2–12 hours and found to be safe and to produce stable prolongation of the P-R interval. Verapamil concentration was highest immediately after the bolus administration and was prevented from falling below 67 ng/ml by rapid infusion. The maintenance concentration remained between 77 and 156 ng/ml for all patients and averaged 122 ng/ml. Verapamil produced transient slight decreases in brachial BP and sinus cycle length coincident with the maximum verapamil concentration. Maximal P-R prolongation occurred slightly later than peak plasma concentration, but it was sustained for the duration of the infusion. Prolongation of the P-R interval was not significantly different at the end of the infusion from the 90 minutes after the start of the regimen. No patient had serious side effects, arrhythmia, or clinically important hypotension. These data demonstrate that infusion regimens can be developed that will produce plasma concentrations adequate to alter hemodynamics and chronotropic responses.

A symposium on calcium channel blockers appeared in the January 1982 issue of *Circulation* (Part II) and in the July 1982 issue of *Chest* (supplement).

Effect of hypotension on hepatic blood flow and lidocaine disposition

In comparison to other highly vascular organs, the liver has a limited ability to autoregulate blood flow in the presence of systemic hypotension. This may have important consequences for the clearance of drugs that are highly extracted by the liver, such as lidocaine, meperidine, morphine, and certain beta blockers whose systemic elimination is dependent on hepatic blood flow. Thus, in CHF, in which hepatic blood flow falls in proportion to the reduction in cardiac output, the clearance of lidocaine is markedly reduced. Since these drugs are commonly given to patients with hypotension and shock, Feely and associates[44] from Nashville, Tennessee, examined the influence of hypotension on liver blood flow and the disposition of lidocaine in 5 patients with idiopathic orthostatic hypotension. Their studies suggest that both hepatic blood flow and lidocaine clearance fall in proportion to the degree of hypotension. Furthermore, the tissue distribution of lidocaine is altered by hypotension, and this alteration results in markedly elevated lidocaine concentrations. With the increasing use of drugs that are highly extracted by the liver, including propranolol and dihydroergotamine, in patients with autonomic dysfunction, it should be recognized that plasma levels of these drugs may be markedly influenced by changes in BP; a given dose of lidocaine may be therapeutic when the patient is in the supine position, but toxic when the patient is seated or upright. These results also may have therapeutic implications for the use of other drugs extracted by the liver in patients with shock or systemic hypotension.

Ethanol potentiation of aspirin-induced prolongation of the bleeding time

The template bleeding time is a sensitive and reproducible measure of primary hemostasis. It is influenced by platelet function, vascular tone, and platelet number. Usually after a normal person ingests 325 mg of aspirin the bleeding time is moderately prolonged, reaching its peak of about twice baseline values within 12 hours and returning to about baseline levels by 24 hours. In 2 subjects who had taken 325 mg of aspirin, Deykin and associates[45] from Boston, Massachusetts, observed a second rise in the bleeding time, at 36 hours after ingestion in 1 and 60 hours in the other, to levels that exceeded the prior peak effect of aspirin. Inquiry revealed that both subjects had consumed ethanol 4 hours before the unexpectedly prolonged bleeding time was measured. Since the authors had not previously observed an effect of moderate ethanol consumption (<50 g) on the bleeding time of normal subjects, the hypothesis that ethanol might potentiate the effect of aspirin on the bleeding time was tested. The data confirmed that ethanol alone has no effect on bleeding time but showed that it enhanced the effect of aspirin when given simultaneously or up to at least 36 hours after aspirin ingestion.

Deykin and associates gave 300 mg of aspirin to 9 subjects and determined bleeding time, platelet counts, and platelet aggregation before aspirin ingestion and at intervals for 5 days afterward. After another 5 days, the subjects were given either 50 g of ethanol or 50 g of ethanol plus 325 mg of aspirin and the studies were repeated. After 5 more days those who had received ethanol alone were given the combination of ethanol and aspirin; those who had received the combination were given ethanol alone. The mean bleeding-time responses were different. The big response to aspirin alone occurred at 12 hours. At 48 hours the bleeding time was not significantly different from the value before aspirin. The simultaneous ingestion of aspirin and ethanol increased both the magnitude and the duration of the bleeding time response.

Peak ethanol levels occurred 2 hours after ingestion of ethanol alone or with aspirin. There was no difference in the peak values after ethanol alone (50 ± 23 mg/dl) and after ethanol plus aspirin (59 ± 29 mg/dl). Similarly, peak salicylate levels occurred at 2 hours and were not different after aspirin alone (1.7 ± 0.4 mg/dl) and after aspirin plus ethanol (1.3 ± 0.4 mg/dl). Platelet counts were unaffected by aspirin, ethanol, or the combination. Ethanol alone had minimal effects on platelet aggregation induced by adenosine diphosphate, epinephrine, or arachidonic acid, and ethanol did not augment the impairment in aggregation caused by aspirin.

All 9 subjects had an ethanol-induced potentiation of the effect of aspirin on the bleeding time, but the magnitude and the duration of the responses varied. There was no correlation between the response to aspirin alone and blood salicylate levels, nor was there a correlation between the response to aspirin plus ethanol and either blood salicylate levels or blood alcohol levels.

Acute myocardial injury after phenylpropanolamine ingestion

Phenylpropanolamine is a sympathomimetic amine used widely as a decongestant and appetite suppressant. It is freely available either over the counter or on prescription. Its effects are largely the result of alpha adrenergic agonist activity resulting from both direct stimulation of adrenergic receptors and release of neuronal norepinephrine. The principal adverse effect of phenylpropanolamine is dose-related systemic hypertension and ventricular arrhythmia. In rats, it can cause myocardial necrosis, but the latter has not been reported in humans after acute ingestion. Pentel and associates[46] from Minneapolis, Minnesota, described 3 patients who developed clinical evidence of myocardial injury after ingestion of phenylpropanolamine. Increases in the serum creatine kinase and MB isoenzyme levels, ventricular arrhythmias, and ECG repolarization abnormalities were seen.

CARDIAC SURGICAL TOPICS

Extent of myocardial damage after open heart surgery: 1975 -vs- 1980

Perioperative myocardial damage caused by cardiac surgery in 32 patients operated on in 1980 was compared by Davids and associates[47] from Maastricht, The Netherlands, with 32 patients operated on in 1975 in terms of total quantity of alpha hydroxybutyrate dehydrogenase released from the heart into the circulation (Fig. 9-1). In the 5-year period between 1975 and 1980, obviously, various changes in anesthesia, pharmacologic treatment, and myocardial preservation techniques took place. Comparison of calculated myocardial damage in 1980 with that in 1975 showed a general reduction of about 40% in the patients having CAGB, 75% in patients having AVR, and 10% in patients having MVR.

Electrolyte -vs- blood cardioplegia

In 1978, Follette and associates (*J Thorac Cardiovasc Surg* 76:604, 1978) reported improved myocardial protection with cold blood cardioplegia compared to cold electrolyte cardioplegia. Singh and colleagues[48] from Providence, Rhode Island, tested this hypothesis in 40 consecutive patients undergoing CABG. Myocardial protection was provided using 1 of 2 cardioplegic solutions in a randomized fashion. Patients in group A received an electrolyte solution with 30 mEq/liter of potassium (K^+) added and a hematocrit of zero. In group B blood from the perfusate was added to the cardioplegic solution attaining a hematocrit of 16% and a K^+ concentration of 30 mEq/liter. The groups were comparable except for intramyocardial temperature. In group A patients it was 17°C, and in group B it was 20°C ($p < 0.001$). At the conclusion of the bypass, LA pressure was 12 ± 0.67 torr in group A and 8 ± 0.49 torr in group B ($p < 0.001$). Creatine phosphokinase (CPK)-MB was elevated in 45% of group A patients and in 15% of group B patients ($p < 0.05$) (Fig. 9-2). Morphometric electron microscopy was performed on LV biopsy specimens obtained before perfusion, immediately after cardioplegia, and 30 minutes after reperfusion. Cross-clamp time in group A patients was 68 ± 4 minutes, and in group B patients, 68 ± 4 minutes; the number of distal anastomoses did not differ (2.4 ± 0.1 -vs- 2.5 ± 0.1). Group A had marked intracellular edema, mitochondrial swelling, pronounced depletion of glycogen stores, and focal myofibrillar disorganization. Group B had near normal myocardial ultrastructure with increased glycogen stores and minimal mitochondrial swelling. The frequency of enzymatic evidence of myocardial necrosis by CPK-MB analysis was higher in group A than in group B. The initial mean postoperative CPK-MB was 59 IU/liter in group A -vs- 35 IU/liter in group B. The authors suggested that the higher mean LA pressure in group A was evidence for more importantly altered cardiac function after electrolyte cardioplegia -vs- blood cardioplegia.

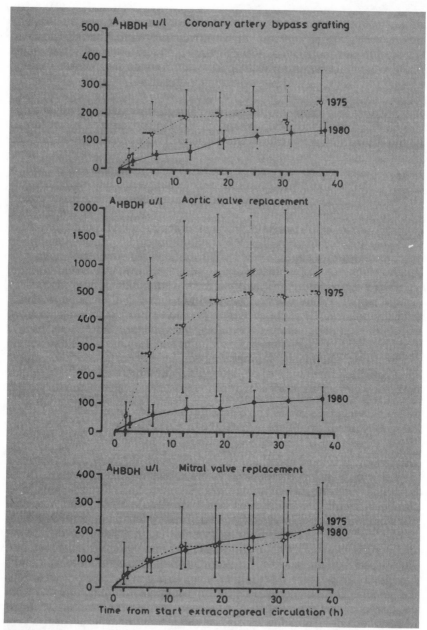

Fig. 9-1. Time course of calculated quantity of alpha hydroxybutyrate dehydrogenase (HBDH) released per liter plasma (A_{HBDH} μ/l) in patients operated upon in 1975 (O) and 1980 (●) for CABG (n = 15 in each year), aortic valve replacement (n = 10 in each year), and mitral valve replacement (n = 7 in each year). Indicated are medians ± 95% confidence limits. Differences between 1975 and 1980 are tested with a 2-tailed Wilcoxon rank test: ■p < 0.05 and ■■p < 0.01. Reproduced with permission from Davids et al.[47]

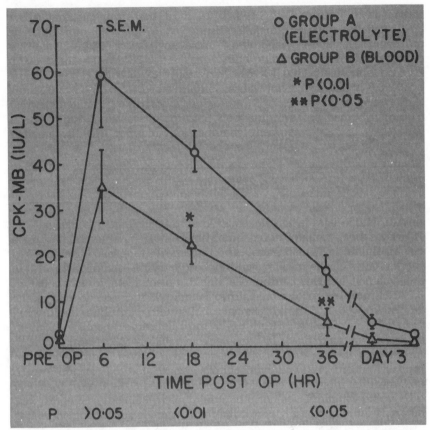

Fig. 9-2. Mean CPK-MB (IU/L) before and after operation (time in hours after release of cross-clamp). Reproduced with permission from Singh et al.[48]

In group A there was an average increase of 51% in mitochondrial size from the preperfusion to the postperfusion biopsies, reflecting an increased propensity toward mitochondrial swelling. In group B, there was a 5% decrease in average mitochondrial swelling. These results were highly significant (p < 0.001).

At the temperature utilized, that is 16° and 20°C, blood cardioplegia resulted in better preservation of myocardial ultrastructure, lower LV filling pressure, and less CPK-MB release. Although frequent reinfusions of the cardioplegic solution were utilized, septal temperatures were higher than in some other studies.

Neuronal and adrenomedullary catecholamine release in response to cardiopulmonary bypass

Marked increases in norepinephrine (NE) and epinephrine (E) concentrations in arterial blood during cardiopulmonary bypass have been demonstrated. Most reports concerned operations done in an era that preceded myocardial protection using cold potassium cardioplegia. Reves and associates[49] from Birmingham, Alabama, studied 28 adults and described the temporal increase in NE and E in relation to the abnormal hemodynamic and biochemical events during cardiopulmonary bypass. Bypass was conducted at a mean perfusate temperature of 28°C. Perfusion flows were between 1.3 and 2.2 liters/min/M². Aortic cross-clamping and cold cardioplegic preservation were utilized. A 9-fold increase in arterial E (from 75 ± 13– 708 ± 117 pg/ml) occurred from prebypass measurements to the end of aortic cross-clamping (Fig. 9-3). The E decreased rapidly after myocardial and pulmonary reperfusion. Arterial NE increased 2-fold from preaortic cross-clamping to 30 minutes of aortic cross-clamping and was associated with an increase in mean BP (Fig. 9-4). The peak increases in catecholamines occurred when the heart and lungs were excluded from the circulation, suggesting that either or both contributed to the increase perhaps by a chemoreceptor reflex located in either or both organs. Thus, elevated levels of catecholamines might be responsible for postoperative hypertension. Also, elevated levels of E and NE may be potentially detrimental to the myocardium and myocardial function after release of the aortic cross-clamp and reperfusion.

Fig. 9-3. Mean plasma levels of epinephrine (Epi) during cardiac anesthesia and surgery. Bars indicate SEM. Reproduced with permission from Reves.[49]

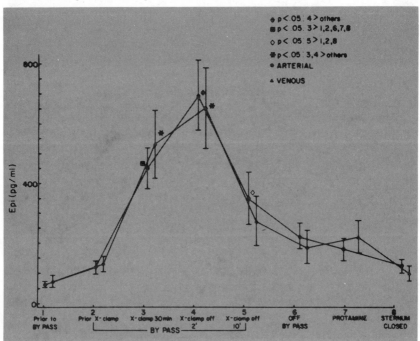

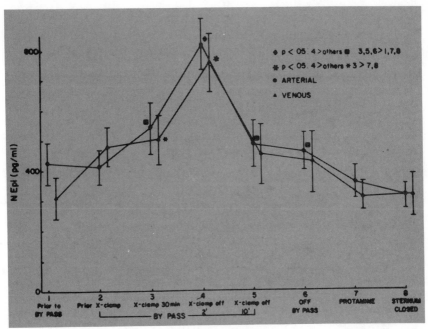

Fig. 9-4. Mean plasma levels of norepinephrine (NEpi) during cardiac anesthesia and surgery. Bars indicate SEM. Reproduced with permission from Reves.[49]

Pulmonary capillary wedge pressure -vs- left atrial pressure in the early postsurgical period

Simultaneous measurements of mean pulmonary capillary wedge (PCW) pressure and mean LA pressure were obtained before and after cardiopulmonary bypass and for a period of 16 hours postoperatively in 20 consecutive patients undergoing elective cardiac operation. In contrast to several previous reports that mean PCW pressure accurately reflected left-sided hemodynamics, Mammana and colleagues[50] from Chicago, Illinois, found that mean PCW pressure significantly exceeded the mean LA pressure in the early period after bypass and was most significantly in error at 4, 8, and 12 hours after operation ($p < 0.02$) (Fig. 9-5). The authors suggested that the disparity between mean PCW and LA pressures may be due to an increase in lung interstitial water or it may be related to the differing effects of afterload reducing agents on the pulmonary -vs- the systemic circulation. They suggested that mean LA pressure more accurately reflected LV filling and performance in the early postoperative period and should be used instead of Swan-Ganz monitoring to assess the hemodynamics of postsurgical patients.

Cardiac and pulmonary transplantation

Due to the pioneering, persistent, and outstanding work of Shumway and associates in Stanford, California, cardiac transplantation should become an

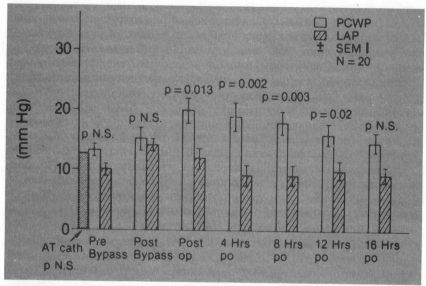

Fig. 9-5. Pulmonary capillary wedge pressure (PCWP) compared to left atrial pressure (LAP) (all patients), expressed as mean ± SEM, at all intervals studied. Analysis by 2 throw t test. Reproduced with permission from Mammana.[50]

accepted modality of treatment in a few patients with terminal cardiac disease. Pennock and associates[51] from Stanford reported the outcome of 227 cardiac transplant procedures performed in 206 patients from January 1968 to April 1981 (Fig. 9-6). Postoperative survival rates by the actuarial method were 63% for 1 year, 51% for 3 years, and 39% at 5 years after transplantation. Infection remained the primary cause of death following transplantation (76 of 131 patients, 58%), followed by acute rejection (24 of 181, 18%), graft arteriosclerosis (14 of 131, 11%), and malignancy (6 of 131, 5%). Most patients were treated with conventional immunosuppressive medications, including RATG, azathioprine, and prednisone. Monitoring for rejection was based on clinical parameters, ECG voltage, T lymphocyte counts, and liberal use of transvenous RV endomyocardial biopsy. Many deaths from infection occurred during augmented immunosuppressive therapy for acute rejection which accounted for 22%–27% of deaths during various time intervals from operation to the end of the second postoperative year. After 2 years, only 1 death was due to acute rejection. During the period under review, infection caused 65% of early deaths, 40% of total deaths.

Of 85 surviving 1 year, 21 had graft arteriosclerosis. In 11 patients, the arteriosclerosis resulted in graft failure. The authors found that incompatibility at HLA-A2 locus was associated with a higher incidence of graft arteriosclerosis than was apparent for all other A locus incompatibilities, and they have included HLA-A2 compatibility as part of the selection criteria for recipient and donor matching. In 148 recipients who were at risk ≥3 months

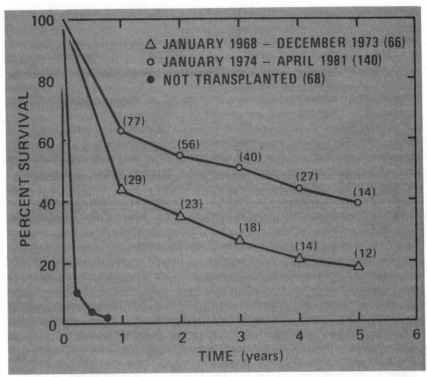

Fig. 9-6. Actuarial survival curves for Stanford cardiac transplantation program. Triangles include all patients treated January 1968–December 1973. Open circles include all patients treated January 1974–April 1981. Closed circles include patients chosen as potential recipients but not receiving heart transplant. Reproduced with permission from Pennock et al.[51]

after transplantation, 19 developed cancer. Three independent variables were shown to be significantly associated with the development of lymphoma: idiopathic cardiomyopathy, age of recipient, and second transplant procedure.

The remarkable achievement of cardiac transplantation can be inferred by the fact that 97% of 106 patients surviving ≥1 year after cardiac transplantation achieved New York Heart Association class I status, and most of them have returned to employment. The average duration of hospitalization was 65 days. The average cost was $83,432.00. Cardiac transplantation should be reserved for terminally ill patients with class IV cardiac disability. The present report documents satisfactory medium-term survival and excellent functional rehabilitation.

Since the first cardiac transplant 15 years ago, the survival has improved to 70% at 1 year and 50% at 5 years after transplantation at the Stanford Medical Center. These results and those from other centers were reviewed by Reitz and Stinson[52] from Stanford, California. The total number of cardiac transplant procedures per year is now about 100. The new interest in cardiac transplantation of course is based on the advances occurring during the last decade (Fig. 9-7). Most patients undergoing cardiac transplantation have CAD and the second largest group have idiopathic dilated cardiomyopathy. Most patients having cardiac transplants today return to a normal, functional capacity. Limitations are usually due to chronic immunosuppression, particularly with conventional therapy, including osteoporosis, myopathy, weight gain, and increased susceptibility to unusual infections. At Stanford, the overall patient survival at 1 year is 65%, and 45% at 5 years. The longest survivor at Stanford is now 12 years. Late complications after transplantation include increased frequency of malignancy, primarily lymphoproliferative disorders, and the development of CAD in the transplanted heart. In the 1980s cardiac transplantation has been combined with bilateral lung transplantation for some patients with severe pulmonary vascular disease, either primary or secondary to congenital heart disease. Reitz and Stinson, since March 1981, have performed transplantation on 5 patients with a combined heart and bilateral lung graft; 4 are alive and markedly improved.

Reitz and associates[53] from Stanford, California, described their initial

Fig. 9-7. Cardiac transplantation activity worldwide (black dots) and at Stanford Medical Center (white dots). Early worldwide enthusiasm gave way to reality of difficult management of rejection and complications (early 1970s). Improved patient selection, earlier and more specific diagnosis of rejection, and better immunosuppression management have yielded better results and recent wider application. Dash lines in 1981 data reflect incomplete year (up to October 1981). Reproduced with permission from Reitz and Stinson.[52]

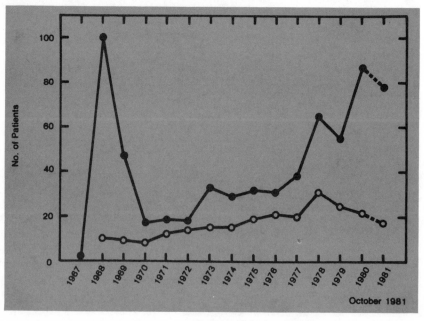

experience with 3 patients who received both heart and lung transplants. The primary immunosuppressive agent used was cyclosporin A. In the first patient, a 45-year-old woman with primary pulmonary hypertension, acute rejection of the transplant was diagnosed 10 and 25 days after surgery but was treated successfully; this patient still had normal exercise tolerance 10 months later. The second patient, a 30-year-old man, underwent transplantation for Eisenmenger's syndrome due to ASD and VSD. His graft was not rejected, and his condition was markedly improved 8 months after surgery. The third patient, a 29-year-old woman with TGA, died 4 days postoperatively of renal, hepatic, and pulmonary complications. The authors attribute their success to experience with heart-lung transplantation in primates, to the use of cyclosporin A, and to the anatomic and physiologic advantages of combined heart-lung replacement. It is hoped that such transplants may ultimately provide an improved outlook for selected terminally ill patients with pulmonary vascular disease and certain other intractable cardiopulmonary disorders.

Donor sinus node function was studied in 10 patients from day 4–24 after cardiac transplantation by Mackintosh and associates[54] from Cambridge, England. Cycle length, atrial arrhythmias, corrected sinus node recovery time, and estimated sinoatrial conduction time were recorded daily. Five patients had at least 2 sets of results suggesting sinus node dysfunction (group A) and 5 patients had no such abnormalities (group B). The prognosis in group A was poor, with 4 of the 5 patients dying within 4 months of the operation; 1 unexpected death from arrhythmias was recorded by ambulatory ECG monitoring. All 5 patients in group B survived ≥8 months. In 9 patients, sinus node function varied from day to day, with corrected sinus node recovery time reaching a peak at 11–18 days after operation. The longest corrected sinus node recovery time was 11,160 ms. Neither the differences between the patients, nor the day to day variation, could be explained solely by the degree of rejection as assessed by biopsy or by the ischemia time of the heart during procurement. Sinus node dysfunction soon after transplantation is associated with a poorer prognosis and might be the terminal event in some cases.

The electrophysiologic characteristics of ventricular muscle and Purkinje fiber from the hearts of 5 patients undergoing cardiac transplantation were examined by Dangman and associates[55] from New York City. All 5 patients had experienced CHF and CAD before surgery and were receiving digitalis. Ventricular muscle demonstrated a maximal diastolic potential (MDP) of −78 mV, action potential amplitude (APA) of 104 mV, a phase O upstroke velocity of 297 V/sec and action potential duration (APD) at 50% repolarization of 190 ms. Purkinje fibers had a MDP of −80 mV, and APA of 107 mV, a V_{max} of 388 V/second, and APD at 50% repolarization of 195 ms. Fibers examined from infarcted sections of the heart revealed significantly longer APD than those from noninfarcted tissue, which resulted in marked dispersion of APD in infarcted and adjacent zones. Both epinephrine and ouabain induced delayed after depolarizations in Purkinje fibers and this suggested that delayed after depolarizations and resultant triggered activity can occur in the human ventricle.

Cytomegalovirus, herpes simplex virus, and varicella zoster virus cause serious infection in immunosuppressed patients. Herpes simplex produces prolonged and severe oral and genital lesions in renal and cardiac transplant recipients. Herpes zoster is also common in these patients, although visceral dissemination is rare. Cytomegalovirus infections cause significant mortality and morbidity, particularly in cardiac and renal transplant recipients with primary cytomegalovirus infection. Pulmonary infections also are common. Transplant recipients have severe and prolonged infections with herpes viruses, despite high titers of circulating antibody. Specific deficits in cell-mediated immunity, however, to herpes simplex virus, cytomegalovirus, and varicella zoster virus have been demonstrated in patients following cardiac transplantation. Pollard and colleagues[56] from Stanford, California, studied prospectively in 36 cardiac transplant recipients immune responses and infections with herpes viruses. Specific lymphocyte transformation and interferon production in response to viral antigens, viral culture results, antibody levels, responses to phytohemagglutinin, and T cell numbers were determined. Responses to phytohemagglutinin and T cell numbers were depressed for 6–12 weeks. Cytomegalovirus infection occurred in 100% of seropositive patients and in 62% of seronegative patients. Primary infection was more frequently symptomatic. Heart implantation from a seropositive patient was significantly correlated with subsequent infection in seronegative patients. Depression of transformation in response to cytomegalovirus correlated with prolonged shedding. Herpes simplex infection occurred in 95% of seropositive patients but decreased after 12 weeks. Asymptomatic shedding was rare, and primary infection did not occur. Return of transformation in response to herpes simplex was associated with decreased infection. Herpes zoster occurred in 22% during the first year, and transformation responses to varicella zoster returned thereafter. Depression of interferon production in response to viruses did not correlate with infection as well as did lymphocyte transformation.

C-reactive protein measurements in infective complications following cardiac operation

Studies on acute phase protein levels have shown C-reactive protein (CRP) to rise more rapidly than the other proteins following inflammation and tissue damage. A report by Ghoneim and associates[57] from Leeds, England, described the time course of CRP levels in patients following uncomplicated open heart operations, and its behavior in patients in whom serious infections developed in the early postoperative period (Fig. 9-8). There were 100 patients studied who had uncomplicated cardiac operation. Seventeen other patients were studied in whom serious infections, including prosthetic valve endocarditis, developed early in the postoperative period, and there were 11 patients with late onset of prosthetic valve endocarditis. The CRP levels were measured by single radial immunodiffusion. Patients without postoperative infective complications showed a rapid increase in CRP levels that reached a peak within 72 hours after operation, followed by a

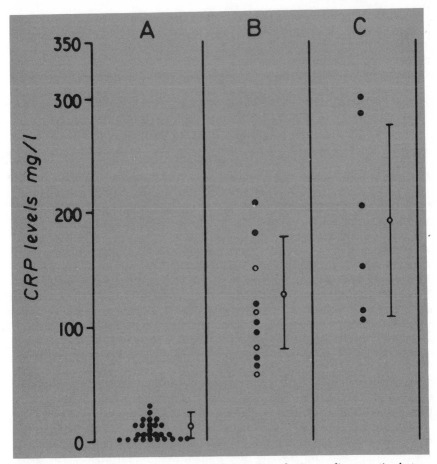

Fig. 9-8. Serum C-reactive protein (CRP) levels in patients having cardiac operation but no infection (A), patients with late onset of prosthetic valve endocarditis and infective endocarditis (B), and patients with early prosthetic valve endocarditis (C). The levels shown represent serum levels when first tested after clinical diagnosis of endocarditis had been made, and each measurement represents 1 patient. In section B, the open circles represent patients with late onset of prosthetic valve endocarditis while closed circles are those with endocarditis of native valves. Mean and standard deviation are indicated for each group. Reproduced with permission from Ghoneim et al.[57]

progressive decline. A mean peak rise, attained by the third day, was 420 mg/liter. This was followed by progressive decline until levels <30 mg/liter were reached by the third postoperative week. Levels of ≥200 mg/liter in the second postoperative week or ≥100 mg/liter during the third postoperative week were always associated with infection. The differences between the CRP levels in infected and uninfected patients were significant (p < 0.01). Serial measurements were of prognostic value in evaluating the response to chemotherapy, and in predicting the outcome of the disease. The authors suggest embarking on an intensive investigation for a focus of infection in any patient with a high CRP level (> 100 mg/liter) in the third postoperative week even in the absence of pyrexia.

OPERATIVE TREATMENT OF CERTAIN AORTIC AND PERIPHERAL ARTERIAL CONDITIONS

Gelatin-resorcin-formol biologic glue in aortic dissection

Bachet and colleagues[58] from Paris, France, reported 25 patients operated on from January 1977 to September 1980 in whom gelatin-resorcin-formol (GRF) biologic glue was used for tissue reinforcement during operations for acute dissection of the ascending aorta. Results in these patients (GRF group) were compared with results of 25 patients operated on between 1970 and 1976 with "classical techniques" (CT group). The aortic valve was replaced in 3 cases in the GRF group and in 12 cases in the CT group. The coronary arteries were bypassed or reimplanted in 20% of patients in each group. Average volume of intraoperative blood transfusion was 5,800 ml in the CT group and 2,100 ml in the GRF group ($p < 0.01$). There were 4 intraoperative deaths in the CT group and none in the GRF group. Postoperative renal failure, cerebral ischemia, persisting peripheral ischemia, and infection were more frequent in the CT group, being responsible for 8 hospital deaths in this group and for 2 in the GRF group ($p < 0.01$). Hospital mortality was therefore reduced from 48% (CT group) to 8% (GRF group) ($p < 0.01$).

The authors concluded that the use of GRF glue significantly reduces the necessity for AVR, the amount of intraoperative and postoperative bleeding, and the frequency and severity of postoperative complications. The long-term survival rate at 4 years was raised from 40%–91%. The authors admit that the results in the GRF group have certainly benefited from the general progress in preoperative and postoperative management, better radiologic techniques, and better myocardial protection during the operation. They stress, however, that the operative procedures were much more simple with the GRF glue. They further suggest that the quality and tightness of the adhesion of the 2 layers of the dissection after operation with GRF glue may reduce the risk of persisting or recurrent dissection.

Ascending aortic aneurysm: replacement or repair?

The Robicsek method of handling dilation of the ascending aorta is discussed by Egloff and colleagues[59] from Zurich, Switzerland. Between 1971 and 1980, 100 patients underwent operation for ascending aortic aneurysm. Acute dissection was present in 29, chronic dissection in 11, dilation only in 56, and inflammatory disease in 4. Four different operative procedures were applied independent of the type of disease: repair and reduction aortoplasty (21 patients), reduction aortoplasty reinforced by nylon net (17 patients), supracoronary graft replacement (42 patients), and composite graft replacement with reimplantation of both coronary ostia (20 patients). Early mortality was 10%, and late mortality was 12% after a mean follow-up of 45 months. The authors concluded that reduction aortoplasty (partial aortic resection) supported by a tightly wrapped synthetic net is a suitable method in patients with normal sinuses of Valsalva and without dissection or inflammatory disease. They drew particular attention to the use of proximal anchor stitches generally passed from the aortic valve prosthesis through the aortic wall, then anchored to the external Dacron material. Compared with a supracoronary or composite graft replacement, this method carried a lower complication rate, particularly in regard to cerebral vascular accidents and AMI. For patients with acute and chronic dissection with intact aortic root, supracoronary graft replacement was preferred, whereas in those with anuloaortic ectasia with dilated sinus of Valsalva and in all patients with Marfan's syndrome, composite graft replacement has become the procedure of choice.

Profound hypothermia and circulatory arrest for aneurysm of the aortic arch

Experience with profound hypothermia and circulatory arrest in the treatment of aneurysms of the aortic arch is reported by Ergin and associates[60] from New York City. In 21 consecutive patients, the aortic arch, varying portions of the ascending aorta and descending aorta, and in some the aortic valve were replaced with the aid of a standard method of profound total body hypothermia and circulatory arrest. Fourteen patients underwent elective, and 7 patients emergency arch replacement for aortic dissection. Replacement of the aortic arch was performed during a single period of circulatory arrest using surface cooling before core cooling with the patient on cardiopulmonary bypass to produce an average core temperature of 120–15°C. During the period of cooling, suspension or AVR and replacement of the ascending aorta are carried out. Thereafter, the head vessels are clamped and replacement of the arch is accomplished during a single period of circulatory arrest. Cardiopulmonary bypass is then resumed to warm the patient and resuscitate the heart. Myocardial preservation is provided with cold potassium cardioplegia and topical profound hypothermia. After termination of cardiopulmonary bypass, protamine is administered, and all patients are given fresh frozen plasma, platelet concentrates, and freshly drawn autologous blood to restore the coagulation mechanism. Intravenous steroids are administered for 48 hours. The average cerebral ischemic time was 37 ± 14 minutes. The average core temperature was $13.7° \pm 1.8°C$. Average myocardial ischemic time was 79 ± 28 minutes, and the average duration of cardiopulmonary bypass was 130 ± 32 minutes. There were 3 deaths among the 14 patients undergoing elective operation, and 3 deaths among the 7 patients undergoing emergency operation. Among the survivors, there were no neurologic sequelae; however 1 of the deaths was accompanied by cerebral dysfunction. The authors stress the use of surface cooling. They emphasize that excessive coagulopathy was not a problem using bolus administration of blood components and discontinuing cardiopulmonary bypass only when normothermia had been fully achieved.

These excellent results in a difficult group of patients attest not only to the simplicity and reproducibility of the method, but also to the focused interest and attention to detail.

Chronic traumatic thoracic aneurysm

The natural history of chronic, traumatic thoracic aneurysm was analyzed by Finkelmeier and associates[61] from Charlottesville, Virginia. They collected 401 cases reported during 1950–1980 with an additional 12 cases from their own institution. Of the patients, 42% developed signs or symptoms of aneurysm expansion within 5 years of injury; 85% within 20 years. Pain was the most frequent symptom, followed by serial enlargement on chest roentgenogram. Of the 60 patients followed without operative intervention, 20 died of their aortic lesions (Fig. 9-9). For these patients, the combined risk of dying or developing signs or symptoms was 41% at 5 years. Of the 401 patients, 332 underwent operative repair of the aneurysm with an operative mortality of 5%. The major cause of operative death was bleeding (2%), cardiac problems (2%), and renal failure (1%). Thirty-two patients (11%) had a major complication: bleeding (5%), cardiac failure (1%), renal failure (1%), spinal cord injury (1%), cerebral vascular accident (1%), and pulmonary insufficiency (1%). Damage to the recurrent laryngeal nerve occurred in 7% of patients.

In 60 nonoperative and in 94 operative patients adequate follow-up information was available. Five years after injury, 93% of the operative patients were alive, and only 71% of the nonoperative patients ($p = 0.0006$). At 10 years, the survival was 85% in the operative group and 66% in the nonoperative group; at 15 years after injury, 15% of the operative patients and 34% of the nonoperative patients had died.

Although this retrospective study includes only cases drawn from the "literature" and which might have been reported to prove 1 or another biases or illustrate a technique, they documented the natural history of nonoperative and operative treatment of post-traumatic thoracic aneurysm, and they showed that survival was improved by operation. The 1.4% incidence of paraplegia is appreciably less than the generally reported incidence of paraplegia subsequent to operations on the thoracic aorta as a whole. They argue appropriately that chronic, traumatic aneurysm results from an injury to the aorta at a discreet point, as contrasted to atherosclerotic aneurysms that complicates a condition involving many systemic arteries and in which aneurysmal repair may require interruption or obliteration of a large part of the descending thoracic aorta.

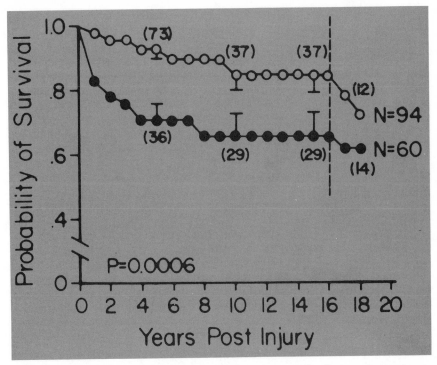

Fig. 9-9. Probability of surviving chronic traumatic aneurysm. O—O, Operative treatment. ●—●, Nonoperative treatment. Reproduced with permission from Finkelmeier et al.[61]

Spinal cord injury after cross-clamping descending thoracic aorta

Operations on the descending thoracic aorta for surgical correction of coarctation, repair of traumatic injury, or resection of an aneurysm, usually necessitate cross-clamping of the aorta. This procedure may cause irreversible ischemic damage by compromising blood flow to the spinal cord resulting in paraplegia. The risk varies between 0.5% and 10%. Berendes and colleagues[62] from Leiden, The Netherlands, monitored lumbar spinal fluid pressure during operation on the descending aorta in 8 patients. One patient incurred ischemic damage of the spinal cord, resulting in paraparesis, and in that patient spinal fluid pressure increased to such high levels that it may have caused tamponade of the spinal cord. The lumbar spinal fluid pressure increase resulted from expansion of cerebral vessels caused by an acute rise of arterial pressure after aortic clamping, probably aggravated by the administration of a vasodilating drug. In 7 patients not developing paraparesis, the mean spinal fluid pressure was 14 mmHg during aortic cross-clamping, while mean femoral artery pressure was 41 mmHg. In the 1 patient developing paraparesis, mean spinal fluid pressure was 41 mmHg, while mean femoral artery pressure during aortic cross-clamping was 38 mmHg. The authors presented additional experimental information to suggest that the cerebrospinal fluid space has limited compliance after an incremental change of approximately 50 ml of fluid. They suggest that proximal arterial hypertension plus cerebral vasodilation may cause an excessive increase in spinal fluid pressure. In addition, reduction of BP below the aortic clamp results in a tamponade effect, seriously diminishing the driving pressure in the radicular arteries and causing spinal cord ischemia. The authors suggest monitoring aortic pressure distal to the clamp, monitoring cerebrospinal fluid pressure in the lumbar region, and using a shunting procedure, should arterial pressure and lumbar spinal fluid pressure become nearly equal.

Spinal cord injury after operations on the descending thoracic aorta is a danger constantly facing patients with lesions of the descending thoracic aorta. Monitoring of cerebrospinal fluid pressure and the recently described assessment of somatosensory evoked potentials have been shown to be helpful in a retrospective analysis of patients who have developed paraparesis or paraplegia. The best method to prevent neurologic injury has yet to be determined.

Platelet deposition on Dacron aortic bifurcation grafts

Stratton and colleagues[63] from Seattle, Washington, assessed the interaction between platelets and chronically implanted prosthetic arterial graft surfaces in man by imaging indium-111 labeled platelet deposition in 15 patients with Dacron aortic bifurcation grafts. The grafts had been in place for 9–120 months. These results were compared with those obtained by platelet imaging of the aortofemoral vessels of 13 normal young adults without grafts. Quantitative evaluation was performed in both groups by graft/blood ratio that compared indium-111 platelet activity in the aortofemoral vascular region to whole blood activity over a 96 hour imaging time. In addition, blinded qualitative visual interpretation was performed on all studies by comparing aortofemoral area activity with that in adjacent native arteries. Reproducibility of the technique was evaluated by repeat imaging and quantitative analysis of 6 patients with grafts. Quantitative evaluation of the normal subjects revealed that the mean vessel/whole blood activity ratio was 2 at 24 hours after platelet injection and remained constant for the duration of the study. In contrast, patients with grafts had a mean graft/blood ratio of 3 at 24 hours, which increased progressively to 8 at 96 hours, documenting ongoing platelet deposition in patients with vascular grafts. Independent qualitative visual interpretation of the aortofemoral region disclosed no abnormal uptake in normal subjects, whereas 13 of 15 patients with grafts had platelet deposition. The 6 reproducibility studies in patients with grafts were quantitatively unchanged and remained visually positive.

Thus, platelet deposition in chronically implanted Dacron arterial grafts was consistently present, progressive over 96 hours, quantifiable, and reproducible. The results of this investigation imply absent or incomplete endothelial cell coverage of the new graft flow surface, and, furthermore, the techniques may be useful in assessing prosthetic material, thrombogenicity, and the efficacy of platelet-inhibitory drugs in man.

Pentoxifylline in treatment of intermittent claudication

The efficacy, safety, and tolerance of pentoxifylline in the treatment of intermittent claudication associated with chronic occlusive arterial disease were evaluated by Porter and colleagues[64], in a double-blind, placebo-controlled, parallel-group, multicenter (7 institutions in the USA) clinical trial involving a total of 128 outpatients. The response to treatment was ascertained at regular intervals during the trial by measuring the distance walked prior to the onset of claudication when patients were subjected to a standardized treadmill test. Pentoxifylline given orally in dosages up to 1,200 mg/day was significantly more effective than placebo in increasing both the initial and absolute claudication distances in patients with chronic occlusive arterial disease. Reduction of lower limb paresthesias also suggested greater clinical improvement in the pentoxifylline-treated patients. These results support the hypothesis that pentoxifylline reduces blood viscosity by improving red cell flexibility, and thereby enhances blood flow in patients with chronic occlusive arterial disease. Although the precise mode of therapeutic action requires clarification, pentoxifylline was well tolerated with minimal untoward effects.

UNCATEGORIZABLE

Left ventricular function in trained and untrained healthy subjects

Bar-Shlomo and colleagues[65] from Ontario, Canada, compared LV function in 18 normal sedentary controls (mean age, 28 years) and 9 endurance trained athletes (mean age, 19 years) at rest and during supine bicycle exercise. Heart rate (HR) BP, LV EF, and relative changes in LV end-diastolic (EDV) and end-systolic (ESV) volumes were assessed at rest and at each level of graded exercise using gated RNA. Athletes attained a much greater work load than controls (mean, 22.1 kpm/kg body weight -vs- 13 kpm/kg). Both groups achieved similar increases in HR, BP, and EF. In the control, the mean EDV increased to 124% of that at rest and the mean ESV increased to 81% of the rest level. In contrast, the mean EDV did not significantly change during exercise in athletes and the mean ESV decreased to 64% of rest. Although trained and untrained healthy subjects had similar increases in the LV EF during exercise, different mechanisms were used to achieve these increases. Untrained subjects increased EDVs, whereas trained subjects decreased ESVs. Thus, the ability of athletes to exercise without increasing preload may be an effect of training and might have important implications in reducing myocardial oxygen demand during exercise.

Left ventricular diastolic capacity

The ventricles even during normal volemia and in the supine position maintain a reserve capacity to enlarge beyond the normal end-diastolic volume (EDV) and augment stroke output by the Frank-Starling mechanism. Flessas and Ryan[66] in Boston, Massachusetts, used plasma volume expansion with 500 ml of low molecular weight dextran in 9 normal subjects, 13 patients with CAD, 4 with AS, and 1 with cardiomyopathy. The LV EDV increased from a control value of 12–23 mmHg and EDV from 84–98 ml/M^2. The EDV/LV EDP curve constructed for the 12 patients from multiple angiograms at progressively increasing filling pressures during plasma volume expansion showed an initial part where EDV increased in parallel with LV EDP and a final steep or perpendicular portion of the curve where EDV increased minimally or not at all as LV EDP exceeded 20 mmHg. Exponential equations were used to fit diastolic volume pressure data obtained with catheter-tip manometers in 7 patients. The exponential constant, k, ranged from 0.012–0.044 ml^{-1} and was inversely related to EDV. For comparable EDV, there were no differences in k values between normal subjects and patients with a variety of heart diseases.

Plasma catecholamines, platelet aggregation, and associated thromboxane formation after physical exercise, smoking, or norepinephrine infusion in healthy men

To study the possible role of catecholamines in platelet activation, Siess and associates[67] from Munich, West Germany, measured platelet aggregation stimulated by adenosine diphosphate (ADP), collagen, arachidonic acid, and 1-epinephrine, thromboxane B_2 (TXB_2) formation, and plasma levels of catecholamines and renin in healthy men both before and after 6 days of propranolol treatment (40 mg 3 times/day) under control conditions and during sympathoadrenergic stimulation by physical exercise or smoking. Exercise markedly increased plasma norepinephrine and plasma renin activity. Smoking predominately increased plasma epinephrine. Propranolol did not consistently influence these variables, but blunted the circulatory response to exercise and smoking. Despite the marked increases of plasma catecholamines after both stimuli and without beta blockade, platelet aggregation stimulated by ADP, 1-epinephrine, collagen, and arachidonic acid and associated TXB_2 formation was not enhanced. Moreover, plasma norepinephrine levels in the same range due to infusion significantly reduced platelet aggregation with low dose collagen, 1-epinephrine, and ADP. These data do not support a role of endogenous catecholamines in inhibiting platelet activation and TXB_2 formation.

Cardiovascular responses to exercise after 10 days of bed rest

In assessing the reduced effort tolerance of patients recovering from AMI it is difficult to separate the role of cardiac damage from that of bed rest deconditioning. Although studies have been performed on the effects of prolonged bed rest, these studies often involve healthy, young subjects who are not comparable in age to those often afflicted with AMI. Convertino and associates[68] from Moffett Field, California, assessed the cardiorespiratory response to 10 days of continuous recumbancy in 12 healthy men aged 50 years who underwent supine and upright graded maximal exercise testing before and after bed rest. They found that the decrease in peak oxygen uptake after bed rest was greater during upright exercise than during supine exercise. Also, the decrease in submaximal work was greater in the upright than in the supine position. Ventilation volume also was found to be significantly elevated after bed rest during maximal and submaximal effort in both supine and upright positions. After bed rest, the peak heart rate increased 5% during supine and upright testing. The increases in rate-pressure product after bed rest were significantly larger during upright and supine exercise. Thus, these results indicate that orthostatic stress is the most important factor limiting exercise tolerance after bed rest in normal middle-aged men. These investigators confirm the clinical approach of Levine and Lown who introduced armchair treatment of acute coronary thrombosis in 1952 and further suggest that intermittent exposure to gravitational stress in the bed rest stage of convalescence from AMI may obviate much of the deterioration of cardiovascular performance.

Myocardial fiber disarray in normal hearts

In his original necropsy description of HC, Teare described disorganization of myocardial fibers in the ventricular septum. Subsequently, it has been demonstrated by Maron and associates and others they myocardial fiber disarray is not specific for HC, but may occur in other conditions. If the amount of disarray is quantified, however, the amount of disarray of myocardial fibers in the ventricular septum is far greater in patients with HC than in any other condition. In a report entitled "Myocardial Disarray, a Critical Review," Becker and Caruso[69] from Amsterdam, The Netherlands, described histologic observations in 5 hearts and gross observations in 5 other hearts of patients aged 1 day to 75 years, and these patients died of diseases unrelated to the cardiovascular and/or pulmonary systems. In the 5 patients in whom histologic studies were performed, 12 full-thickness blocks were removed for study, including 2 blocks from the ventricular septum. Each block was cut sequentially in 3 different planes, reembedding being necessary for each of the 3 cuts. Becker and Caruso were able to distinguish subepicardial, middle, and subendocardial layers by their gross fiber orientations and they also found many regions of interdigitating myocardial fibers by the gross dissection method. Of the 180 histologic sections studied, only 42 showed a parallel fiber arrangement or only 23% of the sections were judged to show normal histology; 79 sections (44%) showed a minor deviation of normal, whereas disorganization was present in 59 sections (33%). Changing the orientation of the block produced a change in the dominant microscopic appearance in 52 of the 60 blocks; in only 8 blocks were the same results produced irrespective of the plane of section. Thus, the authors did not find a strictly parallel arrangement in any block when sectioned in all 3 planes. In 15 blocks, they found a different histology in each of the 3 planes, and in the remaining 37 blocks a change in histology was found when sections were studied in 2 planes.

The authors have made some fairly strong conclusions based on study of only 5 hearts histologically, including patients with a large age scatter (1 day, 4 months, and 4, 9, and 21 years), none of whom had HC. It is hazardous to apply, as they did, their observations to patients with HC. These authors apparently have not studied at necropsy patients HC.

Cardiac catheterization and cardiac surgical facilities in a single county in Minnesota compared with nationwide facilities

Cardiac catheterization and cardiac operations were evaluated by Kennedy and associates[70] from Rochester, Minnesota, in the population of Olmsted County, Minnesota, from 1973 through 1980, and trends in this region were compared with nationwide trends based on data from several sources. The medical service area of Olmsted County possessed characteristics necessary to study actual use of health services in a defined population because it is a stable population of approximately 90,000 persons and 98% of all residents therein receive their hospital-based care at local hospitals. This fact is especially true for cardiac care, for the only facilities for cardiac catheterization and cardiac surgery in southern Minnesota are located in one of the hospitals affiliated with the Mayo Clinic. The rates of coronary angiography and CABG operations in Olmsted County increased over time but overall the rates of catheterization and operation appeared to be leveling off. For the country as a whole, the data appeared to show similar trends but there are wide differences among regions in the rates of operation and catheterization (Table 9-3). In 1980, 40% of hospitals with cardiac catheterization laboratories and 55% of those with facilities for open heart surgery were doing fewer than the suggested minimum numbers of these procedures necessary to achieve optimum results. The data support the view that further growth in the number of cardiac centers should be avoided. The authors suggested that there was a need for continued evaluation of the use of cardiac services if quality was to be protected and cost controlled.

Thrombosis complicating pulmonary artery catheterization via the internal jugular vein

The clinical diagnosis of deep vein thrombosis has been shown to be unreliable. Chastre and associates[71] from Paris, France, prospectively determined by angiography the frequency of internal jugular vein thrombosis in

TABLE 9-3. *Cardiac catheterization procedures and open heart operations and hospitals providing such services, according to region, 1980. Reproduced with permission from Kennedy et al.*[70]

| REGION* | CARDIAC CATHETERIZATION† | | | | OPEN HEART OPERATION | | | |
| | PROCEDURES | | HOSPITALS | | OPERATIONS | | HOSPITALS | |
	thousands	*rate‡*	*no.*	*rate§*	*thousands*	*rate‡*	*no.*	*rate§*
New England	19.3	157	45	3.6	6.6	53	26	2.1
Middle Atlantic	66.0	179	118	3.2	22.9	62	69	1.9
South Atlantic	66.1	179	129	3.5	20.5	55	83	2.2
East South-Central	35.9	245	51	3.5	13.0	89	35	2.4
West South-Central	71.5	301	105	4.4	19.8	83	81	3.4
East North-Central	91.9	221	173	4.2	31.2	75	111	2.7
West North-Central	38.2	222	74	4.3	13.5	79	53	3.1
Mountain	25.9	228	51	4.5	8.7	76	37	3.3
Pacific	71.3	224	167	5.3	24.7	78	110	3.5
Total	*486.1*	*215*	*913*	*4.0*	*160.9*	*71*	*605*	*2.7*

* For a few individual states, only 1979 or 1978 figures were available. Geographic regions of the United States as defined for the federal census are as follows: *New England*—Connecticut, Maine, Massachusetts, New Hampshire, Rhode Island, and Vermont; *Middle Atlantic*—New Jersey, New York, and Pennsylvania; *South Atlantic*—Delaware, District of Columbia, Florida, Georgia, Maryland, North Carolina, South Carolina, Virginia, and West Virginia; *East South-Central*—Alabama, Kentucky, Mississippi, and Tennessee; *West South-Central*—Arkansas, Louisiana, Oklahoma, and Texas; *East North-Central*—Illinois, Indiana, Michigan, Ohio, and Wisconsin; *West North-Central*—Iowa, Kansas, Minnesota, Missouri, Nebraska, North Dakota, and South Dakota; *Mountain*—Arizona, Colorado, Idaho, Montana, Nevada, New Mexico, Utah, and Wyoming; *Pacific*—Alaska, California, Hawaii, Oregon, and Washington. † Includes coronary arteriography, left ventriculography, and cardiac catheterization. ‡ Number of cases per 100,000 population per year. The lack of information on age, sex, and race precluded an adjustment of the rates for these factors. § Number of hospitals per million population.

33 consecutive critically ill patients who had temporary monitoring with Swan-Ganz catheters via the internal jugular vein. Of them, 22 patients (66%) had venographic or autopsy evidence of internal jugular vein thrombosis. Thus, venous thrombosis is a frequent complication of temporary monitoring with the Swan-Ganz catheter, especially in patients whose circulatory function has been impaired for a prolonged period.

Effect of weight loss on sleep-disordered breathing and oxygen desaturation in extreme obesity

Four morbidly obese men who had been found to have significant sleep-disordered breathing and oxygen desaturation were restudied by Harman and associates[72] from Gainesville, Florida, after an average weight loss of 108 kg (range, 53–155 kg). In all subjects, weight loss was accompanied by a significant reduction in the number of episodes per hour of sleep-disordered breathing events. In 3, there was improvement in the severity of desaturation accompanying abnormal breathing. The 2 subjects with daytime somnolence and hypercapnia before weight loss showed the most dramatic improvement in desaturation. This suggests that obesity is a cause, rather than an effect, of the sleep apnea syndrome.

Atrial pacing, epinephrine infusion, and autonomic blockade in asymptomatic men with normal coronary arteries

Taggart and associates[73] from London and Oxford, England, studied 20 asymptomatic men, aged 17–57 years, with an abnormal resting ECG but normal epicardial coronary arteries and normal LV angiograms. Echoes in all 20 also were normal. Sixteen had flat or inverted T waves in the lateral leads, 2 had ST depression, and 2 had mixed patterns. T-wave abnormalities and, to a lesser extent, ST changes returned to normal or regressed after an overnight rest. Subsequent atrial pacing to 160 beats/minute reproduced or increased the respective ECG abnormalities. When epinephrine was infused in low doses just sufficient to produce discernible effects on the ST-T segment and atrial pacing was repeated, the effect of the latter was enhanced. Both epinephrine and atrial pacing influenced the ST-T segment in the same direction. Intravenous propranolol blocked the effect of epinephrine and its synergistic effect with pacing but exerted little if any influence on the effect of pacing alone. Atropine given intravenously after propranolol reduced the effect of atrial pacing on the ST-T configuration. Treadmill exercise tests were positive in 9 and borderline in 1 patient. After beta blockade (oral oxprenolol), all tests were negative. Since beta blockade did not prevent pacing-induced ST depression but normalized the false positive exercise test, the latter does not appear to be rate related but more probably the result of the direct influence of catecholamines. Isolated T-wave changes and ST depression in the resting ECG differ in that they are influenced both by the heart rate and catecholamines acting synergistically.

Cardiac damage in suspected cardiac contusion

Although cardiac damage may be frequently associated with trauma to the chest, the true incidence of nonpenetrating trauma to the heart is difficult due to lack of specificity of available cardiac techniques. Nevertheless, the clinical diagnosis of cardiac damage in this setting remains important. Potkin and associates[74] from Seattle, Washington, evaluated noninvasive tests for detecting myocardial damage in 100 patients with severe nonpenetrating chest trauma. Noninvasive tests included serial ECG, serial total creatine phosphokinase (CPK) and CPK-MB enzymes, continuous Holter monitoring recording to detect arrhythmia, and technetium-99 pyrophosphate scintigraphy. Peak CPK-MB elevations occurred in 72 patients, ECG abnormalities were observed in 70 patients, and 27 patients had Lown grade ≥3 arrhythmias. Fifteen patients died and were autopsied. The noninvasive abnormalities were nonspecific and thus did not reflect myocardial contusion that led to clinically important cardiac complications.

Effects of hemodialysis and renal transplantation on left ventricular size and function

Ikaheimo and associates[75] from Oulu, Finland, investigated 13 patients with chronic renal failure by echo preoperatively before and after hemodialysis and again after a successful renal transplantation to evaluate the cardiac changes caused by the transplantation. After renal transplantation, the LV end-diastolic and end-systolic diameters and cardiac index decreased, probably because the LV filling pressure decreased. The LV wall thickness and mass decreased, apparently because of a decrease in LV preload and afterload, because the systolic BP decreased. The LA diameter decreased presumably in response to the decreased LV preload and wall hypertrophy. The changes in the indexes of LV function as a result of hemodialysis appear to predict the changes seen after renal transplantation. Thus, renal transplantation appears to result in normal LV and LA volume, to lessen LV hypertrophy, without significantly improving LV function.

Morphologic evidence for coronary artery spasm in eclampsia

Bauer and associates[76] from Baltimore, Maryland, examined the role of vascular spasm as a component of the eclamptic state. They hypothesized if abnormal vascular reactivity affects the coronary arteries in eclampsia, one might expect to find areas of myocardial contraction band necrosis, a lesion secondary to coronary reflow after periods of no flow. The investigators reviewed the cardiac findings in 34 patients with fatal eclampsia characterized by hypertension, edema, proteinuria, and convulsions without evident cause. Each was compared with the next pregnant or puerperal nontoxemic autopsied patient. The eclamptic patients ranged in age from 15–45 years (mean, 27). Convulsions began ante partum in 21 patients, intrapartum in 8, and postpartum in 5. Heart weights ranged from 200–407 g (mean, 312). One patient had rheumatic valvular disease and 1, myocarditis. Histologic study of heart sections showed the presence of contraction band necrosis in 12 patients (35%). The control cases included 2 patients with rheumatic valvular disease, 2 with endocarditis, 2 with myocarditis, 2 with pericarditis, 1 with leukemia. Only 1 (3%) control patient had contraction band necrosis. Thus, the frequent occurrence of myocardial contraction band necrosis suggested that coronary artery spasm may be common in patients who die with eclampsia.

References

1. WADA T, HONDA M, MATSUYAMA S: Extra echo spaces-ultrasonographic and computerized tomography correlations. Br Heart J 47:430–438, May 1982.
2. GINZTON LE, LAKS MM: The differential diagnosis of acute pericarditis from the normal variant: new ECG criteria. Circulation 65:1004–1009, May 1982.

3. ARMSTRONG WF, SCHILT BF, HELPER DJ, DILLON JC, FEIGENBAUM H: Diastolic collapse of the right ventricle with cardiac tamponade: an echo study. Circulation 65:1491–1496, June 1982.

4. GROSE R, GREENBERG M, STEINGART R, COHEN MV: LV volume and function during relief of cardiac tamponade in man. Circulation 66:149–155, July 1982.

5. KERBER RE, GASCHO JA, LITCHFIELD R, WOLFSON P, OTT D, PANDIAN NG: Hemodynamic effects of volume expansion and nitroprusside compared with pericardiocentesis in patients with acute cardiac tamponade. N Engl J Med 307:929–931, Oct 7, 1982.

6. ALCAN KE, ZABETAKIS PM, MARINO ND, FRANZONE AJ, MICHELIS MF, BRUNO MS: Management of acute cardiac tamponade by subxiphoid pericardiotomy. JAMA 247:1143–1148, Feb 26, 1982.

7. MAISCH B, MAISCH S, KOCHSIEK K: Immune reactions in tuberculous and chronic constrictive pericarditis. Am J Cardiol 50:1007–1013, Nov 1982.

8. KUTCHER MA, KING SB, ALIMURUNG BN, CRAVER JM, LOGUE RB: Constrictive pericarditis as a complication of cardiac surgery: recognition of an entity. Am J Cardiol 50:742–748, 1982.

9. NICOLOSI GL, BORGIONI L, ALBERTI E, BURELLI C, MAFFESANTI M, MARINO P, SLAVICH G, ZANUTTINI D: M-mode and two-dimensional echocardiography in congenital absence of the pericardium. Chest 81:610–613, May 1982.

10. ADENLE AD, EDWARDS JE: Clinical and pathologic features of metastatic neoplasms of the pericardium. Chest 81:166–169, Feb 1982.

11. WAGENVOORT CA, WAGENVOORT N: Smooth muscle content of pulmonary arterial media in pulmonary venous hypertension compared with other forms of pulmonary hypertension. Chest 81:581–585, May 1982.

12. COLLINS FS, ORRINGER EP: Pulmonary hypertension and cor pulmonale in the sickle hemoglobinopathies. Am J Med 73:814–821, Dec 1982.

13. PACKER M, GREENBERG B, MASSIE B, DASH H: Deleterious effects of hydralazine in patients with pulmonary hypertension. N Engl J Med 306:1326–1331, June 3, 1982.

14. KADOWITZ PJ, HYMAN AL: Hydralazine and the treatment of primary pulmonary hypertension. N Engl J Med 306:1357–1358, June 3, 1982.

15. LUPI-HERRERA E, SANDOVAL J, SEOANE M, BIALOSTOLZKY D: The role of hydralazine therapy for pulmonary arterial hypertension of unknown cause. Circulation 65:645–650, Apr 1982.

16. KRONZON I, COHEN M, WINER HE: Adverse effect of hydralazine in patients with primary pulmonary hypertension. JAMA 247:3112–3114, June 11, 1982.

17. RUBIN LJ, HANDEL F, PETER RH: The effects of oral hydralazine on RV end-diastolic pressure in patients with RV failure. Circulation 65:1369–1373, June 1982.

18. RICH S, MARTINEZ J, LAM W, ROSEN KM: Captopril as treatment for patients with pulmonary hypertension. Problem of variability in assessing chronic drug treatment. Br Heart J 48:272–277, Sept 1982.

19. IKRAM H, MASLOWSKI AH, NICHOLLS MG, ESPINER EA, HULL FTL: Hemodynamic and hormonal effects of captopril in primary pulmonary hypertension. Br Heart J 48:541–555, Dec 1982.

20. RUBIN LJ, GROVES BM, REEVES JT, FROSOLONO M, HANDEL F, CATO AE: Prostacyclin-induced acute pulmonary vasodilation in primary pulmonary hypertension. Circulation 66:334–337, Aug 1982.

21. TIRLAPUR VG: Nocturnal hypoxemia and associated electrocardiographic changes in patients with chronic obstructive airways disease. N Engl J Med 306:125–130, Jan 21, 1982.

22. BRENT BN, BERGER HJ, MATTHAY RA, MAHLER D, PYTLIK L, ZARET BL: Physiologic correlates of right ventricular ejection fraction in chronic obstructive pulmonary disease: a combined radionuclide and hemodynamic study. Am J Cardiol 50:255–262, Aug 1982.

23. BRENT BN, MAHLER D, BERGER HJ, MATTHAY RA, PYTLIK L, ZARET BL: Augmentation of right ventricular performance in chronic obstructive pulmonary disease by terbutaline: a combined radionuclide and hemodynamic study. Am J Cardiol 50:313–319, Aug 1982.

24. HOOPER WW, SLUTSKY RA, KOCIENSKI DE, WITZTUM KF, SPRAGG RG, ASHBURN WL, MOSER KM:

Right and left ventricular response to subcutaneous terbutaline in patients with chronic obstructive pulmonary disease: radionuclide angiographic assessment of cardiac size and function. Am Heart J 104:1027–1032, Nov 1982.

25. MATTHAY RA, BERGER HJ, DAVIES R, LOKE J, GOTTSCHALK A, ZARET BL: Improvement in cardiac performance by oral long-acting theophylline in chronic obstructive pulmonary disease. Am Heart J 104:1022–1026, Nov 1982.

26. BELL WR: Pulmonary embolism: progress and problems. Am J Med 72:181–183, Feb 1982.

27. GOLDHABER SZ, HENNEKENS CH, EVANS DA, NEWTON EC, GODLESKI JJ: Factors associated with correct antemortem diagnosis of major pulmonary embolism. Am J Med 73:822–826, Dec 1982.

28. IWASAKI T, TANIMOTO M, YAMAMOTO T, MAKIHATA S, KAWAI Y, YORIFUJI S: Echocardiographic abnormalities of tricuspid valve motion in pulmonary embolism. Br Heart J 47:454–460, May 1982.

29. JARDIN F, FARCOT JC, BOISANTE L, PROST JF, GUERET P, BOURDARIAS JP: Mechanism of paradoxic pulse in bronchial asthma. Circulation 66:887–894, Oct 1982.

30. RASMUSSEN S, CORYA BD, PHILLIPS JF, BLACK MJ: Unreliability of M-mode left ventricular dimensions for calculating stroke volume and cardiac output in patients without heart disease. Chest 81:614–619, May 1982.

31. STAMM RB, CARABELLO BA, MAYERS DL, MARTIN RP: Two-dimensional echocardiographic measurement of left ventricular ejection fraction: prospective analysis of what constitutes an adequate determination. Am Heart J 104:136–144, July 1982.

32. SCHNITTGER I, FITZGERALD PJ, DAUGHTERS GT, INGELS NB, KANTROWITZ NE, SCHWARZKOPF A, MEAD CW, POPP RL: Limitations of comparing left ventricular volumes by two dimensional echocardiography, myocardial markers and cineangiography. Am J Cardiol 50:512–519, Sept 1982.

33. WATANABE T, KATSUME H, MATSUKUBO H, FURUKAWA K, IJICHI H: Estimation of right ventricular volume with two dimensional echocardiography. Am J Cardiol 49:1946–1953, June 1982.

34. KERBER RE, LITCHFIELD R: Postoperative abnormalities of interventricular septal motion: two-dimensional and M-mode echocardiographic correlations. Am Heart J 104:263–268, Aug 1982.

35. LINKS JM, BECKER LC, SHINDLEDECKER JG, GUZMAN P, BURROW RD, NICKOLOFF EL, ALDERSON PO, WAGNER HN: Measurement of absolute left ventricular volume from gated blood pool studies. Circulation 65:82–91, Jan 1982.

36. TOBIS J, NACIOGLU O, JOHNSTON WD, SEIBERT A, ISERI LT, ROECK W, ELKAYAM U, HENRY WL: Left ventricular imaging with digital subtraction angiography using intravenous contrast injection and fluoroscopic exposure levels. Am Heart J 104:20–27, July 1982.

37. DEHMER GJ, FIRTH BG, HILLIS LD, NICOD P, WILLERSON JT, LEWIS SE: Nongeometric determination of right ventricular volumes from equilibrium blood pool scans. Am J Cardiol 49:78–84, Jan 1982.

38. KORR KS, GANDSMAN EJ, WINKLER ML, SHULMAN RS, BOUGH EW: Hemodynamic correlates of right ventricular ejection fraction measured with gated radionuclide angiography. Am J Cardiol 49:71–77, Jan 1982.

39. RATIB O, HENZE E, SCHON H, SCHELBERT HR: Phase analysis of radionuclide ventriculograms for the detection of coronary artery disease. Am Heart J 104:1–12, July 1982.

40. BRANTIGAN CO, BRANTIGAN TA, JOSEPH N: Effect of beta blockade and beta stimulation on stage fright. Am J Med 72:88–94, Jan 1982.

41. SMITH TW, BUTLER VP JR, HABER E, FOZZARD H, MARCUS FI, BREMNER WF, SCHULMAN IC, PHILLIPS A: Treatment of life-threatening digitalis intoxication with digoxin-specific Fab antibody fragments. N Engl J Med 307:1357–1362, Nov 25, 1982.

42. KLEIN HO, LANG R, WEISS E, DESEGNI E, LIBHABER C, GUERRERO J, KAPLINSKY E: The influence of verapamil on serum digoxin concentration. Circulation 65:998–1003, May 1982.

43. Reiter MJ, Shand DG, Aanonsen LM, Wagoner R, McCarthy E, Pritchett ELC: Pharmacokinetics of verapamil: experience with a sustained intravenous infusion regimen. Am J Cardiol 50:716–721, Oct 1982.

44. Feely J, Wade D, McAllister CB, Wilkinson GR, Robertson D: Effect of hypotension on liver blood flow and lidocaine disposition. N Engl J Med 307:866–869, Sept 30, 1982.

45. Deykin D, Janson P, McMahon L: Ethanol potentiation of aspirin-induced prolongation of the bleeding time. N Engl J Med 306:852–854, Apr 8, 1982.

46. Pentel PR, Mikell FL, Zavoral JH: Myocardial injury after phenylpropanolamine ingestion. Br Heart J 47:51–54, Jan 1982.

47. Davids HA, Hermens WTH, Hollaar L, van der Laarse A, Huysmans HA: Extent of myocardial damage after open-heart surgery assessed from serial plasma enzyme levels in either of two periods (1975 and 1980). Br Heart J 47:167–172, Feb 1982.

48. Singh AK, Farrugia R, Teplitz C, Karlson KE: Electrolyte versus blood cardioplegia: randomized clinical and myocardial ultrastructural study. Ann Thorac Surg 33:218–227, March 1982.

49. Reves JG, Karp RB, Buttner EE, Tosone S, Smith LR, Samuelson PN, Kreusch GR, Oparil S: Neuronal and adrenomedullary catecholamine release in response to cardiopulmonary bypass in Man. Circulation 66:49–55, July 1982.

50. Mammana RB, Hiro S, Levitsky S, Thomas PA, Plachetka J: Inaccuracy of pulmonary capillary wedge pressure when compared to left atrial pressure in the early postsurgical period. J Thorac Cardiovasc Surg 84:420–425, Sept 1982.

51. Pennock JL, Oyer PE, Reitz BA, Jamieson SW, Bieber CP, Wallwork J, Stinson EB, Shumway NE: Cardiac transplantation in perspective for the future. J Thorac Cardiovasc Surg 83:168–177, Feb 1982.

52. Reitz BA, Stinson EB: Cardiac transplantation-1982. JAMA 248:1225–1227, Sept 10, 1982.

53. Reitz BA, Wallwork JL, Hunt SA, Pennock JL, Billingham ME, Oyer PE, Stinson EB, Shumway NE: Heart-lung transplantation. Successful therapy for patients with pulmonary vascular disease. N Engl J Med 306:557–563, March 11, 1982.

54. Mackintosh AF, Carmichael DJ, Wren C, Cory-Pearce R, English TAH: Sinus node function in first three weeks after cardiac transplantation. Br Heart J 48:584–588, Dec 1982.

55. Dangman KH, Danilo P, Jr., Hordoff AJ, Mary-Rabine L, Reder RF, Rosen MR: Electrophysiologic characteristics of human ventricular and Purkinje fibers. Circulation 65:362–368, Feb 1982.

56. Pollard RB, Arvin AM, Gamberg P, Rand KH, Gallagher JG, Merigan TC: Specific cell-mediated immunity and infections with herpes viruses in cardiac transplant recipients. Am J Med 73:679–687, Nov 1982.

57. Ghoneim ATM, McGoldrick J, Ionescu MI: Serial c-reactive protein measurements in infective complications following cardiac operation: evaluation and use in monitoring response to therapy. Ann Thorac Surg 34:166–175, Aug 1982.

58. Bachet J, Gigou F, Laurian C, Bical O, Goudot B, Guilmet D, Dubost C: Four-year clinical experience with the gelatin-resorcin-formol biological glue in acute aortic dissection. J Thorac Cardiovasc Surg 83:212–217, Feb 1982.

59. Egloff L, Rothlin M, Kugelmeier J, Senning A, Turina M: The ascending aortic aneurysm: replacement or repair? Ann Thorac Surg 34:117–124, Aug 1982.

60. Ergin MA, O'Connor J, Guinto R, Griepp RB: Experience with profound hypothermia and circulatory arrest in the treatment of aneurysms of the aortic arch. J Thorac Cardiovasc Surg 84:649–655, Nov 1982.

61. Finkelmeier BA, Mentzer RM, Kaiser DL, Tegtmeyer CJ, Nolan SP: Chronic traumatic thoracic aneurysm: influence of operative treatment on natural history—an analysis of reported cases, 1950–1980. J Thorac Cardiovasc Surg 84:257–266, Aug 1982.

62. Berendes JN, Bredee JJ, Schipperheyn J, Mashhour YAS: Mechanisms of spinal cord injury after cross-clamping of the descending thoracic aorta. Circulation 66:I112–I116, Aug 1982.

63. STRATTON JR, THIELE BL, RITCHIE JL: Platelet deposition on Dacron aortic bifurcation grafts in man: quantitation with indium 111 platelet imaging. Circulation 66:1287–1293, Dec 1982.

64. PORTER JM, CUTLER BS, LEE BY, REICH T, REICHLE FA, SCOGIN JT, STRANDNESS DE: Pentoxifylline efficacy in the treatment of intermittent claudication: multicenter controlled double-blind trial with objective assessment of chronic occlusive arterial disease patients. Am Heart J 104:66–72, July 1982.

65. BAR-SHLOMO BZ, DRUCK MN, MORCH JE, JABLONSKY G, HILTON JD, FEIGLIN DHI, McLAUGHLIN PR: Left ventricular function in trained and untrained healthy subjects. Circulation 65:484–488, March 1982.

66. FLESSAS AP, RYAN TJ: LV diastolic capacity in man. Circulation 65:1197–1203, June 1982.

67. SIESS W, LORENZ R, ROTH P, WEBER PC: Plasma catecholamines, platelet aggregation and associated thromboxane formation after physical exercise, smoking or norepinephrine infusion. Circulation 66:44–48, July 1982.

68. CONVERTINO V, HUNG J, GOLDWATER D, DeBUSK R: Cardiovascular responses to exercise in middle-aged men after 10 days of bed rest. Circulation 65:134–140, Jan 1982.

69. BECKER AE, CARUSO G: Myocardial disarray: a critical review. Br Heart J 47:527–538, June 1982.

70. KENNEDY RH, KENNEDY MA, FRYE RL, GIULIANI ER, McGOON DC, PLUTH JR, SMITH HC, RITTER DG, NOBREGA FT, KURLAND LT: Cardiac-catheterization and cardiac-surgical facilities. Use, trends, and future requirements. N Engl J Med 307:986–993, Oct 14, 1982.

71. CHASTRE J, CORNUD F, BOUCHAMA A, VIAU F, BENACERRAF R, GIBERT C: Thrombosis as a complication of pulmonary-artery catheterization via the internal jugular vein. Prospective evaluation by phlebography. N Engl J Med 306:278–282, Feb 4, 1982.

72. HARMAN EM, WYNNE JW, BLOCK AJ: The effect of weight loss on sleep-disordered breathing and oxygen desaturation in morbidly obese men. Chest 82:291–294, Sept 1982.

73. TAGGART P, DONALDSON R, GREEN J, JOSEPH SP, KELLY HB, MARCOMICHELAKIS J, NOBLE D, WHITE J: Interrelation of heart rate and autonomic activity in asymptomatic men with unobstructed coronary arteries: studies with atrial pacing, adrenaline infusion, and autonomic blockade. Br Heart J 47:19–25, Jan 1982.

74. POTKIN RT, WERNER JA, TROBAUGH GB, CHESTNUT CH III, CARRICO CJ, HALLSTROM A, COBB LA: Evaluation of noninvasive tests of cardiac damage in suspected cardiac contusion. Circulation 66:627–631, Sept 1982.

75. IKAHEIMO M, LINNALUOTO M, HUTTUNEN K, TAKKUNEN J: Effects of renal transplantation on left ventricular size and function. Br Heart J 47:155–160, Feb 1982.

76. BAUER TW, MOORE GW, HUTCHINS GM: Morphologic evidence for coronary artery spasm in eclampsia. Circulation 65:255–258, Feb 1982.

Author Index

Korr KS, 440
Kostiainen E, 28
Kostis JB, 28
Kotler MN, 288, 327
Kotlyarov EV, 87
Kouchoukos NT, 15, 76, 178, 202
Kramer BL, 410
Kramer JR, 302
Kramer RJ, 175
Kramer-Fox R, 293
Krebber HJ, 142
Krebs W, 141, 299
Kreigel DE, 94
Kren A, 131
Kreusch GR, 448
Kreutzer EA, 393
Kreutzer GO, 393
Krivokapich J, 144
Krneta A, 282
Król RB, 295
Kromhout D, 34
Krone RJ, 128
Kronzon I, 429
Kruse I, 230
Kuber MT, 120
Kubler W, 13, 138, 140, 306, 325
Kuck KJ, 141, 142
Kugelmeier J, 456
Kugler JD, 362, 410, 411
Kulbertus HE, 115, 165
Kullman S, 281
Kuo PT, 28
Kupersmith J, 203
Kuramoto K, 414
Kurland LT, 464
Kutcher MA, 426
Kutsche LM, 323
Kuwajima I, 414
Kwok KL, 17

L'Abbate A, 42, 54
LaBlanche JM, 61
Lacina SJ, 356
Laddu AR, 46, 198
LaFollette L, 3
Lakatta EG, 402
Lakier JR, 24
Laks H, 78, 321
Laks MM, 423

Lalor C, 254
Lam W, 192, 225, 430
Lamas GA, 108
Lamb IH, 66
Lamb P, 155
Lambertz H, 141
Landa DW, 47
Landmark K, 346
Lang P, 382
Lang R, 188, 442
Lange D, 306
Laragh JH, 243, 293, 408, 411
Larosa JC, 26
Latson TW, 14
Laura JP, 393
Laurenceau JL, 190
Laurent JM, 61
Laurian C, 456
Lawrie GM, 88
Layton C, 5
Leahy M, 401
Leanage R, 379
Leatham A, 226
Lebwohl MG, 298
Lee BY, 461
Lee DCS, 401
Lee G, 139
Lee K, 139
Lee KL, 11, 190
Lee PK, 415
Lee PS, 45
Lee W, 368
Leech G, 226
LeFree M, 44
Legha SS, 352
Legrand V, 165
Leier CV, 353, 404
Leino U, 28
LeJemtel TH, 53, 410, 411, 414
Lell W, 76
Lemann J, 253
Lemire J, 45
Lenox CC, 392
Leon MB, 53
Leong K, 9
Leppert J, 281
Leppo J, 11
Lerberg DB, 370
Lerner B, 42
Lesch M, 344

Lesperance J, 68, 71, 127
Lester RM, 1, 132
Lever HM, 302
Levin DC, 5
Levine AS, 357
Levine HJ, 310
Levine TB, 411, 416, 418
Levinson PD, 269
Levitsky LL, 356
Levitsky S, 449
Levy MJ, 389
Levy PS, 195
Levy RA, 158
Levy RI, 19
Lewis B, 18, 25
Lewis RP, 14, 353
Lewis SE, 118, 439
Libersa C, 61
Liberthson RR, 91
Libhaber C, 442
Lichstein E, 125
Lichtenberg R, 9
Lichtenthal PR, 210
Lie JT, 340
Lie KI, 112, 125, 151
Liebau G, 417
Liem KL, 253
Lijnen P, 278
Lilienfeld A, 147
Lim YL, 85
Lincoln C, 383
Linden CV, 29
Linden RJ, 41
Lindholm J, 30
Lindsay J, 233
Lindsay J Jr, 87
Links JM, 438
Linnaluoto M, 467
Lipinska I, 22
Lipson LC, 16, 53, 69, 71
Lister G, 364
Litchfield RL, 160, 425, 438
Little WC, 6
Littler WA, 282
Litwak R, 203
Livelli F Jr, 222
Livelli FD, 192
Llewellyn M, 49
Lock JE, 394
Lockhart C, 368
Loeb H, 151

Subject Index